Handbook of Muscle Variations and Anomalies in Humans

Handbook of Muscle Variations and Anomalies in Humans

A Compendium for Medical Education, Physicians, Surgeons, Anthropologists, Anatomists, and Biologists

Eve K. Boyle
Department of Anatomy
Howard University College of Medicine
Washington, District of Columbia

Vondel S. E. Mahon
R Adams Cowley Shock Trauma Center
University of Maryland Medical Center
Baltimore, Maryland

Rui Diogo
Department of Anatomy
Howard University College of Medicine
Washington, District of Columbia
and
Center for the Advanced Study of Human Paleobiology
The George Washington University
Washington, District of Columbia

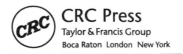

CRC Press
Taylor & Francis Group
Boca Raton London New York

CRC Press is an imprint of the
Taylor & Francis Group, an **informa** business

First edition published 2022
by CRC Press
6000 Broken Sound Parkway NW, Suite 300, Boca Raton, FL 33487-2742

and by CRC Press
2 Park Square, Milton Park, Abingdon, Oxon, OX14 4RN

CRC Press is an imprint of Taylor & Francis Group, LLC

ISBN: 978-0-367-53862-0 (hbk)
ISBN: 978-0-367-53863-7 (pbk)
ISBN: 978-1-003-08353-5 (ebk)

DOI: 10.1201/9781003083535

Typeset in Times
by codeMantra

Contents

Preface

Most textbooks and atlases of human anatomy describe only a few cases of variations in the "normal" population and/or of anomalies of the muscles. These variations and anomalies are also often excluded from the curricula in colleges of medicine and dentistry in the U.S.A. and in many other countries. However, it is known that each person within the "normal" population has at least a few muscle variations, and there are millions of individuals born globally every year with muscle anomalies. It is highly likely that during their careers, almost all medical professionals working with any aspect related to muscles—including muscle physiology, gross anatomy, physiotherapy, and surgery—will be faced with at least a few cases of muscle variations and/or anomalies. There are therefore crucial gaps of knowledge between what teachers of medical and dentistry schools teach, what students learn, what textbooks and atlases show, and the reality that medical professionals will face in practice during their careers.

This is the first textbook and anatomical atlas to be exclusively focused on the variations and anomalies of human muscles. It is based on the authors' own work—our lab has been particularly focused on human variations and defects in many species of animals—and a comprehensive review of the literature. This book combines three important goals: (1) provide a comparative context, based on evolutionary thinking and comparative zoological anatomy, for the existence of variations and defects in humans, particularly for medical students, professors, and students of human gross anatomy; (2) summarize the major types of variations and anomalies found in the skeletal muscles of humans; and (3) include schematic figures for an easy visualization of these variations and anomalies. This approach dovetails with classical and contemporary approaches to medical instruction and clinical practice.

This book may be of interest to students of medical and other health sciences—such as dentistry, physiotherapy, and orthopedics—instructors, teaching assistants, professors, and other medical researchers and pathologists; students and teachers at nonmedical colleges, universities, and high schools where human gross anatomy is also taught; and scientists and research students in biological fields including biological anthropology, comparative anatomy, functional morphology, zoology, and evolutionary and developmental biology.

Acknowledgments

We would all like to thank Boyani Moikobu, Latonya Aaron, Tah-jai Sharpe, Rowan Sherwood, and Brandon Wallace for their assistance in formatting references. We all also want to thank Chuck Crumly for always thinking a step ahead and inviting us to do this book for Taylor & Francis, and for helping us define key aspects about the organization of the book. Many thanks also to Ana Lucia Eberhart.

Eve K. Boyle would like to thank the many mentors and academic advisors who have facilitated her understanding of musculoskeletal anatomy and provided opportunities to teach and conduct research. Special thanks to Drs. Kirsten Brown, Jeremy DeSilva, Sergio Almécija, Bernard Wood, Briana Pobiner, and Shiloh Jones. Thank you also to the students, staff, and faculty of the George Washington University School of Medicine and Health Sciences and the Georgetown University School of Medicine.

Vondel S. E. Mahon would like to thank God, Lovon Mahon, Nancy Welsh, Mary Klunk, Izel Glover, Ann Brown, Janet Carlile, Dan Thompson, the University of Maryland Medical Center R. Adams Cowley Shock Trauma Center, the Johns Hopkins University School of Medicine Department of Art as Applied to Medicine, the CUNY Baccalaureate for Unique and Interdisciplinary Studies, the Thomas W. Smith Academic Fellowship, The Art Students League of New York, the Medgar Evers College of the City University of New York, the AMI, and his beloved family, mentors, and friends.

Rui Diogo would like to thank the numerous colleagues that have worked with him on the subjects covered in this book, as well as to the institutions that have funded those works, and to Howard University, where he teaches anatomy and undertakes research about a plethora of anatomical, evolutionary, and societal topics.

About the Authors

Eve K. Boyle is an evolutionary anthropologist with expertise in informal science education, public engagement, project management, and broadening participation initiatives. She received her Ph.D. from the Center for the Advanced Study of Human Paleobiology of George Washington University in 2019. As a postdoctoral fellow at Howard University from 2019 to 2020, she was the first project manager for the Visible Ape Project. She served as an AAAS Science & Technology Policy Fellow at the National Science Foundation from 2020 to 2022.

Vondel S. E. Mahon is a Medical Illustrator at Mahon Illustrations LLC and at a private enterprise. He received his M.A. in Medical and Biological Illustration from the Department of Art as Applied to Medicine at the Johns Hopkins University School of Medicine. For his master's thesis, he developed a novel tool for orthopedic trauma education with the Johns Hopkins University Computer Aided Medical Procedures Laboratory and the Johns Hopkins Medicine Technology Innovation Center. He holds an interest in the use of Extended Reality (XR) technology in healthcare and medical education. He is also a proud member of the Association of Medical Illustrators (AMI).

Rui Diogo is a multi-awarded researcher, speaker, and writer who is renowned worldwide for addressing broader scientific questions and societal issues using state-of-the-art empirical data from many different fields of science. He obtained his Bachelor's degree in Biology from the University of Aveiro, Portugal, and later did a Ph.D. at the University of Liege, Belgium, a postdoc at the King's College of London, and then a master's and a Ph.D. at the Department of Biology of George Washington University, U.S.A. A wonderer and a wanderer, he has done research, gave speeches, or traveled in more than 120 countries. He is the author of more than 150 papers in top journals and 20 books, including *Learning and Understanding Human Anatomy and Pathology*—used at several medical schools worldwide; *Evolution Driven by Organismal Behavior*—often listed among the ten best evolutionary books in 2017; and the already highly-acclaimed *Meaning of Life, Human Nature, and Delusions*.

Contributors

Warrenkevin Henderson
Boston University
Boston, Massachusetts

Hannah Jacobson
George Washington University
Washington, District of Columbia

Noelle Purcell
George Washington University
Washington, District of Columbia

Rowan Sherwood
Department of Anthropology
University of Michigan
Ann Arbor, Michigan

Kylar Wiltz
Howard University College of Medicine
Washington, District of Columbia

Malynda Williams
Howard University College of Medicine
Washington, District of Columbia

1 Introduction

Eve K. Boyle
Howard University College of Medicine

Vondel S. E. Mahon
University of Maryland Medical Center

Rui Diogo
Howard University College of Medicine

CONTENTS

Portions of this introduction are reproduced by permission from John Wiley and Sons: Diogo, R., Smith, C.M. and Ziermann, J.M. 2015. Evolutionary developmental pathology and anthropology: A new field linking development, comparative anatomy, human evolution, morphological variations and defects, and medicine. *Dev Dyn* 244:1357–1374. © 2015 Wiley Periodicals, Inc.

WHY DO HUMANS HAVE ANATOMICAL VARIATIONS AND ANOMALIES?

When Charles Darwin wanted to convince a highly skeptical scientific community and general public that we evolved from other primates in *The Descent of Man* (1871), he started by discussing human anatomical variations and anomalies. Why? Because he knew that a strong way to show that we descend from other animals is to highlight the commonalities we share with them and particularly, the commonalities that are only present in some humans, as a reminder of the nonhuman ancestors we had several millions of years ago. Our anatomical variations and anomalies, in particular those that are related to the presence of evolutionary reversions, are indeed the most direct, strong evidence of our evolutionary past. This is because there are features that are present in adults of other species that are typically absent in humans, but for some reason can still be found in some human adults. The most likely scientific explanation, Darwin argued, is that such features were present in our adult ancestors and then were evolutionary lost but evolutionarily "re-acquired." Not only that: even for some anatomical features that appear in humans that have nothing to do with traits typically present in other animals, these usually also show that we share evolutionary and developmental commonalities with them because such variations and anomalies are also present in some cases within other species. For instance, one of the more severe malformations in humans is cyclopia, the presence of a single eye. We never had an ancestor that was truly a cyclops, but many other mammals also have cyclopic malformations.

This phenomenon is now known as Alberch's (1989) ill-named "logic of monsters." According to this theory, which has been strongly supported by a plethora of empirical data, there is a parallel between the variation/anomalies in normal/abnormal individuals of a certain taxon and the fixed diversity observed in wildtype individuals of other taxa. According to Alberch (1989), this parallel might be achieved through regulation of a conserved developmental program (i.e., a set of genetic and/or epigenetic interactions) such that the structure of these internal interactions constrains the realm of possible variation upon which selection can operate. This program may lead to the breakdown in the evolution of some clades, but within most clades this would lead to death of the embryos. This leads us to distinguish between variant features and anomalies. By definition, anatomical variants are structures present in the common population, that is, the population that is karyotypically normal and that does not have severe congenital malformations, or so-called "birth defects." Anatomical anomalies are precisely often the result of genetic mutations or severe congenital malformations, such as cyclopia, a feature that is never found in the common population. However, this does not mean that anatomical anomalies are always more severe than variants. For instance, a certain limb muscle missing in an individual from the common population would be seen as a variant, while the very same feature seen in, let's say, a person with Down syndrome, would be seen as an anatomical anomaly. According to the "logic of monsters," this parallel between the variation and anomalies in so-called "normal" vs "abnormal" individuals of a certain taxon is exactly to be often expected.

As noted by Diogo et al. (2015), such a parallel between the more common phenotypic variations seen in the normal human population and malformations seen in birth defects is also to be expected according to Shapiro et al.'s (1983) "lack of homeostasis" model. This model was in large part formulated based on observations of human trisomic individuals and states that the presence of a whole extra functioning chromosome or of a large chromosome segment causes a disruption of evolved genetic balance. Because of the obligatory integration of the entire genotype, this disruption affects the products of the trisomic chromosome and other chromosomes. This results in decreased physiological and developmental buffering against genetic and environmental forces, which leads to decreased developmental and physiological homeostasis where the pathways and processes that will be the most often and seriously affected are those that are more unstable. This instability thus leads to variations in the normal population. An illustrative example predicted by both the "logic of monsters" and "lack of homeostasis" hypotheses is the presentation of palmaris longus. The absence of palmaris longus (see Fig 3.14) is a common human polymorphism. Polymorphisms are different from variations, because although they are also present in the "normal" population as variants are, they are present in more than 2% of the "normal" population, while variations are present in less than 2%. So, within the "normal" population there are *variants*—present in less than 2% of the population; *polymorphisms*—present between 2% and 50% of the population; and the *common phenotype*—present in more than 50% of the population. In the case of the palmaris longus, this *absence* of muscle is a polymorphism because the muscle is absent in about ~15%–20% of the "normal" human population. Interestingly, the absence of the muscle is often amplified in humans with severe congenital malformations. For example, palmaris longus was reported to be absent in 74% (105) of 141 defective upper limbs reviewed by Smith et al. (2015), further reinforcing that variants and polymorphisms are often amplified in people with congenital malformations.

However, with exception to this similarity between the "logic of monsters" and the "lack of homeostasis" models, they differ fundamentally in their assumptions and predictions. The "lack of homeostasis" model argues that defects are mostly random and disorganized due to a general lack of homeostasis. The "logic of monsters" predicts, instead, that defects are mostly "logical" and "constrained" because developmental constraints are kept intact by internal homeostasis, even when things go "wrong" in both evolution and embryonic development. That is why the "logic of monsters" model predicts—contrary to the "lack of homeostasis" model—that congenital malformations mirror, or amplify, variations, and that both of them further mirror evolutionary events that occurred in other taxa at completely different geological times. This prediction has been supported by studies demonstrating that similar patterns of intra-specific diversity within a taxon (plasticity) and inter-specific diversity among different taxa usually

result from similar developmental mechanisms (Hodin 2000). The "logic of monsters" is thus framed in an "internalist" view of evolution and development that contrasts with the more "externalist" view of adaptationists, who maintain that selection by the external environment is the main evolutionary force. For example, frogs and salamanders tend to exhibit loss of digit one and reduction of digit five due to developmental constraints. This pattern is found in frogs living in different environments that are exposed to different external factors (Alberch and Gale 1985). That is, the recurrent loss/reduction of such digits in frogs seems to have much more to do with internal mechanisms than with specific external conditions, although of course the latter might play some role in the specific frog groups and/or geological time in which those loses/reductions happen.

The works of Alberch, as well as of his colleague Stephen Jay Gould and various other authors in the 1970s and 1980s, have led to the rise of evolutionary developmental biology (Evo-Devo), which has revived interest in comparative anatomy, particularly of soft tissues, and of "teratology," now designated as the study of congenital malformations. These are fields that were somewhat dormant for many years after having a prominent role in anatomical and biological studies in the 18th, 19th, and early 20th centuries, with only a few notable works in the latter half of the 20th century (e.g., Willis 1958). Following this trend, one of us (RD) has created, with other colleagues a new subfield within Evo-Devo: *Evolutionary Developmental Pathology (Evo-Devo-Path)*, which is exactly focused on understanding the evolutionary and developmental basis of human variations and anomalies (Diogo et al. 2015; Diogo and Wood 2016). This new subfield—which was specifically applied to human anatomy, by Diogo et al. (2016)—is in a way a comeback to the study of the links between normal and abnormal development and pathologies, which began to be intensively undertaken centuries ago by authors such as St. Geoffroy St. Hilaire, but that were then somewhat neglected for decades during the 20th century. Fortunately, more and more authors are realizing the importance of investigating these links, although with Evo-Devo they have been mainly studied by focusing principally on osteological or superficial features (e.g., absence of a certain bone, shape of head), with fewer studies being done about the muscular system of both humans and nonhuman animals with anatomical variations or anomalies. However, now that we understand the developmental—including both genetic and epigenetic—and evolutionary basis for why we have anomalies and variations, it is time to develop Evo-Devo-Path to the detailed study of soft tissues such as muscles.

For instance, we now know that evolutionary reversions did play a substantial role in primate/human evolution. In a phylogenetic work about muscle evolution in primates, Diogo and Wood (2012b) have shown that 28 out of the 220 (12.7%) evolutionary changes unambiguously optimized in the most accepted primate phylogenetic tree are reversions to a plesiomorphic (ancestral) state. Of those 28 reversions, six were directly related to our own evolution because they occurred at nodes that lead to the origin of modern humans. Nine of these reversions go against Dollo's law, which states that once a complex structure is lost, it is unlikely to be regained. Our Evo-Devo-Path studies support the idea that reacquisition of morphological structures in adults that have been absent for long periods of time is possible because the associated developmental pathways were maintained in the members of that taxon.

For example, chimpanzees display a reversion of a synapomorphy of the Hominidae (great apes and modern humans) that was acquired at least 15.4 million years ago. Adult chimpanzees have two contrahentes digitorum muscles (see Figure 3.18) in addition to adductor pollicis (see Figure 3.19), which is the only contrahens muscle present in the typical phenotype in adults of other apes. Chimpanzees thus have contrahentes muscles going to digit four and the other to digit five. Developmental studies of hand muscles show that karyotypically normal human embryos do exhibit contrahentes going to various fingers, but these muscles usually are reabsorbed or incorporated within other structures during later embryonic development (Cihak 1972). In karyotypically abnormal humans, such as those with trisomies 13, 18, or 21, the contrahentes often persist after birth as "atavisms" (see Figure 3.18), which are structures that present as developmental anomalies or variations and resemble the common adult character state of the ancestors of the taxon to which the individual belongs. Cihak (1972) showed that intermetacarpales muscles of the hand are also present as discrete muscles in early stages of karyotypically normal human embryonic development but later join with flexor breves profundi muscles to form the dorsal interossei (see Figure 3.18). Therefore, the evolutionary reversions that result in the presence of contrahentes and intermetacarpales muscles in chimpanzees are likely related to heterochronic (specifically paedomorphic) events in the chimpanzee lineage (Diogo and Wood 2012b). So, it is very likely that many variants and anomalies that are present in adult humans and that were present in our adult ancestors are structures that were always present in the embryos of our ancestors, but that then became absent, or fused with other structures, in later stages of development. But, for some reason, either genetic or epigenetic, they persist until later stages of development in certain people as variations or anomalies. That is precisely what happens to features such as the presence of various hand or foot contrahentes muscles, or a platysma cervicale muscle of the head (see Figure 2.3).

We have been studying cadaveric material from fetal, neonatal, and adult humans with trisomies and from mouse models for Down syndrome (e.g., Ts65Dn) to investigate the developmental mechanisms related to the atypical development of muscles. Research on the skeletons of trisomic individuals has supported the idea that for some features there is in fact a developmental delay. For example, some nasal bones develop after the 24th week in cases of trisomy 21, while in karyotypically normal humans the developmental onset is the 10th week (e.g., Keeling et al. 1997). Interestingly, these studies provided examples of different phenotypic patterns often seen in different trisomies, for instance regarding the axial skeleton in fetuses with trisomy 18 vs fetuses with trisomy 21 (Keeling et al. 1997), further supporting the ill-named "logic of monsters." One hypothesis we aim to test in future works is that the disappearance of certain muscles during early developmental stages of karyotypically normal humans is related to apoptosis, and that the persistence of these atavistic muscles later in ontogeny in individuals with trisomies 13, 18, and 21 is associated with delayed development specifically due to decreased muscle apoptosis. Some authors suggest that humans with DS show an increase of apoptosis in structures such as neurons, granulocytes, and lymphocytes (e.g., Elsayed and Elsayed 2009). If our studies support the hypothesis that these individuals have decreased muscle apoptosis that leads to the presence of additional muscles in later ontogenetic stages, this will imply a more nuanced pattern of apoptosis (i.e., a mosaic scenario where apoptosis is increased in some tissues and decreased in others). Within the numerous Down syndrome cases listed in the tables of Dunlap et al. (1986), there are 12 supernumerary muscles, as opposed to two absences. Therefore, Down syndrome individuals seem to present with more accessory muscles in general, supporting our hypothesis these individuals may have decreased apoptosis in skeletal muscles. Bersu (1980) also suggested that the persistence of some embryonic muscles in later stages of development of trisomic individuals likely has to do with failure of normal cell death or some other process of involution. If there is indeed a contrast in apoptosis between the nervous system (e.g. more apoptosis of nerve cells) and muscular system (i.e. less apoptosis and presence of extra muscles), our hypothesis might also shed light on the etiology of hypotonia (low muscle tone) that is present in individuals with Down syndrome.

Some authors suggest that cases in which complex structures are formed early in "normal" ontogeny but later become lost/indistinct during development (so-called "hidden variation"), may allow organisms to have greater ontogenetic potential early in development. If faced with external perturbations (e.g., climate change, habitat occupied by new species), evolution can use that potential (adaptive plasticity: e.g., West-Eberhard 2003). However, authors such as Gould (1977, 2002) and Alberch (1989) suggested that these cases support instead a "constrained" (internalist) rather than an "adaptationist" (externalist) view of evolution. This is because it is not likely that the persistence of some muscles in later developmental stages of karyotypically abnormal humans is due to natural selection and adaptive evolution. This corresponds with the idea defended by Galis and Metz (2007: 415–416): "without denying the evolutionary importance of phenotypic plasticity and genetic assimilation, we think that for the generation of macroevolutionary novelties the evidence for the impact of hidden variation is limited" (see also Levinton 2001).

Further studies are needed to determine if hidden variation plays a role as important in generating evolutionary novelties, and they seem to play in the reappearance of some traits associated with these novelties, as in anatomical reversions that violate Dollo's law. In this sense, it is important to emphasize that "atavistic" muscles of karyotypically normal human embryos do not correspond to the muscles of adult primates or of other adult mammals. These muscles instead correspond to the embryonic muscles of these latter taxa (Diogo and Wood 2012a,b). The developmental pathways resulting in the presence of these muscles in adults were not completely lost in modern humans, even after several million years of evolution, likely because these pathways are recruited in the formation of other structures that are present and functional in modern human adults.

However, it should also be noted there is still some confusion about the use of the term "atavism." Darwin and other 19th century authors considered the presence of a tail-like appendage at the height of the coccyx or lumbar spine in some human newborns to be an "atavism," a position subscribed to by us. Indeed, some authors have described muscles associated with these structures that they suggest do resemble caudal muscles of other animals (Wiedersheim 1895). But it is also clear that many features considered to be "atavisms" in trisomic humans (e.g., Barash et al. 1970; Dunlap et al. 1986) cannot actually be atavisms, because those features were never present in our direct ancestors. However, some muscle variants and anomalies that we will describe in this book are atavistic by definition (e.g., dorsoepitrochlearis, epitrochleoanconeus, levator claviculae, opponens hallucis). What is not so clear is whether their presence is due to a developmental delay, but that is not a requirement to consider a feature as an "atavism." This short discussion highlights the need for more research on the ontogeny of these structures in humans and other primates, which is crucial to clarify these issues.

According to Hall (1984), the presence of atavistic features as human variations might represent the maintenance of structures that were adult polymorphisms in the past, within the normal human population and/or their ancestors. For instance, as mentioned above, palmaris longus (see Figure 3.14) is present in ~80%–85% of the normal human population. Since this muscle is present in about 100% of the normal population of primates, including most apes, there is apparently a trend toward a decreased frequency of palmaris longus along human evolutionary history (Diogo and Wood 2012a,b). If this is indeed the case, it is likely that in future generations, palmaris longus may become present in a very small percentage of normal adult humans and would therefore be considered a rare, "atavistic" variation. If in the future palmaris longus will be present in most human embryos/fetuses but typically absent in adults, those embryonic/fetal stages will indeed somewhat mirror what happens today in the normal adult human population. However, although in this case currently the late fetal and adult configurations of the palmaris longus are essentially the same in humans (Bardeen 1906), one has to stress again that the embryonic palmaris longus of those future humans would not directly correspond to the adult palmaris longus seen in most humans living today, but instead to the embryonic palmaris longus of those humans, and of nonhuman primates.

Regarding all the muscles of the head and upper and lower limbs as a whole, within the 1540 cases of human muscle congenital malformations that we have compiled (Smith et al. 2015), 257 (17%) are potential atavisms and 352 (23%) can potentially be due to developmental delay. Therefore, if more detailed comparative developmental studies confirm that these numbers, or even just a substantial portion of them, are truly atavistic and/or due to developmental delay, these would be significant proportions. Interestingly, within those 1540 cases, 650 (42%) concern the presence of abnormal structures (e.g., muscle heads/slips or tendons) and 590 (38%) concern the complete absence, while only 145 (9%) concern fusions and 66 (4%) concern complete duplications of muscles usually present in the normal human population. Despite the substantial proportions of potential atavisms and/or developmental delays mentioned above, those cases are a minority among all cases of birth defects/anomalies we have compiled so far. This supports other research that suggests many other factors are probably involved in leading to anatomical defects found in these individuals, apart from developmental retardation. Such factors can include, for instance, the aberrant organization of primordia and misdirected morphogenetic movements (Barash et al. 1970).

In a nutshell, it can thus be said that there are likely many different reasons why humans have anatomical variations and anomalies. It is likely that variations are more often cases of imprints of our past (Boyle et al. 2020) than are anomalies, because, as noted above, variations and anomalies can sometimes refer to the very same feature, but in general the former are not as severe as some of the most severe anomalies. Simply put, people can't survive and be part of the common population with a cyclopia. Cyclopia is exclusively an anomaly, not a thing of our evolutionary past, and moreover—and likely precisely because of that—it concerns only embryos/fetuses in general and never a variation within the common adult human population. It should be noted that in this book we are interested in anomalies and variations *after* embryonic development, and therefore we do include information on fetal musculature, when available. There is much we still do not know, both about the specific developmental mechanisms and about the anatomical patterns, of muscle variations and anomalies. Much more work is done, and one of the aims of the present book is precisely to pave the way for such works in the future by providing an atlas of several variants/anomalies found in all body regions of current human individuals of all non-embryonic ages.

TOWARD A MORE HOLISTIC APPROACH TO HUMAN ANATOMY AND EVOLUTION

A second and related primary aim of this book is to pave the way for a more holistic approach to human anatomy and human evolution. Here we contribute to that goal by gathering and presenting the result of a 20 year-long comparison of the muscle variants and anomalies of humans, and between them and those of other animals, in particular our closest relatives, the nonhuman primates. Our Evo-Devo-Path research includes more traditional Evo-Devo lines of research but also pays special attention to data obtained from chordate comparative, developmental, and evolutionary anatomy and from the direct study of normal/abnormal human development (using, e.g., cadaveric collections of hospitals, museums, and other institutions), with a primary focus on soft tissues like muscles (e.g., Diogo 2004a,b, 2005, 2007; Diogo and Abdala 2007, 2010; Diogo et al. 2008a,b, 2009a,b, 2018, 2019), including primates (e.g., Diogo and Wood 2011, 2012b, 2016; Diogo et al. 2010, 2012, 2013a,b, 2017). We hope this work will pave the way for a more holistic approach to human anatomy and evolution, as well as help physicians and surgeons, medical students, and biologists and anthropologists to better understand where the structures of our body come from, and why they are as they are. As noted above, this applies to features that (1) have a so-called "normal" configuration and are present in more than 50% of the common population; (2) are polymorphisms, and as such, are present in less than 50% and more than 2%; (3) are variations, which are traits present in up to 2% of the common population; or (4) anomalies, which are found in people with severe malformations or genetic syndromes. The former item was discussed Diogo et al. (2016), *Learning and understanding human anatomy and pathology: an evolutionary and developmental guide for medical students*. That book paved the way not only for a more comprehensive understanding of the human body informed by evolution and development, but also for us to compare the common phenotype of our internal structures, including muscles, to our anatomical polymorphisms, variants, and anomalies, which are precisely the subject of the present book. We provide here an illustrative example to explain how they are linked, and how physicians and surgeons, students, teachers, and scientists in general can benefit from such a broader, more holistic approach.

This example concerns non-pentadactyly, a topic that has long attracted researchers' attention because this is the most common human limb birth defect. We have studied alterations in muscle attachments found in congenital non-pentadactyl human limbs and evaluated whether these changed patterns are similar to those found in wildtype nonhuman tetrapods with non-pentadactyl limbs (Smith et al. 2015). The most significant conclusion of those studies was that the non-pentadactyl limbs of wildtype taxa (e.g., frogs, salamanders, crocodilians, chickens, humans) with birth defects exhibit a consistent "nearest neighbor" pattern. In other words, the identity and attachments of the distal forelimb and hindlimb muscles seem to be mainly related to the physical (topological) position, and not to the number of the anlage or the homeotic identity of the digits to which the muscles are attached. Topological position refers to the adult relationship with other structures, and not to the position of the developmental anlagen.

Hinchliffe and Johnson (1980: pp. 96–97) described a "nearest-neighbor" model for limb muscle to bone relationships, as well as for muscle to nerve connections. These authors argued that such a dynamic, flexible model ensures correspondence between these tissues during dramatic evolutionary changes and in congenital malformations. Wolpert's "positional information" model is similar and suggests that the positional value of a cell/structure (e.g., the skeleton) can be recognized by and affect the typical patterning/morphogenesis of another cell/structure (e.g., muscles), without changing the overall phenotype/shape of that other cell/structure (Wolpert 1969, 2011). According to this model, muscle cells of limbs do not have positional values, so it would be reasonable to assume that they are affected by and follow the positional values of the skeleton, conforming to the expectations of the "nearest neighbor" model.

Our soft-tissue studies of humans supported our "nearest neighbor" model. As predicted by our model, in a trisomy 18 fetus with a six-digit hand (partial duplication of thumb) and a four-digit hand (no thumb), the hand with no thumb presented all thumb muscles but these muscles went to the most radial digit, which was digit two. As also anticipated by our model, in the hand with partial thumb duplication there was no duplication of the thumb muscles. This finding supports the results of experimental studies on mouse models demonstrating that limb skeletal and connective/muscle tissue patterning can be uncoupled (e.g., Li et al. 2010). The number of thumb muscles did not change, but their insertions varied according to the adult topological position of the two thumbs. The muscles that typically go to the radial (e.g., abductor pollicis brevis) and ulnar (e.g., adductor pollicis) aspects of the thumb now attach onto the radial side of the most radial thumb and ulnar side of the most ulnar thumb, respectively. Recent comparative studies indicate that the developmental factors for skeletal morphological identity in vertebrates reside less in the embryonic cell lineages, and more in the topological position in the embryo, which allows the relative position of bony elements to be highly conserved in evolution (Hirasawa and Kuratani 2015).

Our recent Evo-Devo-Path studies and comparisons have supported, so far, the idea that internal constraints play a central role in both normal and abnormal human development. Our research thus provides support for Alberch's "logic of monsters," because there are consistent patterns seen in both individuals with different genetic syndromes and variations of the normal human population. For example, Wood (1867a,b, 1868) found that muscle variations are much more frequent in the upper limb than in the lower limbs of the normal human population (292 vs 119 cases in his sample, i.e., 71% vs 29%, or almost 2.5 times more upper than lower limb variations). In our sample of 316 head, upper, and lower limb defects compiled from studies of severe congenital malformations (see Smith et al. 2015), the proportion was exactly the same: 158 upper limb defects (50%), 94 head defects (30%), and 64 lower limb defects (20%), so almost 2.5 times more upper than lower limb defects. Interestingly, most of the defects found in the upper limbs (65%) and lower limbs (84%) are also found in the autopods and zeugopods, which are mainly evolutionary innovations of tetrapods. This makes sense within an internalist view of evolution, because these phylogenetically more recent innovations are also the last limb regions to form during development and more prone to developmental changes, variations, and defects. It also makes sense within an externalist view of evolution, since the more distal limb regions are in closer contact with prey, substrates, and objects, and are thus more prone to evolutionary adaptive changes.

This connection between development (ontogeny), the order in which morphological structures appear in evolution (phylogeny), interactions with the environment (ecomorphology), and evolvability (adaptation) supports the "logic of monsters" since it predicts a parallel between the variant phenotypes of normal populations and defects in abnormal individuals. Within the 64 limb muscle defects reviewed by Smith et al. (2015) that involve changes of attachment (origin and insertion), the changes of insertion tended to be toward more proximal limb regions, while the changes of origin tended to be toward more distal regions. Overall, most of the attachment changes involved insertion changes. This finding parallels phylogeny, because in primate and human evolution, more changes involve the insertion sites of limb muscles than origin sites. Furthermore, this finding makes sense both within an externalist framework—as insertions are more distal by definition and are in closer contact with the outside—and within an internalist framework—as the origin of limb muscles tends to form first in ontogeny, so terminal changes would more likely affect their insertion (Diogo and Tanaka 2014; Diogo and Ziermann 2014). Lastly, as noted above, it appears that the upper limb is most prone to phenotypic changes and defects among the head and limb regions of the body. Again, more studies are needed to clarify if these patterns are seen concerning other soft tissues such as arteries, veins, nerves, and even internal organs, and the information provided in the present book will be hopefully useful to motivate researchers to undertake, and pave the way for, such future works.

BRIEF NOTES ABOUT OUR METHODOLOGY

As noted above, we include information on variations and anomalies present in human muscles after embryonic development. For each muscle, we provide the Latin name, with the common English name shown in parentheses, when they are slightly different. We then include the synonyms of the muscle that we encountered over the course of our research, not meant to be an exhaustive list. In some cases, this section also includes synonyms we believe should be attributed to that muscle based on anatomical descriptions.

Next, we describe the typical presentation of each muscle. For most muscles, this section provides the typical presentation as described by Standring (2016). Some muscles

are only present in humans as variations and/or anomalies, and therefore have no typical or "normal" presentation to be compared with. For most muscles, this section provides the typical innervation also described by Standring (2016). For muscles that are present only as variations and/or anomalies, the innervation is listed under "Variations." Innervation may shed light about a muscle's developmental origins and is often clinically relevant for variations.

Then, we provide descriptions of the comparative anatomy of each muscle. For most muscles, this section describes the typical presentation and significant variations in the apes, the closest living relatives of humans. The apes include gibbons (*Hylobates*), orangutans (*Pongo*), gorillas (*Gorilla*), common chimpanzees (*Pan troglodytes*), and bonobos (*Pan paniscus*). When relevant, we included anatomical information for other primates or, in some cases, non-primate animals. "N/A" in this section indicates that, to our knowledge, the muscle has not been observed or described in the apes.

We then include information on each muscle's variations in humans. For most muscles, this section details variations on the typical presentation that have been described in the literature. For accessory or supernumerary muscles that are present as variations, this section describes its presentation when it is found in humans. Accessory muscles received their own entries—and were not just listed as variations of other muscles—when enough information was available to fill out more than only the "Description" portion of the "Variations" section.

For the variations, the prevalence section provides the prevalence of the variations as listed in the literature. In general, as noted above, a "typical" configuration is present in more than 50% of the common population, polymorphisms are features present in less than 50% and more than 2%, and variations present in up to 2% of the common population. However, as you will see throughout the text, prevalence for some presentations that are considered variations often exceed 2% and should perhaps be more aptly considered as polymorphisms. "N/A" in this section indicates that, to our knowledge, no prevalence data on variations are available.

We first included variations described by anatomists in the 19th century such as Hallett (1848), Macalister (1867a,b; 1875), Knott (1880, 1883a,b), and Wood (1864, 1865, 1866, 1867a,b, 1868, 1870). We then referred to comprehensive works such as Mori (1964), Sato (1968a,b,c, 1969, 1970), Rickenbacher et al. (1985), Bergman et al. (1988), and *Bergman's Comprehensive Encyclopedia of Human Anatomic Variation* (2016, edited by Tubbs, Shoja, and Loukas) to double-check the information listed in earlier texts and to better understand the breadth of variations that exist for each muscle. Lastly, we conducted an exhaustive search for journal articles published through early 2021 to provide additional information on rare variations, variation prevalence, and clinical implications of variations.

Next, we describe each muscle's anomalous presentations in humans. For most muscles, this section details anatomical anomalies found in individuals with chromosomal conditions, developmental defects of the musculoskeletal system, or other congenital disorders. "N/A" in this section indicates that, to our knowledge, no anomalies of that muscle have been described. We also include the prevalence of the anomalies as listed in the literature, mostly provided by Smith et al. (2015). "N/A" in this section indicates that, to our knowledge, no prevalence data on anomalies are available.

Lastly, in the clinical implications section, we include information on the clinical relevance of variations and/or anomalies. "N/A" in this section indicates that we did not easily find clinical implications of the variations.

2 Head and Neck Muscles

Eve K. Boyle
Howard University College of Medicine

Vondel S. E. Mahon
University of Maryland Medical Center

Rui Diogo
Howard University College of Medicine

Warrenkevin Henderson
Boston University

Hannah Jacobson
George Washington University

Noelle Purcell
George Washington University

Kylar Wiltz
Howard University College of Medicine

CONTENTS

DOI: 10.1201/9781003083535-2

FACIAL MUSCLES

OCCIPITOFRONTALIS (FIGURES 2.1, 2.3)

Synonyms

The occipital and frontal components of occipitofrontalis may be referred to as two separate muscles: occipitalis and frontalis.

Typical Presentation

Description

Occipitofrontalis consists of the occipitalis and frontalis muscles, connected by the epicranial aponeurosis (Standring 2016). Occipitalis extends from the highest nuchal line and mastoid region to attach to the epicranial aponeurosis (Standring 2016). Frontalis extends from the superficial fascia of the eyebrows to attach to the epicranial aponeurosis, having connections with other forehead muscles (Standring 2016).

Innervation

Occipitofrontalis is innervated by the facial nerve, the occipital portion via the posterior auricular branch and the frontal portion via the temporal branches (Standring 2016).

Comparative Anatomy

Frontalis has a similar typical presentation in the apes, extending from the skin of the eyebrow and nose to the epicranial aponeurosis (Raven 1950; Miller 1952; Gibbs 1999; Diogo et al. 2010, 2012, 2013a,b, 2017). Occipitalis typically presents similarly to humans in common chimpanzees, bonobos, and gorillas, extending from the occipital and mastoid regions to the epicranial aponeurosis (Gibbs 1999; Diogo et al. 2010, 2013a, 2017). In gibbons, occipitalis is typically differentiated into a main portion (occipitalis proprius) and a cervico-auriculo-occipitalis portion (Deniker 1885; Lightoller 1928; Loth 1931; Diogo et al. 2012). A vestigial cervico-auriculo-occipitalis bundle may be present rarely in common chimpanzees (Seiler 1976) and gorillas (Ruge 1887). In orangutans, occipitalis is split into a pars profunda and pars superficialis (Sullivan and Osgood 1925; Diogo et al. 2013b).

Variations

Description

The muscular portions of occipitofrontalis may fuse or decussate across the midline (Macalister 1875; Knott 1883a, Bergman et al. 1988; Watanabe 2016; Raveendran and Anthony 2021). Either the occipital or frontal portion may be absent (Macalister 1875; Bergman et al. 1988; Watanabe 2016). The muscle fibers of the frontalis and occipitalis may directly connect (Macalister 1875). Both the occipitalis and frontalis may be divided into fascicles instead of presenting as continuous sheets (Macalister 1875; Knott 1883a). When fasciculated, occipitalis may split into superior and inferior parts (Macalister 1875). Occipitalis may join with auricularis posterior or receive fibers from sternocleidomastoid (Macalister 1875). Frontalis can vary in its extent and at the level where it attaches to the epicranial aponeurosis (Macalister 1875; Knott 1883a). It may have attachments directly to the nasal or maxillary bones (Macalister 1875; Bergman et al. 1988). It may send a slip to levator labii superioris alaeque nasi, or more rarely, the medial palpebral ligament (Macalister 1875; Knott 1883a). Temporoparietalis is occasionally present between frontalis, auricularis anterior, and auricularis superior (Standring 2016).

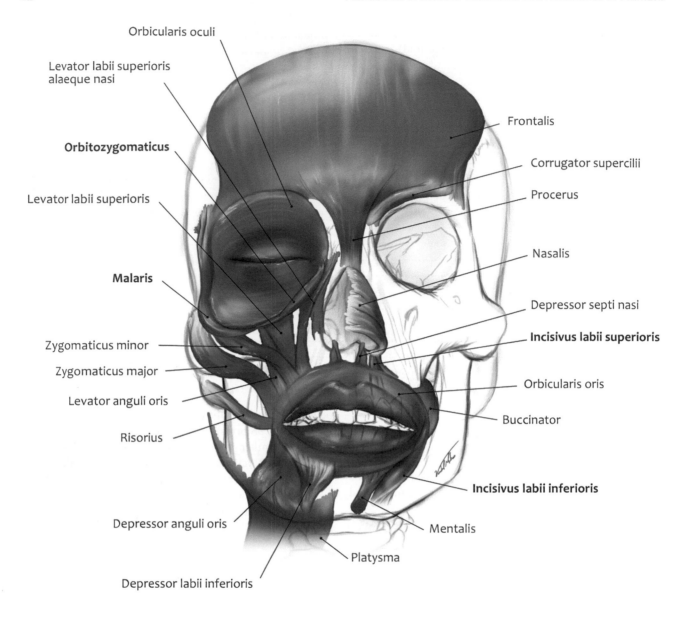

FIGURE 2.1   Muscles of the face in anterior view. In all figures, muscles that are present as variations and/or anomalies are bolded.

Prevalence

In a sample of 26 cadavers, Raveendran and Anthony (2021) found that fibers of the frontalis muscles decussated only near the eyebrows before diverging in seven cases (26.9%), decussated up to the middle of the muscles before diverging in 12 cases (46.2%), and did not decussate at all in seven cases (26.9%).

Anomalies

Description

In a fetus with craniorachischisis, the frontalis was situated deep to a layer of fatty tissue, and the occipitalis was missing, bilaterally (Alghamdi et al. 2017). In a female fetus with trisomy 18, the left and right frontalis muscles were fused at the midline (Alghamdi et al. 2018). Occipitofrontalis may also be hypoplastic in individuals with trisomy 18 (Bersu and Ramirez-Castro 1977).

Prevalence

Occipitofrontalis was hypoplastic in all eight cases of trisomy 18 (100%) examined by Bersu and Ramirez-Castro (1977).

Clinical Implications

Understanding variations in frontalis decussation is helpful for administering botulinum toxin type A therapies (Raveendran and Anthony 2021).

ORBICULARIS OCULI (FIGURE 2.1)

See also: Malaris, Orbitozygomaticus

Synonyms

This muscle may also be referred to as orbicularis palpebrarum (Macalister 1875).

Typical Presentation

Description

Orbicularis oculi is comprised of orbital, palpebral, and lacrimal parts and a ciliary bundle (Standring 2016). The fibers of the orbital part form complete ellipses around the orbit and originate from the nasal part of the frontal bone, the frontal process of the maxilla, and the medial palpebral ligament (Standring 2016). These fibers form depressor supercilii (Macalister 1875; Standring 2016). The fibers of the palpebral part originate from the medial palpebral ligament, course across the eyelids, and end as the lateral palpebral raphe (Standring 2016). The fibers of the lacrimal part originate from the lacrimal bone and insert into the tarsi of the eyelids and the lateral palpebral raphe (Standring 2016).

Innervation

Orbicularis oculi is innervated by the temporal and zygomatic branches of the facial nerve (Standring 2016).

Comparative Anatomy

Orbicularis oculi has a similar typical presentation in the apes, as it is divided into orbital, palpebral, and lacrimal parts with a ciliary bundle, depressor supercilii, bony attachments around the orbit, and an origin from the medial palpebral ligament (Deniker 1885; Sullivan and Osgood 1925; Lightoller 1928; Raven 1950; Miller 1952; Seiler 1976; Gibbs 1999; Burrows et al. 2006; Diogo et al. 2010, 2012, 2013a,b, 2017). It may send a tendon to the zygomatic bone in orangutans (Sullivan and Osgood 1925; Diogo et al. 2013b).

Variations

Description

Orbicularis oculi connects variably with frontalis, corrugator supercilii, zygomaticus minor, levator labii superioris, and levator labii superioris alaeque nasi (Macalister 1875; Standring 2016; Watanabe 2016). It may send a slip to levator palpebrae superioris (Knott 1883a). Zygomaticus minor may originate entirely from orbicularis oculi (Macalister 1875; Knott 1883a). Platysma may reach orbicularis oculi (Macalister 1875; Bergman et al. 1988; Watanabe 2016). The orbicularis oculi muscles may connect via a transversus glabellae muscle (Burkitt and Lightoller 1926; Bergman et al. 1988; Watanabe 2016). There may be a fascicle that surrounds the lacus lacrimalis (Macalister 1875). The orbital part may be absent (Bergman et al. 1988; Watanabe 2016). The peripheral fibers may be absent (Macalister 1875). The orbital and palpebral parts may be completely separate (Macalister 1875; Bergman et al. 1988; Watanabe 2016). Orbicularis oculi is associated with two variable muscles: malaris and the orbitozygomatic muscle (see the entries for these muscles) (Henle 1858, 1871; Lightoller 1925; Hwang et al. 2002; Park et al. 2011, 2012; Zufferey 2013; Standring 2016; Watanabe 2016; Kampan et al. 2018).

Prevalence

Sato (1968a) found orbicularis oculi present in all 190 facial sides (100%) in Kyushu-Japanese males and present in all 121 sides (100%) in females.

Anomalies

Description

In a boy with trisomy 13q, the orbicularis oculi muscles covered most of the midface and their lower borders lay below the level of the nostrils (Pettersen 1979). In a fetus with trisomy 18 and cyclopia, the orbicularis oculi muscles appeared to converge at the midline and expand laterally (Smith et al. 2015). On the left side of this specimen, orbicularis oculi blended with auricularis anterior. In individuals with trisomy 21, Bersu (1980) observed that the superficial muscles in the midface region were poorly differentiated and replaced by a sheet of muscle that was continuous laterally with the orbital part of orbicularis oculi.

Prevalence

Bersu (1980) found that the midface muscles were replaced by a single muscle sheet that was continuous with orbicularis oculi in five out of five individuals with trisomy 21 (100%).

Clinical Implications

N/A

CORRUGATOR SUPERCILII (FIGURE 2.1)

Synonyms

N/A

Typical Presentation

Description

Corrugator supercilii originates from the medial aspect of the superciliary arch and attaches to the skin over the middle part of the supraorbital margin (Standring 2016). It is situated deep to, and mingles with, orbicularis oculi and the frontal portion of occipitofrontalis (Standring 2016).

Innervation

Corrugator supercilii is innervated by the temporal branches of the facial nerve (Standring 2016).

Comparative Anatomy

Corrugator supercilii has a similar typical presentation in the apes, extending from the medial end of the superciliary arch to the eyebrow region (Deniker 1885; Lightoller 1928; Miller 1952; Seiler 1976; Gibbs 1999; Diogo et al. 2010, 2012, 2013a,b, 2017).

Variations

Description

Corrugator supercilii may be completely separate from, or completed fused with, orbicularis oculi (Macalister 1875;

Watanabe 2016). It may be split into several fasciculi or arise from two or three tendinous slips (Macalister 1875). It may be bilaminar (Macalister 1875). It may vary in its superior and lateral extents (Janis et al. 2007). Corrugator supercilii may be absent (Macalister 1875; Sato 1968a; Watanabe 2016).

Prevalence

Sato (1968a) found corrugator supercilii present in 269 out of 328 facial sides (82.01%) in Kyushu-Japanese males and present in 181 out of 220 sides (82.27%) in females.

Anomalies

Description

Corrugator supercilii was absent in a fetus with trisomy 18 and cyclopia (Smith et al. 2015) and a fetus with craniorachischisis (Alghamdi et al. 2017).

Prevalence

N/A

Clinical Implications

Understanding variability in the extent of corrugator supercilii and its varied relationships with the supraorbital nerve is important for successfully performing complete resection of this muscle (Janis et al. 2007, 2008).

MALARIS (FIGURE 2.1)

See also: Orbicularis oculi

Synonyms

This muscle may be referred to as the lateral muscular band of orbicularis oculi (Park et al. 2011) or the lateral bundle of the malaris muscle (Henle 1858, 1871; Lightoller 1925).

Typical Presentation

This muscle is only present as a variation.

Comparative Anatomy

A "pars orbicularis malaris" of orbicularis oculi was described in orangutans as being similar to zygomaticus minor and blended with zygomaticus major (Sullivan and Osgood 1925; Diogo et al. 2013b). Pellatt (1979) reported the presence of malaris in common chimpanzees, and some authors designate malaris as a bundle of zygomaticus major in this species (Burrows et al. 2006; Diogo et al. 2013a).

Variations

Description

When present, malaris is a thin band of muscle that originates from the superficial temporal fascia lateral to orbicularis oculi and is continuous with the inferolateral margin of that muscle (Henle 1858, 1871; Lightoller 1925; Park et al. 2011; Zufferey 2013; Standring 2016; Watanabe 2016). Its extent varies and it may end at the zygomatic arch, in the cheek region, or at the

angle of the mouth (Henle 1858, 1871; Lightoller 1925; Park et al. 2011; Standring 2016; Watanabe 2016). It may blend with zygomaticus major, zygomaticus minor, levator labii superioris, and/or orbicularis oris (Lightoller 1925; Standring 2016). Kampan et al. (2018) found a suspending bundle between the attachments of malaris (lateral bundle) and the orbitozygomatic muscle (medial bundle) and suggest all three bundles are part of the same malaris muscle complex.

Innervation

Malaris is innervated by the temporal branches of the facial nerve (Kampan et al. 2018).

Prevalence

In a sample of 61 hemifaces, Park et al. (2011) found malaris present in 33 cases (54.1%). It ended at the zygomatic arch in 17 cases (27.9%), in the cheek region in 11 cases (18%), and at the angle of the mouth in five cases (8.2%). In a sample of 22 head halves, Kampan et al. (2018) found lateral bundles of orbicularis oculi in all cases (100%).

Anomalies

N/A

Clinical Implications

Understanding variations in the presence and presentation of malaris is helpful for planning and administering periorbital botulinum toxin type A (Botox) injections (Park et al. 2011; Zufferey 2013).

ORBITOZYGOMATICUS (FIGURE 2.1)

See also: Orbicularis oculi

Synonyms

This muscle may be referred to as the medial muscular band of orbicularis oculi (Park et al. 2012), the medial bundle of the malaris muscle (Henle 1858, 1871; Lightoller 1925), zygomatico-orbicularis muscle (Diogo et al. 2013a,b, 2017), or malar levator (Snider et al. 2017).

Typical Presentation

This muscle is only present as a variation.

Comparative Anatomy

Diogo et al. (2013a,b) state that "zygomatico-orbicularis" is absent in orangutans and common chimpanzees.

Variations

Description

Hwang et al. (2002) used "orbitozygomatic muscle" to refer to a muscle easily separated from orbicularis oculi that originated from the medial palpebral ligament and inserted into the zygomaticus muscles and the skin of the cheek. Park et al. (2012) found that it may originate from the frontal portion of occipitofrontalis without an origin from the medial palpebral ligament. Park et al. (2012) also found that the muscle may end above the inferior border of orbicularis oculi. Snider et al. (2017) describe a "malar levator" situated between orbicularis oculi and levator labii superioris alaeque nasi that inserted into the malar fat pad. Kampan et al. (2018) found a suspending bundle between the attachments of malaris (lateral bundle) and the orbitozygomatic muscle (medial bundle) and suggest all three bundles are part of the same malaris muscle complex.

Innervation

The orbitozygomatic muscle is innervated by the zygomatic branches of the facial nerve (Kampan et al. 2018).

Prevalence

In a sample of 42 hemifaces, Hwang et al. (2002) found the orbitozygomatic muscle present in 17 cases (40.5%). In a sample of 22 head halves, Kampan et al. (2018) found medial bundles of orbicularis oculi in nine cases (40.9%). Snider et al. (2017) found a malar levator in all 12 cadavers they dissected (100%). In a sample of 61 hemifaces, Park et al. (2012) found the orbitozygomatic muscle present in 40 cases (65.6%). It attached to the frontal portion of occipitofrontalis without an attachment to the medial palpebral ligament in 14 cases (23%). It extended between the medial palpebral ligament and the skin of the cheek in 14 cases (23%). It inserted into the cheek skin and attached to the frontal portion of occipitofrontalis without an attachment to the medial palpebral ligament in 12 cases (19.7%). In 14 cases (23%), the insertion of the muscle did not pass the inferior border of orbicularis oculi. In 12 cases (19.7%), the insertion of the muscle was beyond the inferior border of orbicularis oculi.

Anomalies

N/A

Clinical Implications

As neurovascular structures travel in the deep surface of the orbitozygomatic muscle, it may be a useful landmark to avoid injury when performing a subciliary incision (Hwang et al. 2002).

Zygomaticus minor (Figure 2.1)

Synonyms

N/A

Typical Presentation

Description

Zygomaticus minor originates from the zygomatic bone and ends in the muscles of the upper lip, where it merges with levator labii superioris (Standring 2016).

Innervation

Zygomaticus minor is innervated by the buccal and zygomatic branches of the facial nerve (Standring 2016).

Comparative Anatomy

Zygomaticus minor has a similar typical presentation in the apes, extending from the zygomatic bone and orbicularis oculi to the upper lip and corner of the mouth (Raven 1950; Miller 1952; Gibbs 1999; Diogo et al. 2010, 2012, 2013a,b, 2017). It may occasionally fuse with zygomaticus major, forming a muscle mass that decussates with nearby muscles (Gibbs 1999).

Variations

Description

Zygomaticus minor may receive a slip from risorius or orbicularis oculi (Macalister 1875; Watanabe 2016). It may also originate entirely from orbicularis oculi (Macalister 1875; Knott 1883a). It may be fused with zygomaticus major (Macalister 1875; Bergman et al. 1988; Watanabe 2016). Macalister (1875) notes that Eustachius described a rare case in which zygomaticus minor joined with frontalis. Zygomaticus minor may end before it reaches the upper lip (Macalister 1875). It may have an additional attachment to the lateral alar region of the nose (Choi et al. 2014). It may be doubled or, more rarely, tripled upon insertion (Macalister 1875; Bergman et al. 1988; Watanabe 2016). Zygomaticus minor may also be absent (Macalister 1875; Sato 1968a; Bergman et al. 1988; Pessa et al. 1998; Watanabe 2016).

Prevalence

Sato (1968a) found zygomaticus minor absent in 8 out of 378 facial sides (2.12%) in Kyushu-Japanese males and absent in 13 out of 242 sides (5.37%) in females. Pessa et al. (1998) found zygomaticus minor present only in 18 out of 50 (36%) hemifacial cadaver dissections. Farahvash et al. (2010) found zygomaticus minor present in 31 out of 52 (59.6%) hemifacial cadaver dissections. Choi et al. (2014) classified the anatomy of zygomaticus minor into three types based on dissections of 54 hemifaces from 30 cadavers. Zygomaticus minor attached to the upper lip only in 34 cases (type A, 63%). In 17 of these cases, the muscle was straight (31.5%), and in the 17 other cases (31.5%), the muscle was curved. Zygomaticus minor attached to the upper lip and the lateral alar region in 15 cases (type B, 27.8%). Zygomaticus minor was poorly developed or absent in five cases (type C, 9.2%).

Anomalies

Description

In a fetus with craniorachischisis, zygomaticus minor was absent on the right side (Alghamdi et al. 2017). In an infant with mandibulofacial dysostosis, zygomaticus minor was absent and replaced with connective tissue (Herring et al. 1979). In a neonate with trisomy 13, zygomaticus major and minor formed a continuous sheet of muscle on the right side (Aziz 1980). In two neonates with trisomy 18, a continuous sheet of muscle fibers extended from the cheek to the nose and the fibers of zygomaticus minor, zygomaticus major, and levator labii superioris could not be differentiated (Aziz 1979, 1981). Similarly, in a female fetus with trisomy 18, zygomaticus major, zygomaticus minor, levator labii superioris, levator labii superioris alaeque nasi, and levator anguli oris were fused bilaterally and formed a single muscle sheet that extended from the zygomatic bone and inferior margin of orbicularis oculi to the upper lip (Alghamdi et al. 2018). These authors describe this muscle sheet as the "complex triangle." Individuals with trisomy 21 also show poor differentiation of the midface muscles, as the zygomaticus muscles and levator labii superioris are not distinct and are replaced by a muscle sheet that extends between orbicularis oculi and orbicularis oris (Bersu 1980).

Prevalence

Replacement of distinct zygomaticus muscles and levator labii superioris with a single sheet of muscle was found in five out of five (100%) individuals with trisomy 21 (Bersu 1980).

Clinical Implications

The attachment of zygomaticus minor into the nose ala could aggravate nasal flaring and action of other muscles in this region and may also form a protrusion next to the nose ala during certain facial expressions (Choi et al. 2014).

Zygomaticus major (Figure 2.1)

Synonyms

N/A

Typical Presentation

Description

Zygomaticus major originates from the zygomatic bone and ends at the angle of the mouth, where it merges with levator anguli oris and orbicularis oris (Standring 2016).

Innervation

Zygomaticus major is innervated by the buccal and zygomatic branches of the facial nerve (Standring 2016).

Comparative Anatomy

Zygomaticus major has a similar typical presentation in the apes, extending from the zygomatic bone and the temporalis fascia to the corner of the mouth (Raven 1950; Miller 1952; Gibbs 1999; Diogo et al. 2010, 2012, 2013a,b, 2017). It may occasionally fuse with zygomaticus minor, forming a muscle mass that decussates with nearby muscles (Gibbs 1999). Zygomaticus major may be divided into two bundles in gibbons, gorillas, and common chimpanzees (Deniker 1885; Sonntag 1923; Raven 1950; Burrows et al. 2006; Diogo et al. 2010, 2012, 2013a).

Variations

Description

Zygomaticus major may fuse with zygomaticus minor or risorius (Macalister 1875; Bergman et al. 1988; Watanabe

2016). It may connect with orbicularis oculi or platysma (Macalister 1875).

It may originate from the masseteric fascia (Macalister 1875). Zygomaticus major may fuse with depressor anguli oris at its insertion (Macalister 1875). It may be absent (Macalister 1875; Sato 1968a; Bergman et al. 1988). Zygomaticus major may be doubled throughout or at its insertion, and this latter presentation is often referred to as bifid zygomaticus major (Macalister 1875; Bergman et al. 1988; Watanabe 2016).

Prevalence

Sato (1968a) found zygomaticus major present in 376 out of 386 facial sides (97.41%) in Kyushu-Japanese males and present in 245 out of 248 sides (98.79%) in females. In a sample of 50 hemifaces, Pessa et al. (1998) found a single zygomaticus major in 33 cases (66%) and a double or bifid zygomaticus major in 17 cases (34%). In a sample of 70 cadavers, Hu et al. (2008) found a bifid zygomaticus major in 28 cases (40%). In a sample of 52 hemifaces, Farahvash et al. (2010) found a single zygomaticus major in 42 cases (80.8%) and a bifid zygomaticus major in ten cases (19.2%). In a sample of 29 sides from 15 heads, Elvan et al. (2020) found a bifid zygomaticus major on four sides (13.8%). In a meta-analysis of seven studies (including some detailed here), Phan and Onggo (2019) found that the overall prevalence of bifid zygomaticus major is 22.7%.

Anomalies

Description

In a fetus with craniorachischisis, zygomaticus major was absent on the right side (Alghamdi et al. 2017). In a fetus with trisomy 18 and cyclopia, zygomaticus major originated from orbicularis oculi and the zygomatic process and spread wider than is typical (Smith et al. 2015). It also received fibers from platysma. In an infant with mandibulofacial dysostosis, zygomaticus major originated from the zygomatic process of the frontal bone (Herring et al. 1979).

In a neonate with trisomy 13, zygomaticus major and minor formed a continuous sheet of muscle on the right side (Aziz 1980). In two neonates with trisomy 18, a continuous sheet of muscle fibers extended from the cheek to the nose and the fibers of zygomaticus minor, zygomaticus major, and levator labii superioris could not be differentiated (Aziz 1979, 1981). Similarly, in a female fetus with trisomy 18, zygomaticus major, zygomaticus minor, levator labii superioris, levator labii superioris alaeque nasi, and levator anguli oris were fused bilaterally and formed a single muscle sheet that extended from the zygomatic bone and inferior margin of orbicularis oculi to the upper lip (Alghamdi et al. 2018). These authors describe this muscle sheet as the "complex triangle." Individuals with trisomy 21 also show poor differentiation of the midface muscles, as the zygomaticus muscles and levator labii superioris are not distinct and are replaced by a muscle sheet that extends between orbicularis oculi and orbicularis oris (Bersu 1980).

Prevalence

Replacement of distinct zygomaticus muscles and levator labii superioris with a single sheet of muscle was found in five out of five (100%) individuals with trisomy 21 (Bersu 1980).

Clinical Implications

Understanding variations of zygomaticus major is important for planning and performing facial reanimation surgery (Hu et al. 2008).

LEVATOR LABII SUPERIORIS (FIGURE 2.1)

Synonyms

This muscle may also be referred to as levator labii superioris proprius (Macalister 1875).

Typical Presentation

Description

Levator labii superioris originates from the maxilla and zygomatic bone and inserts into the muscles of the upper lip (Standring 2016).

Innervation

Levator labii superioris is innervated by the buccal and zygomatic branches of the facial nerve (Standring 2016).

Comparative Anatomy

Levator labii superioris has a similar typical presentation in the great apes, extending from the infraorbital region to the upper lip (Miller 1952; Gibbs 1999; Diogo et al. 2010, 2013a,b, 2017). In gibbons, the muscle runs posteroanteriorly and mediolaterally from the infraorbital region to the nose, with only a few fibers attaching near the upper lip, thus having a presentation similar to that found in non-catarrhine primates (Deniker 1885; Diogo et al. 2012).

Variations

Description

Levator labii superioris may be fused with levator labii superioris alaeque nasi (Macalister 1875). It may also be fused in rare cases with zygomaticus minor (Macalister 1875). It may send a slip to nasalis or have a connection to levator anguli oris (Macalister 1875; Watanabe 2016). Levator labii superioris may be doubled or tripled (Macalister 1875). It may also have two or three heads, with the outer head arising from the zygomatic bone or orbicularis oculi (Macalister 1875; Knott 1883a; Watanabe 2016). Levator labii superioris may be absent (Macalister 1875; Sato 1968a; Watanabe 2016).

Prevalence

Macalister (1875) states that levator labii superioris may be fused with levator labii superioris alaeque nasi in about one out of every three subjects. Sato (1968a) found levator labii superioris present in 230 out of 240 facial sides (95.83%) in Kyushu-Japanese males and present in 158 out of 162 sides (97.53%) in females.

Anomalies

Description

In an infant with mandibulofacial dysostosis, levator labii superioris was absent and replaced with connective tissue (Herring et al. 1979). In a fetus with craniorachischisis, levator labii superioris was absent on the right side (Alghamdi et al. 2017). It was also absent in a neonate with trisomy 13 (Aziz 1980). Bersu and Ramirez-Castro (1977) noted that in infants with trisomy 18, levator labii superioris and levator labii superioris alaeque nasi were more extensively fused than usual. In two neonates with trisomy 18, a continuous sheet of muscle fibers extended from the cheek to the nose and the fibers of zygomaticus minor, zygomaticus major, and levator labii superioris could not be differentiated (Aziz 1979, 1981). Similarly, in a female fetus with trisomy 18, zygomaticus major, zygomaticus minor, levator labii superioris, levator labii superioris alaeque nasi, and levator anguli oris were fused bilaterally and formed a single muscle sheet that extended from the zygomatic bone and inferior margin of orbicularis oculi to the upper lip (Alghamdi et al. 2018). These authors describe this muscle sheet as the "complex triangle." Individuals with trisomy 21 also show poor differentiation of the midface muscles, as the zygomaticus muscles and levator labii superioris are not distinct and are replaced by a muscle sheet that extends between orbicularis oculi and orbicularis oris (Bersu 1980).

Prevalence

Replacement of distinct zygomaticus muscles and levator labii superioris with a single sheet of muscle was found in five out of five (100%) individuals with trisomy 21 (Bersu 1980).

Clinical Implications

N/A

LEVATOR LABII SUPERIORIS ALAEQUE NASI (FIGURE 2.1)

Synonyms

This muscle may also be referred to as levator alae nasi (Pessa et al. 1998).

Typical Presentation

Description

Levator labii superioris alaeque nasi originates from the frontal process of the maxilla (Standring 2016). Its medial slip inserts into the nose, on the perichondrium, and skin over the lateral wall of the major alar cartilage (Standring 2016). Its lateral slip ends in the upper lip where it merges with levator labii superioris and orbicularis oris (Standring 2016).

Innervation

Levator labii superioris alaeque nasi is innervated by the superior buccal and zygomatic branches of the facial nerve (Standring 2016).

Comparative Anatomy

Levator labii superioris alaeque nasi has a similar typical presentation in the apes, extending from the maxilla and region of the medial palpebral ligament to the ala of the nose and upper lip (Gratiolet and Alix 1866; Miller 1952; Gibbs 1999; Burrows et al. 2006; Diogo et al. 2010, 2012, 2013a,b, 2017).

Variations

Description

Levator labii superioris alaeque nasi may only have one slip (Macalister 1875). The medial slip may be doubled or separated from the lateral slip (Macalister 1875; Watanabe 2016). Levator labii superioris alaeque nasi may be fused with levator labii superioris (Macalister 1875). It may receive a slip from frontalis or procerus (Macalister 1875; Watanabe 2016). It may send fibers to nasalis (Macalister 1875; Hur et al. 2010). It may also be absent (Sato 1968a; Watanabe 2016).

This muscle is associated with anomalous nasi, also known as the musculus anomalous of Albinus or the rhomboideus of Santorini (Macalister 1875; Standring 2016). It originates from the frontal process of the maxilla and ends near the canine fossa (Macalister 1875; Standring 2016). Its origin may connect to the medial slip of levator labii superioris alaeque nasi, and its insertion may fuse with levator anguli oris (Macalister 1875).

Prevalence

Macalister (1875) states that levator labii superioris alaeque nasi may be fused with levator labii superioris in about one out of every three subjects. Sato (1968a) found levator labii superioris alaeque nasi present in 217 out of 230 facial sides (94.35%) in Kyushu-Japanese males and present in 175 out of 184 sides (95.11%) in females. In a sample of 40 cadavers, Hur et al. (2010) found that the medial slip of levator labii superioris alaeque nasi sent fibers to the transverse part of nasalis in 36 cases (90%).

Anomalies

Description

Levator labii superioris alaeque nasi may be absent in individuals with cleft lip defects (Standring 2016). In an infant with mandibulofacial dysostosis, levator labii superioris alaeque nasi inserted onto the wing of the nose but not the upper lip (Herring et al. 1979). In a fetus with craniorachischisis, levator labii superioris alaeque nasi was absent bilaterally (Alghamdi et al. 2017). Bersu and Ramirez-Castro

(1977) noted that in infants with trisomy 18, levator labii superioris and levator labii superioris alaeque nasi were more extensively fused than usual.

In a fetus with trisomy 18 and cyclopia, levator labii superioris alaeque nasi seemed to originate from the maxilla and insert into orbicularis oris (Smith et al. 2015). In a female fetus with trisomy 18, zygomaticus major, zygomaticus minor, levator labii superioris, levator labii superioris alaeque nasi, and levator anguli oris were fused bilaterally and formed a single muscle sheet that extended from the zygomatic bone and inferior margin of orbicularis oculi to the upper lip (Alghamdi et al. 2018). These authors describe this muscle sheet as the "complex triangle."

Prevalence

N/A

Clinical Implications

N/A

LEVATOR ANGULI ORIS (FIGURE 2.1)

Synonyms

This muscle may also be referred to as musculus caninus (Macalister 1875) or levator anguli oris facialis (Diogo and Abdala 2010).

Typical Presentation

Description

Levator anguli oris originates from the canine fossa of the maxilla and inserts into the angle of the mouth, where it blends with other muscles that contribute to the modiolus (Standring 2016).

Innervation

Levator anguli oris is innervated by the buccal and zygomatic branches of the facial nerve (Standring 2016).

Comparative Anatomy

Levator anguli oris has a similar typical presentation in the apes, extending from the canine fossa to the angle of the mouth, often blending with nearby muscles (Raven 1950; Miller 1952; Gibbs 1999; Diogo et al. 2010, 2012, 2013a,b, 2017).

Variations

Description

Levator anguli oris may be divided (Macalister 1875). It may be connected with nasalis (Macalister 1875). It may be continuous with levator labii superioris or depressor anguli oris (Macalister 1875; Watanabe 2016).

Prevalence

N/A

Anomalies

Description

Levator anguli oris was absent bilaterally in a fetus with craniorachischisis (Alghamdi et al. 2017). In a female fetus with trisomy 18, zygomaticus major, zygomaticus minor, levator labii superioris, levator labii superioris alaeque nasi, and levator anguli oris were fused bilaterally and formed a single muscle sheet that extended from the zygomatic bone and inferior margin of orbicularis oculi to the upper lip (Alghamdi et al. 2018). These authors describe this muscle sheet as the "complex triangle." In an infant with mandibulofacial dysostosis, levator anguli oris originated medially, near the medial corner of the eye (Herring et al. 1979).

Prevalence

N/A

Clinical Implications

N/A

Risorius (Figure 2.1)

Synonyms

This muscle may also be referred to as risorius of Santorini (Macalister 1875).

Typical Presentation

Description

Risorius originates from one or more structures in the region near the parotid gland and attaches to the modiolus (Standring 2016).

Innervation

Risorius is innervated by the buccal branches of the facial nerve (Standring 2016).

Comparative Anatomy

Risorius is typically absent in gibbons (Diogo et al. 2012), orangutans (Diogo et al. 2013b), and bonobos (Miller 1952; Diogo et al. 2017). It is often present in gorillas (Deniker 1885; Ruge 1887; Raven 1950; Seiler 1976; Diogo et al. 2010) and in common chimpanzees (Sonntag 1923; Seiler 1976; Burrows et al. 2006; Diogo et al. 2013a). When present, it extends from the superior margin of platysma to the angle of the mouth (Gibbs 1999; Diogo et al. 2010, 2013a).

Variations

Description

Risorius may present as a wide fan of fibers or one or more fascicles (Macalister 1875; Bergman et al. 1988; Sekine et al. 1988; Standring 2016). Risorius may also be absent (Sato 1968a; Bergman et al. 1988; Pessa et al. 1998; Farahvash et al. 2010; Watanabe 2016). Typical origins of risorius include the parotid fascia, fascia over the masseter, fascia over

platysma, fascia over the mastoid process, and/or the zygomatic arch (Macalister 1875; Knott 1883a; Standring 2016; Watanabe 2016). The muscle may also arise from the skin over the superior third of sternocleidomastoid or the external ear (Macalister 1875; Knott 1883a; Watanabe 2016). It can also originate from the masseter tendon (Macalister 1875; Eisler 1912; Sekine et al. 1988). Risorius may receive a slip from or fuse with transversus nuchae (Macalister 1875; Knott 1883a; Jovanovski et al. 2020). It may send a slip to zygomaticus minor or fuse with zygomaticus major (Macalister 1875; Watanabe 2016). It may blend with orbicularis oris (Knott 1883a). At its insertion, it may join with depressor anguli oris (Macalister 1875; Sekine et al. 1988; Kim et al. 2015a; Watanabe 2016).

Some authors have classified risorius into three types depending on its orientation and direction of insertion: platysma risorius (inserts into the modiolus horizontally), zygomaticus risorius (inserts into the modiolus from above horizontal), and triangularis risorius (inserts into the modiolus from below horizontal) (Lightoller 1925; Loth 1931; Sekine et al. 1988; Kim et al. 2015a). According to Kim et al. (2015a), the layer at which risorius inserts into the modiolus can also be classified into three types, ranging from superficial to, flush with, or deep to depressor anguli oris.

Prevalence

Sato (1968a) found risorius absent in 39 out of 386 facial sides (10.1%) in Kyushu-Japanese males and absent in 32 out of 240 sides in females (13.3%). Ito et al. (2006) found risorius absent in 4 out of 10 cadavers (40%). Pessa et al. (1998) found risorius present in only 3 out of 50 (6%) hemifacial cadaver dissections. Farahvash et al. (2010) found risorius present in 16 out of 52 (30.8%) hemifacial cadaver dissections. In a sample of 80 cadavers, Kim et al. (2015a) found platysma risorius in 36 cases (45%), triangularis risorius in 28 cases (35%), and zygomaticus risorius in 16 cases (20%). The insertion level of risorius was superficial in 45 cases (56.3%), flush in 25 cases (31.2%), and deep in 10 cases (12.5%).

Anomalies

Description

Risorius has been found absent bilaterally in both a neonate with trisomy 18 (Aziz 1979) and a neonate with trisomy 13 (Aziz 1980). In a fetus with craniorachischisis, the right risorius was absent (Alghamdi et al. 2017). In individuals with trisomy 21, Bersu (1980) found that platysma cervicale merged with risorius upon insertion. In an infant with mandibulofacial dysostosis, risorius originated from the fascia over the masseter and was distinguished completely from platysma (Herring et al. 1979).

Prevalence

In their literature review, Smith et al. (2015) found that risorius was absent in 1 out of 20 individuals with trisomy 13 (5%) and 1 out of 17 individuals with trisomy 18 (5.9%).

Clinical Implications

As risorius can cover different parts of the masseter depending on its attachments, injection of botulinum toxin type A into the masseter may affect risorius (Bae et al. 2014). Vector of attachment (platysma risorius, zygomaticus risorius, or triangularis risorius) may affect the function of risorius and how it acts on the lips (Kim et al. 2015a).

BUCCINATORIUS (BUCCINATOR) (FIGURE 2.1)

Synonyms

N/A

Typical Presentation

Description

Buccinator originates from the maxilla, mandible, and the pterygomandibular raphe and inserts into the modiolus (Standring 2016).

Innervation

Buccinator is innervated by the buccal branch of the facial nerve (Standring 2016).

Comparative Anatomy

Buccinator has a similar typical presentation in the apes, extending from the maxilla, mandible, and pterygomandibular raphe to the angle of the mouth and lips (Raven 1950; Miller 1952; Gibbs 1999; Diogo et al. 2010, 2012, 2013a,b, 2017).

Variations

Description

Buccinator may vary in the extent of its maxillary and mandibular attachments (Macalister 1875; Hur et al. 2011a). An inferior bundle (fourth band) of the buccinator may be present, which extends from the mandible and passes under orbicularis oris, ending beyond the modiolus (Hur et al. 2011a). Macalister (1875) reports that it may be thin and underdeveloped in its center. It may be bilaminar (Bergman et al. 1988). It may fuse with masseter or connect to the buccopharyngeal part of the superior pharyngeal constrictor (Macalister 1875; Bergman et al. 1988). It may receive a slip from tensor veli palatini or the parotid duct (Macalister 1875; Knott 1883a; Patel and Loukas 2016).

Ullah and Khan (2006) report the presence of an accessory muscle in the infratemporal fossa that they term the zygobuccinator muscle, which originated from the posterior surface of the frontal process of the zygomatic bone and inserted into the buccinator. This muscle likely corresponds to the temporobuccinator band described by Gaughran (1957) (Buck 2007).

Prevalence

In a sample of 40 hemifaces, Hur et al. (2011a) found a fourth band of the buccinator on 14 sides (35%).

Anomalies

Description

Bersu et al. (1976) describe a male infant with Hanhart syndrome. The buccinator muscles were comprised of fibers that attached to the lateral surface of the maxilla with some fibers blended with the anomalous portion of the superior pharyngeal constrictor. In a fetus with craniorachischisis, both buccinator and masseter were undifferentiated muscle tissues situated medial to the ears (Alghamdi et al. 2017).

Prevalence

N/A

Clinical Implications

The fourth band of buccinator may affect the alveolar bone of the mandible or occlusion during muscular movements (Hur et al. 2011a).

ORBICULARIS ORIS (FIGURE 2.1)

See also: Incisivus labii superior, Incisivus labii inferior

Synonyms

Some authors have described parts of orbicularis oris as separate muscles: protractor labii superioris, protractor labii inferioris, co-angustator labii inferioris, constrictor labii inferioris, constrictor labii superioris, levator prolabii superioris, and nasalis labii superioris (Macalister 1875; Knott 1883a).

Typical Presentation

Description

Orbicularis oris encircles the mouth and is comprised of four parts that each contain a pars peripheralis (superficial or extrinsic) and pars marginalis (deep or intrinsic) (Standring 2016). The fibers of orbicularis oris originate from the modiolus and receive contributions from buccinator, levator anguli oris, and depressor anguli oris (Standring 2016). The fibers have submucosal, fascial, and dermal attachments around the lips (Standring 2016).

Innervation

Orbicularis oris is innervated by the buccal and mandibular branches of the facial nerve (Standring 2016).

Comparative Anatomy

Orbicularis oris has a similar typical presentation in the apes, but it is possible that this muscle is not differentiated into peripheral and marginal portions (Diogo et al. 2010, 2012, 2013a,b, 2017).

Variations

Description

Orbicularis oris may vary in its development and in the amount and extent of accessory bands from the alveolar arches (Macalister 1875). Orbicularis oris is associated with incisivus labii superioris and incisivus labii inferioris, two bundles that are considered accessory bundles of the orbicularis oris complex (see the entries for these muscles) (Standring 2016; Iwanaga et al. 2017).

Prevalence

N/A

Anomalies

Description

Fibers of orbicularis oris are affected by cleft lip defects (Bersu et al. 1977; De Mey et al. 1989; Wijayaweera et al. 2000). In incomplete clefts, the intrinsic portion of the muscle ends in the submucosa of the vermilion border of the lip while the extrinsic portion crosses the cleft and is distorted (De Mey et al. 1989; Wijayaweera et al. 2000). In complete clefts, the intrinsic portion is again interrupted, and fibers of the extrinsic portion are horizontally oriented on the medial side and deviate along the margin of the cleft on the lateral side (De Mey et al. 1989; Wijayaweera et al. 2000). In an infant with trisomy 18 and a bilateral cleft lip, the fibers of orbicularis oris ended at the medial border of each maxillary process (Bersu et al. 1977).

In a neonate with trisomy 13, orbicularis oris was absent (Aziz 1980). In a fetus with trisomy 18 and cyclopia, the inferior part of orbicularis oris was comprised of only the deep (marginal) portion (Smith et al. 2015).

Prevalence

N/A

Clinical Implications

N/A

DEPRESSOR ANGULI ORIS (FIGURE 2.1)

Synonyms

This muscle may also be referred to as triangularis (Huber and Hughson 1926).

Typical Presentation

Description

Depressor anguli oris is continuous with platysma, originating from the mental tubercle and from along the oblique line of the mandible (Standring 2016). It ends at the angle of the mouth, having connections to risorius, orbicularis oris, and levator anguli oris (Standring 2016).

Innervation

Depressor anguli oris is innervated by the marginal mandibular branch and the buccal branch of the facial nerve (Standring 2016).

Comparative Anatomy

Depressor anguli oris has a similar typical presentation in the apes, extending from the angle of the mouth to the fascia of platysma, with connections to nearby muscles (Miller 1952; Gibbs 1999; Diogo et al. 2010, 2012, 2013a,b, 2017). It may be differentiated into two or more bundles in gorillas (Ruge 1887; Diogo et al. 2010). It is fused with platysma cervicale and orbicularis oris in bonobos (Miller 1952; Diogo et al. 2017). Transversus menti has been noted as a variation in common chimpanzees (Gratiolet and Alix 1866; Loth 1931; Diogo ct al. 2013a) and in onc fetal gorilla (Dcnikcr 1885).

Variations

Description

Depressor anguli oris may not always have a continuous origin from platysma and can originate entirely from the mandible (Macalister 1875; Watanabe 2016). It may be split by the facial artery into three bundles (Macalister 1875). Its fibers may be continuous with levator labii superioris or zygomaticus major (Macalister 1875; Watanabe 2016). Its medial fibers may pass deep to depressor labii inferioris, enabling connections to incisivus labii inferioris, mentalis, and/or the inferior border of the mandible (Hur et al. 2014). It may be absent in some cases (Sato 1968a).

Transversus menti is a variation that occurs when fibers of depressor anguli oris cross the midline and interdigitate with those of its counterpart below the mental symphysis (Hallett 1848; Macalister 1875; Sato 1968a; Weaver 1978; Bergman et al. 1988; Sripanidkulchai et al. 2013; Standring 2016; Watanabe 2016). It may also be referred to as transversalis menti (Santorini), faisceau sous-symphysien (Cruveilhier), or the mental sling (Macalister 1875; Knott 1883a; Standring 2016). When transversus menti is present, its fibers may interdigitate with fibers of platysma, such that they may be mistaken for fibers of platysma that cross the midline (Hallett 1848).

Prevalence

Hur et al. (2014) studied depressor anguli oris in 40 hemifaces from cadavers. Medial fibers of depressor anguli oris that pass deep to depressor labii inferioris were found in 18 specimens (45%). These fibers connected to incisivus labii inferioris and the inferior border of the mandible in 14 specimens (35%), connected to incisivus labii inferioris and fibers of mentalis in two specimens (5%), connected to incisivus labii inferioris only in one specimen (2.5%), and blended with mentalis only in one specimen (2.5%).

Sato (1968a) found depressor anguli oris present in 366 out of 372 facial sides (98.39%) in Kyushu-Japanese males and present in 230 out of 240 sides (95.83%) in females. Sato (1968a) found transversus menti present in 206 out of 330 facial sides (62.42%) in Kyushu-Japanese males and present in 116 out of 206 sides (56.31%) in females. Knott (1883a) found transversus menti in 3 out of 11 cases (27.3%). Weaver (1978) found transversus menti in 9 out of 16 (56.25%) cadaveric heads.

Anomalies

Description

In a fetus with trisomy 18 and cyclopia, depressor anguli oris was partially fused with mentalis and depressor labii inferioris (Smith et al. 2015). It also received fibers from platysma (Smith et al. 2015). In descriptions of other specimens with trisomy 18, both Bersu and Ramirez-Castro (1977) and Aziz (1979) noted that depressor anguli oris was poorly differentiated and partially blended with depressor labii inferioris and platysma.

Congenital hypoplasia or agenesis of depressor anguli oris is a primary cause of asymmetric crying facies (ACF) (Pasick et al. 2013; Akcan et al. 2016; Watanabe 2016). This anomaly is often associated with other congenital anomalies throughout the body and has been observed in individuals with 22q11.2 deletion syndrome and infants born after in vitro fertilization (Alexiou et al. 1976; Pasick et al. 2013; Akcan et al. 2016; Watanabe 2016).

Prevalence

Alexiou et al. (1976) found hypoplasia of depressor anguli oris in 44 out of 6487 neonates (0.68%).

Clinical Implications

Understanding variations in depressor anguli oris is helpful for administering botulinum toxin type A therapies (Hur et al. 2008, 2014). Weaver (1978) suggests that transversus menti could be used in reconstructive surgery in cases where depressor anguli oris and/or depressor labii inferioris are damaged.

Depressor labii inferioris (Figure 2.1)

Synonyms

N/A

Typical Presentation

Description

Depressor labii inferioris originates from the oblique line of the mandible and inserts into the mucosa and skin of the lower lip (Standring 2016). It is continuous with platysma, merges with orbicularis oris, and decussates with its counterpart (Standring 2016).

Innervation

Depressor labii inferioris is innervated by the mandibular branch of the facial nerve (Standring 2016).

Comparative Anatomy

Depressor labii inferioris has a similar typical presentation in the apes, extending from the mandible and platysma to the lower lip and blending with its counterpart and other nearby muscles (Deniker 1885; Sonntag 1923; Raven 1950; Miller 1952; Seiler 1976; Pellatt 1979; Gibbs 1999; Burrows et al. 2006; Diogo et al. 2010, 2012, 2013a,b, 2017).

Variations

Description

Depressor labii inferioris may be divided into two or more fascicles (Macalister 1875).

Prevalence

N/A

Anomalies

Description

In a fetus with trisomy 18 and cyclopia, depressor labii inferioris was partially fused with mentalis and depressor anguli oris (Smith et al. 2015). In the female fetus with trisomy 18 dissected by Alghamdi et al. (2018), depressor labii inferioris was fused with mentalis bilaterally. In descriptions of other specimens with trisomy 18, both Bersu and Ramirez-Castro (1977) and Aziz (1979) noted that depressor labii inferioris was poorly differentiated and partially blended with depressor anguli oris and platysma. In a fetus with craniorachischisis, depressor labii inferioris was also poorly differentiated, primarily connected to fat-like tissue, and had only a few muscle fibers on the anterior surface of the chin (Alghamdi et al. 2017).

Prevalence

N/A

Clinical Implications

N/A

Procerus (Figure 2.1)

Synonyms

This muscle may also be referred to as pyramidalis nasi (Macalister 1875).

Typical Presentation

Description

Procerus originates from the nasal bone, the lateral nasal cartilage, and the transverse portion of nasalis (Standring 2016). It inserts into the skin of the glabella and is partially blended with occipitofrontalis (Standring 2016).

Innervation

Procerus is typically innervated by the lower zygomatic and temporal branches of the facial nerve but may be innervated by the buccal branch of the facial nerve in some cases (Standring 2016).

Comparative Anatomy

Procerus has a similar typical presentation in the apes, extending from frontalis to the dorsomedial region of the nose, blending with frontalis and/or levator labii superioris alaeque nasi (Gratiolet and Alix 1866; Miller 1952; Seiler 1976; Pellatt 1979; Gibbs 1999; Burrows et al. 2006; Diogo et al. 2010, 2012, 2013a,b, 2017).

Variations

Description

The portion of procerus closest to the orbit or the entire muscle may be absent (Macalister 1875; Bergman et al. 1988; Watanabe 2016). The procerus muscles may present as a single slip that continues onto the bridge of the nose (Macalister 1875; Watanabe 2016). In rare cases, it may be continuous with the inner border of levator labii superioris alaeque nasi (Macalister 1875). It may be separate from occipitofrontalis (Macalister 1875).

Prevalence

N/A

Anomalies

Description

Procerus may be absent in individuals with cleft lip defects (Standring 2016). Procerus was absent bilaterally in a fetus with trisomy 18 and cyclopia (Smith et al. 2015). In a fetus with craniorachischisis, procerus was represented by a thin sheet of fibers between the eyes (Alghamdi et al. 2017).

Prevalence

N/A

Clinical Implications

N/A

NASALIS (FIGURE 2.1)

Synonyms

The transverse part of nasalis may be referred to as compressor naris or compressor nasi (Macalister 1875; Standring 2016). The alar part of nasalis may be referred to as dilator naris posterior (Macalister 1875; Standring 2016).

Typical Presentation

Description

The transverse part of nasalis originates from the maxilla superior and lateral to the incisive fossa and merges with its counterpart along the bridge of the nose (Standring 2016). The alar part of nasalis originates from the maxilla superior to the lateral incisor and canine teeth and inserts into the skin and cartilage of the ala (Standring 2016).

Innervation

Nasalis is typically innervated by the buccal branch of the facial nerve but may also be innervated by the zygomatic branch in some cases (Standring 2016).

Comparative Anatomy

Nasalis has a similar typical presentation in the apes, extending from the maxilla to the lateral margin and ala of the nose (Raven 1950; Miller 1952; Gibbs 1999; Diogo et al. 2010, 2012, 2013a,b, 2017).

Variations

Description

Nasalis may continue into procerus (Bergman et al. 1988; Watanabe 2016). The transverse part of nasalis may be split into fascicles or upper and lower bands (Macalister 1875). The transverse parts may present as a single sheet of muscle (Macalister 1875). The muscle may be poorly developed or absent (Macalister 1875). It may be fused with levator anguli oris (Macalister 1875). The transverse part may receive fibers from levator labii superioris alaeque nasi (Macalister 1875; Hur et al. 2010). It may also have an origin from the upper half of the alar facial crease (Hur et al. 2010). The alar part of nasalis may be absent (Macalister 1875). It may merge with a slip of orbicularis oris (Macalister 1875).

Prevalence

In a sample of 40 cadavers, Hur et al. (2010) found that the medial slip of levator labii superioris alaeque nasi sent fibers to the transverse part of nasalis in 36 cases (90%). The transverse part of nasalis originated from the maxilla only in 26 cases (65%) and from both the maxilla and the alar facial crease in 14 cases (35%).

Anomalies

Description

Nasalis may be absent in individuals with cleft lip defects (Standring 2016). In some specimens with trisomy 18, nasalis was not identifiable (Bersu and Ramirez-Castro 1977). In a fetus with trisomy 18 and cyclopia, a muscle possibly corresponding to nasalis was found on the superior portion of the maxilla, situated where the nose typically lies (Smith et al. 2015). It originated from the lateral maxilla and inserted along the midline prominence below the orbit, with a partial insertion into levator labii superioris alaeque nasi (Smith et al. 2015). Similarly, in a fetus with craniorachischisis, a possible nasalis was identified on the left side spanning the region between the nose and mouth (Alghamdi et al. 2017).

Prevalence

Nasalis was not identifiable in two out of four cases of trisomy 18 (50%) (Bersu and Ramirez-Castro 1977).

Clinical Implications

N/A

DEPRESSOR SEPTI NASI (FIGURE 2.1)

Synonyms

This muscle may be referred to as depressor septi (Standring 2016), depressor septi mobilis narium, nasolabialis, depressor apicis naris, or nasalis labii superioris (Macalister 1875; Knott 1883a).

Typical Presentation

Description

Depressor septi nasi may be considered a septal attachment of orbicularis oris (Knott 1883a). It originates from the maxilla above the incisors and from orbicularis oris and inserts into the columella, medial crus of the major alar cartilage, and nasal septum (Standring 2016).

Innervation

Depressor septi nasi is typically innervated by the buccal branch of the facial nerve but may be innervated by the zygomatic branch in some cases (Standring 2016).

Comparative Anatomy

Depressor septi nasi has a similar typical presentation in the apes, situated deep to orbicularis oris and extending from the maxilla to the inferior region of the nose (Raven 1950; Burrows et al. 2006; Diogo et al. 2010, 2012, 2013a,b, 2017).

Variations

Description

Depressor septi nasi may be absent or poorly developed (Rohrich et al. 2000; Ebrahimi et al. 2012; Standring 2016; Kikuta et al. 2020). It may also be hypertrophic (Ohtsuka 2005; Watanabe 2016). It may be indistinguishable from orbicularis oris (Macalister 1875). The origin from the maxilla may be absent (Rohrich et al. 2000; Ebrahimi et al. 2012; Kikuta et al. 2020). Kikuta et al. (2020) found that it originated from orbicularis oris and incisivus labii superioris, without an origin directly from the maxilla. Slips may extend between the medial crura and the tip of the nose (Standring 2016).

Prevalence

In a sample of 55 cadavers, Rohrich et al. (2000) found that depressor septi nasi originated completely from orbicularis oris in 34 cases (61.8%). It originated from the periosteum of the maxilla and partially from orbicularis oris in 12 cases (21.8%). Depressor septi nasi was rudimentary or absent in nine cases (16.4%). In a sample of 82 muscles from 41 cadavers, Ebrahimi et al. (2012) found that depressor septi nasi originated from the periosteum of the maxilla in 36 cases (44%) and from orbicularis oris in 32 cases (39%). The muscles were diminutive or floating and comprised of fibrous tissue in 14 cases (17%). In a sample of 20 sides, Kikuta et al. (2020) found depressor septi nasi present on 18 sides (90%). On 6 of these 18 sides (33%), depressor septi nasi was difficult to separate completely from orbicularis oris.

Anomalies

Description

Depressor septi nasi may be absent in individuals with cleft lip defects (Standring 2016).

Prevalence

N/A

Clinical Implications

Hypertrophy of depressor septi nasi may present as a swelling or mass of the columella (Ohtsuka 2005).

INCISIVUS LABII SUPERIORIS (FIGURE 2.1)

Synonyms

This muscle may be referred to as cuspidator oris or labialis superior profundus (Seiler 1976; Diogo et al. 2010, 2012, 2013a,b, 2017), accessory fasciculi or skeletal head of orbicularis oris, facial portion of orbicularis oris, incisive bundle of orbicularis oris, or incisive Cowper (Iwanaga et al. 2017).

Typical Presentation

This muscle is present only as a variation or anomaly.

Comparative Anatomy

Incisivus labii superioris has a similar typical presentation in the apes, extending between the incisive fossa of the maxilla and orbicularis oris (Seiler 1976; Iwanaga et al. 2021).

Variations

Description

Incisivus labii superioris is considered an accessory muscle of orbicularis oris (Iwanaga et al. 2017). It arises deep to the superior portion of orbicularis oris, below the alar portion of nasalis, lateral to depressor septi, and medial to levator anguli oris (Lightoller 1925; Standring 2016; Iwanaga et al. 2017; Hur 2018). It originates from the incisive fossa of the maxilla above the eminence of the lateral incisor (Standring 2016). Its bony attachment extends mediolaterally between the areas above the central incisor and the canine and superoinferiorly between the attachment of nasalis and the mucogingival junction (Iwanaga et al. 2017). Its fibers course laterally, interdigitate with orbicularis oris, and divide into superficial and deep parts that attach to the modiolus (Lightoller 1925; Standring 2016; Iwanaga et al. 2017). Hur (2018) notes that it may not divide into superficial and deep parts in some cases. It blends with other muscles at the angle of the mouth, particularly levator anguli oris (Lightoller 1925; Standring 2016; Iwanaga et al. 2017; Hur 2018).

Innervation

N/A

Prevalence

In a sample of 52 facial sides, Hur (2018) found incisivus labii superioris present in all cases (100%). It divided into superficial and deep parts upon insertion in 48 cases (92.3%) and did not divide in four cases (7.7%). In a sample of 20 facial sides, Kikuta et al. (2020) found incisivus labii superioris present in all cases (100%).

Anomalies

Description

In an adult cadaver with an incomplete isolated cleft palate on the right maxilla, incisivus labii superioris was incompletely divided by two fistulae (Kikuta et al. 2019).

Prevalence

N/A

Clinical Implications

Understanding the anatomy of incisivus labii superioris is important for planning and performing surgical procedures and injections in the upper lip region (Iwanaga et al. 2017).

INCISIVUS LABII INFERIORIS (FIGURE 2.1)

Synonyms

This muscle may be referred to as labialis inferior profundus (Seiler 1976; Diogo et al. 2010, 2012, 2013a,b, 2017).

Typical Presentation

This muscle is present only as a variation.

Comparative Anatomy

Incisivus labii inferioris has a similar typical presentation in the apes, extending from the incisive fossa of the mandible to orbicularis oris and the skin of the chin region (Seiler 1976; Iwanaga et al. 2021).

Variations

Description

Incisivus labii inferioris is considered an accessory muscle of orbicularis oris situated lateral to mentalis (Hur et al. 2011a; Standring 2016). It originates from the incisive fossa of the mandible below the eminence of the lateral incisor (Hur et al. 2011a; Standring 2016). Its fibers course laterally, interdigitate with orbicularis oris, and divide into superficial and deep bundles that attach to the modiolus (Lightoller 1925; Hur et al. 2011a; Standring 2016). It may also have connections to buccinator, mentalis, or depressor anguli oris (Hur et al. 2011a, 2013, 2014).

Innervation

N/A

Prevalence

In a sample of 40 hemifaces, Hur et al. (2011a) found that incisivus labii inferioris was present on 39 sides (97.5%). It blended with mentalis on 10 sides (25%), merged into buccinator on 36 sides (90%), and merged into orbicularis oris on three sides (7.5%). In a sample of 40 hemifaces, Hur et al. (2013) found that fibers of incisivus labii inferioris

intermingled with the upper lateral portion of mentalis in all cases (100%) and with the lower or middle portions of mentalis in 22 cases (55%). In a sample of 40 hemifaces, Hur et al. (2014) fibers of depressor anguli oris connected to incisivus labii inferioris and the inferior border of the mandible in 14 specimens (35%), connected to incisivus labii inferioris and fibers of mentalis in two specimens (5%), and connected to incisivus labii inferioris only in one specimen (2.5%).

Anomalies

N/A

Clinical Implications

N/A

MENTALIS (FIGURE 2.1)

Synonyms

This muscle may also be referred to as levator menti (Macalister 1873).

Typical Presentation

Description

Mentalis originates from the incisive fossa of the mandible and inserts into the skin of the chin (Standring 2016).

Innervation

Mentalis is innervated by the marginal mandibular branch of the facial nerve (Standring 2016).

Comparative Anatomy

Mentalis has a similar typical presentation in the apes, descending from the region of the anterior teeth into the skin at the inferior edge of the mandible (Raven 1950; Gibbs 1999; Diogo et al. 2010, 2012, 2013a, 2017). In all apes, it may interdigitate with its counterpart on the other side of the body (Lightoller 1928; Raven 1950; Gibbs 1999; Diogo et al. 2010, 2012, 2013a,b, 2017). It may also blend with platysma or depressor labii inferioris in some cases (Gibbs 1999; Diogo et al. 2012, 2013a).

Variations

Description

Mentalis may be connected with platysma (Bergman et al. 1988; Lee and Yang 2016). It may be split into two bundles (Watanabe 2016). The direction of its lateral fibers may vary (Hur et al. 2013). It may have connections to orbicularis oris, depressor anguli oris, or incisivus labii inferioris (Hur et al. 2013, 2014).

Prevalence

In a sample of 40 hemifaces, Hur et al. (2013) found that the lateral fibers of mentalis coursed inferomedially in 38 cases (95%) and inferolaterally in two cases (5%).

The upper fibers of mentalis interlaced with the inferior border of orbicularis oris in all cases (100%). Fibers of incisivus labii inferioris intermingled with the upper lateral portion of mentalis in all cases (100%) and with the lower or middle portions of mentalis in 22 cases (55%). In a sample of 40 hemifaces, Hur et al. (2014) found that fibers of depressor anguli oris connected to incisivus labii inferioris and fibers of mentalis in two specimens (5%) and blended with mentalis only in one specimen (2.5%).

Anomalies

Description

In a fetus with trisomy 18 and cyclopia, mentalis was partially fused with depressor anguli oris and depressor labii inferioris (Smith et al. 2015). In a female fetus with trisomy 18, mentalis was fused with depressor labii inferioris bilaterally (Alghamdi et al. 2018). In a fetus with craniorachischisis, mentalis presented as a thin muscle layer deep to a poorly differentiated depressor labii inferioris (Alghamdi et al. 2017).

Prevalence

N/A

Clinical Implications

N/A

PLATYSMA MYOIDES (PLATYSMA) (FIGURE 2.1)

Synonyms

N/A

Typical Presentation

Description

Platysma originates from the fascia over pectoralis major and deltoideus (Standring 2016). It courses over the clavicle and along the anterior aspect of the neck to connect to the lower border of the mandible, skin and subcutaneous tissue of the lower face, the lower lip, and the muscles near the mouth (Standring 2016). Some fibers decussate across the midline (Bergman et al. 1988; Standring 2016; Watanabe 2016).

Innervation

Platysma is innervated by the cervical branch of the facial nerve (Standring 2016).

Comparative Anatomy

Platysma has a similar typical presentation in the apes, arising from the pectoral fascia and inserting onto the mandible and near the mouth (Diogo et al. 2010, 2012, 2013a, b, 2017). Sphincter colli profundus is typically not present in the apes, but Diogo et al. (2017) identify some fibers in one adolescent bonobo that run ventrally from the ear region and may correspond to a vestigial auricular portion of sphincter colli profundus.

Variations

Description

The development of platysma may vary, presenting in some cases as a well-developed sheet of muscle and in other cases as multiple detached bundles (Macalister 1875; Bergman et al. 1988; Standring 2016; Lee and Yang 2016; Watanabe 2016). It may also be absent unilaterally, bilaterally, or in the lower half only (Macalister 1875; Sato 1968b; Bergman et al. 1988; Lee and Yang 2016). It may have a high origin directly from the clavicle or a low origin from the level of the third or fourth rib (Macalister 1875).

Platysma may have connections to risorius, mentalis, depressor anguli oris, depressor labii inferioris, zygomaticus minor, zygomaticus major, auricularis anterior, orbicularis oculi, or transversus nuchae (Macalister 1875; Bergman et al. 1988; Bakkum and Miller 2016; Lee and Yang 2016; Watanabe 2016). Its fibers can extend to the mastoid process or the concha of the auricle (Macalister 1875). Some fibers can also join with serratus anterior, infraspinatus, latissimus dorsi, or trapezius (Macalister 1875). It may connect via slips to the occipital bone, the skin of the forehead, the midline of the back of the neck, the skin over the upper lobes of the mammary gland, the tendon of latissimus dorsi, or the skin over deltoideus (Macalister 1875; Lee and Yang 2016; Watanabe 2016). The degree to which the fibers of both platysma muscles interlace may vary (Mori 1964; de Castro 1980; Kim et al. 2001; Lee and Yang 2016; Watanabe 2016). When transversus menti is present, its fibers may interdigitate with fibers of platysma, such that they may be mistaken for fibers of platysma that cross the midline (Hallett 1848).

Sphincter colli profundus is a variable sheet of muscle that may originate from the clavicle deep to platysma and insert into the fascia of the auricle (Bergman et al. 1988; Lee and Yang 2016). Beattie and Horsfall (1930) describe a variant muscle situated immediately below the skin that originated from the posterior border of the mandible, the sheath of the masseter, and the sheath of the medial pterygoid muscle. This muscle inserted into the superficial fascia and skin over the mastoid. They conclude that this muscle was derived from sphincter colli profundus.

Prevalence

Sato (1968b) found platysma absent on 2 out of 168 sides (1.19%) in Kyushu-Japanese females. In a sample of 128 cadavers, Mori (1964) found that the lower border of platysma ended on the first intercostal space in 76 cadavers (59.4%) and on the second intercostal space in 52 cadavers (40.6%). The fibers of the platysma muscles did not intersect in 16 cadavers (12.5%). The fibers of the platysma muscles intersected under the chin in 84 cadavers (65.6%), in the neck above the laryngeal prominence in three cadavers (2.3%), in the neck below the laryngeal prominence in 19 cadavers (14.8%), and at the sternum in six cadavers (4.6%).

de Castro (1980) studied platysma in 50 cadavers. Fibers of the platysma muscles interlaced just below the chin (within 1–2 cm) in 75% of cadavers and at the level of the thyroid cartilage in 15% of cadavers. The fibers did not interlace in the remaining 10% of cases. Kim et al. (2001) studied platysma in 70 Korean cadavers. Fibers of the platysma muscles interlaced just below the mandibular border (within 20 mm) in 30 cadavers (42.8%) and interlaced more than 20 mm from the border in 30 cadavers (42.8%), The fibers did not interlace in the remaining 10 cases (14.3%). In 29 cadavers (41.4%), both the left and right fibers interlaced with each other. In 20 cases (28.6%), the right platysma fibers covered the left fibers. In 11 cadavers (15.7%), the left platysma fibers covered the right fibers.

Anomalies

Description

In a female anencephalic fetus, platysma was abnormally well-developed and extended along the surface of the thorax (Windle 1893). In a fetus with craniorachischisis, platysma was a thin layer of fibers that passed distally from the latero-inferior borders of the mouth (Alghamdi et al. 2017). On the left side of one infant with trisomy 13, sternocleidomastoid sent slips to platysma (Pettersen et al. 1979). In a neonate with trisomy 13, platysma was comprised of two small bundles on both sides of the chin that merged anteriorly (Aziz 1980). Summarizing four cases of trisomy 18, Bersu and Ramirez-Castro (1977) found that the facial muscles were poorly differentiated and depressor anguli oris, depressor labii inferioris, and platysma were more fused than usual at the angle of the mouth. In another infant with trisomy 18, platysma originated above the clavicle bilaterally (Aziz 1979). In a fetus with trisomy 18 and cyclopia, platysma had a strong fascial connection to sternocleidomastoid and sent fibers to zygomaticus major and depressor anguli oris (Smith et al. 2015).

Prevalence

In their literature review, Smith et al. (2015) found that platysma was anomalous in 2 out of 20 (10%) individuals with trisomy 13 (left and right sides separated, absent cervical portion). In 1 out of 17 individuals with trisomy 18 (5.9%), platysma originated above the clavicles.

Clinical Implications
N/A

Platysma cervicale (Figure 2.3)

Entry adapted by permission from Springer Nature Customer Service Centre GmbH: Springer Current Molecular Biology Reports, Muscles Lost in Our Adult Primate Ancestors Still Imprint in Us: on Muscle Evolution, Development, Variations, and Pathologies. E. Boyle, V. Mahon, R. Diogo, 2020.

Synonyms

This muscle is also referred to as the transversus nuchae (Futamura 1906; Lewis 1910), transversalis nuchae (Blodget and Blatt 1966), occipital platysma (Gasser 1967), occipitalis minor or the occipital transverse muscle (Bergman et al. 1988), or the querer Halsmuskel (Bakkum and Miller 2016).

Typical Presentation

This muscle is only present as a variation or anomaly.

Comparative Anatomy

Platysma cervicale is often present in adult nonhuman mammals (Smith et al. 2015). Among nonhuman apes, platysma cervicale is only present as a distinct muscle in gibbons and orangutans, sometimes absent in gorillas, and typically absent in common chimpanzees and bonobos. When the muscle is present in common chimpanzees, bonobos, and gorillas, it is often diminutive and resembles the presentation of this muscle in humans (Diogo et al. 2010, 2012, 2013a,b, 2017).

Variations

Description

Platysma cervicale is present in normal human development, as the occipital lamina that gives rise to this muscle is established during the sixth week of embryonic growth (Lewis 1910; Sataloff and Selber 2003). It typically disappears in early embryonic developmental stages and is therefore often absent in normal adult humans (Futamura 1906; Lewis 1910; Gasser 1967; Smith et al. 2015). Gasser (1967) notes that between CR58 and CR80 mm (crown-rump length of 58–80 mm) "occipital platysma" is present as a distinct band that runs between the platysma muscle and the occipital region, but this muscle was not identified in a CR 142 mm fetus. Gasser (1967) also observes the occasional presence of "transversus nuchae" laying dorsal to auricularis posterior in the lower occipital or upper cervical region between CR58 and CR80 mm. Later, these muscles were still observed in 210 mm and 270 fetuses and were blended with auricularis posterior (Gasser 1967).

When present, platysma cervicale often extends from the region of auricularis posterior to the external occipital protuberance or superior nuchal line (Macalister 1875; Knott 1883a; Blodget and Blatt 1966; Sato 1968a; Bergman et al. 1988; Bakkum and Miller 2016; Standring 2016; Watanabe 2016). It may connect with auricularis posterior, auricularis superior, splenius capitis, or sternocleidomastoid (Macalister 1875; Knott 1883a; Blodget and Blatt 1966; Bergman et al. 1988; Bakkum and Miller 2016; Standring 2016). Blodget and Blatt (1966) describe a "pencil-shaped" transversalis nuchae muscle that arises from the surface of splenius capitis and inserts onto the anterior border of sternocleidomastoid.

Hallett (1848) describes what is likely platysma cervicale as a variation of the lower fascicle of auricularis posterior. Hallett (1848) states that the lower fascicle formed a round-bellied muscle that attached to the occipital protuberance and superior nuchal line at one end and the concha auris at the other end. The muscle was sheathed and situated between the tendons of occipitofrontalis and sternocleidomastoid.

Its presentation can also resemble the condition seen in anomalous cases, in which the muscle can originate from near the mouth or parotid fascia to insert near the occipital region (Wood 1864; Schmidt 1982; Bergman et al. 1988; Lei et al. 2010; Bakkum and Miller 2016; Jovanovski et al. 2020). Wood (1864) notes that it may extend from the parotid fascia and risorius to trapezius and occipitofrontalis. Jovanovski et al. (2020) found that transversus nuchae fused with risorius bilaterally. Lei et al. (2010) observed fibers extending to the zygomatic region. Platysma cervicale may have two bellies (Schmidt 1982; Lei et al. 2010; Jovanovski et al. 2020).

Innervation

Platysma cervicale may be innervated by a branch of the facial nerve (Blodget and Blatt 1966; Jovanovski et al. 2020), or from anastomoses of facial nerve branches and great auricular nerve branches (Schmidt 1982).

Prevalence

The variation described by Hallett (1848) was observed in 3 out of 105 subjects (2.9%). In a sample of 28 bodies, Knott (1883a) found transversus nuchae bilaterally in five bodies (17.9%) and unilaterally in two bodies (7.1%). Sato (1968a) found that transversus nuchae was present in 105 out of 300 facial sides (35%) in Kyushu-Japanese males and present in 62 out of 196 sides (31.6%) in females. Bergman et al. (1988) cite studies that state that "occipitalis minor" is present frequently in Malaysian individuals, present in 56% of Black individuals, present in 50% of Japanese individuals, present in 36% of European individuals, and typically absent in Khoisan peoples and Melanesians. Lei et al. (2010) found "transversus nuchae" on 12 out of 20 sides (60%) from a total sample of 10 cadavers (seven male and three female). The muscle was absent in the females. Standring (2016) suggests that "transversus nuchae" is present in 25% of individuals.

Watanabe et al. (2017) found "transversus nuchae" in 40 out of 124 sides (32.2%) from a total sample of 62 cadavers (present in 26 cadavers, bilaterally in 14 and unilaterally in 12).

Watanabe et al. (2017) observed that this muscle extended from the external occipital protuberance to insert onto the mastoid process (43% of cases) or originated from the external occipital protuberance and curved around the mastoid process to join with platysma (58% of cases).

Anomalies

Description

Platysma cervicale frequently presents as an anomaly in individuals with trisomy 13, 18, or 21. When present, platysma cervicale is a discrete bundle of the platysma complex that extends from the mouth to the nuchal region (Smith et al. 2015). It can either originate from the posterior platysma myoides and insert with sternocleidomastoideus onto

the mastoid process, or it can originate from the corner of the mouth and/or parotid fascia and insert with trapezius onto the occipital bone (Bersu and Ramirez-Castro 1977; Colacino and Pettersen 1978; Pettersen 1979; Pettersen et al. 1979; Bersu 1980; Aziz 1981; Urban and Bersu 1987; Smith et al. 2015).

It was also present bilaterally in both a female fetus with triploidy (Moen et al. 1984) and a male neonate with Meckel syndrome (Pettersen 1984). Mieden (1982) describes an infant with median cleft lip, hypotelorism, and alobar holoprosencephaly. Transversus nuchae was present on the left side, extending over trapezius in between the occipital protuberance and the posterior border of sternocleidomastoid (Mieden 1982).

Prevalence

In their literature review, Smith et al. (2015) found that platysma cervicale was present in 5 out of 20 individuals with trisomy 13 (25%), 13 out of 17 individuals with trisomy 18 (76.5%), and 5 out of 5 individuals with trisomy 21 (100%).

Clinical Implications

Platysma cervicale may present as a painful swelling or mass in the neck (Blodget and Blatt 1966).

MUSCLES OF MASTICATION

MASSETER (FIGURE 2.2)

Synonyms

N/A

Typical Presentation

Description

Masseter is comprised of three layers (Standring 2016). The superficial layer originates from the maxillary process of the zygomatic bone and from the zygomatic arch (Standring 2016). The middle and deep layers also originate from the zygomatic arch (Standring 2016). The superficial layer inserts onto the lower mandibular ramus and angle of the mandible, the middle layer inserts into the middle of the mandibular ramus, and the deep layer inserts into the upper portion of the mandibular ramus and the coronoid process (Standring 2016).

Innervation

Masseter is innervated by the masseteric nerve, a branch of the anterior division of the mandibular nerve (Standring 2016).

Comparative Anatomy

Masseter has a similar typical presentation in the apes, extending from the zygomatic arch to the mandible (Raven 1950; Miller 1952; Gibbs 1999; Diogo et al. 2010, 2012, 2013a,b, 2017).

Masseter can send fibers to the tendon of temporalis in gorillas (Diogo et al. 2010) and to the medial pterygoid in

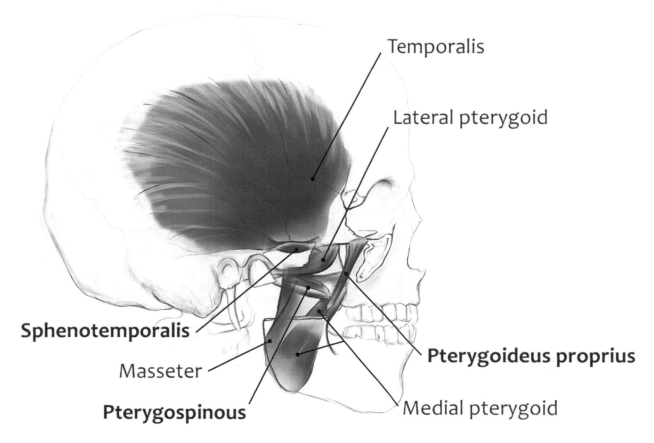

FIGURE 2.2 Muscles of mastication in lateral view. Masseter is only partially shown.

gibbons (Diogo et al. 2012). The superficial and deep portions are well separated in chimpanzees (Sonntag 1923; Miller 1952), while there is no strong fascia or aponeurosis between these layers in the other apes (Sonntag 1924; Boyer 1939; Gibbs 1999; Diogo et al. 2010, 2012, 2013b). Zygomatico-mandibularis—an accessory muscle superficial to temporalis that extends from the deep surface of the zygomatic process to the coronoid process of the mandible—has been found as an accessory bundle of the masseter in common chimpanzees (Gratiolet and Alix 1866; Starck 1973; Göllner 1982; Diogo et al. 2013a) and in a few orangutans (Boyer 1939; Saban 1968) and gorillas (Göllner 1982).

Variations

Description

Macalister (1875) notes that the muscles of mastication have few variations aside from individual variations in size. Most authors describe masseter as having a superficial and deep head (e.g., Macalister 1875; Bergman et al. 1988; Watanabe 2016), not the three-layered configuration deemed typical by Standring (2016). Connections between the muscles of mastication may occur and reflect these muscles' shared origin from the same muscular mass (Bergman et al. 1988). For example, the deep layer of the masseter may send fibers to temporalis and masseter may receive a slip from the medial pterygoid (Macalister 1875; Knott 1883a; Bergman et al. 1988; Watanabe 2016). Masseter may also fuse with

buccinator (Macalister 1875). The deep layer of the masseter may originate in part from the temporomandibular ligament (Macalister 1875). There is no consensus regarding whether masseter sends fibers to the articular disc of the temporomandibular joint (Standring 2016). Bergman et al. (1988) note that both the masseter and temporalis muscles may send fibers to this articular disc.

Prevalence

N/A

Anomalies

Description

The presentation of the masseter muscle is often affected by congenital malformations, cephalic disorders, and various syndromes. Macalister (1875) notes that Dumeril found the masseter muscles absent in a specimen with phocomelia. The masseter can be underdeveloped in cases of hemifacial microsomia (e.g., Takashima et al. 2003) or hypertrophic in cases of congenital hemifacial hyperplasia (e.g., Rončević 1986; Tsuneki et al. 2019).

On the right side of a male infant with Hanhart syndrome, Bersu et al. (1976) found that the right mandible was represented by a small bone. The fibers of the masseter were oriented obliquely downward and posteriorly and had a restricted insertion on the angle of the mandible. In an infant with mandibulofacial dysostosis, there was one superficial layer and three deeper layers of the masseter muscle (Herring et al. 1979). In a neonate with trisomy 13, the right anterior belly of the digastric was quadrupled, with the fourth belly inserting onto the masseter (Aziz 1980).

Mieden (1982) describes two male fetuses with cyclopia and alobar holoprosencephaly. In one specimen, the muscles of mastication were absent on the right side and temporalis and masseter were small on the left side. In an otocephalic fetus examined by Lawrence and Bersu (1984), the mandible was represented by two separate bony masses located within the middle ear cavities. Due to this anomaly, temporalis and masseter fused at the midline into a muscle mass that formed the floor of the oral cavity. In a fetus with craniorachischisis, Alghamdi et al. (2017) found that both masseter and buccinator were undifferentiated muscle tissues situated medial to the ears.

Prevalence

N/A

Clinical Implications

N/A

TEMPORALIS (FIGURE 2.2)

Synonyms

Some authors have referred to the anteromedial/deep portion of temporalis as a separate muscle, sphenomandibularis (Dunn et al. 1996), but there is little evidence to support designating this portion as an independent muscle (e.g., Türp et al. 1997; Schön Ybarra and Bauer 2001; Geers et al. 2005; Akita et al. 2019).

Typical Presentation

Description

Temporalis originates from the deep temporal fascia and from the temporal fossa (Standring 2016). It ends in a tendon that inserts onto the coronoid process and anterior margin of the mandibular ramus (Standring 2016).

Innervation

Temporalis is innervated by the deep temporal branches of the anterior division of the mandibular nerve (Standring 2016).

Comparative Anatomy

Temporalis has a similar typical presentation in the apes, extending from the temporal fossa and temporal fascia to the coronoid process and anterior margin of the mandibular ramus (Boyer 1939; Raven 1950; Miller 1952; Gibbs 1999; Diogo et al. 2010, 2012, 2013a,b, 2017). A "pars suprazygomatica" of the temporalis is typically present in many primates including several genera of monkeys (Diogo and Wood 2011) and has been observed in some gorillas (Raven 1950; Göllner 1982; Diogo et al. 2010), common chimpanzees, and bonobos (Göllner 1982; Diogo et al. 2017).

Variations

Description

Macalister (1875) notes that the muscles of mastication have few variations aside from individual variations in size. Temporalis can vary in the extent of its origin on the cranium and its insertion along the mandible (Macalister 1875; Bergman et al. 1988; Watanabe 2016). Temporalis may send fibers to the articular disc of the temporomandibular joint (Zenker 1955; Bergman et al. 1988; Standring 2016). Connections between the muscles of mastication may occur and reflect these muscles' shared origin from the same muscular mass (Bergman et al. 1988). For example, temporalis may receive fibers from the deep layer of the masseter and temporalis may be connected to the lateral pterygoid (Macalister 1875; Bergman et al. 1988; Watanabe 2016).

Temporalis minor was termed by Henle (1871) to refer to an accessory muscle that originated from the anterior portion of temporalis and inserted onto the mandibular notch (Bergman et al. 1988; Watanabe 2016). Ullah and Khan (2006) report the presence of an accessory muscle in the infratemporal fossa that they term the zygobuccinator muscle, which originated from the posterior surface of the frontal process of the zygomatic bone and inserted into the buccinator. This muscle likely corresponds to the temporobuccinator band described by Gaughran (1957) (Buck 2007).

Prevalence

N/A

Anomalies

Description

The presentation of the temporalis may be affected by congenital malformations and cephalic disorders. Temporalis can be underdeveloped in cases of hemifacial microsomia (e.g., Takashima et al. 2003). Mieden (1982) describes two male fetuses with cyclopia and alobar holoprosencephaly. In one specimen, the muscles of mastication were absent on the right side and temporalis and masseter were small on the left side. In an otocephalic fetus examined by Lawrence and Bersu (1984), the mandible was represented by two separate bony masses located within the middle ear cavities. Due to this anomaly, temporalis and masseter fused at the midline into a muscle mass that formed the floor of the oral cavity. Temporalis also sent fibers to the bony masses that represented the coronoid process of each mandible. In a fetus with craniorachischisis, Alghamdi et al. (2017) found that temporalis was absent on the right side and was represented by undifferentiated muscle tissue between the eye and the ear on the left side.

Bersu et al. (1976) describe a male infant with Hanhart syndrome in which the right mandible was represented by a small bone. On the right side, the insertion of temporalis was diffuse and most of the muscle attached to the coronoid process. Smaller portions of the muscle inserted onto the articular mass and condylar process or blended with the superior fascicle of pterygoideus lateralis. In an infant with mandibulofacial dysostosis, temporalis was divided into superficial, middle, and deep parts (Herring et al. 1979). On both sides of a fetus with trisomy 18 and cyclopia, the insertion of temporalis reached the angle of the mandible (Smith et al. 2015).

Prevalence
N/A

Clinical Implications
Variations in the dimensions of the medial portion of temporalis may contribute to maxillary nerve compression, headaches, and tic douloureux (Schön Ybarra and Bauer 2001). Temporalis hypertrophy may occur in tandem with masseter hypotrophy (e.g., Legg 1880; Graziano et al. 2016) or without associated hypertrophy of the masseter (e.g., Wilson and Brown 1990; Wang et al. 2013; Watanabe 2016; Tuncel et al. 2017).

PTERYGOIDEUS LATERALIS (LATERAL PTERYGOID) (FIGURE 2.2)

Synonyms
This muscle may be referred to as pterygoideus externus (Macalister 1875).

Typical Presentation
Description
The lateral pterygoid has two heads (Standring 2016). The upper head originates from the infratemporal crest of the greater wing of the sphenoid, and the lower head originates from the lateral pterygoid plate of the sphenoid (Standring 2016). The two heads merge and insert onto the pterygoid fovea on the neck of the mandible (Standring 2016).

Innervation
The upper head and the lateral portion of the lower head of lateral pterygoid are innervated by a branch of the buccal nerve (Standring 2016). The medial portion of the lower head is innervated by a branch of the anterior division of the mandibular nerve (Standring 2016).

Comparative Anatomy
The lateral pterygoid has a similar typical presentation in the apes, arising via two heads from the lateral pterygoid plate and sphenoid to the capsule of the temporomandibular joint and the neck of the mandible (Gratiolet and Alix 1866; Sonntag 1923, 1924; Boyer 1939; Raven 1950; Miller 1952; Wall et al. 1994; Gibbs 1999; Diogo et al. 2010, 2012, 2013a,b, 2017).

Variations
Description
Macalister (1875) notes that the muscles of mastication have few variations aside from individual variations in size. The degree of separation between the upper and lower heads may vary (Macalister 1875; Bergman et al. 1988). The lateral pterygoid may alternatively be comprised of one or three heads (Bertilsson and Ström 1995; Fujita et al. 2001; Watanabe 2016). When present, the third head may be referred to as an inner or medial head that originates from the greater wing of the sphenoid and inserts into the pterygoid fovea and/or the medial part of the temporomandibular joint disc-capsule complex (Bertilsson and Ström 1995; Fujita et al. 2001; Pompei Filho et al. 2009; Kiliç et al. 2010; Dergin et al. 2012; Antonopoulou et al. 2013).

Connections between the muscles of mastication may occur and reflect these muscles' shared origin from the same muscular mass (Bergman et al. 1988). For example, the lateral pterygoid may join with temporalis or digastricus (Macalister 1875; Bergman et al. 1988; Watanabe 2016). A portion of the upper head may insert into the articular capsule and/or articular disc of the temporomandibular joint (Bertilsson and Ström 1995; Naidoo 1996; Fujita et al. 2001; Mazza et al. 2009; Kiliç et al. 2010; Dergin et al. 2012; Antonopoulou et al. 2013; Standring 2016; Watanabe 2016). The upper head may exclusively insert into the articular capsule and disc (Naidoo 1996; Mazza et al. 2009; Kiliç et al. 2010; Dergin et al. 2012; Antonopoulou et al. 2013). The lower head may also send fibers to the disc or joint capsule (Naidoo 1996; Kiliç et al. 2010; Fujita et al. 2001).

The pterygoid muscles are associated with several accessory muscles. Sphenotemporalis was termed by Mack (1984) to describe a small muscle in the infratemporal fossa situated superior and deep to the upper head of the lateral pterygoid (see the entry for this muscle). The pterygospinous or pterygospinsosus muscle extends between the posterior margin of the lateral pterygoid plate and the spine of the sphenoid (see the entry for this muscle) (Macalister 1875; Poland 1890; Nathan 1989; von Lüdinghausen et al. 2006; Watanabe 2016). Pterygoideus proprius extends between the infratemporal crest and the tuber palati or the lateral pterygoid plate (see the entry for this muscle) (Macalister 1875; Poland 1890; Tubbs et al. 2007; Watanabe 2016).

Prevalence
Bertilsson and Ström (1995) conducted a comprehensive review of 89 research articles on the anatomy of the lateral pterygoid. These authors found that 65% of the articles report lateral pterygoid having two heads, 20% of the articles report lateral pterygoid presenting as a single head, and 15% of the articles report lateral pterygoid having three heads. Furthermore, 60% of the articles report an insertion onto the mandible, articular disc, and joint capsule of the temporomandibular joint; 30% report an insertion into the mandible with only a few fibers inserting into the disc; and 10% found an insertion exclusively into the mandible.

Naidoo (1996) studied the insertions of the lateral pterygoid in 40 cadaveric specimens. In 26 specimens (65%), the upper head inserted into the pterygoid fovea, capsule, and disc. In 11 specimens, the upper head inserted into the condyle only. In two cases, it inserted into the disc only (5%). In one case, the lower head had an additional insertion into the meniscus (2.5%). Fujita et al. (2001) studied the lateral pterygoid in 20 cadaveric specimens. Two heads of the muscle (upper and lower) were found in 13 specimens (65%), while seven specimens had a third inner head (35%). All 20 upper heads (100%), all seven inner heads (100%), and two lower heads (10%) had an insertion into the disc-capsule complex of the temporomandibular joint.

Mazza et al. (2009) studied the insertion of the upper head in 193 temporomandibular joint specimens. In 63 cases (32.6%), the upper head inserted via a single bundle onto the joint capsule and mandible. In 76 cases (39.4%) the upper head inserted via two bundles, one onto the disc and one onto the mandible. In 54 cases (28%), the upper head inserted via a single bundle onto the disc. Pompei Filho et al. (2009) evaluated 178 MRI to determine the prevalence of the third head of the lateral pterygoid. The third head was found in 36 cases (20.2%), and these heads inserted entirely onto the disc of the temporomandibular joint.

Kiliç et al. (2010) examined the lateral pterygoid in 49 temporomandibular joint specimens from 26 cadavers. Two heads were present in 32 specimens (65.3%), and three heads were present in 17 specimens (34.7%). In 18 specimens (36.7%), the upper head inserted into the disc-capsule complex and the mandible, and the lower head inserted into the mandible. In 14 specimens (28.6%), the upper head inserted into the disc-capsule complex and the lower head inserted into the mandible. In 13 specimens (26.5%), both the upper head and the lower head inserted into the mandible only. In four specimens (8.2%), the upper head inserted into the disc-capsule complex and the lower head inserted into the complex and into the mandible.

Dergin et al. (2012) examined the lateral pterygoid in 98 temporomandibular joint specimens from 49 patients using MRI. In 29 cases (29.6%), the upper head inserted into the disc and the lower head inserted into the mandible. In 40 cases (40.8%), the upper head inserted into the disc and the mandible, and the lower head inserted into the mandible. In 29 cases (29.6%), the upper head inserted into the disc and both the lower head and third head inserted into the mandible. Antonopoulou et al. (2013) studied the attachment of the upper head of the lateral pterygoid in 36 sides from 18 cadavers. These authors found that the upper head inserted into the pterygoid fovea and the disc-capsule complex of the temporomandibular joint in 20 cases (55.5%). It inserted into the pterygoid fovea only in 10 cases (27.8%) and into the disc-capsule complex only in six cases (16.7%). A third medial head was found in eight cases (22.2%).

Stöckle et al. (2019) conducted a comprehensive review of 11 research articles on the anatomy of the lateral pterygoid. In an overall sample of 521 subjects, the relative frequency of one-headed lateral pterygoid muscles was between 7.7% and 26.7%, the relative frequency of two-headed lateral pterygoid muscles was between 61.4% and 91.1%, and the relative frequency of three-headed lateral pterygoid muscles was between 4% and 35%.

Anomalies

Description

Bersu et al. (1976) describe a male infant with Hanhart syndrome in which the right mandible was represented by a small bone. On the right side, the pterygoid muscles were partially fused and difficult to separate from one another. The well-developed superior fascicle of the lateral pterygoid received a contribution from temporalis and inserted completely onto the temporomandibular articular mass. Fibers from the inferior fascicle extended beyond the condylar process on its medial side and attached along the medial aspect of the sphenomandibular ligament and to the petrotympanic fissure.

Mieden (1982) describes two male fetuses with cyclopia and alobar holoprosencephaly. In one specimen, the muscles of mastication were absent on the right side, and the medial and lateral pterygoid muscles were fused on the left side. In the second specimen, the medial and lateral pterygoid muscles were fused bilaterally. In an otocephalic fetus examined by Lawrence and Bersu (1984), the mandible was represented by two separate bony masses located within the middle ear cavities. The lateral pterygoid was represented by a fused muscle mass on both sides.

In an infant with mandibulofacial dysostosis, the lateral pterygoid had three heads of origin that joined to insert onto the anterior and lateral aspects of the medial condyle (Herring et al. 1979). In a fetus with craniorachischisis, the lateral pterygoid muscles were missing on both sides (Alghamdi et al. 2017).

In one neonate with trisomy 13, an accessory muscle slip extended from the upper head of the lateral pterygoid to the lower part of the medial pterygoid near its insertion point (Pettersen et al. 1979). On both sides of one neonate with trisomy 18, the lateral pterygoid inserted onto the deep aspect of the temporomandibular joint and adjacent part of the temporal bone, with no fibers extending to the mandible (Aziz 1979). In a fetus with trisomy 18 and cyclopia, the lateral pterygoid was mostly normal but had an origin that extended more superiorly and posteriorly on the cranium (Smith et al. 2015).

Prevalence

In their literature review, Smith et al. (2015) found that a slip from the lateral pterygoid to the medial pterygoid was only present in the case described by Pettersen et al. (1979), thus having a prevalence of 1 out of 20 individuals (5%) with trisomy 13. These authors also found that an insert exclusively onto the temporomandibular joint and adjacent temporal bone was only observed in the case described by Aziz (1979), thus having a prevalence of 1 out of 17 individuals (5.9%) with trisomy 18.

Clinical Implications

It is unclear whether an insertion of the upper head entirely into the articular disc increases risk of anterior disc displacement (Taskaya-Yilmaz et al. 2005; Mazza et al. 2009; Dergin et al. 2012; Antonopoulou et al. 2013). Valenzuela et al. (2020) suggest that cases where the upper belly inserts only into the disc and a third head is present may have the most risk of developing symptoms related to temporomandibular dysfunction.

Pterygoideus medialis (Medial pterygoid) (Figure 2.2)

Synonyms

This muscle may be referred to as pterygoideus internus (Macalister 1875).

Typical Presentation

Description

The medial pterygoid has two heads (Standring 2016). The deep head originates from the medial surface of the lateral pterygoid plate of the sphenoid (Standring 2016). The superficial head originates from the maxillary tuberosity and the pyramidal process of the palatine (Standring 2016). It inserts onto the medial surface of the mandibular ramus and angle of the mandible (Standring 2016).

Innervation

The medial pterygoid is innervated by the medial pterygoid branch of the mandibular nerve (Standring 2016).

Comparative Anatomy

The medial pterygoid has a similar typical presentation in the apes, originating from the medial surface of the lateral pterygoid plate and sometimes the pterygoid fossa to insert onto the medial side of the mandible (Raven 1950; Miller 1952; Gibbs 1999; Diogo et al. 2010, 2012, 2013a,b, 2017). It may also have origins from the pyramidal process of the palatine, the maxillary tuberosity, and/or the pterygomandibular raphe in orangutans (Boyer 1939; Gibbs 1999; Diogo et al. 2013b).

Variations

Description

Macalister (1875) notes that the muscles of mastication have few variations aside from individual variations in size. Connections between the muscles of mastication may occur and reflect these muscles' shared origin from the same muscular mass (Bergman et al. 1988). For example, the medial pterygoid may send a slip to the masseter (Bergman et al. 1988; Watanabe 2016). It may also give origin to styloglossus or send a slip to tensor veli palatini (Macalister 1875; Bergman et al. 1988; Watanabe 2016). The medial pterygoid may originate in part from the pterygoid fossa or the lateral surface of the medial pterygoid plate (Bhojwani et al. 2017).

An accessory medial pterygoid muscle or accessory bundle of the muscle may be present (Koritzer and Suarez 1980; Abe et al. 1997; Sakamoto and Akita 2004). Koritzer and Suarez (1980) report the presence of an accessory medial pterygoid muscle that had a broad origin spanning from the posterior superior margin of the lateral pterygoid plate to the anterior margin of the carotid canal, medial to the foramen spinosum and foramen ovale. The muscle coursed inferiorly and narrowed to an insertion onto the medial surface and/or the superior border of the medial pterygoid muscle about a centimeter below its exit from the pterygoid fossa. A small, independent accessory muscle bundle may be present with attachments below or posterior to the retromolar pad, or into the fascia of the mylohyoid muscle (Abe et al. 1997; Sakamoto and Akita 2004).

The pterygoid muscles are associated with several other accessory muscles. Sphenotemporalis was termed by Mack (1984) to describe a small muscle in the infratemporal fossa situated superior and deep to the upper head of the lateral pterygoid (see the entry for this muscle). The pterygospinous or pterygospinsosus muscle extends between the posterior margin of the lateral pterygoid plate and the spine of the sphenoid (see the entry for this muscle) (Macalister 1875; Poland 1890; Nathan 1989; von Lüdinghausen et al. 2006; Watanabe 2016). Pterygoideus proprius extends between the infratemporal crest and the tuber palati or the lateral pterygoid plate (see the entry for this muscle) (Macalister 1875; Poland 1890; Penhall et al. 1998; Tubbs et al. 2007; Watanabe 2016).

Prevalence

In a sample of 39 head halves, Bhojwani et al. (2017) found that the deep head of the medial pterygoid originated from the medial surface of the lateral pterygoid plate and the pterygoid fossa in seven specimens (17.9%). In 28 specimens (71.8%), the origin from these two structures was expanded onto the lateral surface of the medial pterygoid plate. In one specimen (2.6%), the origin was from the medial pterygoid plate and the pterygoid fossa.

In a sample of 84 medial pterygoid muscle specimens from 42 cadavers, Abe et al. (1997) found a small, independent accessory muscle bundle in ten specimens (11.9%) from five cadavers. The bundle inserted posterior to the retromolar pad in five specimens (6%), below the retromolar pad in three specimens (3.6%), and into the fascia of mylohyoid in two specimens (2.4%). In a sample of 24 head halves from 12 cadavers, Sakamoto and Akita (2004) found an accessory muscle bundle of the medial pterygoid in ten head halves (41.7%) from five cadavers.

Anomalies

Description

Bersu et al. (1976) describe a male infant with Hanhart syndrome in which the right mandible was represented by a small bone. On the right side, the pterygoid muscles were partially fused and difficult to separate from one another. The attachments of the medial pterygoid were extensive, with some fibers inserting onto the angle of the mandible, others blending with the lateral pterygoid fibers that joined with the sphenomandibular ligament, and other fibers passed into the neck deep to styloglossus and blended with the tongue muscles and middle pharyngeal constrictor.

Mieden (1982) describes two male fetuses with cyclopia and alobar holoprosencephaly. In one specimen, the muscles of mastication were absent on the right side, and the medial and lateral pterygoid muscles were fused on the left side. In the second specimen, the medial and lateral pterygoid muscles were fused bilaterally. In an infant with mandibulofacial dysostosis, the medial pterygoid arose from the lower orbital bar and pterygoid process and inserted just above the mylohyoid line and onto the medial condyle and the skull (Herring et al. 1979). In an otocephalic fetus examined by Lawrence and Bersu (1984), the mandible was represented by two separate bony masses located within the middle ear cavities. The medial pterygoid was represented by a fused muscle mass on both sides.

In a fetus with craniorachischisis, the medial pterygoid was absent on the right side (Alghamdi et al. 2017). On the left side, it seemed to be represented by fibers that extended between the maxilla and the mandible. In one neonate with trisomy 13, an accessory muscle slip extended from the upper head of the lateral pterygoid to the lower part of the medial pterygoid near its insertion point (Pettersen et al. 1979).

Prevalence

In their literature review, Smith et al. (2015) found that a slip from the lateral pterygoid to the medial pterygoid was only present in the case described by Pettersen et al. (1979), thus having a prevalence of 1 out of 20 individuals (5%) with trisomy 13.

Clinical Implications

N/A

SPHENOTEMPORALIS (FIGURE 2.2)

See also: Pterygoideus lateralis, Pterygoideus medialis

Synonyms

N/A

Typical Presentation

This muscle is present only as a variation.

Comparative Anatomy

Mack (1984) states that it is possible that sphenotemporalis is a vestigial remnant of a muscle situated between the alisphenoid and squamosal, which is found in some bats and wombats.

Variations

Description

Sphenotemporalis was termed by Mack (1984) to describe a small muscle in the infratemporal fossa situated superior and deep to the upper head of the lateral pterygoid. It is attached to the cranium on either side of the sphenotemporal suture. It originated from the greater wing of the sphenoid, with its attachment extending as far laterally as the infratemporal crest. The muscle coursed horizontally to insert onto the anterior aspect of the articular eminence

on the squamous portion of the temporal bone (Mack 1984; Watanabe 2016). Mack (1984) notes that sphenotemporalis is distinct from the lateral pterygoid and should not be considered a slip of this muscle.

Innervation

Sphenotemporalis is innervated by a nerve arising directly from the trigeminal ganglion (Mack 1984).

Prevalence

Mack (1984) found sphenotemporalis in 2 out of 30 half heads (6.7%).

Anomalies

N/A

Clinical Implications

N/A

PTERYGOSPINOUS (FIGURE 2.2)

See also: Pterygoideus lateralis, Pterygoideus medialis

Synonyms

This muscle was originally named the pterygospinosus muscle (Thane) (Poland 1890). This muscle may also be referred to as pterygotympanicus (Saban) (Mack 1984). A variant of pterygospinous is the pterygofascialis muscle (Poland 1890).

Typical Presentation

This muscle is present only as a variation.

Comparative Anatomy

Diogo et al. (2013a,b, 2017) note that pterygotympanicus has not been observed in the apes.

Variations

Description

The pterygospinous muscle may replace the pterygospinous ligament or course along the ligament (Macalister 1875; Poland 1890; Standring 2016; Watanabe 2016). When present, it often replaces the pterygospinous ligament, originating from the posterior margin of the lateral pterygoid plate between the two pterygoid muscles and inserting onto the spine of the sphenoid (Macalister 1875; Poland 1890; Nathan 1989; von Lüdinghausen et al. 2006; Watanabe 2016). von Lüdinghausen et al. (2006) also observed an additional insertion into the capsule and articular disc of the temporomandibular joint in some cases. These authors suggest that due to its innervation and location, it could be designated as a third head of the lateral pterygoid. In cases where the pterygospinous muscle is present with a fibrous or ossified pterygospinous ligament, the upper attachment of the muscle varies and is associated with an abnormal arrangement of the sphenomandibular ligament (Poland 1890). In some cases, muscle may insert into the petrotympanic fissure and blend with the sphenomandibular ligament (Poland 1890).

Van Dongen (1968) observed that the pterygospinous muscle was present in a fetus at CR80mm (crown-rump length 80mm). Mérida Velasco et al. (1994) examined this muscle in five human fetuses and found that it originated from the posterior border of the lateral pterygoid plate and inserted into Meckel's cartilage. These authors suggest that it is a remnant of the masticatory muscle group.

Poland (1890) considers pterygofascialis to be a variant of the pterygospinous muscle. In one case, pterygofascialis arose from the sphenomandibular ligament and attached to the posterior edge and outer aspect of the medial pterygoid (Poland 1890; Watanabe 2016). In a second case, it had the same origin and attached onto both the posterior edge and outer aspect of the medial pterygoid and the lateral pterygoid plate (Poland 1890). In these cases, the sphenomandibular ligament did not attach to the spine of the sphenoid but to the petrotympanic fissure (Poland 1890).

Innervation

Nathan (1989) observed that the pterygospinous muscle is innervated by a branch of the inferior alveolar nerve. von Lüdinghausen et al. (2006) observed that this muscle is innervated by a small twig of the pterygoid branch of the mandibular nerve.

Prevalence

In a sample of ten sides from five fetuses, Mérida Velasco et al. (1994) found the pterygospinous muscle on eight sides (80%). In a sample of 54 cadaveric specimens, von Lüdinghausen et al. (2006) found a pterygospinous muscle in five cases (9.3%). In three cases, the muscle had an attachment into the medial surface of the temporomandibular joint capsule and articular disc. The muscle was present alongside a pterygospinous osseous bar in one case and alongside a pterygospinous ligament in two cases.

Anomalies

N/A

Clinical Implications

When the pterygospinous muscle is present, it may affect the distribution pattern of the mandibular nerve (von Lüdinghausen et al. 2006).

PTERYGOIDEUS PROPRIUS (FIGURE 2.2)

See also: Pterygoideus lateralis, Pterygoideus medialis

Synonyms

N/A

Typical Presentation

This muscle is present only as a variation.

Comparative Anatomy

N/A

Variations

Description

When present, the pterygoideus proprius (Henle 1858) typically originates from the infratemporal crest of the greater wing of the sphenoid, courses superficially over the lateral pterygoid muscle, and inserts onto the lower part of posterior edge of the lateral pterygoid plate (Wagstaffe 1871; Macalister 1875; Knott 1880, 1883a; Poland 1890; Eisler 1912; Barker 1981; Bergman et al. 1988; Penhall et al. 1998; Akita et al. 2001; Tubbs et al. 2007; Watanabe 2016). Macalister (1875) describes it as a nearly vertical slip. The muscle may also originate from the anteromedial portion of temporalis (Poland 1890; Akita et al. 2001). In some cases, it inserts onto the tuber palati (Macalister 1875), either referring to the pyramidal process of the palatine bone (Tubbs et al. 2007) or the maxillary tuberosity (Knott 1880).

Pterygoideus proprius may be entirely tendinous or be comprised of both muscular and tendinous fibers (Wagstaffe 1871; Poland 1890; Tubbs et al. 2007; Watanabe 2016). The posterior fibers of the muscle may join with those of the medial pterygoid muscle (Wagstaffe 1871; Tubbs et al. 2007). The lateral pterygoid may partially originate from the pterygoideus proprius (Wagstaffe 1871; Macalister 1875; Poland 1890; Penhall et al. 1998; Watanabe 2016).

Penhall et al. (1998) propose three potential scenarios for the development of pterygoideus proprius. First, some deep muscle fibers of the temporalis anlage may attach to the lateral pterygoid plate before temporalis attaches onto the coronoid, thus persisting as a separate, vertical band of fibers. Second, this muscle may be formed by fibers of the lateral pterygoid that fail to attach to the articular disc and/or the mandible and elongate with growth into a vertical slip that retains an attachment to the sphenoid. Third, the muscle could be formed by fibers of lateral pterygoid that fail to join the upper or lower head of this muscle during development.

Innervation

Akita et al. (2001) found that pterygoideus proprius is innervated by twigs of the anterior deep temporal nerve.

Prevalence

Knott (1883a) found three cases of pterygoideus proprius in a sample of 112 bodies (2.7%). Penhall et al. (1998) found three cases of pterygoideus proprius in a sample of about 150 cadavers (~2%). Akita et al. (2001) found the muscle in 3 out of 66 head halves (3%).

Anomalies

N/A

Clinical Implications

Tubbs et al. (2007) suggest that pterygoideus proprius has the potential to impinge upon the lingual or alveolar nerve branches of the trigeminal nerve or compress the maxillary artery.

EXTRINSIC MUSCLES OF THE EAR AND MIDDLE EAR MUSCLES

Auricularis anterior (Figure 2.3)

Synonyms

This muscle may also be referred to as attrahens aurem (Macalister 1875).

Typical Presentation

Description

Auricularis anterior originates from the epicranial aponeurosis and attaches to the auricle at the spine of the helix (Standring 2006).

Innervation

Auricularis anterior is innervated by a temporal branch of the facial nerve (Standring 2016).

Comparative Anatomy

Diogo et al. (2010, 2012, 2013a,b, 2017) consider auricularis anterior to be a bundle of the auriculo-orbitalis muscle present in the apes, which extends from the anterior aspect of the ear to the region of frontalis.

Variations

Description

Auricularis anterior and superior may blend to form a continuous sheet of muscle (Macalister 1875; Knott 1883a). Auricularis anterior may originate from the zygomatic arch and insert into the tragus, and in this case would be referred to as musculus auricularis anterior profundus (Macalister 1875; Knott 1883a). It may be doubled, with one part inserting into the helix and the other inserting into the concha (Macalister 1875). Its lower border may connect to platysma (Macalister 1875). Auricularis anterior may be absent more often than the other extrinsic ear muscles (Macalister 1875; Bergman et al. 1988; Watanabe 2016). It may be reduced and comprised of a single bundle or numerous unconnected fasciculi (Macalister 1875; Watanabe 2016).

Prevalence

N/A

Anomalies

Description

On the left side of a fetus with trisomy 18 and cyclopia, auricularis anterior was present and partially fused with auricularis superior and orbicularis oculi (Smith et al.

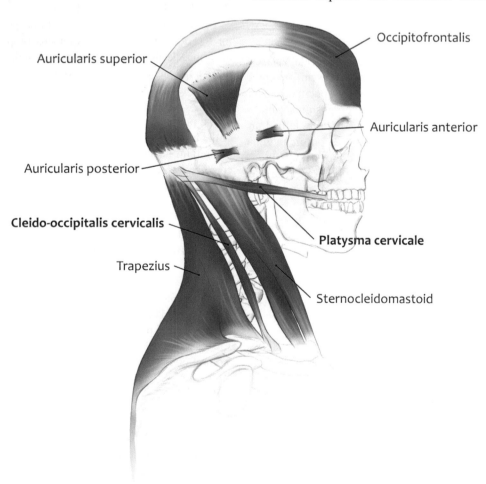

FIGURE 2.3 Extrinsic muscles of the ear and posterolateral neck muscles in lateral view.

2015). On the right side, auricularis anterior was not a distinct muscle. Auricularis anterior was absent bilaterally in a neonate with trisomy 18 (Aziz 1979) and in a fetus with craniorachischisis (Alghamdi et al. 2017).

Prevalence

In their literature review, Smith et al. (2015) found that auricularis anterior was absent in 1 out of 17 cases of trisomy 18 (5.9%).

Clinical Implications

N/A

Auricularis superior (Figure 2.3)

Synonyms

This muscle may also be referred to as attollens aurem (Macalister 1875).

Typical Presentation

Description

Auricularis superior originates from the epicranial aponeurosis and attaches to the superior part of the auricle (Standring 2006).

Innervation

Auricularis superior is innervated by a temporal branch of the facial nerve (Standring 2016).

Comparative Anatomy

Auricularis superior has a similar typical presentation in the apes, extending from the epicranial aponeurosis to the superior aspect of the ear, with occasional origins from, or connections to, the temporal fascia in orangutans and gorillas (Raven 1950; Miller 1952; Gibbs 1999; Diogo et al. 2010, 2012, 2013a,b, 2017).

Variations

Description

Auricularis superior and anterior may blend to form a continuous sheet of muscle (Macalister 1875; Knott 1883a). Auricularis superior may connect with transversus nuchae (Macalister 1875; Bergman et al. 1988). It may be divided into multiple fascicles (Macalister 1875). It may have a lower origin, from the temporal aponeurosis (Macalister 1875). Its fibers may not reach the auricle and instead end in the temporal aponeurosis (Macalister 1875). It may be absent in rare cases (Macalister 1875; Bergman et al. 1988; Hoogbergen et al. 1996; Watanabe 2016).

Prevalence

N/A

Anomalies

Description

On the left side of a fetus with trisomy 18 and cyclopia, auricularis superior was present and partially fused with auricularis anterior (Smith et al. 2015). Auricularis superior presented as a thin sheet of muscle in a neonate with trisomy 18 (Aziz 1979). In a fetus with craniorachischisis, auricularis superior was found only on the left side, presenting as a thin sheet of muscle extending between the superior aspect of the ear and the superior side of the left eye (Alghamdi et al. 2017). In an infant with mandibulofacial dysostosis, auricularis superior had two bellies that fused into an intermediate tendon (Herring et al. 1979). The tendon became muscular again and the muscle ended in the fascia of the neck.

Prevalence

N/A

Clinical Implications

N/A

Auricularis posterior (Figure 2.3)

Synonyms

This muscle may also be referred to as retrahens aurem (Macalister 1875).

Typical Presentation

Description

Auricularis posterior originates from the mastoid portion of the temporal bone and attaches to the auricle at the ponticulus (Standring 2016).

Innervation

Auricularis posterior is innervated by the posterior auricular branch of the facial nerve (Standring 2016).

Comparative Anatomy

Auricularis posterior is typically not present as a distinct muscle in orangutans (Ruge 1887; Sullivan and Osgood 1925; Lightoller 1928; Miller 1952; Diogo et al. 2013b). In bonobos, it extends from the mastoid region of the temporal bone to the posterior aspect of the ear, as in humans (Gibbs 1999; Miller 1952; Diogo et al. 2017). In gibbons, common chimpanzees, and gorillas, it extends from the occipital region to the posterior aspect of the ear (Raven 1950; Gibbs 1999; Diogo et al. 2010, 2012, 2013a).

Variations

Description

Auricularis posterior may be comprised of two or three fascicles (Macalister 1875; Knott 1883a; Standring 2016). In rare cases, it may have four or more fascicles, or present as a continuous sheet of muscle (Macalister 1875). One of the fascicles may be replaced by a tendinous band (Macalister 1875; Knott 1883a). The lower fascicle may arise from the cervical fascia (Macalister 1875). Hallett (1848) describes a variation of the lower fascicle that is likely platysma cervicale or transversus nuchae (see the entry for this muscle). Auricularis posterior may have connections to sternocleidomastoid, occipitofrontalis, platysma, or transversus nuchae (Macalister 1875; Knott 1883a; Bergman et al. 1988). It may be doubled (Macalister 1875). It may also be absent in some cases (Macalister 1875; Bergman et al. 1988; Sato 1968a; Hoogbergen et al. 1996; Watanabe 2016).

Prevalence

Sato (1968a) found auricularis posterior present in 312 out of 342 facial sides (91.23%) in Kyushu-Japanese males and present in 194 out of 226 sides (85.84%) in females.

Anomalies

Description

In a fetus with craniorachischisis, auricularis posterior was found only on the left side, presenting as a thin band of fibers extending from the posterior-superior aspect of the ear to the posterior neural tissue (Alghamdi et al. 2017). Auricularis posterior was absent in an infant with mandibulofacial dysostosis (Herring et al. 1979).

Prevalence

N/A

Clinical Implications

N/A

TENSOR TYMPANI (NOT ILLUSTRATED)

Synonyms

N/A

Typical Presentation

Description

Tensor tympani originates from the greater wing of the sphenoid, the pharyngotympanic tube, and from the bony canal it occupies (Standring 2016). It inserts via a tendon onto the manubrium of the malleus (Standring 2016).

Innervation

Tensor tympani is innervated by a branch of the trigeminal nerve (Standring 2016).

Comparative Anatomy

Tensor tympani has a similar typical presentation in the apes, extending from the pharyngotympanic tube and adjacent regions of the neurocranium to insert onto the malleus (Diogo et al. 2010, 2012, 2013a,b, 2017).

Variations

Description

Tensor tympani may be doubled (Macalister 1875; Le Double 1897; Rodríguez-Vázquez 2016). It may also be split into lateral and medial parts, with the lateral belly having a typical presentation and the medial belly traveling with the facial nerve in the facial canal (Wright and Etholm 1973; Rodríguez-Vázquez 2016). Some fibers of tensor veli palatini may be continuous with tensor tympani

(Barsoumian et al. 1998; Abe et al. 2004; Rodríguez-Vázquez 2016; Standring 2016). Tensor tympani may be absent and replaced by a fibrous band (Kelemen 1943; Rodríguez-Vázquez 2016).

Prevalence

In a sample of 496 ears with normal development, Wright and Etholm (1973) found that tensor tympani was split into medial and lateral parts in one ear (0.2%).

Anomalies

Description

Tensor tympani has been noted as absent bilaterally in a fetus with craniorachischisis (Alghamdi et al. 2017) and in an otocephalic fetus (Lawrence and Bersu 1984). In one infant with trisomy 13–15 and another infant with trisomy 18, tensor tympani bifurcated into medial and lateral parts unilaterally (Wright and Etholm 1973). In both cases, the medial part traveled with the facial nerve in the facial canal, to just above the oval window, where it exited the canal and blended with stapedius.

On the right side of a male infant with Hanhart syndrome, some lateral pterygoid fibers attached to the petrotympanic fissure and formed a separate muscle bundle that was about half the size of a typical tensor tympani (Bersu et al. 1976). It passed through the fissure and inserted via a tendon onto the malleus. On the left side of an infant with CHARGE syndrome, the manubrium of the malleus was absent and tensor tympani instead attached to the head of the malleus (Wright et al. 1986). In the right ear of a fetus with trisomy 18, tensor tympani was anomalous and its tendon inserted onto one side of the malleus (Tadaki et al. 2003).

Prevalence

In their literature review, Tadaki et al. (2003) found that anomalies of tensor tympani or its tendon were found in 5 out of 16 cases of trisomy 18 (31.25%). In a sample of 13 temporal bones from children with the Pierre Robin sequence, Gruen et al. (2005) found that the middle ear muscles were anomalous in five bones.

Clinical Implications

Bifurcation of tensor tympani into medial and lateral parts was found in an individual who also had chronic otitis media (Wright and Etholm 1973).

STAPEDIUS (NOT ILLUSTRATED)

Synonyms

N/A

Typical Presentation

Description

Stapedius originates from the pyramidal eminence of the tympanic cavity and inserts via a tendon onto the neck of the stapes (Standring 2016).

Innervation

Stapedius is innervated by a branch of the facial nerve (Standring 2016).

Comparative Anatomy

Information about stapedius in the apes is scarce, but it likely has a typical presentation similar to that in humans and inserts on the stapes (Diogo et al. 2010, 2012, 2013a,b, 2017).

Variations

Description

Stapedius may be doubled (Macalister 1875; Le Double 1897; Wright and Etholm 1973; Bergman et al. 1988; Rodríguez-Vázquez 2016). The length of the stapedius tendon may vary (Hough 1958; Zawawi et al. 2014; Rodríguez-Vázquez 2016). Ectopic muscle tissue may be present in the middle ear and is often closely associated with the facial nerve (Hoshino and Paparella 1971; Wright and Etholm 1973; Rodríguez-Vázquez 2016). Hypoplasia or absence of stapedius, and/or absence of its tendon, may occur (Kelemen 1943; Hough 1958; Hoshino and Paparella 1971; Wright and Etholm 1973; Bergman et al. 1988; Kopuz et al. 2006; Rodríguez-Vázquez et al. 2010; Rodríguez-Vázquez 2016; Dalmia and Behera 2017).

Prevalence

Out of 500 middle ear surgeries, Hough (1958) found stapedius completely absent in five cases (1%). In a sample of 195 temporal bones from 141 individuals, hypoplasia of stapedius and absence of its tendon was found in two bones (1%) and ectopic muscle tissue was present in 12 bones (6.2%) (Hoshino and Paparella 1971). In a sample of 496 ears with normal development, stapedius was doubled in two ears (0.4%) and absent in two ears (0.4%), the stapedius tendon was absent in four ears (0.8%), and ectopic muscle tissue was present in 18 ears (3.6%) (Wright and Etholm 1973).

Anomalies

Description

Stapedius has been noted as absent bilaterally in a fetus with craniorachischisis (Alghamdi et al. 2017) and in an otocephalic fetus (Lawrence and Bersu 1984). In two infants with CHARGE syndrome, stapedius was absent bilaterally (Wright et al. 1986). In an infant with mandibulofacial dysostosis, stapedius was located posterosuperior to the jaw articulation (Herring et al. 1979). In the right ear of a fetus with trisomy 18, stapedius lacked a tendon and connected to the head of the stapes via funicular tissue (Tadaki et al. 2003). Wright and Etholm (1973) found ectopic muscle tissue in the middle ear of an infant with 13–15 trisomy.

Prevalence

In their literature review, Tadaki et al. (2003) found that anomalies of stapedius or its tendon were found in 5 out of 18 cases of trisomy 18 (27.8%). In a sample of 13 temporal bones from children with the Pierre Robin sequence, Gruen et al. (2005) found that the middle ear muscles were anomalous in five bones.

Clinical Implications

Ectopic muscle tissue in the middle ear has been found in individuals who also exhibit chronic otitis media, presbycusis, or sensorineural deafness (Wright and Etholm 1973). A shortened stapedius tendon may cause conductive hearing loss (Zawawi et al. 2014).

MUSCLES OF THE TONGUE

INTRINSIC MUSCLES OF THE TONGUE (NOT ILLUSTRATED)

Synonyms

N/A

Typical Presentation

Description

There are four paired intrinsic muscles of the tongue (Standring 2016). The superior longitudinal muscle courses from the submucous fibrous tissue of the posterior tongue and the medial lingual septum to the margins of the tongue (Standring 2016). The inferior longitudinal muscle courses from the root of the tongue and the body of the hyoid to the apex of the tongue, blending with styloglossus (Standring 2016). The transverse muscle blends with palatopharyngeus as it extends from the median fibrous septum to the submucous tissue at the lateral lingual margin (Standring 2016). The vertical muscle is situated just under the superior longitudinal muscle with fibers that extend dorsoventrally (Standring 2016).

Innervation

The intrinsic muscles of the tongue are innervated by the hypoglossal nerve (Standring 2016).

Comparative Anatomy

N/A

Variations

Description

Patel and Loukas (2016) note that there are no variations of the intrinsic muscles of the tongue. However, variable slips associated with the extrinsic muscles may affect the external anatomy of the tongue (see the entries for these muscles below) (Macalister 1875; Patel and Loukas 2016).

Prevalence

N/A

Anomalies

Description

Congenital malformations that affect the intrinsic muscles of the tongue are often associated with other birth defects or clinical syndromes and include aglossia (complete absence), microglossia or hypoglossia (reduction), and macroglossia

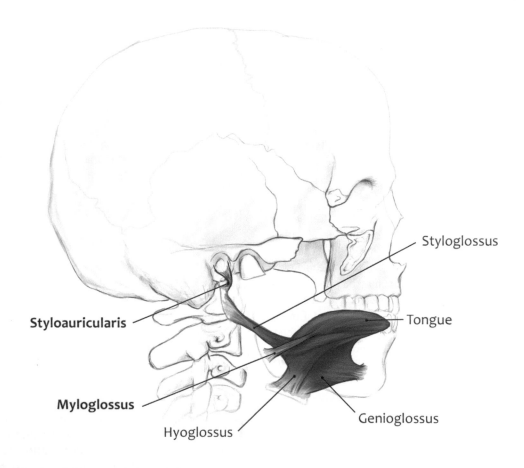

FIGURE 2.4 Muscles of the tongue in lateral view.

(enlargement), bifid tongue (anterior separation of the tongue along the midline), and an accessory tongue (Stevenson 2006; Kumar et al. 2009; Patel and Loukas 2016). Agrawal et al. (2014) describe an individual with a congenital trilobe tongue associated with partial cleft palate.

Other anomalies of the tongue include occupying a position in the pharynx and an extended connection with the mandible (Mieden 1982; Lawrence and Bersu 1984; Pettersen 1984). Mieden (1982) describes two male fetuses with cyclopia and alobar holoprosencephaly. In one fetus, the oral cavity was reduced and separated from the pharynx by the buccopharyngeal membrane. A small tongue filled the pharynx and compressed the epiglottis. In an otocephalic fetus examined by Lawrence and Bersu (1984), the oral cavity was reduced and separated from the pharynx by a membrane deemed to be the buccopharyngeal membrane. A small tongue was situated posterior to the membrane and filled the pharynx. The dorsal surface of the tongue faced the posterior pharyngeal wall, and the tip of the tongue was oriented inferiorly. The tongue was connected via muscle fibers to the body of the hyoid. In a male neonate with Meckel syndrome, Pettersen (1984) found that the anterior two-thirds of the tongue were malformed, and the tongue was united with the mandible on the left side. The tongue was very thin anteriorly along the midline. The posterior third of the tongue was normal.

Prevalence

In a sample of 2301 patients from the United States, McCarthy (1941) found macroglossia in one individual. In a sample of 1,906 Chilean individuals, Witkop and Barros (1963) found macroglossia in one individual (0.05%) and a bifid tongue in two individuals (0.1%). In a sample of 956 African American patients, Schaumann et al. (1970) found macroglossia in one individual (0.1%) and a bifid tongue in another individual (0.1%).

Clinical Implications

N/A

GENIOGLOSSUS (FIGURE 2.4)

Synonyms

This muscle may also be referred to as geniohyoglossus (Macalister 1875).

Typical Presentation

Description

Genioglossus originates from the superior mental spine on the posterior surface of the mental symphysis (Standring 2016). Its superior fibers insert along the length of the ventral surface of the tongue and blend with the intrinsic tongue muscles (Standring 2016). Its intermediate fibers insert into the posterior tongue (Standring 2016). Its inferior fibers insert into the body of the hyoid and have an additional attachment into constrictor pharyngis medius (Standring 2016). Genioglossus muscles on each side of the body decussate across the midline anteriorly (Standring 2016).

Innervation

Genioglossus is innervated by the hypoglossal nerve (Standring 2016).

Comparative Anatomy

Genioglossus has a similar typical presentation in the apes, extending from the mandible to the tongue and the hyoid (Deniker 1885; Sonntag 1923; Gibbs 1999; Diogo et al. 2010; 2012, 2013a,b, 2017). In a gorilla dissected by Diogo et al. (2010), the connection of genioglossus to the hyoid seemed to be loose or absent.

Variations

Description

Genioglossus may fuse with geniohyoid or receive fibers from styloglossus (Macalister 1875; Knott 1883a; Lee and Yang 2016; Standring 2016). Genioglossus may send a slip to the stylohyoid ligament (Macalister 1875; Bergman et al. 1988). The muscle may also be tripled (Macalister 1875). Genioglossus is also associated with several named accessory slips. A slip from genioglossus to the epiglottis is referred to as levator epiglottidis (Bergman et al. 1988; Patel and Loukas 2016) or genioepiglotticus (Luschka) (Macalister 1875). The central muscle of Bochdalek refers to a small muscle in the posterior quarter of the tongue where the genioglossus muscles meet along the midline (Macalister 1875). A slip from genioglossus to constrictor pharyngis superior is referred to as geniopharyngeus (Winslow) (Macalister 1875; Knott 1883a; Bergman et al. 1988; Patel and Loukas 2016). An isolated bundle of genioglossus that passes between the superior mental spine and the apex of the tongue is referred to as longitudinalis linguae inferior medius (Bergman et al. 1988; Patel and Loukas 2016). A separate deep slip of genioglossus that originates from the most inferior part of the genial tubercle and inserts into the hyoid is referred to as genioglossus accessorius (Luschka) (Macalister 1875; Knott 1883a).

Prevalence

Knott (1883a) found genioglossus accessorius separated from the other fibers of genioglossus in one out of seven subjects (14.3%).

Anomalies

Description

Shortness of genioglossus, a highly attached genioglossus, or fibrosis of the genioglossus along with the frenulum can contribute to ankyloglossia, or tongue-tie (Choi et al. 2011; Sharma et al. 2013; Patel and Loukas 2016).

Bersu et al. (1976) describe a male infant with Hanhart syndrome in which the right mandible was represented by a small bone. In this infant, the right genioglossus muscle was absent. It was replaced by a muscle mass that passed from the inferior margin of the right mandible to the deep surface of the left hyoglossus muscle. On the left side of a fetus with craniorachischisis, genioglossus was fused with geniohyoid (Alghamdi et al. 2017).

In a male neonate with Meckel syndrome, auriculoglossus was present on each side of the body, originating from the region of the external auditory meatus and blending with hyoglossus at its insertion (Pettersen 1984). The left muscle was more prominent and had a slip that continued from the association with hyoglossus to blend with genioglossus. Additionally, the genioglossus muscles were separated a bit more than usual in the midline which gave the impression of two distinct tongue halves. An accessory muscle slip was also present in the frenulum between the two genioglossus muscles.

Prevalence

In a sample of 956 African American patients, Schaumann et al. (1970) found partial ankyloglossia in 21 individuals (2.2%). In 17 of the cases, the degree of ankyloglossia was minor. In four of the cases, both the frenulum and the fibers of genioglossus were markedly fibrosed.

Clinical Implications

Partial myotomy of the genioglossus muscle can be used with other surgical methods to correct ankyloglossia (Choi et al. 2011).

HYOGLOSSUS (FIGURE 2.4)

Synonyms

N/A

Typical Presentation

Description

Hyoglossus originates from the greater horn and the body of the hyoid and inserts into the lateral aspect of the tongue between styloglossus and the inferior longitudinal muscle (Standring 2016).

Innervation

Hyoglossus is innervated by the hypoglossal nerve (Standring 2016).

Comparative Anatomy

In the apes, hyoglossus is differentiated into ceratoglossus, which connects the greater horn of the hyoid to the tongue, and chondroglossus, which primarily connects the body of the hyoid to the tongue (the lesser horn is often reduced or absent) (Kohlbrügge 1890–1892; Saban 1968; Diogo et al. 2010, 2012, 2013a,b, 2017).

Variations

Description

The origin of hyoglossus may be continuous with a slip from thyrohyoid (Macalister 1875). Geniohyoid may originate from hyoglossus (Bergman et al. 1988; Patel and Loukas 2016). Wood (1868) observed a case in which the superior belly of the omohyoid was doubled and the upper belly fused with hyoglossus and the middle pharyngeal constrictor. The bundles that comprise hyoglossus may vary in their development and how separated they are from one another (Macalister 1875; Bergman et al. 1988; Ogata et al. 2002; Standring 2016). When the fibers of hyoglossus that originate from the greater horn are distinct from the fibers that originate from the body of the hyoid, the former comprise a bundle referred to as ceratoglossus and the latter form a bundle referred to as basioglossus (Bergman et al. 1988; Patel and Loukas 2016). Chondroglossus is a bundle that originates from the lesser horn and body of the hyoid and inserts into the intrinsic muscles of the tongue (Bergman et al. 1988; Ogata et al. 2002; Standring 2016). It may be considered as the third part of hyoglossus but is typically partitioned from it by fibers of genioglossus (Le Double 1897; Ogata et al. 2002; Standring 2016). Triticeoglossus (Bochdalek) is a bundle that originates from the cartilago triticea and inserts into the tongue with the posterior fibers of hyoglossus (Macalister 1875; Knott 1883a; Bergman et al. 1988; Patel and Loukas 2016; Standring 2016). It may be considered as the fourth part of hyoglossus and is often present when the posterior fibers of hyoglossus lie posterior to the lingual artery (Macalister 1875).

Prevalence

Macalister (1875) notes that Bochdalek found triticeoglossus in 8 out of 22 subjects (36.4%). Macalister (1875) found triticeoglossus as a bundle with connections to hyoglossus in one out of six subjects (16.7%) and as a completely distinct muscle in 1 out of 30 subjects (3.3%). Knott (1883a) found triticeoglossus in 4 out of 44 cases (11.4%). In a sample of 100 tongue halves from 50 cadavers, Ogata et al. (2002) found chondroglossus in all specimens (100%) but observed that the chondroglossus muscle fibers were sparse and poorly developed in 14% of specimens.

Anomalies

Description

In a fetus with trisomy 13, the right posterior belly of the digastric inserted into the hyoid bone and had an extended attachment into the posterior aspect of hyoglossus (Pettersen et al. 1979). Furthermore, the right hyoglossus muscle was comprised of two distinct muscle sheets that were separated by a gap. Bersu et al. (1976) describe a male infant with Hanhart syndrome in which the right mandible was represented by a small bone. In this infant, the right hyoglossus was substantially reduced. An accessory muscle was present that sent a slip between the geniohyoid muscles to have a diffuse insertion onto the deep aspect of the left geniohyoid

and the hyoglossus muscles. Furthermore, the right genioglossus muscle was absent and replaced by a muscle mass that passed from the inferior margin of the right mandible to the deep surface of the left hyoglossus muscle.

Mieden (1982) describes two male fetuses with cyclopia and alobar holoprosencephaly. In one case, auriculoglossus was present on the left side, originating from the tympanic bone and attaching to hyoglossus (Mieden 1982). In a male neonate with Meckel syndrome, Pettersen (1984) found an auriculoglossus muscle on each side of the body originating from the region of the external auditory meatus and blending with hyoglossus at its insertion. The left muscle was more prominent and had a slip that continued from the association with hyoglossus to blend with genioglossus.

In an otocephalic fetus examined by Lawrence and Bersu (1984), the oral cavity was reduced and separated from the pharynx by a membrane deemed to be the buccopharyngeal membrane. A small tongue was situated posterior to the membrane and filled the pharynx. The dorsal surface of the tongue faced the posterior pharyngeal wall and the tip of the tongue was oriented inferiorly. The tongue was connected via muscle fibers to the body of the hyoid. Hyoglossus was the only extrinsic tongue muscle present in this specimen. In a fetus with craniorachischisis, the attachment of hyoglossus was more medial than normal on the right side, and hyoglossus was fused with styloglossus on the left side (Alghamdi et al. 2017).

Prevalence

In their literature review, Smith et al. (2015) found that hyoglossus was anomalous in only 1 out of 20 individuals with trisomy 13 (5%).

Clinical Implications

N/A

STYLOGLOSSUS (FIGURE 2.4)

Synonyms

N/A

Typical Presentation

Description

Styloglossus originates from the styloid process and from the stylomandibular ligament (Standring 2016). It inserts along the lateral length of the tongue, blending with the inferior longitudinal muscle, and has an oblique insertion that blends with hyoglossus (Standring 2016).

Innervation

Styloglossus is innervated by the hypoglossal nerve (Standring 2016).

Comparative Anatomy

Styloglossus has a similar typical presentation in the apes, originating from the styloid process and/or the temporal bone and inserting into the tongue with some fibers blending with hyoglossus (Kohlbrügge 1890–1892; Dean 1984; Gibbs 1999; Diogo et al. 2010, 2012, 2013a,b, 2017). In one bonobo, Diogo et al. (2017) found that styloglossus was fused with the superior pharyngeal constrictor and stylopharyngeus.

Variations

Description

Styloglossus may be doubled, comprised of either two parallel bellies or two superimposed layers (Macalister 1875; Bergman et al. 1988; Patel and Loukas 2016). It may originate from the medial pterygoid (Macalister 1875; Bergman et al. 1988; Patel and Loukas 2016). It may send fibers to genioglossus or to the pharynx (Macalister 1875; Patel and Loukas 2016). An accessory head of styloglossus may originate from the stylomandibular ligament (Macalister 1875; Knott 1883a; Patel and Loukas 2016).

Styloglossus may also be absent (Macalister 1875; Knott 1883a; Bergman et al. 1988; Patel and Loukas 2016). When absent, styloglossus may be replaced by myloglossus (Wood), which originates from the inner aspect of the angle of the mandible and inserts into the lateral aspect of the tongue (see the entry for this muscle) (Wood 1867b; Macalister 1875; Knott 1883a; Valenti 1926; Bergman et al. 1988; Nakajima and Nakamura 2008; Patel and Loukas 2016; Buffoli et al. 2017). Myloglossus can present as a slip or second head of styloglossus instead of a distinct muscle (Macalister 1875; Patel and Loukas 2016).

Styloglossus may connect to the accessory muscle stylo-auricularis (Hyrtl) which originates from the styloid process and attaches to the cartilage of the external auditory meatus (see the entry for this muscle) (Macalister 1875; Knott 1883a; Patel and Loukas 2016; Touré and Anzouan-Kacou 2016). Styloglossus may also connect to auriculoglossus (Gruber), a slip that may pass from the ear to the tongue (Macalister 1875). A slip from genioglossus to the epiglottis is referred to as levator epiglottidis (Bergman et al. 1988) or genioepiglotticus (Luschka) and may be continuous with styloglossus (Macalister 1875; Patel and Loukas 2016).

Prevalence

As noted in Mérida-Velasco et al. (2006), Barnwell (1977) studied the origin of styloglossus in 14 fetuses. Styloglossus originated from the styloid process and the stylomandibular ligament in 10 fetuses (71.4%) and from the stylomandibular ligament only in one fetus (7.1%). Mérida-Velasco et al. (2006) studied the origin of styloglossus in 18 sides of nine fetuses. In all cases (100%), styloglossus originated in Reichert's cartilage, the structure from which the styloid process arises during development. On 12 sides (66.7%), styloglossus had an accessory head that originated from the angle of the mandible. The authors note that this accessory head likely does not correspond to myloglossus as it attaches to the main belly of styloglossus before reaching the tongue. On four sides (22.2%), styloglossus was connected to the angle of the mandible by fibrous tracts. On two sides (11.1%) of one specimen, an accessory bundle was present that originated from the fibrous tract connecting the angle of the mandible to Reichert's cartilage.

Anomalies

Description

Bersu et al. (1976) describe a male infant with Hanhart syndrome. In this infant, the right styloglossus was substantially reduced. Mieden (1982) describes two male fetuses with cyclopia and alobar holoprosencephaly. On the left side of one specimen, styloglossus was absent.

On the right side of one infant with trisomy 18, an accessory styloglossus muscle originated from the temporal bone (Bersu and Ramirez-Castro 1977). The accessory styloglossus muscle blended with hyoglossus just below the fibers from the normal styloglossus muscle. In a male neonate with Meckel syndrome, Pettersen (1984) found that both styloglossus muscles originated anterior to the styloid process. On the right side of this specimen, the muscle had an additional origin from an aponeurotic attachment to the stylohyoid ligament. In a fetus with craniorachischisis, Alghamdi et al. (2017) found that the right styloglossus originated from an enlarged styloid process and from the "temporo-occipital" bone. It inserted into the outer side of the mandible lateral to hyoglossus. The left styloglossus was absent.

Prevalence

N/A

Clinical Implications

N/A

MYLOGLOSSUS (FIGURE 2.4)

See also: Styloglossus

Synonyms

This muscle may also be referred to as mandibuloglossus (Valenti 1926; Bergman et al. 1988).

Typical Presentation

This muscle is only present as a variation.

Comparative Anatomy

N/A

Variations

Description

Myloglossus originates from the inner surface of the angle of the mandible and inserts into the lateral aspect of the tongue (Wood 1867b; Macalister 1875; Knott 1883a; Valenti 1926; Bergman et al. 1988; Nakajima and Nakamura 2008; Patel and Loukas 2016; Buffoli et al. 2017). Knott (1883a) attributes its name to Rolfincius but other authors (e.g., Valenti 1926; Bergman et al. 1988) credit Wood. It may present as a slip or second head of styloglossus instead of a distinct muscle (Macalister 1875; Patel and Loukas 2016). In these cases, it often joins with styloglossus before reaching the tongue (Buffoli et al. 2017). Myloglossus may be associated with a rudimentary styloglossus or replace styloglossus when it is absent (Macalister 1875; Nakajima and Nakamura 2008; Patel and Loukas 2016; Buffoli et al. 2017).

Myloglossus may join with hyoglossus upon reaching the tongue (Wood 1867b; Valenti 1926; Buffoli et al. 2017). In the cases observed by Nakajima and Nakamura (2008), myloglossus bifurcated around hyoglossus just before inserting into the tongue. One bundle passed to the apex of the tongue while the other blended with hyoglossus, thus having an insertion similar to a normal styloglossus muscle. According to Nakajima and Nakamura (2008), styloglossus typically develops as a bicipital muscle with the head from the angle of the mandible disappearing before birth, so myloglossus represents the persistence of this muscular head. Buffoli et al. (2017) suggest a different mechanism of development and argue that myloglossus forms from some bundles of the medial pterygoid muscle that fuse with the inferolateral portion of styloglossus.

Innervation

In the bilateral presentation of myloglossus described by Nakajima and Nakamura (2008), one side was innervated by both the hypoglossal and the mandibular nerve while the other side was innervated by the hypoglossal nerve only. Innervated was supplied by both the hypoglossal nerve and/or the mandibular nerve (via the buccal or mylohyoid nerves) in the cases described by Buffoli et al. (2017).

Prevalence

In a sample of 21 sides from 11 heads, Buffoli et al. (2017) found "myloglossal structures" on 13 sides (61.9%). Out of these 13 cases, a myloglossus muscle was found in five cases (38.5%), a myloglossal ligament was found in three cases (23%), and a myloglossal ligament that had some muscular fibers was found in five cases (38.5%). The myloglossus muscles were associated with a normal-sized styloglossus muscle in one out of five cases (20%) and a rudimentary styloglossus in four cases (80%). The myloglossal ligaments were associated with a normal-sized styloglossus muscle in seven out of eight cases (87.5%) and a rudimentary styloglossus muscle in one case (12.5%). Out of the 13 cases, the myloglossal structures inserted into hyoglossus (lingual insertion) in four cases (30.8%) and into styloglossus in nine cases (69.2%). All the myloglossal ligaments inserted into styloglossus (100%) while four out of five myloglossus muscles (80%) inserted into hyoglossus.

Mérida-Velasco et al. (2006) studied the origin of styloglossus in 18 sides of nine fetuses. In all cases (100%), styloglossus originated in Reichert's cartilage, the structure from which the styloid process arises during development. On 12 sides (66.7%), styloglossus had an accessory head that originated from the angle of the mandible. The authors note that this accessory head likely does not correspond to myloglossus as it attaches to the main belly of styloglossus before reaching the tongue. However, this accessory head would be considered a myloglossal structure according to the classification used by Buffoli et al. (2017). On four sides (22.2%), styloglossus was connected to the angle of the mandible by fibrous tracts. On two sides (11.1%) of one specimen, an accessory bundle was present that originated from the fibrous tract connecting the angle of the mandible to Reichert's cartilage.

Anomalies
N/A

Clinical Implications
N/A

STYLOAURICULARIS (FIGURE 2.4)

See also: Styloglossus

Synonyms
This muscle may also be referred to as depressor auriculae (Lauth) (Macalister 1875; Knott 1883a).

Typical Presentation
This muscle is only present as a variation or anomaly.

Comparative Anatomy
Styloauricularis may be the homologue of the mandibulo-auricularis muscle, which is typically absent in most primates but found in other mammals (Huber and Hughson 1926; Diogo et al. 2018).

Variations

Description
Styloauricularis (Hyrtl) originates from the styloid process and inserts into the cartilage of the external auditory meatus (Macalister 1875; Knott 1883a; Patel and Loukas 2016; Touré and Anzouan-Kacou 2016). It is described here along with the tongue muscles as it is considered an auricular slip of styloglossus (Macalister 1875). A variant of styloauricularis is auriculoglossus (Gruber), a slip that may pass from the ear to the tongue (Macalister 1875). Styloauricularis may have tendinous or fleshy attachments (Macalister 1875; Touré and Anzouan-Kacou 2016). It may be comprised of one or two bellies, have two heads, have two tendons, or may be replaced by a fibrous cord (Macalister 1875; Knott 1883a).

Innervation
Styloauricularis is innervated by the facial nerve (Touré and Anzouan-Kacou 2016).

Prevalence
N/A

Anomalies

Description

Styloauricularis is present in the form of auriculoglossus in some individuals with congenital malformations. Mieden (1982) describes two male fetuses with cyclopia and alobar holoprosencephaly. In one case, auriculoglossus was present on the left side, originating from the tympanic bone and attaching to hyoglossus (Mieden 1982). In a male neonate with Meckel syndrome, Pettersen (1984) found an auriculoglossus muscle on each side of the body originating from the region of the external auditory meatus and blending with hyoglossus at its insertion. The left muscle was more prominent and had a slip that continued from the association with hyoglossus to blend with genioglossus.

Prevalence

N/A

Clinical Implications

Styloauricularis can be a landmark for the facial nerve (Touré and Anzouan-Kacou 2016).

MUSCLES OF THE SOFT PALATE

Tensor veli palatini (Figure 2.5)

Synonyms

This muscle may also be referred to as tensor palati (Macalister 1875).

Typical Presentation

Description

Tensor veli palatini originates from the scaphoid fossa of the pterygoid process and from the medial surface of the sphenoidal spine (Standring 2016). It also has an origin from the pharyngotympanic tube (Eustachian tube or auditory tube) (Standring 2016). Its fibers end in a tendon that courses around the pterygoid hamulus to insert into the palatine aponeurosis (Standring 2016). Some researchers may use the name dilator tubae to refer to the portion of tensor veli palatini that originates from the pterygoid hamulus and has attachments to the pharyngotympanic cartilage, connective tissue lateral to the tubal wall, and Ostmann's fat pad (Standring 2016).

Innervation

Tensor veli palatini is innervated by the medial pterygoid branch of the mandibular nerve (Standring 2016).

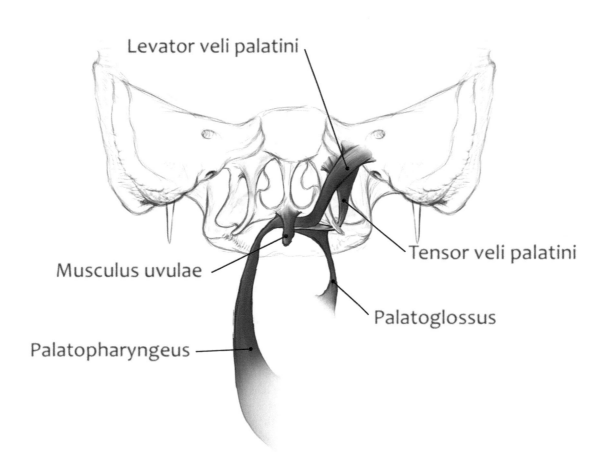

FIGURE 2.5   Muscles of the soft palate in posterior view.

Comparative Anatomy

Tensor veli palatini has a similar typical presentation in the apes, extending from the Eustachian tube cartilage and adjacent regions of the cranium (e.g., scaphoid fossa) to the pterygoid hamulus and soft palate (Gratiolet and Alix 1866; Sonntag 1923; Dean 1985; Gibbs 1999; Diogo et al. 2010, 2012, 2013a,b, 2017). As the palate is closer to the roof of the nasopharynx in adult apes than it is in adult humans, tensor veli palatini in the apes does not pass as distinctly downward to reach the palate as it does in humans (Aiello and Dean 1990; Gibbs 1999; Diogo et al. 2010, 2012, 2013a,b, 2017).

Variations

Description

Tensor veli palatini may be longitudinally divided (Macalister 1875; Patel and Loukas 2016). The portion designated as dilator tubae may vary in its development and connections to the rest of the muscle (Barsoumian et al. 1998). The attachment to the pharyngotympanic tube cartilage varies with age (Suzuki et al. 2003). Tensor veli palatini may have an insertion into the palatine bone (Macalister 1875; Standring 2016). It may also have additional insertions into the maxillary tuberosity, or the submucosal tissue close to the palatoglossal arch (Abe et al. 2004; Patel and Loukas 2016). Muscular fibers may be present in the tendon near its insertion, giving tensor veli palatini a digastric appearance (Macalister 1875). Tensor veli palatini may receive an accessory slip from the medial pterygoid or from the outer margin of the scaphoid fossa (Macalister 1875; Patel and Loukas 2016). It may send a slip to the buccinator muscle (Macalister 1875; Patel and Loukas 2016). Some fibers of tensor veli palatini may be continuous with fibers of tensor tympani (Barsoumian et al. 1998; Standring 2016).

Prevalence

Barsoumian et al. (1998) examined tensor veli palatini and dilator tubae on 20 sides from 16 heads. On 13 sides (65%) from 11 heads, most of dilator tubae was distinct from tensor veli palatini and the two only shared connective tissue and some fibers. On five sides (25%) from five heads, dilator tubae was strongly intermingled with tensor veli palatini. On two sides (10%), dilator tubae was deficient.

Abe et al. (2004) studied tensor veli palatini on 119 sides from 77 heads. The muscle originated from the auditory tube and cranial base in all cases. On 29 sides (24.4%), the auditory tube and cranial base origins were equal in width. On eight sides (6.7%), the auditory tube origin was wider than the cranial base origin. On 41 sides (34.5%), the auditory tube origin was narrower than the cranial base origin. On 37 sides (31.1%), the auditory tube origin was narrower than the cranial base origin and the latter was shifted anteromedially toward the pharyngeal opening of the auditory tube. On four sides (3.4%), the origins did not overlap and were separated posterolaterally. In addition to the primary insertion into the palatine aponeurosis, Abe

et al. (2004) found additional insertions into the maxillary tuberosity on 40 sides (33.6%) and into the submucosal tissue near the palatoglossal arch on 45 sides (37.8%). Overall, a palatine insertion only was found on 54 sides (45.4%), a palatine and pharyngeal insertion were found on 25 sides (21%), a palatine and maxillary insertion were found on 20 sides (16.8%), and a palatine insertion with both secondary insertions was found on 20 sides (16.8%).

Anomalies

Description

The morphology of tensor veli palatini often varies in individuals with cleft palate (e.g., Matsune et al. 1991; Arnold et al. 2005; Heidsieck et al. 2016; George et al. 2018). Matsune et al. (1991) measured the ratio of the length of the Eustachian tube cartilage with insertion of tensor veli palatini to its total length (nasopharyngeal end to tubal isthmus). In cleft palate cases, this ratio was smaller than in control cases and the insertions had fewer muscular and tendinous fibers (Matsune et al. 1991; Heidsieck et al. 2016). These results demonstrate an abnormal insertion into the Eustachian tube cartilage in cleft palate patients. Arnold et al. (2005) examined a fetus with bilateral cleft palate and found that tensor veli palatini was situated under the auditory tube and inserted at the lateral wall of the auditory tube. George et al. (2018) found that tensor veli palatini was shorter and less voluminous in adults with repaired cleft palate than in adults without cleft palate.

It can also vary in individuals with other congenital defects (Herring et al. 1979; Lawrence and Bersu 1984; Pettersen 1984; Alghamdi et al. 2017; Perry et al. 2020). In an infant with mandibulofacial dysostosis, tensor veli palatini was enlarged (Herring et al. 1979). In an otocephalic fetus examined by Lawrence and Bersu (1984), muscle fibers were present in the soft palate, but individual palatal muscles could not be identified. In a male neonate with Meckel syndrome, Pettersen (1984) found that the right tensor veli palatini traveled lateral to the lateral pterygoid plate and its tendon blended with the lower portion of it. Tensor veli palatini was absent in the fetus with craniorachischisis described by Alghamdi et al. (2017). Perry et al. (2020) found that tensor veli palatini was shorter, thinner, and less voluminous in children with 22q11.2 deletion syndrome (DiGeorge syndrome) relative to control subjects.

Prevalence

Using histology, Matsune et al. (1991) measured the ratio of the length of the Eustachian tube cartilage with insertion of tensor veli palatini to its total length (nasopharygneal end to tubal isthmus) in 20 control cases and in ten individuals with cleft palate. In all 20 controls (100%) and six cleft palate cases (60%), tensor veli palatini inserted into the tip of the lateral lamina of the Eustachian tube cartilage. Four cleft palate cases (40%) lacked an insertion. Overall, the ratio of tensor veli palatini insertion on the Eustachian tube cartilage to the total length of this cartilage was smaller in the cleft palate cases.

Clinical Implications

An abnormal attachment or variation in size or length of tensor veli palatini in individuals with cleft palate likely contributes to recurrent otitis media with effusion (Matsune et al. 1991; Arnold et al. 2005; Heidsieck et al. 2016; George et al. 2018).

Levator veli palatini (Figure 2.5)

Synonyms

This muscle may also be referred to as levator palati (Macalister 1875).

Typical Presentation

Description

Levator veli palatini originates via a tendon from the inferior surface of the petrous temporal bone, the cartilage of the pharyngotympanic tube (Eustachian tube or auditory tube), and from the vaginal process of the sphenoid (Standring 2016). It inserts into the palatine aponeurosis between the two fasciculi of palatopharyngeus (Standring 2016). Levator veli palatini intermingles with its counterpart at the midline (Standring 2016).

Innervation

Levator veli palatini is innervated by the pharyngeal plexus (Standring 2016).

Comparative Anatomy

Levator veli palatini has a similar typical presentation in the apes, extending from the Eustachian tube and the apex of the petrous temporal bone to the soft palate (Gratiolet and Alix 1866; Kohlbrügge 1890–1892; Sonntag 1923; Dean 1985; Gibbs 1999; Diogo et al. 2010, 2012, 2013a,b, 2017). As the palate is closer to the roof of the nasopharynx in adult apes than it is in adult humans, levator veli palatini is more horizontal in the apes and does not pass as distinctly downward to reach the palate as it does in humans (Gratiolet and Alix 1866; Sonntag 1923; Aiello and Dean 1990; Gibbs 1999; Diogo et al. 2010, 2012, 2013a,b, 2017).

Variations

Description

Levator veli palatini may be longitudinally divided with the fibers from the Eustachian tube and the fibers from the petrous bone remaining separated (Macalister 1875; Patel and Loukas 2016). The portion of the muscle that originates from the Eustachian tube may be referred to as salpingostaphylinus (Macalister 1875; Patel and Loukas 2016). Levator veli palatini may entirely arise from the cartilage of the Eustachian tube or this tubal origin may be reduced (Macalister 1875; Patel and Loukas 2016). The portion of the muscle that originates from the petrous bone may be split at its origin (Macalister 1875; Patel and Loukas 2016). Levator veli palatini may also have a single origin with a doubled insertion (Macalister 1875; Patel and Loukas 2016).

Prevalence

N/A

Anomalies

Description

The morphology of levator veli palatini may vary in individuals with cleft palate or other palatal anomalies (e.g., Pettersen 1984; Lindman et al. 2001; Senoo et al. 2001; Arnold et al. 2005; Kotlarek et al. 2017; Trudel et al. 2018). In a male neonate with Meckel syndrome, Pettersen (1984) observed that the right levator veli palatini split around the hamulus of the medial pterygoid plate and attached onto the periosteum of the partial palatal shelf. The left muscle traveled medial to the hamulus and attached to the small flap of the soft palate. Kotlarek et al. (2017) found that levator veli palatini had smaller circumference, diameter, and volume in adults with repaired cleft palate than in adults without cleft palate.

Lindman et al. (2001) found that levator veli palatini had a smaller mean muscle fiber diameter and greater variability in fiber size and form in sample of infants with cleft palate compared to normal adults. Arnold et al. (2005) examined a fetus with bilateral cleft palate and found that levator veli palatini originated only from the auditory tube, ran parallel and medial to the auditory tube, and inserted into the dorsomedial edge of the palatal cleft.

Senoo et al. (2001) describe a case of congenital unilateral soft palate aplasia in which palatoglossus and levator veli palatini were absent on the right side. In a child with palatal anomaly associated with 8q22.1–22.2 microduplication, levator veli palatini had an insertion into the hard palate bilaterally (Trudel et al. 2018). There were also thin, membranous gaps between levator veli palatini and palatoglossus on both sides.

Prevalence

N/A

Clinical Implications

An aberrant insertion of levator veli palatini may contribute to hypernasal speech (Seif and Dellon 1978).

Musculus uvulae (Figure 2.5)

Synonyms

This muscle may also be referred to as azygos uvulae or motor uvulae (Harrison 1848; Macalister 1875).

Typical Presentation

Description

Musculus uvulae originates from the posterior nasal spine of the palatine bone and from the palatine aponeurosis (Standring 2016). It courses posteriorly to insert beneath the uvular mucosa (Standring 2016). It merges with its counterpart along the majority of its length (Standring 2016).

Innervation

Musculus uvulae is innervated by the pharyngeal plexus (Standring 2016).

Comparative Anatomy

There is no information on musculus uvulae in bonobos (Diogo et al. 2017). It is well-developed in gibbons (Kohlbrügge 1890–1892; Diogo et al. 2012). In gorillas, it originates from the soft palate and courses posterior to insert onto or near to the uvula (Diogo et al. 2010). In orangutans and common chimpanzees, it is present but may end in a membrane without attaching to the uvula (Gratiolet and Alix 1866; Chapman 1880; Sonntag 1923, 1924; Gibbs 1999; Diogo et al. 2013a,b).

Variations

Description

The degree of separation between the two uvular muscles on either side of the midline can vary from complete fusion to complete separation (Macalister 1875). Macalister (1875) describes a patient that exhibited an unusual action of musculus uvulae on the uvula and concludes that the muscle was inserted into the extreme tip of the uvula.

Prevalence

N/A

Anomalies

Description

The morphology of musculus uvulae may vary in individuals with cleft palate (Lewin et al. 1980; Shprintzen et al. 1985; Todd and Krueger 1992; Perry et al. 2019). In cases of classic or occult submucous cleft palate, musculus uvulae is often absent, is deficient, or shows some degree of diastasis (Lewin et al. 1980; Shprintzen et al. 1985). Todd and Krueger (1992) described cases of what they termed miniscule submucous cleft palate that exhibited reduced bulk of musculus uvulae. Perry et al. (2019) found that musculus uvulae was reduced in volume in adults with repaired cleft palate than in adults without cleft palate. In an otocephalic fetus examined by Lawrence and Bersu (1984), muscle fibers were present in the soft palate but most individual palatal muscles could not be identified. The only muscle clearly present was musculus uvulae.

Prevalence

In 29 patients with occult submucous cleft palate, Lewin et al. (1980) found that ten patients (34.5%) had an absent or hypoplastic musculus uvulae and 19 patients (65.5%) showed signs of deficient muscular fusion. In a sample of 25 children with bifid uvulae, Shprintzen et al. (1985) found that musculus uvulae was absent in 19 children (76%). Of the remaining six children, two exhibited a musculus uvulae with a deep midline groove, two had a small uvular muscle mass, and two had a moderate uvular muscle mass.

Clinical Implications

N/A

PALATOGLOSSUS (FIGURE 2.5)

See also: Muscles of the tongue

Synonyms

N/A

Typical Presentation

Description

Palatoglossus originates from the palatine aponeurosis of the soft palate (Standring 2016). It inserts into the side of the posterior tongue, with some fibers attaching to the dorsal surface of the tongue and other fibers blending with the intrinsic transverse muscle (Standring 2016). At its origin, palatoglossus is continuous with its counterpart on the other side of the body (Standring 2016). Though it is considered one of the extrinsic muscles of the tongue, palatoglossus is described in this section as its innervation and function are more similar to the soft palate muscles.

Innervation

Palatoglossus is innervated by the pharyngeal plexus (Standring 2016).

Comparative Anatomy

There is no information on palatoglossus in orangutans (Gibbs 1999; Diogo et al. 2013b). In the other apes, palatoglossus corresponds to muscle fibers within the palatoglossal fold that connect the soft palate to the supero-posterior portion of the tongue (Gibbs 1999; Diogo et al. 2010, 2012, 2013a, 2017). The muscle is most distinct in common chimpanzees and bonobos (Diogo et al. 2013a, 2017).

Variations

Description

Palatoglossus may send some fibers to palatopharyngeus or be connected with this muscle by a slip (Macalister 1875). Its origin may vary, with potential attachments closer to the uvula or the rim of the hard palate (Kuehn and Azzam 1978; Patel and Loukas 2016). Palatoglossus is in close proximity to an accessory slip, the amygdaloglossal muscle (Broca), which extends between the muscles of the tongue and the capsule of the palatine tonsil (Patel and Loukas 2016).

Prevalence

N/A

Anomalies

Description

Senoo et al. (2001) describe a case of congenital unilateral soft palate aplasia in which palatoglossus and levator veli palatini were absent on the right side. In a fetus with craniorachischisis, palatoglossus was the only soft palate/pharyngeal muscle that was present (Alghamdi et al. 2017). Bersu et al. (1976) describe a male infant with Hanhart syndrome. On the right side of this infant, the muscles of the soft palate were underdeveloped and displaced. A muscle descended from the cartilage of the auditory tube and split into two portions at the level of the soft palate. The anterior portion of this muscle inserted onto the side of the tongue forming the right palatoglossal arch. The posterior portion blended with the superior pharyngeal constrictor and the stylopharyngeus muscles forming the palatopharyngeal arch. In an otocephalic fetus examined by Lawrence and Bersu (1984), muscle fibers were present in the soft palate, but most individual palatal muscles could not be identified. In a male neonate with Meckel syndrome, Pettersen (1984) found that palatoglossus and palatopharyngeus originated from the medial aspect of the medial pterygoid plate on each side, instead of originating from the soft palate.

Prevalence

N/A

Clinical Implications

Ma et al. (1999) suggest that a short palatoglossus is associated with hypernasal or nasal emissive speech.

PALATOPHARYNGEUS (FIGURE 2.5)

See also: Salpingopharyngeus

Synonyms

This muscle may also be referred to as pharyngopalatinus (Whillis 1930).

Typical Presentation

Description

Palatopharyngeus is comprised of two fasciculi (Standring 2016). The anterior fasciculus originates from the posterior margin of the hard palate and from the palatine aponeurosis (Standring 2016). The posterior fasciculus has a connection with the mucosa of the pharyngeal region of the palate (Standring 2016). The two fasciculi join in the posterolateral margin of the soft palate and receive a contribution from salpingopharyngeus (Standring 2016). Palatopharyngeus inserts with stylopharyngeus into the posterior border of the thyroid cartilage (Standring 2016). It also partially inserts into pharyngeal fibrous tissue and decussates with the fibers of its counterpart (Standring 2016).

Innervation

Palatopharyngeus is innervated by the pharyngeal plexus (Standring 2016).

Comparative Anatomy

There is no information on this muscle in orangutans (Diogo et al. 2013b). Though there is also little information on this muscle in the other apes, palatopharyngeus seems to have a similar typical presentation as it connects the palatine region to the pharyngeal wall (Kohlbrügge 1890–1892; Diogo et al. 2010, 2012, 2013a, 2017). In a gorilla dissected by Diogo et al. (2010), palatopharyngeus was blended with the inferior pharyngeal constrictor.

Variations

Description

The extent of the origin from the nasal side of the palatine aponeurosis may vary (Okuda et al. 2008; Sumida et al. 2012). Sumida et al. (2012) argued that palatopharyngeus has two additional fasciculi of origin, the first being a posterior fasciculus that originated from the uvula and the second being salpingopharyngeus (see the entry for this muscle). The nature of its insertions into the thyroid cartilage, hypopharynx, and posterior pharynx can also vary (Sumida et al. 2012). Palatopharyngeus may receive some fibers from palatoglossus or be connected with this muscle by a slip (Macalister 1875).

Palatopharyngeus may be split into two or three parts (Macalister 1875). Macalister (1875) notes that Winslow found the muscle divided into three portions including peristaphylo-pharyngeus (velum to pharynx), pharyngo-staphylinus (uvula to pharynx), and thyro-staphylinus (uvula to the posterior margin of the thyroid cartilage). Macalister (1875) also notes that Luschka divided the muscle into a pars thyreo-palatina and a pars pharyngo-palatina.

Palatopharyngeus is associated with Passavant's muscle (palatopharyngeal sphincter) (Whillis 1930; Standring 2016; Sakamoto 2016a; Sumida et al. 2017). Its existence is debated in the literature (Standring 2016; Sumida et al. 2017). Some consider Passavant's muscle to be a portion of the superior pharyngeal constrictor and/or palatopharyngeus muscles, perhaps due to the difficulty in distinguishing it from the former (Whillis 1930; Sumida et al. 2012; Sakamoto 2015; Standring 2016; Sumida et al. 2017). Others recognize it as a distinct, sphincter-like muscle that originates from the nasal aspect of the lateral palatine aponeurosis and passes dorsolateral to levator veli palatini to surround the pharynx (Standring 2016; Sumida et al. 2017).

Palatopharyngeus is also in close proximity to several rare accessory pharyngeal muscles, including petropharyngeus (see the entry for this muscle), occipitopharyngeus, mastoidopharyngeus, sphenopharyngeus, pterygopharyngeus externus, azygospharyngeus, and tympanopharyngeus (Bergman et al. 1988; Knott 1883a; Sakamoto 2016a). Some of these muscles may be considered variants of the same accessory muscle, cephalo-pharyngeus (Macalister 1875; Knott 1883a).

Prevalence

Okuda et al. (2008) studied palatopharyngeus in 20 Japanese cadavers. In all cases (100%), an origin was present from the oral tendinous part of the posterior palatine aponeurosis, and this oral side origin interlaced with the fibers of the contralateral palatopharyngeal muscle. In 14 cases (70%), an origin was present from the nasal tendinous part of the posterior palatine aponeurosis. In 17 cases (85%), this nasal side origin interlaced with the fibers of the contralateral palatopharyngeal muscle.

Sumida et al. (2012) studied palatopharyngeus on 100 sides from 50 Japanese cadavers. These authors found four fasciculi of origin, the typical oral and nasal fasciculi, a posterior fasciculus that originated from the uvula, and salpingopharyngeus. On all sides, the oral fasciculus originated from the posterior border of the palatine aponeurosis. On 86 sides (86%), the oral fasciculus had an additional origin from the median line of the soft palate. In a subsample of 72 sides, the posterior fasciculus was present only on 40 sides (55.6%). In a subsample of 77 sides, the nasal fasciculus was present only on 59 sides (76.6%). From these 59 sides, the nasal fasciculus was well-developed on five sides (8.4%), extended toward the palatine aponeurosis on 27 sides (45.8%), and ended in the nasal mucosa of the soft palate before reaching the aponeurosis on 27 sides (45.8%).

Palatopharyngeus, together with contributions from salpingopharyngeus and stylopharyngeus, also had variable insertions (Sumida et al. 2012). Muscle fibers ending at the posterior pharyngeal insertion were found on only 18 out of the 100 sides (18%). In a subsample of 87 sides, there was an insertion into the thyroid cartilage via two bundles on 37 sides (42.5%) and via one bundle on 50 sides (57.5%). In a subsample of 94 sides, the muscle fibers ended at the level of the cricopharyngeal part of the inferior pharyngeal constrictor and formed an aponeurosis on 63 sides (67%), with two of these sides extending to the upper end of the esophagus. On 11 of these 94 sides (11.7%), the muscle fibers ended at the same level but did not form an aponeurosis, with one of these sides extending to the upper end of the esophagus. In the remaining 20 sides (21.3%), the fibers did not reach the cricopharyngeal part of the inferior pharyngeal constrictor and did not form an aponeurosis.

Anomalies

Description

Hypertrophy of Passavant's muscle may occur in individuals with complete cleft palate (Standring 2016). In an infant with mandibulofacial dysostosis, palatopharyngeus originated from the edge of the cleft soft palate and was closely associated with levator veli palatini (Herring et al. 1979). Furthermore, the superior constrictor and palatopharyngeus were continuous at their posterior and inferior attachments and inserted together into the posterior raphe.

Bersu et al. (1976) describe a male infant with Hanhart syndrome. On the right side of this infant, the muscles of the soft palate were underdeveloped and displaced. A muscle descended from the cartilage of the auditory tube and split into two portions at the level of the soft palate. The anterior portion of this muscle inserted onto the side of the tongue forming the right palatoglossal arch. The posterior portion blended with the superior pharyngeal constrictor and the stylopharyngeus muscles forming the palatopharyngeal arch. In a male neonate with Meckel syndrome,

palatoglossus and palatopharyngeus originated from the medial aspect of the medial pterygoid plate on each side, instead of originating from the soft palate (Pettersen 1984).

Prevalence

N/A

Clinical Implications

Lindman and Stål (2002) found that patients with sleep-disordered breathing demonstrated abnormalities in palatopharyngeus including an increase in connective tissue, an increase in the proportion of smaller-sized muscle fibers, and other variations of fiber type.

Salpingopharyngeus (Not Illustrated)

Synonyms

N/A

Typical Presentation

Description

Salpingopharyngeus originates from the cartilage of the pharyngotympanic tube and merges with palatopharyngeus (Standring 2016).

Innervation

Salpingopharyngeus is innervated by the pharyngeal plexus (Standring 2016).

Comparative Anatomy

There is no information on this muscle in orangutans (Diogo et al. 2013b). In gibbons, the pharyngeal muscles have an origin from the pharyngotympanic tube, which may contain fibers that correspond to salpingopharyngeus (Kohlbrügge 1890–1892; Diogo et al. 2012). In one gorilla, Diogo et al. (2010) were not able to identify fleshy fibers within the salpingopharyngeal fold. Diogo et al. (2013a) state that salpingopharyngeus in common chimpanzees is similar to that of humans. Diogo et al. (2017) were not able to determine if salpingopharyngeus was present as a distinct muscle in bonobos.

Variations

Description

Macalister (1875) considers salpingopharyngeus a detached slip of palatopharyngeus. Knott (1883a) considered it a variant of an accessory cephalo-pharyngeus muscle. Sumida et al. (2012) consider it a fourth fasciculus of origin for palatopharyngeus. Salpingopharyngeus may be absent (Sumida et al. 2012). It may be partially or fully replaced by connective and/or adipose tissue (Sumida et al. 2012).

Prevalence

In a sample of 98 sides from 49 Japanese cadavers, Sumida et al. (2012) found that salpingopharyngeus was present as a distinct muscle bundle on 59 sides (60.2%).

Anomalies

Description

In a male neonate with Meckel syndrome, salpingo-pharyngeus was absent (Pettersen 1984). It was absent bilaterally in an otocephalic fetus (Lawrence and Bersu 1984). In an individual with a completely bony left pharyngotympanic tube that communicated with the sphenoid sinus, salpingopharyngeus was hypoplastic (Khan et al. 2017).

Prevalence

N/A

Clinical Implications

N/A

PHARYNGEAL MUSCLES

CONSTRICTOR PHARYNGIS SUPERIOR (SUPERIOR PHARYNGEAL CONSTRICTOR) (FIGURE 2.6)

See also: Petropharyngeus

Synonyms

N/A

Typical Presentation

Description

Constrictor pharyngis superior originates from the pterygoid hamulus, pterygomandibular raphe, mylohyoid line of the mandible, and side of the tongue (Standring 2016). It inserts into the pharyngeal raphe, which attaches to the pharyngeal tubercle of the occipital bone (Standring 2016).

Innervation

Constrictor pharyngis superior is innervated by the pharyngeal plexus (Standring 2016).

Comparative Anatomy

Constrictor pharyngis superior may be only comprised of the glossopharyngeal part in gibbons and orangutans (Kohlbrügge 1890–1892; Diogo et al. 2012, 2013b). All four parts of the superior constrictor and an insertion into the pharyngeal raphe have been found in gorillas, common chimpanzees, and bonobos (Gibbs 1999; Diogo et al. 2010, 2013a, 2017). Pterygopharyngeus is present as a muscle distinct from the superior constrictor in gibbons, extending between the pterygoid hamulus and the pharyngeal wall (Kohlbrügge 1890–1892; Saban 1968; Diogo et al. 2012).

Variations

Description

Macalister (1875) notes that Luschka considered constrictor pharyngis superior a composite muscle comprised of four parts: pterygo-pharyngeus, bucco-pharyngeus, mylo-pharyngeus, and glosso-pharyngeus. The buccopharyngeal part may connect with buccinator (Macalister 1875; Shimada and Gasser 1989). The extent of the origin from the pterygoid hamulus may vary (Macalister 1875). It may have an origin from the medial pterygoid plate (Standring 2016) or the petrous part of the temporal bone (Bergman et al. 1988; Sakamoto 2009, 2016a). Stylopharyngeus may course transversely and join the superior pharyngeal constrictor (Choi et al. 2020). A portion of the superior constrictor may run longitudinally and pass between the superior and middle constrictors, or merge with the middle constrictor and the contralateral constrictor muscles (Choi et al. 2020). An accessory muscle, petropharyngeus, may also be joined

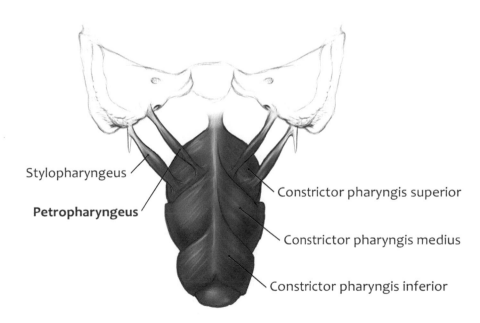

FIGURE 2.6 Pharyngeal muscles in posterior view.

Stylopharyngeus

Petropharyngeus

Constrictor pharyngis superior

Constrictor pharyngis medius

Constrictor pharyngis inferior

with the superior constrictor (Macalister 1875; Knott 1883a; see the entry for this muscle). A slip from genioglossus to constrictor pharyngis superior is referred to as geniopharyngeus (Winslow) (Macalister 1875; Knott 1883a; Bergman et al. 1988; Patel and Loukas 2016). Pterygopharyngeus externus, which attaches to the pterygoid hamulus, may be present as a distinct muscle (Sakamoto 2016a).

Constrictor pharyngis superior is also associated with azygos-pharyngeus (azygos pharyngis or solitarius pharyngis), which originates from the pharyngeal tubercle and inserts into the pharyngeal raphe (Macalister 1875; Knott 1883a; Bergman et al. 1988; Sakamoto 2016a). When present, it overlies the superior and middle constrictors along the midline, and it may be fused with the superior constrictor (Macalister 1875; Knott 1883a). Teixeira et al. (2019) describe a longitudinal bundle that originates bilaterally from the occipital bone near the pharyngeal tubercle and descends to blend with the inferior constrictor. The authors suggest that these are aberrant slips of the superior constrictor. The description of these slips is similar to that of azygos-pharyngeus. Sakamoto (2009) describes longitudinal bundles situated medial to stylopharyngeus that passed over the dorsal surface of the superior constrictor and blended with middle constrictor. Teixeira et al. (2019) state that the bundles found by Sakamoto (2009) do not resemble the bundles described by them.

Additionally, constrictor pharyngis superior is associated with Passavant's muscle (palatopharyngeal sphincter) (Whillis 1930; Sakamoto 2016a; Standring 2016; Sumida et al. 2017). Its existence is debated in the literature (Standring 2016; Sumida et al. 2017). Some consider Passavant's muscle to be a portion of the superior pharyngeal constrictor and/or palatopharyngeus muscles, perhaps due to the difficulty in distinguishing it from the former (Whillis 1930; Sumida et al. 2012; Sakamoto 2015; Standring 2016; Sumida et al. 2017). Others recognize it as a distinct, sphincter-like muscle that originates from the nasal aspect of the lateral palatine aponeurosis and passes dorsolateral to levator veli palatini to surround the pharynx (Sakamoto 2016a; Standring 2016; Sumida et al. 2017).

Prevalence

Knott (1883a) found azygos-pharyngeus in 4 out of 87 subjects (4.6%). In a sample of 110 cadavers, the pterygomandibular raphe was absent on 40 sides (36%), which allowed for complete continuity of the superior constrictor and buccinator muscles. In a sample of 44 sides from 22 cadavers, Sakamoto (2009) found a longitudinal bundle that descended over the superior constrictor to blend with the middle pharyngeal constrictor on six sides (13.6%). Sakamoto (2009) also found that fibers originated from the petrous temporal bone, which passed dorsally to merge with the superior constrictor on eight sides (18.2%) and passed ventrally to attach to the soft palate with the origin of the superior constrictor on five sides (11.4%). In a sample of 44 sides, Choi et al. (2020) found that stylopharyngeus passed transversely and merged with the superior pharyngeal constrictor in one case (2.3%). Furthermore, in five sides (11.4%), a portion of the superior constrictor ran longitudinally and either passed between the superior and middle constrictors or merged with the middle constrictor and the contralateral constrictor muscles.

Anomalies

Description

Bersu et al. (1976) describe a male infant with Hanhart syndrome. In this infant, the inferior parts of both superior pharyngeal constrictors were abnormally thickened. On the right side, some of its fibers inserted into a pterygomandibular raphe while the rest of the fibers inserted into the skull near the pterygoid laminae. On the left side, all fibers inserted onto the skull near the pterygoid laminae. In an infant with mandibulofacial dysostosis, the superior constrictor and palatopharyngeus were continuous at their posterior and inferior attachments and inserted together into the posterior raphe (Herring et al. 1979).

In an infant with trisomy 18, the posterior belly of the digastric sent a slip to the superior constrictor bilaterally (Bersu and Ramirez-Castro 1977). Mieden (1982) describes an infant with median cleft lip, hypotelorism, and alobar holoprosencephaly. This infant had a bilateral accessory slip extending between the intermediate tendon of digastricus and the superior pharyngeal constrictor (Mieden 1982).

In a male neonate with Meckel syndrome, Pettersen (1984) observed that the superior pharyngeal constrictor attached to an aberrant medial extension of the left mandible. Itoh et al. (1991) describe fetal akinesia/hypokinesia sequence in one male and one female infant, each with suite of anatomical anomalies. In the male, the constrictor pharyngis muscles showed irregular but mild atrophy. In an infant with craniorachischisis, the pharyngeal constrictor muscles were absent (Alghamdi et al. 2017).

Prevalence

In a sample of 16 sides from eight infants with trisomy 18, Bersu and Ramirez-Castro (1977) found a slip between the posterior belly of the digastricus and the superior or middle pharyngeal constrictors on four sides (25%).

Clinical Implications

N/A

Stylopharyngeus (Figure 2.6)

Synonyms

N/A

Typical Presentation

Description

Stylopharyngeus originates from the base of the styloid process and ends with attachments to the pharyngeal constrictors, palatopharyngeus, and the thyroid cartilage (Standring 2016).

Innervation

Stylopharyngeus is innervated by the glossopharyngeal nerve (Standring 2016).

Comparative Anatomy

Stylopharyngeus has a similar typical presentation in the apes, extending from the styloid process to the pharyngeal wall, passing between the superior and middle pharyngeal constrictors (Kohlbrügge 1890–1892; Dean 1984; Gibbs 1999; Diogo et al. 2010, 2012, 2013a,b, 2017). In one gibbon, it originated from the tympanic region as no styloid process was present (Diogo et al. 2012). It may be indirectly connected via connective tissue to the greater horn of the hyoid bone in gorillas (Diogo et al. 2010). It may have an insertion into the hyoid bone and/or the thyroid cartilage in common chimpanzees (Gratiolet and Alix 1866; Diogo et al. 2013a). In one bonobo, Diogo et al. (2017) found that stylopharyngeus was fused with styloglossus and the middle constrictor.

Variations

Description

Stylopharyngeus may be doubled or split into two or three slips (Wood 1867b; Macalister 1875; Bergman et al. 1988; Sakamoto 2016a). It may course transversely and join the superior pharyngeal constrictor (Choi et al. 2020). An accessory bundle of stylopharyngeus may either descend parallel to stylopharyngeus and pass between the middle and inferior pharyngeal constrictors or insert into the pharyngeal raphe along the midline with the superior constrictor (Choi et al. 2020). A bundle may also connect it to the intermediate tendon of the digastric (Sakamoto 2009).

Prevalence

In a sample of 44 sides from 22 cadavers, Sakamoto (2009) found a bundle connecting the intermediate tendon of the digastric and stylopharyngeus on one side (2.3%). In a sample of 44 sides, Choi et al. (2020) found that stylopharyngeus passed transversely and merged with the superior pharyngeal constrictor in one case (2.3%). An accessory bundle of stylopharyngeus was present in eight cases (18.2%). In four cases (9.1%), the bundle passed between the middle and inferior pharyngeal constrictors. In four cases (9.1%), the bundle inserted into the pharyngeal raphe with the superior constrictor.

Anomalies

Description

In one neonate with trisomy 13, the right posterior belly of the digastricus split and sent a deep bundle to stylopharyngeus (Colacino and Pettersen 1978). In another neonate with trisomy 13, stylopharyngeus was doubled bilaterally (Pettersen et al. 1979). The extra muscles coursed transversely to the superior pharyngeal constrictor and inserted just lateral to the pharyngeal raphe. In a boy with trisomy 13q, an extra stylopharyngeus muscle was present on the left side and inserted deep into hyoglossus (Pettersen 1979). In an infant with trisomy 18, an abnormal belly of stylopharyngeus coursed posteriorly behind the styloid process and inserted over the superficial surface of the superior constrictor (Bersu and Ramirez-Castro 1977). Stylopharyngeus was absent in a fetus with craniorachischisis (Alghamdi et al. 2017).

Prevalence

In their literature review, Smith et al. (2015) found that a doubled or extra stylopharyngeus muscle was present in 2 out of 20 individuals with trisomy 13 (10%).

Clinical Implications

N/A

PETROPHARYNGEUS (FIGURE 2.6)

Synonyms

Macalister (1875) and Knott (1883a) consider petropharyngeus to be a variant of cephalo-pharyngeus. Sakamoto (2016a) suggests that petropharyngeus with an origin from the vaginal process of the temporal bone would be more aptly named tympanopharyngeus.

Typical Presentation

This muscle is present only as a variation or anomaly.

Comparative Anatomy

Petropharyngeus is not present as a distinct muscle in the apes (Diogo et al. 2010, 2012, 2013a,b, 2017).

Variations

Description

Petropharyngeus originates from the petrous temporal bone and can insert into any of the pharyngeal constrictors (Macalister 1875; Knott 1883a; Shimada et al. 1991; Sakamoto 2009, 2016a; Siddiqui et al. 2017; Choi et al. 2020). It may also originate from the vaginal process of the temporal bone (Knott 1883a; Bergman et al. 1988; Sakamoto 2009, 2016a). It is situated medially, superiorly, and posteriorly to stylopharyngeus (Siddiqui et al. 2017; Choi et al. 2020).

Petropharyngeus may be present bilaterally (Shimada et al. 1991; Sakamoto 2009; Siddiqui et al. 2017). It may be divided into two bundles (Choi et al. 2020). It may present as a thin and small fascicle, a fibromuscular structure, or a well-developed muscular slip (Siddiqui et al. 2017; Choi et al. 2020).

Petropharyngeus often inserts into the superior constrictor (Macalister 1875; Knott 1883a; Sakamoto 2009; Siddiqui et al. 2017; Choi et al. 2020). Shimada et al. (1991) observed that petropharyngeus inserted into the outer surface of the middle pharyngeal constrictor. In the case of a bifurcated petropharyngeus, Choi et al. (2020) found that one bundle passed deep to the superior constrictor and the other inserted into the middle constrictor. Sakamoto (2009) found that petropharyngeus may end over the dorsal surface of the inferior constrictor.

Innervation

Petropharyngeus may be innervated by the glossopharyngeal nerve (Shimada et al. 1991) or the pharyngeal plexus (Sakamoto 2009).

Prevalence

In a sample of 614 Japanese cadavers, Shimada et al. (1991) found petropharyngeus in seven cadavers (1.1%). In a sample of 44 sides from 22 cadavers, Sakamoto (2009) found bundles that correspond to petropharyngeus on both sides of one cadaver (4.5%). In a sample of 24 sides from 12 cadavers, Tubbs et al. (2010) found petropharyngeus on one side (4.2%). In a sample of 44 heads, Siddiqui et al. (2017) found petropharyngeus in three cases (6.8%). In a sample of 44 sides, Choi et al. (2020) found petropharyngeus in 11 cases (25%).

Anomalies

Description

In a child with trisomy 21, petropharyngeus was present bilaterally (Bersu 1980). It extended between the petrous part of the temporal bone and the middle pharyngeal constrictor.

Prevalence

Bersu (1980) found petropharyngeus in one out of five individuals with trisomy 21 (20%).

Clinical Implications

N/A

CONSTRICTOR PHARYNGIS MEDIUS (MIDDLE PHARYNGEAL CONSTRICTOR) (FIGURE 2.6)

See also: Petropharyngeus

Synonyms

N/A

Typical Presentation

Description

Constrictor pharyngis medius originates from the lesser and greater horns of the hyoid, and from the stylohyoid ligament, and inserts into the pharyngeal raphe (Standring 2016).

Innervation

Constrictor pharyngis medius is innervated by the pharyngeal plexus (Standring 2016).

Comparative Anatomy

Constrictor pharyngis medius has an origin only from the greater horn of the hyoid in gibbons and gorillas (Kohlbrügge 1890–1892; Diogo et al. 2010, 2012). It originates from the hyoid in orangutans (Sonntag 1924). It originates from the angle between the greater and lesser horns of the hyoid in common chimpanzees and bonobos (Gratiolet and Alix 1866; Sonntag 1923; Gibbs 1999; Diogo et al. 2013a, 2017). Therefore, it appears that only the ceratopharyngeal part of the middle constrictor is present in the apes. It was fused with stylopharyngeus in one bonobo (Diogo et al. 2017).

Variations

Description

Constrictor pharyngis medius may extend to the base of the cranium along the stylohyoid ligament (Macalister 1875). The origin from the greater horn of the hyoid (ceratopharyngeal part) and the rest of the muscle (chondropharyngeal part) may be distinct (Bergman et al. 1988). If the center portion is deficient, it may appear bipartite (Macalister 1875). Macalister (1875) reports that it may have three parts, with origins from the hyoid, the triticeal cartilage, and the thyrohyoid membrane.

Constrictor pharyngis medius may be fused with the superior belly of omohyoid or sternothyroid (Wood 1868). Its fibers may also connect with hyoglossus, stylohyoid, thyrohyoid, the posterior belly of the digastric, or the triticeal cartilage (Macalister 1875; Sakamoto 2009, 2014). Its fibers may interdigitate with those of stylopharyngeus (Sakamoto 2014). Accessory muscles, such as sphenopharyngeus (Wood 1868) or petropharyngeus (Macalister 1875; see the entry for this muscle), may insert into the middle constrictor. Sakamoto (2009) describes longitudinal bundles situated medial to stylopharyngeus that passed over the dorsal surface of the superior constrictor and blended with the middle constrictor.

Prevalence

In a sample of 44 sides from 22 cadavers, the superior fibers of constrictor pharyngis medius joined with hyoglossus on ten sides (22.7%) and with stylohyoid on five sides (11.4%) (Sakamoto 2009). A longitudinal bundle that descended over the superior constrictor to blend with the middle pharyngeal constrictor was present on six sides (13.6%). In a sample of 82 sides from 41 cadavers, Sakamoto (2014) found fibers of the middle constrictor attached to hyoglossus on 29 sides (35.4%), thyrohyoid on two sides (2.4%), stylohyoid and the posterior belly of the digastric on 33 sides (40.2%), only stylohyoid on seven sides (8.5%), and the triticeal cartilage on one side (1.2%). Fibers of the middle constrictor interdigitated with those of stylopharyngeus on four sides (4.9%).

Anomalies

Description

In an infant with Hanhart syndrome, the right medial pterygoid had extensive attachments and sent fibers to the middle pharyngeal constrictor (Bersu et al. 1976). In an infant with trisomy 18, the posterior belly of the digastric sent a slip to the middle constrictor on the right side (Bersu and

Ramirez-Castro 1977). Itoh et al. (1991) describe fetal akinesia/hypokinesia sequence in one male and one female infant, each with a suite of anatomical anomalies. In the male, the constrictor pharyngis muscles showed irregular but mild atrophy. In an infant with craniorachischisis, the pharyngeal constrictor muscles were absent (Alghamdi et al. 2017).

Prevalence

In a sample of 16 sides from eight infants with trisomy 18, Bersu and Ramirez-Castro (1977) found a slip between the posterior belly of the digastricus and the superior or middle pharyngeal constrictors on four sides (25%).

Clinical Implications

N/A

Constrictor pharyngis inferior (Inferior pharyngeal constrictor) (Figure 2.6)

See also: Petropharyngeus

Synonyms

N/A

Typical Presentation

Description

Constrictor pharyngis inferior has thyropharyngeal and cricopharyngeal parts (Standring 2016). The former originates from the thyroid cartilage and inserts into the pharyngeal raphe (Standring 2016). The latter originates from the cricoid cartilage and merges inferiorly with some fibers of the esophagus (Standring 2016).

Innervation

Constrictor pharyngis inferior is innervated by the pharyngeal plexus (Standring 2016). It may receive additional Innervation from one or more of the laryngeal nerves (Sakamoto 2013).

Comparative Anatomy

Constrictor pharyngis inferior has a similar typical presentation in the apes, as both the thyropharyngeal and cricopharyngeal parts are typically present with insertions into the pharyngeal raphe (Kohlbrügge 1890–1892; Hosokawa and Kamiya 1961–1962; Gibbs 1999; Diogo et al. 2010, 2012, 2013a,b, 2017). It may have an origin from the first tracheal ring in common chimpanzees (Gratiolet and Alix 1866; Gibbs 1999).

Variations

Description

Constrictor pharyngis inferior may have an origin from the trachea (Macalister 1875). The thyropharyngeal and cricopharyngeal parts may be distinct (Bergman et al. 1988). The inferior constrictor may connect with thyrohyoid,

cricothyroid, or sternothyroid (Macalister 1875; Bergman et al. 1988; Sakamoto 2009, 2013, 2016a). Fibers of the lessor constrictor may originate from a tendinous cord that loops over cricothyroid and connects the cricoid cartilage with the inferior thyroid tubercle (Sakamoto 2013, 2016a; Standring 2016). When this tendinous cord is absent or deficient, the inferior constrictor may connect with cricothyroid (Sakamoto 2013, 2016a).

Constrictor pharyngis inferior may receive a slip from the lateral thyrohyoid ligament, which may be referred to as syndesmopharyngeus (Knott 1883a; Bergman et al. 1988; Sakamoto 2016a). Petropharyngeus may end over the dorsal surface of the inferior constrictor (Sakamoto 2009; see the entry for this muscle). Teixeira et al. (2019) describe a longitudinal bundle that originates bilaterally from the occipital bone near the pharyngeal tubercle and descend to blend with the inferior constrictor. The authors suggest that these are aberrant slips of the superior constrictor. The description of these slips is similar to that of the azygos-pharyngeus muscle (Macalister 1875; Knott 1883a; Bergman et al. 1988; Sakamoto 2016a).

Prevalence

Knott (1883a) found syndesmopharyngeus in 2 out of 47 subjects (4.3%). In a sample of 44 sides from 22 cadavers, the tendinous cord connected the two origins of the inferior constrictor on 10 sides (22.7%) (Sakamoto 2009). Fibers of the inferior constrictor connected with thyrohyoid on 13 sides (29.5%), sternothyroid on 29 sides (65.9%), and cricothyroid on 17 sides (38.6%). In a sample of 60 sides from 30 cadavers, the tendinous cord was present on 36 sides (60%) (Sakamoto 2013).

Anomalies

Description

Itoh et al. (1991) describe fetal akinesia/hypokinesia sequence in one male and one female infant, each with a suite of anatomical anomalies. In the male, the constrictor pharyngis muscles showed irregular but mild atrophy. In an infant with craniorachischisis, the pharyngeal constrictor muscles were absent (Alghamdi et al. 2017).

Prevalence

N/A

Clinical Implications

N/A

LARYNGEAL MUSCLES

Cricothyroideus (Cricothyroid) (Figure 2.7)

See also: Ceratocricoid, Thyrotrachealis

Synonyms

N/A

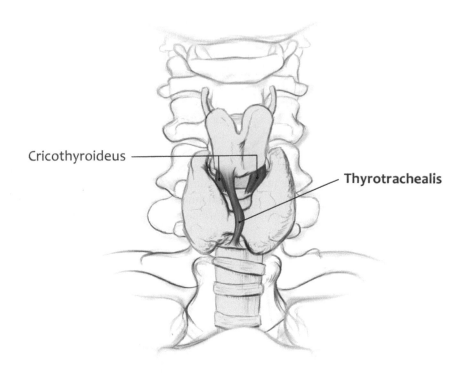

Cricothyroideus

Thyrotrachealis

FIGURE 2.7   Anterior laryngeal muscles in anterior view.

Typical Presentation

Description

Cricothyroid originates from the cricoid cartilage and inserts onto the inferior cornu (oblique part) and lower margin (straight part) of the thyroid cartilage (Standring 2016).

Innervation

Cricothyroid is innervated by the external branch of the superior laryngeal nerve (Standring 2016).

Comparative Anatomy

Cricothyroid has a similar typical presentation in the apes, extending from the cricoid cartilage to the thyroid cartilage (Kohlbrügge 1890–1892; Saban 1968; Gibbs 1999; Diogo et al. 2010, 2012, 2013a,b, 2017). Some authors state that in addition to a straight part and oblique part, a pars interna is also often present in the apes (Gratiolet and Alix 1866; Kohlbrügge 1890–1892; Starck and Schneider 1960; Saban 1968; Gibbs 1999; Diogo et al. 2010, 2012, 2013a,b, 2017). Macalister (1875) states that Eschricht found cricothyroideus superior and a muscle similar to thyroideus transversus anomalus in gibbons.

Variations

Description

Cricothyroid may be bilaminar (Macalister 1875). Mu and Sanders (2008) suggest that cricothyroid has a third, horizontal belly situated deep to the oblique belly. Cricothyroid may have an origin from the first tracheal ring (Macalister 1875; Maranillo and Sanudo 2016). It may connect with thyrohyoid, sternothyroid, or the inferior pharyngeal constrictor (Macalister 1875; Bergman et al. 1988; Sakamoto 2009, 2013, 2016a; Maranillo and Sanudo 2016). The cricothyroid muscles may decussate across the midline (Bergman et al. 1988). If the straight part is separate from the rest of the muscle, it may be referred to as cricothyroideus superior (Macalister 1875; Bergman et al. 1988; Maranillo and Sanudo 2016).

Cricothyroid is associated with several named accessory muscles. Cricothyroid may connect with ceratocricoid, a small bundle that originates from the cricoid cartilage and inserts into the inferior cornu of the thyroid cartilage (see the entry for this muscle). It may connect with thyrotrachealis, which extends from the thyroid cartilage to the trachea (see the entry for this muscle). It may also connect with the internal cricoid muscle, which is situated medial to cricothyroid and has attachments to the cricoid cartilage and thyroid cartilage (Le Double 1897; Maranillo and Sanudo 2016). The deep levator of the thyroid gland may originate from the anteromedial aspect of cricothyroid (Maranillo and Sanudo 2016).

Incisurae mediae obliquus (Gruber) may be present as a small muscle on the inferolateral aspect of the thyroid cartilage (Gruber 1868a; Bergman et al. 1988; Maranillo and Sanudo 2016). It may be present bilaterally (Bergman et al. 1988). It may have a second head that originates from the sternothyroid, and in this case, the muscle would be referred to as incisurae mediae obliquus bicaudatus (Bergman et al. 1988; Maranillo and Sanudo 2016). Thyroideus transversus anomalus (Gruber) extends across the superior portion of the cricothyroid membrane from one side of the inferior border of the thyroid cartilage to another (Macalister 1875; Knott 1883a; Maranillo and Sanudo 2016). It may also be referred to as thyroideus marginalis inferior, incisurae cartilaginis thyroideae mediae transversus, or the transverse thyroid muscle (Macalister 1875; Knott 1883a; Maranillo and Sanudo 2016). Cricohyoid (Zagorsky) extends from the cricoid cartilage to the greater horn or body of the hyoid (Macalister 1875; Bergman et al. 1988; Maranillo and Sanudo 2016). Cricotrachealis originates from the lower margin of the cricoid cartilage, courses behind the isthmus of the thyroid gland, and inserts into the fourth and/or fifth tracheal ring (Macalister 1875; Knott 1883a; Maranillo and Sanudo 2016).

Prevalence

In a sample of 44 sides from 22 cadavers, Sakamoto (2009) found fibers of the inferior constrictor connected with cricothyroid on 17 sides (38.6%).

Anomalies

N/A

Clinical Implications

N/A

THYROTRACHEALIS (FIGURE 2.7)

Synonyms

This muscle may also be referred to as thyrotrachealis profundus (Krause) or thyrotrachealis biceps (Gruber) (Knott 1883a; Bergman et al. 1988).

Typical Presentation

This muscle is present only as a variation.

Comparative Anatomy

Gratiolet and Alix (1866) describe an additional bundle of cricothyroid in one common chimpanzee that could correspond to thyrotrachealis. It originated from the inferior margin of the thyroid cartilage, passed superficial to cricothyroid, and ended in the more anterior tracheal cartilages.

Variations

Description

Thyrotrachealis originates from the lower border of the thyroid cartilage, courses over cricothyroid and the isthmus of the thyroid gland, and inserts into the third, fourth, and/or fifth tracheal rings (Macalister 1875; Knott 1883a; Bergman et al. 1988; Sujata et al. 2013; Maranillo and Sanudo 2016).

It may have medial and lateral heads (Macalister 1875; Bergman et al. 1988; Maranillo and Sanudo 2016). It may be a detached slip of sternothyroid (Macalister 1875). It may merge with cricothyroid or the inferior pharyngeal constrictor (Sujata et al. 2013). Sujata et al. (2013) found an insertion into the fifth through eighth tracheal rings.

Innervation

Thyrotrachealis is innervated by a small twig from the ansa cervicalis (Sujata et al. 2013).

Prevalence

Gruber (1868c) found thyrotrachealis in 21 out of 80 cases (26.3%). Macalister (1875) found five cases of thyrotrachealis in 80 subjects (6.3%). Knott (1883a) found thyrotrachealis in 3 out of 28 subjects (10.7%). Le Double (1897) found thyrotrachealis in 4 out of 60 cases (6.7%).

Anomalies

N/A

Clinical Implications

Thyrotrachealis may lead to the misdiagnosis of thyroid swellings (Sujata et al. 2013).

CERATOCRICOID (FIGURE 2.8)

Synonyms

This muscle may also be referred to as crico-corniculatus (Tourtual), kerato-cricoid (Merkel), Merkel's muscle, or posterior cricothyroid [crico-thyreoideus posticus (Bochdalek)] (Turner 1860; Macalister 1875; Knott 1883a; Hetherington 1934).

Typical Presentation

This muscle is present only as a variation or anomaly.

Comparative Anatomy

Among the primates, ceratocricoid has been observed in guenons (Hetherington 1934). It is not present in the apes (Diogo et al. 2010, 2012, 2013a,b, 2017). In one bonobo, the posterior cricoarytenoid muscle had an attachment onto the inferior cornu of the thyroid cartilage, but these fibers did not form a distinct ceratocricoid muscle (Diogo et al. 2017).

Variations

Description

Ceratocricoid originates from the posterior surface of the cricoid cartilage, behind and below the cricothyroid joint, and inserts into the posterior surface of the inferior cornu of the thyroid cartilage (Turner 1860; Macalister 1875; Hetherington 1934; Bergman et al. 1988; Sharp 1990; Maranillo et al. 2009; Maranillo and Sanudo 2016; Standring 2016). It is situated lateral to, and near the lower border of, cricoarytenoideus posterior (Bergman et al. 1988; Hetherington 1934; Maranillo and Sanudo 2016; Standring 2016). When present, it courses over the recurrent

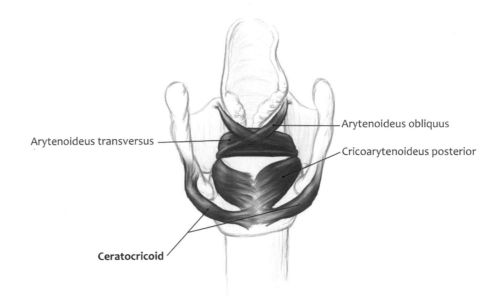

Arytenoideus transversus

Arytenoideus obliquus

Cricoarytenoideus posterior

Ceratocricoid

FIGURE 2.8   Posterior laryngeal muscles in posterior view.

laryngeal nerve (Turner 1860; Hetherington 1934; Sharp 1990; Maranillo et al. 2009; Maranillo and Sanudo 2016). Ceratocricoid is present as a condensation of cells at embryonic stages 22 and 23, at which point it is joined to the posterior cricoarytenoid muscle but extends toward the chondrified inferior cornu (Maranillo et al. 2009). It becomes completely distinct from the posterior cricoarytenoid muscle in the eleventh week of fetal development (Maranillo et al. 2009).

Ceratocricoid may be fused with cricothyroid or the posterior cricoarytenoid muscle (Macalister 1875; Maranillo and Sanudo 2016). It may also have an attachment into the capsule of the cricothyroid joint (Hetherington 1934; Sharp 1990; Maranillo et al. 2009). It may have two bellies (Hetherington 1934; Maranillo et al. 2009). It may also be divided only at its insertion into the thyroid cartilage (Hetherington 1934). It may be present bilaterally (Turner 1860; Macalister 1875; Knott 1883a; Hetherington 1934; Maranillo et al. 2009).

Innervation

Ceratocricoid is innervated by the recurrent laryngeal nerve (Sharp 1990; Maranillo et al. 2009).

Prevalence

Turner (1860) found seven cases of ceratocricoid in 32 subjects (21.9%). Le Double (1897) found five cases of ceratocricoid out of 28 specimens (17.9%). In a review of the literature, Hetherington (1934) reports that the prevalence of ceratocricoid ranges from 10% to 25%. In a sample of 132 subjects, Hetherington (1934) found ceratocricoid in 22 subjects (16.7%). In a sample of 134 hemilarynges, Sharp (1990) found nine cases of ceratocricoid (6.7%). Schweizer and Dörfl (1997) found ceratocricoid in 4 out of 21 larynges (19%). Maranillo et al. (2009) found ceratocricoid present in 8 out of 34 fetal larynges (23.5%) and in 13 out of 90 adult larynges (14.4%).

Anomalies

Description

Ceratocricoid was present in an infant with mandibulofacial dysostosis (Herring et al. 1979).

Prevalence

N/A

Clinical Implications

Ceratocricoid may compress the recurrent laryngeal nerve, and thus be a potential cause of recurrent laryngeal nerve palsy (Maranillo et al. 2009).

CRICOARYTENOIDEUS POSTERIOR (POSTERIOR CRICOARYTENOID) (FIGURE 2.8)

See also: Ceratocricoid

Synonyms

This muscle may also be referred to as cricoarytenoideus posticus (Macalister 1875).

Typical Presentation

Description

Cricoarytenoideus posterior originates from the posterior surface of the cricoid cartilage and inserts into the muscular process of the arytenoid cartilage (Standring 2016). It has three muscular compartments: horizontal (medial), oblique, and vertical (lateral) (Sanders et al. 1994; Maranillo and Sanudo 2016; Standring 2016).

Innervation

Cricoarytenoideus posterior is innervated by the recurrent laryngeal nerve (Standring 2016).

Comparative Anatomy

Cricoarytenoideus posterior has a similar typical presentation in the apes, extending from the dorsal portion of the cricoid cartilage to the arytenoid cartilage (Diogo et al. 2010, 2012, 2013a,b, 2017). The posterior cricoarytenoid muscles may meet at the midline in some gibbons (Kohlbrügge 1890–1892; Starck and Schneider 1960; Diogo et al. 2012), orangutans (Sonntag 1924), and common chimpanzees (Jordan 1971a,b,c; Diogo et al. 2013a). The ceratoarytenoideus lateralis muscle (ceratoarytenoid) is distinctly present in some common chimpanzees (Macalister 1871; Saban 1968). Bundles that potentially correspond to ceratoarytenoid have been described in gibbons (Kohlbrügge 1890–1892; Starck and Schneider 1960; Diogo et al. 2012).

Variations

Description

Cricoarytenoideus posterior (the posterior cricoarytenoid muscle) may be divided (Macalister 1875). It may also be bilaminar (Macalister 1875). It may send a slip to the cricothyroid joint (Macalister 1875; Maranillo and Sanudo 2016). The posterior cricoarytenoid muscle is associated with a few accessory muscles. It may be joined to the ceratocricoid muscle (Macalister 1875; Maranillo and Sanudo 2016; see the entry for this muscle). It may also be associated with ceratoarytenoid (also referred to as posterior thyroarytenoid, accessory thyroarytenoid, or ceratoarytenoideus lateralis), which extends between the inferior cornu of the thyroid cartilage and the muscular process of the arytenoid cartilage (Gruber 1868b; Macalister 1867b, 1875; Knott 1883a; Le Double 1897; Hetherington 1934; Saban 1968; Maranillo and Sanudo 2016). A cricocorniculate muscle may be present that originates from the upper margin of the cricoid cartilage and inserts into the corniculate cartilage (Maranillo and Sanudo 2016).

Wells and Thomas (1927) describe an accessory muscle of posterior cricoarytenoid that is referred to as the superior cricoarytenoid muscle by Maranillo and Sanudo (2016). It originated from the superior part of the left lamina of the cricoid cartilage, just lateral to the median ridge. The muscle coursed superiorly and laterally over the transverse and oblique arytenoid muscles. It inserted on the right side of the larynx into the apex of the arytenoid cartilage and the mucous membrane of the aryepiglottic fold, with some fibers inserting into the transverse arytenoid (Wells and Thomas 1927; Maranillo and Sanudo 2016).

Prevalence

Hetherington (1934) found ceratoarytenoid in 3 out of 66 individuals (4.5%).

Anomalies

Description

In cases of laryngeal cleft, the posterior cricoarytenoid muscles may be deficient or displaced (Lim et al. 1979).

In a fetus with craniorachischisis, the posterior cricoarytenoid muscles were attached at the midline (Alghamdi et al. 2017).

Prevalence

N/A

Clinical Implications

N/A

CRICOARYTENOIDEUS LATERALIS (LATERAL CRICOARYTENOID) (FIGURE 2.9)

Synonyms

N/A

Typical Presentation

Description

Cricoarytenoideus lateralis originates from the upper border of the arch of the cricoid cartilage and inserts into the muscular process of the arytenoid cartilage (Standring 2016).

Innervation

Cricoarytenoideus lateralis is innervated by the recurrent laryngeal nerve (Standring 2016).

Comparative Anatomy

Cricoarytenoideus lateralis has a similar typical presentation in the apes, extending from the anterior portion of the cricoid cartilage to the muscular process of the arytenoid cartilage (Gibbs 1999; Diogo et al. 2010, 2012, 2013a,b, 2017). There may be an additional insertion onto the thyroid cartilage in orangutans and common chimpanzees (Jordan 1971a; Gibbs 1999).

Variations

Description

Cricoarytenoideus lateralis (the lateral cricoarytenoid muscle) may receive a slip from the thyroid cartilage (Macalister 1875). It may be fused with thyroarytenoideus (Bergman et al. 1988). The extent of its attachment on the arytenoid cartilage may vary (Mossallam et al. 1987).

The lateral cricoarytenoid muscle is associated with several accessory muscles. It may be connected with cricoepiglotticus, which originates from the inner surface of the cricoid cartilage near the lateral cricoarytenoid and attaches to the epiglottis (Knott 1883a; Maranillo and Sanudo 2016). A similar slip termed cricomembranosus (cricomembranous muscle) may pass to the quadrangular membrane, which extends between the epiglottis and the arytenoid cartilage (Knott 1883a; Maranillo and Sanudo 2016). The lateral cricoarytenoid muscle may send a bundle to the thyroarytenoid muscle and thyroid cartilage termed the internal lateral cricothyroid muscle (Maranillo and Sanudo 2016). Syndesmoarytenoid may extend from the muscular process of the arytenoid cartilage and the lateral cricoarytenoid to the cricothyroid ligament (Maranillo and Sanudo 2016). Arythyrocricoid may originate from the transverse or oblique arytenoid muscles and insert into lateral cricoarytenoid (Maranillo et al. 2011).

Wells and Thomas (1927) describe an accessory muscle of lateral cricoarytenoid that is referred to as the cricothyrohyoid muscle by Maranillo and Sanudo (2016). It was situated on the lateral aspect of the larynx on the left side of the body. It originated from the superolateral angle of the cricoid cartilage, beneath the lateral cricoarytenoid muscle. The muscle coursed superiorly and anteriorly over thyroarytenoideus and thyroepiglotticus to insert into a band of fascia that was continuous with the median thyrohyoid ligament (Wells and Thomas 1927; Maranillo and Sanudo 2016).

Prevalence

Krause found cricoepiglotticus in 34% of cases, and Knott found this muscle in 3 out of 19 subjects (15.8%) (Knott 1883a).

Anomalies

N/A

Clinical Implications

N/A

ARYTENOIDEUS TRANSVERSUS (TRANSVERSE ARYTENOID) (FIGURE 2.8)

Synonyms

Together with arytenoideus obliquus, this muscle may be referred to as arytenoideus proprius (Macalister 1875) or interarytenoideus (Kanthack 1892).

Typical Presentation

Description

Arytenoideus transversus is a single muscle that extends between the muscular processes and lateral borders of the two arytenoid cartilages (Standring 2016). It is situated deep into the arytenoideus obliquus muscles on the posterior surface of the larynx (Standring 2016).

Innervation

Arytenoideus transversus is innervated by the recurrent laryngeal nerves (Standring 2016).

Comparative Anatomy

In gibbons and bonobos, arytenoideus is present as a single, unpaired muscle that extends between the two arytenoid cartilages, and is not divided into an arytenoideus transversus and arytenoideus obliquus (Kohlbrügge 1890–1892; Starck and Schneider 1960; Diogo et al. 2012, 2017). In orangutans, gorillas, and common chimpanzees, the arytenoideus transversus is present in all cases and the arytenoideus obliquus is present in some cases (Gratiolet and Alix

1866; Sonntag 1923; Starck and Schneider 1960; Gibbs 1999; Diogo et al. 2010, 2013a,b).

Variations

Description

Arytenoideus transversus (the transverse arytenoid) may send fibers to thyroarytenoid (Macalister 1875; Kanthack 1892). The direction of its fibers or the proportion of its fibers relative to the oblique arytenoid may vary (Macalister 1875; Maranillo and Sanudo 2016). The transverse arytenoid may connect with the thyroarytenoid or the lateral cricoarytenoid via a fascicle referred to as the arythyrocricoid (Maranillo et al. 2011). It may also connect with the straight arycorniculate muscle (aryteno-corniculatus rectus), which lies deep to the transverse arytenoid and extends from the base of the arytenoid cartilage to the corniculate cartilage (Luschka 1869; Macalister 1875; Le Double 1897; Maranillo and Sanudo 2016).

Prevalence

Maranillo et al. (2011) found the arythyrocricoid fascicle in 29 out of 30 larynges (96.7%), and due to bilateral presence in some cases, a total of 47 arythyrocricoid fascicles were found. Arythyrocricoid originated from the transverse arytenoid in 16 cases (34%) and from both the transverse and oblique arytenoid muscles in 18 cases (38.3%). Arythyrocricoid inserted into the thyroarytenoid muscle in 18 cases (38.3%), the lateral cricoarytenoid muscle in 5 cases (10.6%), and into both muscles in 24 cases (51.1%).

Anomalies

Description

In cases of laryngeal cleft, the interarytenoid may show partial agenesis (Lim et al. 1979). In an infant with mandibulofacial dysostosis, the transverse arytenoid was enlarged (Herring et al. 1979).

Prevalence

N/A

Clinical Implications

The presence of arythyrocricoid may affect vocal fold position following laryngeal nerve palsy or interfere with electromyographic testing of laryngeal nerve function (Maranillo et al. 2011).

ARYTENOIDEUS OBLIQUUS (OBLIQUE ARYTENOID) (FIGURE 2.8)

Synonyms

Together with arytenoideus transversus, this muscle may be referred to as arytenoideus proprius (Macalister 1875) or interarytenoideus (Kanthack 1892).

Typical Presentation

Description

The arytenoideus obliquus muscles cross each other, extending from the muscular process of one arytenoid cartilage to the apex of the contralateral arytenoid cartilage (Standring 2016). Fibers of oblique arytenoid that extend from the apex of the arytenoid cartilage to the aryepiglottic fold are referred to as aryepiglotticus (Standring 2016) or arytenoepiglottic muscles (Maranillo and Sanudo 2016).

Innervation

Arytenoideus obliquus is innervated by the recurrent laryngeal nerve (Standring 2016).

Comparative Anatomy

In gibbons and bonobos, arytenoideus is present as a single, unpaired muscle that extends between the two arytenoid cartilages, and is not typically divided into an arytenoideus transversus and arytenoideus obliquus (Kohlbrügge 1890–1892; Starck and Schneider 1960; Diogo et al. 2012, 2017). In orangutans, gorillas, and common chimpanzees, the arytenoideus transversus is present in all cases, and the arytenoideus obliquus is present in some cases (Gratiolet and Alix 1866; Sonntag 1923; Starck and Schneider 1960; Gibbs 1999; Diogo et al. 2010, 2013a,b). Arytenoideus obliquus may blend with thyroarytenoideus in chimpanzees (Jordan 1971a; Gibbs 1999).

Variations

Description

One or both of the arytenoideus obliquus muscles (the oblique arytenoid muscles) may be absent (Macalister 1875; Maranillo and Sanudo 2016). Its proportion relative to the transverse arytenoid may vary (Macalister 1875). Some fibers may connect with thyroarytenoid (Macalister 1875; Kanthack 1892). It may also connect to the cricoid cartilage or the corniculate cartilage (Macalister 1875; Maranillo and Sanudo 2016).

The oblique arytenoid muscles are associated with a few accessory muscles. The oblique arytenoids may connect with the thyroarytenoid or the lateral cricoarytenoid via a fascicle referred to as the arythyrocricoid (Maranillo et al. 2011). The oblique arycorniculate muscle (aryteno-corniculatus obliquus) is a fascicle of arytenoideus obliquus that inserts into the corniculate cartilage (Macalister 1875; Le Double 1897; Maranillo and Sanudo 2016). The arymembranous muscle may extend from the arytenoid cartilage to the quadrangular membrane (Maranillo and Sanudo 2016).

Prevalence

Maranillo et al. (2011) found the arythyrocricoid fascicle in 29 out of 30 larynges (96.7%), and due to bilateral presence in some cases, a total of 47 arythyrocricoid fascicles were found. Arythyrocricoid originated from the oblique arytenoid in 13 cases (27.7%) and from both the transverse and oblique arytenoid muscles in 18 cases (38.3%). Arythyrocricoid inserted into the thyroarytenoid muscle in 18 cases (38.3%), the lateral cricoarytenoid muscle in 5 cases (10.6%), and both muscles in 24 cases (51.1%).

Anomalies

Description

In cases of laryngeal cleft, the interarytenoid may show partial agenesis (Lim et al. 1979).

Prevalence

N/A

Clinical Implications

The presence of arythyrocricoid may affect vocal fold position following laryngeal nerve palsy or interfere with electromyographic testing of laryngeal nerve function (Maranillo et al. 2011).

THYROARYTENOIDEUS (THYROARYTENOID) (FIGURE 2.9)

See also: Superior thyroarytenoideus

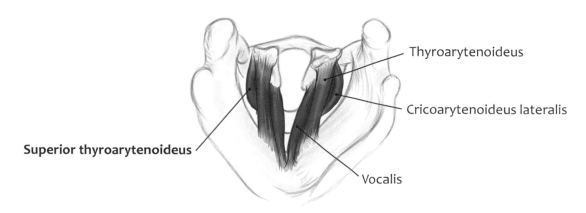

Thyroarytenoideus

Cricoarytenoideus lateralis

Superior thyroarytenoideus

Vocalis

FIGURE 2.9 Laryngeal muscles in superior view.

Synonyms

N/A

Typical Presentation

Description

Thyroarytenoideus originates from the angle of the thyroid cartilage and the cricothyroid ligament and inserts into the arytenoid cartilage (Standring 2016). The deep fibers form vocalis, which is situated between thyroarytenoideus and the vocal ligament, and attach to the vocal process of the arytenoid cartilage (Standring 2016). Some fibers of vocalis insert into the vocal ligament (aryvocalis of Ludwig) (Bergman et al. 1988; Standring 2016). The thyroepiglotticus muscle is formed by fibers of thyroarytenoideus that continue into aryepiglottic fold and end in the margin of the epiglottis (Standring 2016).

Innervation

Thyroarytenoideus is innervated by the recurrent laryngeal nerve (Standring 2016).

Comparative Anatomy

Thyroarytenoideus has a similar typical presentation in the apes, extending from the thyroid cartilage to the arytenoid cartilage (Gibbs 1999; Diogo et al. 2010, 2012, 2013a,b, 2017). In the great apes, both a pars superior (corresponding to thyroarytenoideus) and a pars inferior (or thyroarytenoideus medialis, corresponding to vocalis) seem to be present in most specimens, though the development of the pars inferior may vary (Gibbs 1999; Starck and Schneider 1960; Saban 1968; Diogo et al. 2010, 2013a,b, 2017). Due to conflicting accounts in the literature, it is not clear whether a bundle corresponding to vocalis is typically present in gibbons (Diogo et al. 2012). Thyroepiglotticus may be present in gorillas and common chimpanzees (Gratiolet and Alix 1866; Saban 1968; Gibbs 1999; Diogo et al. 2010, 2013a).

Variations

Description

The extent to which thyroarytenoid and vocalis are distinct may vary (Macalister 1875). The extent of the origin from the thyroid cartilage may also vary (Maranillo and Sanudo 2016).

Thyroarytenoideus may be connected with cricoarytenoideus lateralis, arytenoideus transversus, or arytenoideus obliquus (Macalister 1875; Kanthack 1892; Bergman et al. 1988; Maranillo et al. 2011; Maranillo and Sanudo 2016). Thyroepiglotticus may be present as thyroepiglotticus major (inferior) and thyroepiglotticus minor (superior) (Macalister 1875; Knott 1883a; Le Double 1897; Maranillo and Sanudo 2016). Both insert into the lateral border of the epiglottis (Knott 1883a; Maranillo and Sanudo 2016).

Thyroarytenoideus is associated with several accessory muscles. The superior thyroarytenoideus may be present along its lateral surface (see the entry for this muscle). Thyromembranosus is similar to thyroepiglotticus but inserts into the quadrangular membrane (Maranillo and Sanudo 2016). Fibers of thyroarytenoideus may form ventricularis

(the ventricular muscle), a muscle situated in the vestibular fold with attachments to the angle of the thyroid cartilage and the arytenoid cartilage (Kanthack 1892; Kotby et al. 1991; Maranillo and Sanudo 2016). A fascicle of the superficial fibers of thyroarytenoid referred to as thyreo-corniculatus (thyrocorniculate muscle) may insert into the corniculate cartilage (Knott 1883a; Maranillo and Sanudo 2016). A similar fascicle termed thyreo-cuneiformis (thyrocuneiform muscle) may insert into the cuneiform cartilage (Knott 1883a; Maranillo and Sanudo 2016). Thyroconoid may originate from the thyroarytenoid and thyroid cartilage and insert into the conoid ligament (Maranillo and Sanudo 2016). The inferior thyroid muscle (thyroideus internus or subthyroideus of Krause) may extend from the lower aspect of the angle of the thyroid cartilage to the root of the inferior cornu (Knott 1883a; Le Double 1897; Maranillo and Sanudo 2016).

Prevalence

Knott (1883a) found thyreo-corniculatus in 2 out of 19 cases (10.5%) and the inferior thyroid muscle in 2 out of 43 cases (4.7%). In a sample of 20 larynges, Kotby et al. (1991) found the superior thyroarytenoid muscle bilaterally in 16 larynges (80%) and ventricularis in 19 larynges (95%). In a sample of 100 hemilarynges from 50 cadavers, Lee et al. (2018) found superior thyroarytenoideus in 36 specimens (36%).

Anomalies

N/A

Clinical Implications

N/A

SUPERIOR THYROARYTENOIDEUS (SUPERIOR THYROARYTENOID) (FIGURE 2.9)

See also: Thyroarytenoideus

Synonyms

This muscle may also be referred to as oblique thyroarytenoid (Lee et al. 2018).

Typical Presentation

This muscle is present only as a variation.

Comparative Anatomy

N/A

Variations

Description

The superior thyroarytenoideus is situated lateral to thyroarytenoid, extending from the upper portion of the angle of the thyroid cartilage to the muscular process of the arytenoid cartilage (Zemlin et al. 1984; Kotby et al. 1991; Bergman et al. 1988; Maranillo and Sanudo 2016; Standring 2016; Lee et al. 2018). It may insert into the lateral cricoarytenoid muscle or its superficial fascia (Lee et al. 2018).

Innervation

Superior thyroarytenoideus is likely innervated by the recurrent laryngeal nerve.

Prevalence

Zemlin et al. (1984) found the superior thyroarytenoid muscle in 12 out of 15 larynges (80%). Kotby et al. (1991) found this muscle bilaterally in 16 out of 20 larynges (80%). In a sample of 100 hemilarynges from 50 cadavers, Lee et al. (2018) found this muscle in 36 cases (36%), and it had an insertion into the lateral cricoarytenoid muscle or its fascia in 8 cases (8%).

Anomalies

N/A

Clinical Implications

N/A

INFRAHYOID MUSCLES

STERNOHYOIDEUS (STERNOHYOID) (FIGURE 2.10)

See also: Cleidohyoid

Synonyms

N/A

Typical Presentation

Description

Sternohyoideus originates from the manubrium, medial end of the clavicle, and posterior sternoclavicular ligament and inserts into the inferior margin of the body of the hyoid (Standring 2016).

Innervation

Sternohyoideus is innervated by branches of the ansa cervicalis (Standring 2016).

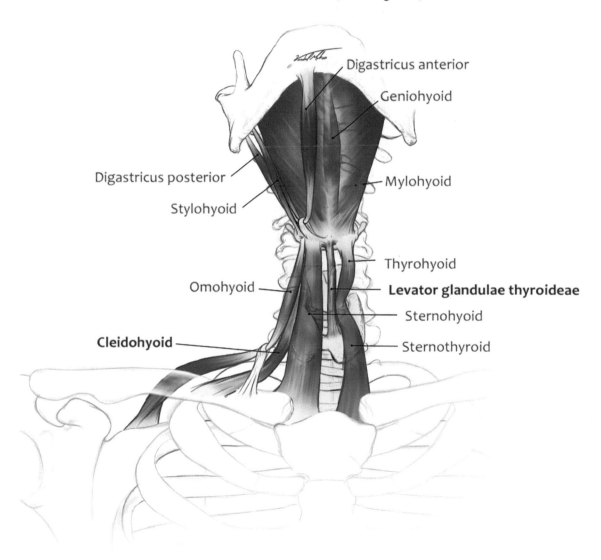

FIGURE 2.10 Suprahyoid and infrahyoid muscles in anterior view.

Comparative Anatomy

Sternohyoideus has a similar typical presentation in the apes, extending from the sternum and adjacent regions to the hyoid (Gratiolet and Alix 1866; Sonntag 1923, 1924; Raven 1950; Miller 1952; Starck and Schneider 1960; Gibbs 1999; Diogo et al. 2010, 2012, 2013a,b, 2017). Tendinous intersections are found in gibbons, common chimpanzees, and bonobos but are not found in gorillas (Gratiolet and Alix 1866; Champneys 1872; Deniker 1885; Kohlbrügge 1890–1892; Starck and Schneider 1960; Diogo et al. 2010, 2012, 2013a, 2017). Sternohyoid may have an additional origin from the first and second ribs in gibbons (Kohlbrügge 1890–1892).

Variations

Description

One or two tendinous intersections may be present in sternohyoid (Hallett 1848; Macalister 1867b, 1875; Mori 1964; Sato 1968b; Standring 2016). The right and left sternohyoid muscles may fuse (Macalister 1875; Sato 1968b; Lee and Yang 2016). Sternohyoid may join with omohyoid or sternothyroid (Hallett 1848; Macalister 1867b, 1875; Wood 1867b, 1868; Kim et al. 2009a; Lee and Yang 2016; Standring 2016; Çetkin et al. 2017). It may also send a slip to mylohyoid (Macalister 1875; Lee and Yang 2016). Sternohyoid may be doubled or absent (Macalister 1875; Lee and Yang 2016; Standring 2016).

The origin of sternohyoid may be confined to just the sternum (Macalister 1875; Mori 1964; Bergman et al. 1988). It may have an additional origin from the first and/or second ribs (Mori 1964; Kim et al. 2009a; Lee and Yang 2016). Macalister (1875) reports a case in which sternohyoid originated from only the posterior sternoclavicular ligament and the cartilage of the first rib. Its clavicular origin may be shifted laterally to the middle of the clavicle (Macalister 1875; Kim et al. 2015b). Sternohyoid may also originate only from the middle of the clavicle (Hallett 1848; Macalister 1875; Bergman et al. 1988; Lee and Yang 2016). This variant may be mistaken for cleidohyoid, an accessory slip that extends from the clavicle to the hyoid bone (Lee and Yang 2016; see the entry for this muscle). An accessory cleidohyoid may fuse with sternohyoid (Leppi 1962; Mori 1964). Sternohyoid is also associated with sternohyoideus azygos, which extends from the manubrium to the hyoid (Bergman et al. 1988; Lee and Yang 2016).

Prevalence

Wood (1868) states that Turner found sternohyoid blended with the superior belly of omohyoid in 4 out of 373 cases (1.1%). In a sample of 86 sides from 43 cadavers, Mori (1964) found that sternohyoid originated from the sternum only on five sides (11.6%); from both the sternum and clavicle on 64 sides (74.4%); from the sternum, clavicle, and first rib on two sides (4.6%); and from the sternum, clavicle, first and second ribs on two sides (4.6%). A tendinous inscription was present on 22 out of 60 sides (36.7%).

Sato (1968b) found at least one tendinous intersection present in 23 out of 338 sides (6.8%) in Kyushu-Japanese males and present in 29 out of 230 sides (12.61%) in females. In males, one intersection was present in 21 out of the 23 sides (91.3%), and two intersections were present in two sides (8.7%). In females, one intersection was present in 19 out of the 29 sides (65.52%) and two intersections were present in ten sides (34.48%). Right and left sternohyoid muscles were fused in 23 out of 169 males (13.61%) and in 5 out of 115 females (4.35%).

Anomalies

Description

In both trisomy 13 and trisomy 18 neonates, Aziz (1979, 1981) found sternohyoideus azygos, a supernumerary slip that arose from the manubrium and inserted near the intermediate tendon of the digastricus. Bersu and Ramirez-Castro (1977) also found sternohyoideus azygos that inserted into the hyoid bone in an infant with trisomy 18. This same infant also had a doubled left sternohyoid. The left sternohyoid was also doubled in a second infant. In the third infant with trisomy 18, two accessory slips were present that originated from the medial ends of the clavicles and inserted into the distal end of the right greater horn of the hyoid (Bersu and Ramirez-Castro 1977).

In a neonate with trisomy 18, the left sternohyoid originated partially behind its counterpart and sent a slip to the deep cervical fascia (Aziz 1979). In addition to this slip and bilateral sternohyoideus azygos muscles, this individual also had two other bilateral supernumerary muscles that ascended from the manubrium to the head (Aziz 1979). In a boy with trisomy 13q, the left sternohyoid was doubled (Pettersen 1979). In a neonate with trisomy 13, sternohyoid and omohyoid fused near their insertions (Aziz 1980). In an individual with craniorachischisis, the sternohyoid muscles were fused with each other and with the proximal portions of the omohyoid muscles (Alghamdi et al. 2017).

Prevalence

In their literature review, Smith et al. (2015) found that sternohyoideus azygos was present in 1 out of 20 individuals with trisomy 13 (5%) and in 2 out of 17 individuals with trisomy 18 (11.8%). They also found that a doubled sternohyoid or a sternohyoid with an accessory slip was found in 1 out of 20 individuals with trisomy 13 (5%) and in 4 out of 17 individuals with trisomy 18 (23.5%).

Clinical Implications

An attachment of sternohyoid to the middle of the clavicle may present as a lateral neck mass, a condition which Kim et al. (2015b) refer to as sternohyoid syndrome.

CLEIDOHYOIDEUS (CLEIDOHYOID) (FIGURE 2.10)

See also: Sternohyoideus, Omohyoideus

Synonyms

This muscle may also be referred to as cleidohyoideus accessorius (Steinbach 1923).

Typical Presentation

This muscle is present only as a variation.

Comparative Anatomy

Common chimpanzees may sometimes exhibit an omohyoid with three bellies including a superior belly, inferomedial belly, and an inferolateral belly (Gratiolet and Alix 1866; Diogo and Wood 2011, 2012a; Diogo et al. 2013a). One of the inferior bellies may correspond to cleidohyoid (Gratiolet and Alix 1866; Sonntag 1923; Diogo et al. 2013a).

Variations

Description

When present, cleidohyoid originates from the middle of the clavicle between the superior belly of omohyoid and the sternohyoid and inserts into the hyoid bone (Macalister 1875; Le Double 1897; Leppi 1962; Mori 1964; Hatipoğlu et al. 2006; Lee and Yang 2016). Its clavicular origin may arise from behind the cleidomastoid head of sternocleidomastoid (Sato et al. 1987; Bergman et al. 1988; Kim et al. 2009a; Stark et al. 2009; Lee and Yang 2016). Cleidohyoid may fuse with either sternohyoid and/or the superior belly of omohyoid (Leppi 1962; Mori 1964; Hatipoğlu et al. 2006). Cleidohyoid may also be used to refer to a variant of sternohyoid that originates only from the middle clavicle, or a variant of omohyoid with an absent inferior belly and a superior belly that originates from the clavicle (Macalister 1875; Knott 1883a; Bergman et al. 1988; Novakov et al. 2012; Lee and Yang 2016).

Innervation

Cleidohyoid is innervated by the ansa cervicalis, specifically branches from the second and/or third cervical nerves (Sato et al. 1987).

Prevalence

Macalister (1875) states that Schwegl found cleidohyoid in 3 out of 100 subjects (3%). Mori (1964) found cleidohyoid present in 8 out of 300 sides (2.7%), fusing with sternohyoid on three sides (1%) and with omohyoid on three sides (1%). Sukekawa and Itoh (2006) found cleidohyoid on 2 out of 67 sides (3%).

Anomalies

This muscle is present only as a variation, though accessory slips in this region occur often in individuals with trisomy 18 (Bersu and Ramirez-Castro 1977; Aziz 1979).

Clinical Implications

The presence of cleidohyoid may complicate surgical approaches in the neck (Leppi 1962).

OMOHYOIDEUS (OMOHYOID) (FIGURE 2.10)

See also: Cleidohyoid

Synonyms

N/A

Typical Presentation

Description

Omohyoideus is comprised of two bellies joined by an intermediate tendon (Standring 2016). The inferior belly originates from the superior margin of the scapula near the scapular notch and ends in the intermediate tendon (Standring 2016). The superior belly arises from the intermediate tendon and inserts into the body of the hyoid (Standring 2016).

Innervation

Omohyoideus is innervated by the ansa cervicalis (Standring 2016).

Comparative Anatomy

Omohyoideus has a similar typical presentation in the apes, extending from the scapula to the hyoid (Deniker 1885; Kohlbrügge 1890–1892; Gibbs 1999; Diogo et al. 2010, 2012, 2013a,b, 2017). The intermediate tendon is poorly developed or absent in gibbons (Deniker 1885; Kohlbrügge 1890–1892; Diogo et al. 2012). The intermediate tendon is absent in most orangutans (Sonntag 1924; Kallner 1956; Diogo et al. 2013b). A well-developed intermediate tendon is present in some gorillas (Macalister 1873; Raven 1950; Diogo et al. 2010). Raven (1950) found an omohyoid with three bellies on one side of a gorilla. The intermediate tendon between the superior and inferior bellies is well-developed in common chimpanzees (Gratiolet and Alix 1866; Macalister 1871; Sonntag 1923; Diogo et al. 2013a). Differing from common chimpanzees, the intermediate tendon is absent in most bonobos, so omohyoid is typically not divided into two bellies in this species (Diogo et al. 2017). In bonobos, the omohyoid may be fused with sternohyoid or the cleidomastoid head of sternocleidomastoid (Miller 1952; Diogo et al. 2017).

Variations

Description

Omohyoid may partially or entirely originate from the superior transverse scapular ligament (Macalister 1875; Mori 1964; Lee and Yang 2016; Standring 2016). Omohyoid may partially or entirely originate from the acromion process (Macalister 1875; Knott 1883a; Bergman et al. 1988; Lee and Yang 2016). It may also originate entirely from the first rib (Macalister 1875) or from the coracoid process (coraco-hyoid of Gruber) (Knott 1880, 1883a). Tubbs et al. (2004a) found an origin of omohyoid from the scapula and an insertion into the transverse process of the sixth cervical vertebra. A partial origin of omohyoid from the clavicle may take the form of an additional head (Hallett 1848; Wood 1864, 1868;

Macalister 1875; Knott 1880; Bergman et al. 1988; Lee and Yang 2016). When the additional head is present, it typically joins with the inferior belly before ending in the intermediate tendon (Hallett 1848; Macalister 1875). The inferior belly may also originate entirely from the clavicle (Hallett 1848; Macalister 1867b, 1875; Bergman et al. 1988; Standring 2016; Singh et al. 2018).

The form of the intermediate tendon is variable, and it may be absent (Hallett 1848; Wood 1868; Macalister 1875; Mori 1964; Bergman et al. 1988; Lee and Yang 2016; Standring 2016). The cervical fascia that surrounds the intermediate tendon may pull the inferior belly of the omohyoid down such that it lies along the clavicle (Hallett 1848; Macalister 1875; Bergman et al. 1988).

Omohyoid may join with sternohyoid (Hallett 1848; Macalister 1867b, 1875; Wood 1867b, 1868; Sukekawa and Itoh 2006; Kim et al. 2009a; Lee and Yang 2016; Standring 2016; Çetkin et al. 2017). It may connect with mylohyoid, stylohyoid, or sternomastoid (Hallett 1848; Macalister 1875; Lee and Yang 2016). It may send a slip to the mandible or the greater horn of the hyoid (Macalister 1875; Lee and Yang 2016). It may also have a tendinous connection to the cartilage of the first rib or the sternoclavicular articulation (Hallett 1848).

One belly or the entire muscle may be doubled (Wood 1864, 1867b; Macalister 1875; Bergman et al. 1988; Rai et al. 2007; Kim et al. 2010; Lee and Yang 2016). In cases of doubling, there are often attachments to sternohyoid (Macalister 1875; Rai et al. 2007; Kim et al. 2020 Lee and Yang 2016). The superior belly may be split into posterior and anterior portions or may present as a lamellar divided structure with three to five bellies (Sukekawa and Itoh 2006). Wood (1868) observed a case in which the superior belly of the omohyoid was doubled. The upper belly fused with hyoglossus and the middle pharyngeal constrictor and received a slip from sternothyroid (Wood 1868).

One belly of omohyoid or the entire muscle may be absent (Hallett 1848; Macalister 1875; Bergman et al. 1988; Zhao et al. 2015; Lee and Yang 2016; Standring 2016). When the superior belly is absent, the inferior belly may end in the cervical fascia and is referred to as the coraco-cervicalis (Hallett 1848; Macalister 1875; Knott 1883a; Lee and Yang 2016). The superior belly may also be replaced by a tendon or undeveloped myofibers (Knott 1880, 1883a; Sukekawa and Itoh 2006). When the inferior belly is absent the superior belly originates from the clavicle (Bergman et al. 1988; Lee and Yang 2016). This variant may be referred to as cleidohyoid, an accessory slip that extends from the clavicle to the hyoid bone (see the entry for this muscle). An accessory cleidohyoid may fuse with omohyoid (Leppi 1962; Mori 1964; Hatipoğlu et al. 2006). A similar slip, cleidothyroid, extends from the clavicle to the thyroid cartilage (Bergman et al. 1988).

Omohyoid is associated with several other accessory slips. Cleidofascialis extends from the clavicle into the cervical fascia (Macalister 1867b; Bergman et al. 1988; Lee and Yang 2016). Omoclavicularis originates from the superior margin of the scapula near the origin of omohyoid and inserts into the middle of the clavicle (Mori 1964; Bakkum and Miller 1964). Cervico-costo-humeralis (Gruber) is considered an aberrant version of omohyoid that originates from the lesser tubercle of the humerus and inserts into the cartilage of the first rib and transverse process of the sixth cervical vertebra (Bergman et al. 1988; Lee and Yang 2016).

Prevalence

Hallett (1848) found that omohyoid had an additional origin from the clavicle in about 1 out of every 15 subjects (6.7%). Macalister (1875) states that an accessory head from the clavicle was found by Wood in 5 out of 70 subjects (7.1%), by Turner in 17 out of 373 cases (4.6%), and by Schwegl in 2 out of 100 cases (2%). Wood (1868) states that Turner found sternohyoid blended with the superior belly of omohyoid in 4 out of 373 cases (1.1%).

In a sample of 94 sides, Mori (1964) found that omohyoid originated from the superior margin of the scapula only on 68 sides (72.3%), from the superior transverse ligament only on two sides (2.1%), and from both on 24 sides (25.5%). In a sample of 240 sides, Mori (1964) found that the intermediate tendon was absent on 26 sides (10.8%). The intermediate tendon was short and narrow on 12 sides (5%) and long and narrow on 76 sides (31.7%). The intermediate tendon did not extend over the entire breadth of the omohyoid and was only present on the medial or lateral side on 108 sides (45%). The intermediate tendon was as wide as the muscle and moderately long on 12 sides (5%) and wide as the muscle but short and wavy on four sides (1.7%). Mori (1964) also found omoclavicularis present on 6 out of 200 sides (3%).

In a sample of 67 sides, Sukekawa and Itoh (2006) found that the superior belly of omohyoid was normal on 43 sides (64.2%), comprised of undeveloped myofibers on four sides (6%), divided into two bellies on seven sides (10.4%), and presented as a lamellar divided belly on five sides (7.5%). The intermediate tendon was absent on one side (1.5%). The superior belly inserted into sternohyoid on one side (1.5%). The superior belly connected to sternohyoid via a supernumerary belly on two sides (3%).

Anomalies

Description

In a female anencephalic fetus, the left superior belly of omohyoid was replaced by a band of fibrous tissue (Windle 1893). Mieden (1982) describes two male fetuses with cyclopia and alobar holoprosencephaly. On the right side of one specimen, fibers from the superior belly of omohyoid joined with fibers of geniohyoid to insert to the mandible. In an individual with craniorachischisis, the intermediate tendons were absent and the proximal portions of the omohyoids fused with the sternohyoid muscles (Alghamdi et al. 2017). There was also an extra slip present deep to the right omohyoid that fused with its distal end and attached proximally to the clavicle (Alghamdi et al. 2017).

The intermediate tendon of omohyoid was poorly developed in all of the specimens with trisomy 18 examined by Bersu and Ramirez-Castro (1977). In one of the cases, bilateral accessory fascicles were present that originated from the clavicle and joined with omohyoid at its midpoint. In another case, the left inferior belly of omohyoid originated entirely from the clavicle and an extra slip from the clavicle was present on the right side. In a third case, the right inferior belly of omohyoideus received an extra slip from the transverse scapular ligament and coracoid process. In the female fetus with trisomy 18 dissected by Alghamdi et al. (2018), omohyoid had an extra head on the left side that arose anterior to its intermediate tendon and ran lateral to the normal head to insert onto the greater horn of the hyoid.

Aziz (1979, 1980, 1981) found that the intermediate tendon of omohyoid was absent bilaterally in two neonates with trisomy 18 and one neonate with trisomy 13. In a neonate with trisomy 13, sternohyoid and omohyoid fused near their insertions (Aziz 1980). In another neonate with trisomy 13, there was an extra superior belly of omohyoid on the right side that extended between sternocleidomastoid and sternohyoid (Pettersen et al. 1979). In a fetus with trisomy 13, the left superior belly of omohyoid was hypoplastic (Pettersen et al. 1979).

Prevalence

In their literature review, Smith et al. (2015) found that anomalies of omohyoid were present in 7 out of 24 individuals with trisomy 13 (29.2%) and in 11 out of 26 individuals with trisomy 18 (42.3%).

Clinical Implications

A doubled omohyoid muscle may cause omohyoid syndrome (Guo-Hua et al. 2009) or progressive dysphagia and dyspnea (Kshirsagar et al. 2019).

STERNOTHYROIDEUS (STERNOTHYROID) (FIGURE 2.10)

See also: Thyrotrachealis

Synonyms
N/A

Typical Presentation
Description
Sternothyroideus originates from the manubrium and cartilage of the first rib and inserts into the oblique line of the thyroid cartilage (Standring 2016).

Innervation
Sternothyroideus is innervated by branches of the ansa cervicalis (Standring 2016).

Comparative Anatomy
Sternothyroideus has a similar typical presentation in the apes, extending from the sternum and adjacent regions to the thyroid cartilage (Gratiolet and Alix 1866; Sonntag 1923; Miller 1952; Gibbs 1999; Diogo et al. 2010, 2012, 2013a,b, 2017). The main body of sternothyroid in the apes

usually passes anteriorly to the posterior portion of the main body of thyrohyoid (Gratiolet and Alix 1866; Deniker 1885; Kohlbrügge 1890–1892; Sonntag 1923; Starck and Schneider 1960; Swindler and Wood 1973; Diogo et al. 2010, 2012, 2013a, 2017). Sternothyroid may be fused with thyrohyoid in gorillas and bonobos (Diogo et al. 2010, 2017). A tendinous intersection may be present in gorillas (Raven 1950) and common chimpanzees (Macalister 1871).

Variations

Description
Sternothyroid may be absent (Macalister 1875; Bale and Herrin 2016). One or more tendinous intersections may be present in the muscle (Hallett 1848; Macalister 1875; Sato 1968b). The right and left sternothyroid muscles may fuse (Wood 1868; Macalister 1875; Sato 1968b; Lee and Yang 2016). The origin of sternothyroid may extend onto the medial half of the first rib (Kim et al. 2009a) or onto the cartilage of the second rib (Macalister 1875). The costal origin may also be absent (Macalister 1875). It may have a second head that arises from the clavicle (Wood 1868; Macalister 1875). Kang et al. (2015) report an accessory belly that originated from the left sternothyroid and pretracheal layer of cervical fascia and inserted into the oblique line of the thyroid cartilage on the right side.

Sternothyroid may be doubled, divided into bundles, or split into two layers (Hallett 1848; Wood 1868; Macalister 1867b, 1875; Bergman et al. 1988; Lee and Yang 2016). Nayak et al. (2009a) report a case in which sternothyroid divided into a lateral belly that inserted into the thyroid cartilage and a medial belly that became tendinous and inserted into the hyoid bone and intermediate tendon of the digastricus. Murugan et al. (2016) report a case in which sternothyroid divided into a medial belly that inserted into the thyroid cartilage and an elongated lateral belly that sent fibers to the carotid sheath, coursed between the internal jugular vein and internal carotid artery, and inserted into the tympanic plate and petrous temporal bone.

Sternothyroid may be joined with sternohyoid, thyrohyoid, omohyoid, levator glandulae thyroideae, cricothyroid, hyoglossus, the middle or inferior pharyngeal constrictors, or the cricoid cartilage (Wood 1868; Macalister 1875; Bergman et al. 1988; Sakamoto 2009; Maranillo and Sanudo 2016; Lee and Yang 2016; Çetkin et al. 2017). Sternothyroid is associated with incisurae mediae obliquus (Gruber), an accessory muscle on the inferolateral aspect of the thyroid cartilage (Gruber 1868a; Bergman et al. 1988; Maranillo and Sanudo 2016). It may have a second head that originates from the sternothyroid, and in this case, the muscle would be referred to as incisurae mediae obliquus bicaudatus (Bergman et al. 1988; Maranillo and Sanudo 2016). It is also associated with thyrotrachealis, which may be a detached slip of sternothyroid (Macalister 1875; see the entry for this muscle).

Prevalence

In a sample of 44 sides from 22 cadavers, Sakamoto (2009) found that fibers of the inferior pharyngeal constrictor connected with sternothyroid on 29 sides (65.9%). Sato (1968b) found at least one tendinous intersection present in 58 out of 362 sides (16.02%) in Kyushu-Japanese males and present in 29 out of 234 sides (12.39%) in females. In males, one intersection was present in 43 out of the 58 sides (74.14%), two intersections were present in nine sides (15.52%), three intersections were present in four sides (6.9%), and five intersections were present in two sides (3.45%). In females, one intersection was present in 25 out of the 29 sides (86.21%) and two intersections were present in 4 sides (13.79%). Right and left sternothyroid muscles were fused in 13 out of 181 males (7.18%) and in 6 out of 117 females (5.13%) (Sato 1968b).

Anomalies

Description

In one neonate with trisomy 13, the posterior belly of the digastric was doubled bilaterally, and the extra belly on the left side received a contribution from sternothyroid (Pettersen et al. 1979).

Prevalence

In their literature review, Smith et al. (2015) found that anomalies of sternothyroid were found in only 1 out of 20 individuals with trisomy 13 (5%, the case described by Pettersen et al. 1979).

Clinical Implications

Variations of sternothyroid may complicate surgical procedures in the anterior neck (Kang et al. 2015).

THYROHYOIDEUS (THYROHYOID) (FIGURE 2.10)

Synonyms

This muscle may also be referred to as the hyothyroid muscle (Hallett 1848).

Typical Presentation

Description

Thyrohyoideus originates from the oblique line of the thyroid cartilage and inserts into the body and greater horn of the hyoid (Standring 2016).

Innervation

Thyrohyoideus is innervated by fibers of the first cervical spinal nerve from the hypoglossal nerve (Standring 2016).

Comparative Anatomy

Thyrohyoideus has a similar typical presentation in the apes, extending from the thyroid cartilage to the hyoid bone (Gibbs 1999; Diogo et al. 2010, 2012, 2013a,b, 2017). Thyrohyoid may be fused with sternothyroid in gorillas and bonobos (Diogo et al. 2010, 2017).

Variations

Description

Thyrohyoid may be continuous with sternothyroid (Macalister 1875; Bergman et al. 1988; Lee and Yang 2016). It may also connect with omohyoid, the middle or inferior pharyngeal constrictors, hyoglossus, levator glandulae thyroideae, cricothyroid, or the cricoid cartilage (Hallett 1848; Macalister 1875; Bergman et al. 1988; Sakamoto 2009, 2014; Lee and Yang 2016; Maranillo and Sanudo 2016). It may be divided into fascicles (Macalister 1875).

Thyrohyoid may connect with hyotrachealis, a slip that originates from the hyoid, passes behind the isthmus of the thyroid gland, and inserts into the perichondrium of the upper rings of the trachea (Macalister 1875). An accessory muscle referred to as thyrohyoideus superior (minor, or azygos) may extend from the upper border of the thyroid cartilage to the hyoid (Macalister 1875). A slip referred to as ceratohyoid or thyrohyoideus lateralis may extend between the superior horn of the thyroid cartilage to the greater horn of the hyoid (Maranillo and Sanudo 2016). Macalister (1875) suggests that variants of ceratohyoid include thyreo-syndesmicus (Sömmerring), which inserts into the posterior thyrohyoid ligament, and a thyreo-triticeal slip, which attaches to the triticeal cartilage.

Prevalence

In a sample of 44 sides from 22 cadavers, Sakamoto (2009) found that fibers of the inferior constrictor connected with thyrohyoid on 13 sides (29.5%). In a sample of 82 sides from 41 cadavers, Sakamoto (2014) found fibers of the middle constrictor attached to thyrohyoid on two sides (2.4%).

Anomalies

Description

In an infant with trisomy 18, the left thyrohyoid was doubled (Bersu and Ramirez-Castro 1977). In a fetus with trisomy 18, there is an accessory slip along the midline between the thyrohyoid muscles (Urban and Bersu 1987). In a fetus with craniorachischisis, thyrohyoid fused with the thyroid cartilage on the right side (Alghamdi et al. 2017).

Prevalence

Doubling of the thyrohyoid was only found in one out of eight infants with trisomy 18 (12.5%) (Bersu and Ramirez-Castro 1977).

Clinical Implications
N/A

LEVATOR GLANDULAE THYROIDEAE (FIGURE 2.10)

Synonyms
N/A

Typical Presentation

This muscle is present only as a variation or anomaly.

Comparative Anatomy

Kohlbrügge (1890–1892) found fibers of the inferior pharyngeal constrictor that attached to the thyroid gland in one gibbon. This structure could correspond to the levator glandulae thyroideae (Diogo et al. 2012).

Variations

Description

Levator glandulae thyroideae originates from the hyoid bone or thyroid cartilage and inserts onto the thyroid gland (Hallett 1848; Macalister 1875; Mori 1964; Sato 1968b; Sultana et al. 2009; Kim et al. 2010; Lee and Yang 2016; Standring 2016; Velasco-Nieves et al. 2020). It may insert into the lobe, pyramidal lobe, isthmus, or sheath of the gland (Hallett 1848; Macalister 1875; Keyes 1940; Mori 1964; Sato 1968b; Bergman et al. 1988; Gregory and Guse 2007; Sultana et al. 2009; Kim et al. 2010; Murugan et al. 2016; Standring 2016). Chaudhary et al. (2013) classify levator glandulae thyroideae as a fibromusculoglandular band.

Levator glandulae thyroideae may be doubled or bifurcated at its origin or insertion (Hallett 1848; Macalister 1875). Pacífico et al. (2019) report a case in which levator glandulae thyroideae had a short bundle that inserted into the cricoid cartilage and a long bundle that inserted into the pyramidal lobe. It may also consist of three slips (Macalister 1875; Loukas et al. 2008a). It may be connected with sternothyroid or thyrohyoid (Hallett 1848; Macalister 1875). This muscle may present as fibers extending from the inferior pharyngeal constrictor to the thyroid gland, in which case it may be referred to as levator glandulae thyroidcac lateralis (Krause) (Knott 1883a; Bergman et al. 1988).

Innervation

Levator glandulae thyroideae may be innervated by a branch from the ansa cervicalis (Loukas et al. 2008a), or more specifically, a branch from the second cervical nerve (Sato et al. 1987). It may also be innervated by the external laryngeal nerve (Keyes 1940; Chaudhary et al. 2013).

Prevalence

Sato (1968b) found levator glandulae thyroideae present in 90 out of 350 sides in males (25.7%) and present in 53 out of 220 sides (24.1%) in females. Lehr (1979) reported one case of this muscle out of 203 cases (0.49%). Sultana et al. (2009) found this muscle in 26 out of 60 cadavers (43.3%). Yadav et al. (2014) found this muscle in 9 out of 26 cadavers (34.6%). In a sample of 52 fetuses, Chaudhary et al. (2016) found levator glandulae thyroideae in 10 fetuses (19.2%).

Mori (1964) found 210 cases of levator glandulae thyroideae in 510 cadavers (41.2%). Mori (1964) classified the muscle into five types. Hyopyramidalis, from the hyoid to the pyramidal lobe, was present in 53 out of the 210 cases (25.2%). Thyreopyramidalis, from the thyroid cartilage to the pyramidal lobe, was present in 18 cases (8.6%). Thyreoglandularis, from the thyroid cartilage to the sheath of the thyroid gland, was present in 115 cases (54.8%). Hyoglandularis, from the hyoid to the sheath of the thyroid gland, was present in 28 cases (13.3%). Tracheoglandularis, from the upper trachea to the capsule of the isthmus, was present in seven cases (3.3%).

Anomalies

Description

In a neonate with trisomy 13, levator glandulae thyroideae extended from the thyroid cartilage to the isthmus of the thyroid gland (Pettersen et al. 1979). In another neonate with trisomy 13, the muscle extended from the hyoid bone to the isthmus of the thyroid gland (Aziz 1980).

Prevalence

In their literature review, Smith et al. (2015) found that levator glandulae thyroideae was present in 2 out of 20 individuals with trisomy 13 (10%).

Clinical Implications

Levator glandulae thyroideae may be mistaken for a tumor or infected thyroglossal duct cyst in medical imaging (Loukas et al. 2008a).

SUPRAHYOID MUSCLES

MYLOHYOIDEUS (MYLOHYOID) (FIGURE 2.10)

Synonyms

N/A

Typical Presentation

Description

Mylohyoid originates from the mylohyoid line of the mandible (Standring 2016). Its posterior fibers insert onto the body of the hyoid bone (Standring 2016). The anterior and middle fibers of mylohyoid on each side insert onto a fibrous median raphe (mylohyoid raphe) (Standring 2016). The mylohyoid raphe extends from the mental symphysis of the mandible to the hyoid (Standring 2016).

Innervation

Mylohyoid is innervated by the nerve to mylohyoid, a branch of the inferior alveolar nerve (Standring 2016).

Comparative Anatomy

Mylohyoideus has a similar typical presentation in the apes, extending from the mylohyoid lines of the mandible to the hyoid bone and the ventral midline (Gibbs 1999; Diogo et al. 2010, 2012, 2013a,b, 2017). The median raphe is absent in orangutans (Sonntag 1924; Brown and Ward 1988) and gorillas (Saban 1968; Göllner 1982; Gibbs 1999; Diogo et al. 2010). The median raphe has been observed in rare cases in gibbons (DuBrul 1958) and common chimpanzees (Göllner 1982). The median raphe is typically present in bonobos (Gibbs 1999; Miller 1952; Diogo et al. 2017).

Variations
Description

Mylohyoid is absent in rare cases (Hallett 1848; Macalister 1875; Bergman et al. 1988; Lee and Yang 2016). Hallett (1848) and Macalister (1875) observed cases in which mylohyoid was completely absent and replaced by an enlarged anterior belly of the digastric muscle. If the median raphe is absent, the two mylohyoid muscles may fuse into a continuous muscle sheet (Zdilla and Lambert 2015; Standring 2016).

Mylohyoid may fuse with, send fibers to, or insert onto the anterior belly of the digastric muscle (Macalister 1875; Malpas 1926; Bergman et al. 1988; Saadeh et al. 2001; Lee and Yang 2016; Standring 2016). It may also join with the intermediate tendon of the digastricus (Hallett 1848). The anterior belly of the digastric may originate from mylohyoid (Lee and Yang 2016). Accessory anterior bellies of the digastric may have attachments to mylohyoid (Sevinç et al. 2009). Mylohyoid may receive a slip from omohyoid, sternohyoid, or stylohyoid (Macalister 1875; Saadeh et al. 2001). The stylohyoid may insert into the outer border of mylohyoid (Macalister 1875). Zdilla and Lambert (2015) report a case in which the mylohyoid muscles did not reach the hyoid bone but inserted into the middle of the geniohyoid musculature via a fibrous "pseudo-hyoid" structure.

The length of the insertion along the hyoid bone may vary (Macalister 1875; Malpas 1926). The sublingual gland and/or fat tissue may partially or entirely herniate through a hiatus in mylohyoideus (Malpas 1926; Gaughran 1963; Nathan and Luchansky 1985; Lee and Yang 2016; Standring 2016; Bender-Heine and Zdilla 2018). Lobes of the submandibular gland may also herniate through mylohyoid and split it into discrete bundles (Macalister 1875; Knott 1883a; Bergman et al. 1988; Lee and Yang 2016). Mylohyoid may also be divided into parts by the submandibular vein (Saadeh et al. 2001). It can also be divided into superficial and deeper layers (Malpas 1926).

Bender-Heine and Zdilla (2018) report a case in which anterior and posterior bellies of mylohyoid were completely separated by fat that herniated from the sublingual space. The anterior bellies inserted into a single-bellied geniohyoid, and the posterior bellies inserted into the intermediate tendons and anterior bellies of the digastric.

Accessory muscles associated with mylohyoid may be present (Sehirli and Çavdar 1996; Lee and Yang 2016; Zdilla et al. 2018). Sehirli and Çavdar (1996) report an accessory mylohyoid situated between the left anterior belly of the digastric and the left mylohyoid. It originated from the left mylohyoid line and inserted into the median raphe and hyoid bone. Zdilla et al. (2018) provide a comprehensive review of the "arrowhead variation," bilateral accessory muscles that extend between the intermediate tendons of the digastric and the median raphe of the mylohyoid musculature (see the entry for digastricus anterior for more information).

Prevalence

Hallett (1848) found that mylohyoideus was connected to the intermediate tendon of the digastricus in one out of five subjects (20%). Mori (1964) found that the median raphe was only clearly present in 45 out of 210 cases (21.4%). In a sample of 19 cadavers, Zdilla et al. (2018) found that the arrowhead variation was present in two cadavers (10.5%).

In a sample of 324 half-heads, Gaughran (1963) found that a process of the sublingual gland herniated through a hiatus in mylohyoideus in 102 cases (31.5%) and fat herniations were present in 15 cases (4.6%). In a sample of 300 half-heads from 150 cadavers, Nathan and Luchansky (1985) found that a part of the sublingual gland and/or fat tissue herniated through a hiatus in mylohyoideus in 82 specimens (27.3%) from 63 cadavers.

Anomalies
Description

Bersu et al. (1976) describe a male infant with Hanhart syndrome in which the right mandible was represented by a small bone. On the right side, mylohyoid had a restricted origin from the distal end of the mandible and inserted along the median raphe. An accessory muscle that was innervated by the mylohyoid nerve originated from the angle of the right mandible and extended across the floor of the mouth to insert onto the middle half of the inferior aspect of the left mandible. A slip from this accessory muscle extended between the geniohyoid muscles to have a diffuse insertion onto the deep aspect of the left geniohyoid and the hyoglossus muscles.

Colacino and Pettersen (1978), Pettersen et al. (1979), and Aziz (1980) report anomalies of mylohyoid in neonates with trisomy 13. In one individual, the mylohyoid muscles were deficient anteriorly (Colacino and Pettersen 1978). In another, the left digastric muscle sent a slip to the left mylohyoid muscle, which was fused with its right counterpart since the median raphe was absent (Pettersen et al. 1979). The mylohyoid raphe was also absent in another neonate (Aziz 1980).

Mylohyoid is also variable in some individuals with trisomy 18 (Bersu and Ramirez-Castro 1977; Aziz 1979; Smith et al. 2015). In one infant, there was an accessory muscle sheet between the bellies of anterior digastric and the mylohyoid musculature (Bersu and Ramirez-Castro 1977). All specimens examined by Bersu and Ramirez-Castro (1977) lacked a median raphe and the left and right mylohyoid muscles were therefore fused in all cases.

The neonate described by Aziz (1979) also lacked a median raphe. In the fetus with trisomy 18 and cyclopia described by Smith et al. (2015), mylohyoid exchanged fibers with the digastric muscle bilaterally. The mylohyoid raphe was absent, so the mylohyoid muscles presented as a continuous muscle sheet. Intermandibularis anterior, a narrow accessory muscle deep to mylohyoideus with transverse fibers that spanned the two halves of the anterior mandible, was present.

Mieden (1982) describes an infant with median cleft lip, hypotelorism, and alobar holoprosencephaly (case I) and two male fetuses with cyclopia and alobar holoprosencephaly (cases II and III). In cases I and III, mylohyoideus was absent bilaterally (Mieden 1982). In a male neonate with Meckel syndrome, Pettersen (1984) found that the anterior belly of the right digastricus sent an accessory slip to the mylohyoideus. In an infant with mandibulofacial dysostosis, mylohyoid was deep but short anteroposteriorly (Herring et al. 1979).

In the fetus with craniorachischisis described by Alghamdi et al. (2017), the right mylohyoid was diminutive and fused with the digastric. The fascia over the left mylohyoid received a tendinous slip from the intermediate tendon of the digastric. The two mylohyoid muscles were fused together.

Prevalence

The median raphe was absent in all nine individuals (100%) with trisomy 18 described by Bersu and Ramirez-Castro (1977) and Aziz (1979). In their literature review, Smith et al. (2015) found that anomalous mylohyoid muscles were present in 2 out of 20 individuals (10%) with trisomy 13.

Clinical Implications

Surgeons and clinicians should be aware of the potential herniation of the sublingual or submandibular glands through mylohyoideus, as well as other variations of this muscle (Gaughran 1963; Nathan and Luchansky 1985; Bender-Heine and Zdilla 2018). Herniation of glandular tissue through mylohyoid (Bender-Heine and Zdilla 2018) or the presence of arrowhead musculature (Zdilla et al. 2018) may affect the spread of infection through the neck.

GENIOHYOIDEUS (GENIOHYOID) (FIGURE 2.10)

Synonyms

N/A

Typical Presentation

Description

Geniohyoid originates from the inferior mental spine on the posterior surface of the mental symphysis (Standring 2016). It inserts onto the body of the hyoid (Standring 2016). It is situated above (deep to) the medial portion of mylohyoid (Standring 2016).

Innervation

Geniohyoid is innervated by a branch of the first cervical spinal nerve that travels with the hypoglossal nerve (Standring 2016).

Comparative Anatomy

Geniohyoid has a similar typical presentation in the apes, extending from the inner surface of the mandible to the hyoid bone (Gratiolet and Alix 1866; Sonntag 1923; Raven 1950; Miller 1952; Gibbs 1999; Diogo et al. 2010, 2012, 2013a,b, 2017). In gibbons and gorillas, the insertion into the hyoid bone bifurcates the posterior portion of hyoglossus (Diogo et al. 2010, 2012). In common chimpanzees and bonobos, the muscle often merges with its counterpart at the midline (Sonntag 1923; Diogo et al. 2013a, 2017).

Variations

Description

Geniohyoid may fuse with its counterpart across the midline and present as a continuous muscle sheet (Hallett 1848; Macalister 1875; Mori 1964; Zdilla and Lambert 2015; Lee and Yang 2016; Standring 2016; Bender-Heine and Zdilla 2018). Zdilla and Lambert (2015) report a case in which the mylohyoid muscles did not reach the hyoid bone but inserted into the middle of the geniohyoid musculature via a fibrous "pseudo-hyoid" structure. Bender-Heine and Zdilla (2018) report a case in which anterior and posterior bellies of mylohyoid were completely separated by fat that herniated from the sublingual space. The anterior bellies inserted into a single-bellied geniohyoid, and the posterior bellies inserted into the intermediate tendons and anterior bellies of the digastric.

Geniohyoid may also fuse with genioglossus or originate from hyoglossus (Macalister 1875; Knott 1883a; Bergman et al. 1988; Lee and Yang 2016; Patel and Loukas 2016; Standring 2016). It may receive an accessory slip from the greater horn of the hyoid (Macalister 1875). In a case where the mylohyoid was deficient, Macalister (1875) observed mentohyoid inserting into geniohyoideus. Geniohyoid may be doubled bilaterally, thus presenting with four geniohyoid muscles (Hallett 1848; Macalister 1875; Bergman et al. 1988). Geniohyoid may also be split into superficial and deep layers (Mori 1964; Mehta et al. 2011b).

Prevalence

N/A

Anomalies

Description

Bersu et al. (1976) describe a male infant with Hanhart syndrome in which the right mandible was represented by a small bone. In this infant, a small portion of the right geniohyoid originated in association with the left geniohyoid on the left mandible and attached to the larger, anomalous part of the muscle that originated from hyoglossus. An accessory muscle was present that sent a slip between the geniohyoid muscles to have a diffuse insertion onto the deep aspect of the left geniohyoid and the hyoglossus muscles.

Mieden (1982) describes an infant with median cleft lip, hypotelorism, alobar holoprosencephaly (case I) and two male fetuses with cyclopia and alobar holoprosencephaly (cases II and III). In case I, geniohyoideus was doubled bilaterally. In case III, both geniohyoideus muscles were divided into superficial and deep heads while the right muscle had a third head that was laterally placed (Mieden 1982). In an infant with mandibulofacial dysostosis, geniohyoid was reduced (Herring et al. 1979). On the left side of a fetus with craniorachischisis, the left geniohyoid was a broad muscle that extended more laterally than is typical (Alghamdi et al. 2017). It originated from the hyoid region and fused with genioglossus. The right geniohyoid was absent.

Prevalence

In their literature review, Smith et al. (2015) found that geniohyoideus was doubled bilaterally in 1 out of 17 individuals with trisomy 18 (5.9%).

Clinical Implications

Understanding variation in the geniohyoid muscle is important for planning and performing operational procedures in the suprahyoid region (Mehta et al. 2011b).

DIGASTRICUS ANTERIOR (ANTERIOR BELLY OF THE DIGASTRIC) (FIGURE 2.10)

See also: Digastricus posterior

Synonyms

This muscle is often referred to as the anterior belly of the digastric (Standring 2016).

Typical Presentation

Description

Digastricus anterior originates from the digastric fossa, a fossa on the inner surface of the inferior margin of the mandible near the midline (Standring 2016). It ends in a tendon (the intermediate tendon) that connects it with digastricus posterior (Standring 2016). The intermediate tendon perforates stylohyoid (Standring 2016).

Innervation

Digastricus anterior is innervated by the nerve to mylohyoid, a branch of the inferior alveolar nerve (Standring 2016).

Comparative Anatomy

Digastricus anterior has a similar typical presentation in most apes, extending from the mandible to the intermediate tendon with occasional attachments to the hyoid (Gratiolet and Alix 1866; Raven 1950; Miller 1952; Gibbs 1999;

Diogo et al. 2010, 2012, 2013a,b, 2017). Digastricus anterior is typically absent in orangutans (Chapman 1880; Sonntag 1924; Cachel 1984; Wall et al. 1994; Gibbs 1999; Diogo et al. 2013b), having only been reported in one specimen by Parsons (1898a). The two digastricus anterior muscles may make contact at the midline in some gibbons (Wall et al. 1994; Gibbs et al. 2002) and gorillas (Bischoff 1880; Hosokawa and Kamiya 1961–1962; Diogo et al. 2010). The anterior belly on each side typically contacts its counterpart in common chimpanzees and bonobos (Wilder 1862; Gratiolet and Alix 1866; Sonntag 1923; Miller 1952; DuBrul 1958; Starck and Schneider 1960; Göllner K. 1982; Diogo et al. 2013a, 2017).

Variations

Description

The anterior and posterior bellies may fail to connect (Bergman et al. 1988). The digastric muscle may have a tendinous inscription (Bergman et al. 1988; Lee and Yang 2016). The muscle may present as trigastric, often with the third head extending between the intermediate tendon and the mandible or midline of the neck (Hallett 1848; Bergman et al. 1988; Lee and Yang 2016). The muscle may also be quadrigastric (Wood 1868; Bergman et al. 1988; Lee and Yang 2016) or even have more than four bellies due to variations in the anterior belly (see below).

Digastricus anterior may cross the midline onto the other side of the body (Macalister 1875; Standring 2016). The anterior bellies on each side of the body may also be connected by fleshy fibers (Macalister 1875; Bergman et al. 1988; Lee and Yang 2016) or via an aponeurotic slip (Venugopal and Mallula 2010). The anterior belly of the digastric may be enlarged as a variation (Çelik et al. 1992; Holibková and Machálek 1999). It may also be absent in rare cases (Sato 1968b; Larsson and Lufkin 1987; Bergman et al. 1988; Sargon et al. 1999; De-Ary-Pires et al. 2003).

The anterior belly of the digastric may fuse with, send fibers to, or originate from mylohyoid (Macalister 1875; Malpas 1926; Bergman et al. 1988; Saadeh et al. 2001; Lee and Yang 2016; Standring 2016). Mylohyoid may join with the intermediate tendon (Hallett 1848). Hallett (1848) and Macalister (1875) observed cases in which mylohyoid was completely absent and replaced by an enlarged digastricus anterior. The anterior belly may send a slip onto the hyoid bone (Macalister 1875) or insert entirely onto this bone when the intermediate tendon is absent (Bergman et al. 1988; Lee and Yang 2016). Stylohyoid may insert onto the intermediate tendon (Macalister 1875; Bergman et al. 1988). The intermediate tendon may pass in front of or behind stylohyoid instead of perforating it (Macalister 1875; Mori 1964; De-Ary-Pires et al. 2003; Harvey et al. 2015). The intermediate tendon may send slips to the lesser horn of the hyoid (Macalister 1875).

Accessory muscles are frequently associated with the anterior belly of the digastric (Macalister 1875; Bergman et al. 1988; Lee and Yang 2016). Mentohyoid refers to a supernumerary muscle situated along the medial margin of digastricus anterior that extends between the hyoid and the mandibular symphysis (Macalister 1867b, 1875; Knott 1883a; Bergman et al. 1988; De-Ary-Pires et al. 2003; Lee and Yang 2016). It may present as a single slip or as two parallel bands (Macalister 1875).

The anterior belly of the digastric may be doubled and may sometimes cross the midline to decussate with its companion and/or find its insertion (Wood 1864, 1867b, 1868; Macalister 1875; Knott 1883a; Bergman et al. 1988; Sargon et al. 1999; Aktekin et al. 2003; Turan-Özdemir et al. 2004; Liquidato et al. 2007; Lee and Yang 2016; Khona et al. 2017; Hsiao and Chang 2019). Unilateral accessory slips of digastricus anterior may also cross the midline (Larsson and Lufkin 1987; Zdilla et al. 2014a; Ortug et al. 2020).

Çelik et al. (1993) report a case in which the right anterior belly is tripled, with all three bellies inserting into the intermediate tendon to join with the right posterior belly. Quadrification of the anterior belly has been found unilaterally with insertion of all bellies into the intermediate tendon (Çelik et al. 2002), and bilaterally with insertion of all bellies into a common tendon that attached to the hyoid (Ozgur et al. 2007). In the latter case, two additional accessory muscles were present on each side near the midline and also inserted into the hyoid, giving each digastricus anterior the appearance of six heads (Ozgur et al. 2007).

Mori (1964) classified the anterior belly of the digastric into nine forms. The normal form refers to an anterior belly that arises from the digastric fossa and becomes continuous with the intermediate tendon. The ape form refers to an anterior belly that extends between the mandible and the intermediate tendon, but also has a connection to the aponeurosis intertendines (aponeurosis interdigastricque). The anterior type refers to an anterior belly comprised of fibers arising from the aponeurosis intertendines that fuse with the fibers arising from the intermediate tendon to form one broad plate. This type is further divided into the continuous type, which demonstrates complete fusion between the two parts, and the discontinuous type, in which there is a boundary between the fibers arising from the aponeurosis intertendines and the normal anterior belly of the digastric. The posterior type refers to when the anterior belly is associated with but distinctly separated from a thin muscle plate that originates from the aponeurosis intertendines and inserts on the mandible. This type is further divided into the continuous form, in which the thin muscle plate passes anteriorly to the inner surface of the mandible and sends fibers to mylohyoideus, and the myloid form, in which the thin muscle plate passes medially to fuse with the mylohyoideus of the opposite side. The biceps form refers to a two-headed anterior belly with a medial head that inserts into the digastric fossa of the opposite side. The sixth form is not named but refers to the presence of an accessory bundle between the mandible and the lateral margin of the anterior belly. The "combinated" form refers to a complicated

presentation of the anterior belly that is comprised of either the coexistence of both the anterior and posterior types or a more intricate form that demonstrates some combination of the six aforementioned types.

De-Ary-Pires et al. (2003) classified the anterior belly of the digastric into five types, the intermediate tendon into three types, and the posterior belly in two types (see the entry for digastricus posterior for more details). A type I anterior belly consists of one belly that originates near the mandibular symphysis. A type II anterior belly is comprised of two bellies with extra slips to the mandible or mylohyoid muscle on either side of the body. A type III anterior belly is comprised of three bellies with extra slips to the mandible or mylohyoid muscle on either side of the body. A type IV anterior belly is comprised of four bellies with extra slips to the mandible or mylohyoid muscle on either side of the body. A type V anterior belly is a normal anterior belly that is present with the mentohyoid muscle. The intermediate tendon was categorized as piercing the stylohyoid muscle (type I), passing superficial to the stylohyoid (type II), or passing deep to the stylohyoid (type III).

Multiple accessory muscles in the submental triangle are common (Wood 1868; Sargon et al. 1999; Peker et al. 2000; Aktekin et al. 2003; Fujimura et al. 2003; Liquidato et al. 2007; Kyung et al. 2011; Yamazaki et al. 2011; Raju et al. 2014; Harvey et al. 2015; Lee and Yang 2016; Hsiao and Chang 2019). These accessory muscles may have attachments to the main anterior belly, intermediate tendon of the digastric, mylohyoid, the mylohyoid raphe, body or digastric fossa of the mandible, and/or the hyoid (Traini 1983; Michna 1989; Sargon and Çelik 1994; Holibková and Machálek 1999; Sargon et al. 1999; Guelfguat et al. 2001; Peker et al. 2000; Aktekin et al. 2003; Fujimura et al. 2003; Turan-Özdemir et al. 2004; Liquidato et al. 2007; Sevinç et al. 2009; Kyung et al. 2011; Yamazaki et al. 2011; Harvey et al. 2015; Raju et al. 2014; Lee and Yang 2016; Khona et al. 2017; Zdilla et al. 2018; Hsiao and Chang 2019; Ortug et al. 2020).

Harvey et al. (2015) report a case in which digastricus anterior on both sides of a cadaver had superficial and deep bellies. In this case, four additional accessory muscle bellies extended across the submental region in a "weave pattern." Zdilla et al. (2014b) report the presence of accessory anterior digastric muscles in the submental region that present in a "fractal" pattern, where two accessory bellies gave origin to two smaller accessory bellies.

Zdilla et al. (2018) provide a comprehensive review of a common presentation of the accessory anterior bellies designated as "arrowhead variations." The arrowhead variation refers to bilateral accessory muscles that extend between the intermediate tendons of the digastric and the median raphe of the mylohyoid musculature (Aktekin et al. 2003; Turan-Özdemir et al. 2004; Zdilla et al. 2018). These accessory arrowhead muscles often send one or two additional accessory bundles to the mandible (Traini 1983; Aktekin et al. 2003; Turan-Özdemir et al. 2004; Zdilla et al. 2018; Hsiao and Chang 2019).

Prevalence

Hallett (1848) found that mylohyoideus was connected to the intermediate tendon of the digastricus in one out of five subjects (20%). Hallett (1848) also found a third belly of the digastric muscle in about 1 in 15 subjects (6.7%). Wood (1868) found that the anterior belly of the digastric was doubled in 5 out of 68 males (7.4%) and 1 out of 34 females (2.9%). Sato (1968b) found that the digastricus muscle was completely absent in 7 out of 324 sides (2.16%) in Kyushu-Japanese males and in 2 out of 232 sides (0.86%) in females.

Mori (1964) classified the anterior belly of the digastric into nine forms (see above for descriptions). Out of a sample of 262 cadavers: the normal form was found in 121 cadavers (46.2%), the ape form was found in five cadavers (1.9%), the continuous form of the anterior type was found bilaterally in 27 cadavers (10.3%) and unilaterally in 18 cadavers (6.9%), the discontinuous form of the anterior type was found bilaterally in one cadaver (0.4%) and unilaterally in five cadavers (1.9%), the continuous form of the posterior type was found in four cadavers (1.5%), the myloid form of the posterior type was found in bilaterally in 12 cadavers (4.6%) and unilaterally in 30 cadavers (11.5%), the biceps form was found in eight cadavers (3.1%), an accessory bundle between the mandible and the anterior belly was found bilaterally in one cadaver (0.4%) and unilaterally in three cadavers (1.1%), the "combined" form was found in a total of 29 cadavers (11.1%), with eight cadavers (3.1%) combining the anterior and posterior types and 21 cadavers (8%) having a more intricate form.

Larsson and Lufkin (1987) examined the anterior belly of the digastric in 40 patients that underwent CT imaging of the oropharynx and 35 patients that underwent MR imaging of the oropharynx. In the CT group, unilateral absence of the anterior belly was observed in one patient (2.5%). In this case, the anterior belly was replaced by a small muscle extending between the mylohyoid raphe and the hyoid. In the MR group, an accessory muscle crossed the midline in one patient (2.9%) with otherwise normal digastric muscles.

Sargon et al. (1999) found variations of the anterior digastric muscle in 5 out of 99 cadavers (5.1%). Accessory bellies of the anterior digastric were found in four cadavers. The absence of the anterior belly on one side and an atypical origin of the muscle on the other side were observed in the fifth cadaver. In a sample of 54 cadavers, Fujimura et al. (2003) found variations of the anterior belly of the digastric in 13 cases (24.1%). In a sample of ten cadavers, Liquidato et al. (2007) found variations of digastricus anterior in four cases (40%). In a sample of 30 cadavers, Khona et al. (2017) found accessory bellies of the anterior digastric in three cadavers (10%). In a sample of 19 cadavers, Zdilla et al. (2018) found that the arrowhead variation was present in two cadavers (10.5%). In a sample of 15 cadavers, Hsiao and Chang (2019) found accessory anterior bellies of the digastric in three cases (20%).

De-Ary-Pires et al. (2003) studied the digastric muscle in 74 cadavers. An anterior belly was absent unilaterally in one cadaver and a posterior belly was absent unilaterally

in another cadaver. Therefore, 146 digastric muscles were studied. These authors classified the anterior belly of the digastric into five types, the intermediate tendon into three types, and the posterior belly in two types (see above for descriptions of the first two structures and the entry for digastricus posterior for description of the latter). They then identified ten patterns exhibited by the 146 muscles. Pattern A—a type I anterior belly, type I intermediate tendon, and type I posterior belly—was present in 96 muscles (65.8%). Pattern B—a type II anterior belly, type I intermediate tendon, and type I posterior belly—was present in eight muscles (5.5%). Pattern C—a type III anterior belly, type I intermediate tendon, and type I posterior belly—was present in one muscle (0.7%). Pattern D—a type IV anterior belly, type I intermediate tendon, and type I posterior belly—was present in one muscle (0.7%). Pattern E—a type V anterior belly, type I intermediate tendon, and type I posterior belly—was present in two muscles (1.4%). Pattern F—a type I anterior belly, type II intermediate tendon, and type I posterior belly—was present in 14 muscles (9.6%). Pattern G—a type I anterior belly, type II intermediate tendon, and type II posterior belly—was present in six muscles (4.1%). Pattern H—a type I anterior belly, type III intermediate tendon, and type I posterior belly—was present in 12 muscles (8.2%). Pattern I—a type II anterior belly, type II intermediate tendon, and type II posterior belly—was present in four muscles (2.7%). Pattern J—a type II anterior belly, type III intermediate tendon, and type II posterior belly—was present in two muscles (1.4%).

Ortug et al. (2020) applied the classifications used by De-Ary-Pires et al. (2003) to examine the digastricus anterior muscles on 80 sides of 40 cadavers. A type I anterior belly was found in 68 sides (85%), a type II anterior belly was found on four sides (5%), a type III anterior belly was found on three sides (3.8%), and a type IV belly was found on two sides (2.5%). A unilateral accessory belly was found in one cadaver (2.5%), and bilateral accessory bellies were found in another cadaver (2.5%).

Anomalies

Description

Bersu et al. (1976) describe a male infant with Hanhart syndrome in which the right mandible was represented by a small bone. On the right side, digastricus posterior had a normal origin and traveled laterally to hyoglossus and inserted by its intermediate tendon onto the body of the hyoid bone at the base of the greater cornu. The anterior digastricus originated from this bony attachment and traveled anterolaterally to attach along the inferior margin of the right mandible.

Colacino and Pettersen (1978), Pettersen (1979), Pettersen et al. (1979), and Aziz (1980) report anomalies of the anterior belly of the digastric in individuals with trisomy 13. In one neonate, the anterior belly of the digastric was doubled bilaterally (Colacino and Pettersen 1978). In another neonate, the left anterior belly had an extra bundle that fused with mylohyoid and decussated across the midline (Pettersen et al. 1979). In a fetus, the anterior bellies of the digastric were doubled bilaterally (Pettersen et al. 1979). The medial anterior belly on the left side originated from the hyoid bone. All anterior bellies inserted into the mandible and had no connections to mylohyoid. In a boy with trisomy 13q, there was an extra belly of the anterior digastric on the left side (Pettersen 1979). In one neonate, the left anterior belly was doubled while the right anterior belly had three bellies that inserted onto the mandible and a fourth belly that inserted onto the masseter (Aziz 1980).

Digastricus anterior is also variable in some individuals with trisomy 18 (Bersu and Ramirez-Castro 1977; Aziz 1979; Smith et al. 2015). On the right side of one infant, the anterior belly was narrow, and an accessory belly extended between the left anterior digastric and the digastric fossa (Bersu and Ramirez-Castro 1977). In another infant, there was an accessory muscle sheet between the bellies of anterior digastric and the mylohyoid musculature, and the anterior belly was doubled on the right side. In two infants, mentohyoideus was present bilaterally. The intermediate tendon was absent bilaterally in all cases examined by Bersu and Ramirez-Castro (1977), and all anterior bellies of the digastric had an insertion into the hyoid. In the neonate described by Aziz (1979), both the left and right anterior bellies of digastric were enlarged. In the fetus with trisomy 18 and cyclopia described by Smith et al. (2015), digastricus anterior had two heads bilaterally. Its medial head decussated with its counterpart across the midline and the lateral head fused with mylohyoid. In a fetus with trisomy 21, there was an accessory anterior digastric belly on the left side (Bersu 1980).

Mieden (1982) describes an infant with median cleft lip, hypotelorism, and alobar holoprosencephaly. This infant had a bilateral accessory slip extending between the intermediate tendon of digastricus and the superior pharyngeal constrictor (Mieden 1982). This author also describes two male fetuses with cyclopia and alobar holoprosencephaly. In one of these cases, the right anterior belly of digastricus was absent, and the left muscle was doubled in size and attached to both sides of the mandibular symphysis.

Moen et al. (1984) found that the anterior bellies of digastricus were doubled on both sides of a male infant with triploidy, and there were extra slips associated with the anterior digastric bellies bilaterally in a female fetus with triploidy. In a male neonate with Meckel syndrome, Pettersen (1984) found that the anterior belly of the right digastricus sent an accessory slip to the mylohyoideus. In an infant with mandibulofacial dysostosis, the anterior belly was fasciculated and these fascicles originated from the body of the hyoid (Herring et al. 1979).

In the fetus with craniorachischisis described by Alghamdi et al. (2017), the right anterior belly of the digastric was fused with mylohyoid. On the left side, the anterior belly was attached to the inferior border of the mandible. The intermediate tendon of the digastric sent a tendinous slip to the fascia over the left mylohyoid.

Prevalence

In their literature review, Smith et al. (2015) found that digastricus anterior was variable in 5 out of 20 individuals with trisomy 13 (25%) and 5 out of 17 individuals with trisomy 18 (29.4%). Mentohyoideus was reported in 4 out of 17 individuals with trisomy 18 (23.5%). The intermediate tendon was absent in all eight infants (100%) with trisomy 18 described by Bersu and Ramirez-Castro (1977).

Clinical Implications

Accessory anterior bellies of the digastric may be mistaken for masses, tumors, or metastatic lymph nodes (Aktekin et al. 2003; Guelfguat et al 2001; Turan-Özdemir et al. 2004; Ozgur et al. 2007; Bonala et al. 2015; Hsiao and Chang 2019).

DIGASTRICUS POSTERIOR (POSTERIOR BELLY OF THE DIGASTRIC) (FIGURE 2.10)

See also: Digastricus anterior

Synonyms

This muscle is referred to as the posterior belly of the digastric (Standring 2016).

Typical Presentation

Description

Digastricus posterior originates from the mastoid notch of the temporal bone (Standring 2016). It courses inferiorly and anteriorly to end in a tendon (the intermediate tendon) that connects it with digastricus anterior (Standring 2016). The intermediate tendon perforates stylohyoid (Standring 2016).

Innervation

Digastricus posterior is innervated by the facial nerve (Standring 2016).

Comparative Anatomy

Digastricus posterior has a similar typical presentation in most apes, extending from the mastoid region of the temporal bone to the intermediate tendon (Raven 1950; Miller 1952; Gibbs 1999; Diogo et al. 2010, 2012, 2013a,b, 2017). Digastricus posterior inserts into the angle of the mandible in orangutans since digastricus anterior is typically absent (Chapman 1880; Sonntag 1924; Cachel 1984; Wall et al. 1994; Gibbs 1999; Diogo et al. 2013b). The origin of the posterior belly of digastricus may extend onto the occipital bone in orangutans (Sonntag 1924), gorillas (Raven 1950; Diogo et al. 2010), and common chimpanzees (Tyson 1699).

Variations

Description

The anterior and posterior bellies may fail to connect (Bergman et al. 1988). The digastric muscle may have a tendinous inscription (Bergman et al. 1988; Lee and Yang

2016). The muscle may present as trigastric, often with the third head extending between the intermediate tendon and the mandible or midline of the neck (Macalister 1875; Hallett 1848; Bergman et al. 1988; Lee and Yang 2016). The muscle may also be quadrigastric (Wood 1868; Bergman et al. 1988; Lee and Yang 2016) or have more than four bellies due to variations in the anterior belly (see the entry for digastricus anterior).

The extent of the origin of the posterior belly may vary, with possible attachments to the mastoid process or the lateral part of the superior nuchal line (Macalister 1875; Bergman et al. 1988; Lee and Yang 2016). It may receive a slip or originate entirely from the styloid process (Macalister 1875; De-Ary-Pires et al. 2003; Standring 2016). It may also receive a slip from the angle of the mandible (Macalister 1875). Splenius may send fibers to its origin (Macalister 1875). An accessory posterior belly of the digastric may originate from the sternohyoid (Lee and Yang 2016) or from the mastoid notch with the normal posterior belly (Ozgursoy and Kucuk 2006; Zhao et al. 2015). If the intermediate tendon is absent, the posterior belly may attach onto the mandible or the styloid process (Macalister 1875; Bergman et al. 1988; Lee and Yang 2016; Standring 2016). The posterior belly may be absent (De-Ary-Pires et al. 2003).

Stylohyoid may fuse with digastricus posterior or insert onto the intermediate tendon (Macalister 1875; Bergman et al. 1988; Lee and Yang 2016). The intermediate tendon may pass in front of or behind stylohyoid instead of perforating it (Macalister 1875; Mori 1964; De-Ary-Pires et al. 2003; Harvey et al. 2015). The intermediate tendon may send slips to the lesser horn of the hyoid (Macalister 1875).

De-Ary-Pires et al. (2003) classified the posterior belly of the digastric into two types, the intermediate tendon into three types, and the anterior belly of the digastric into five types (see the entry for digastricus anterior for more details). A type I posterior belly originated from the mastoid notch. A type II posterior belly originated entirely or partially from the styloid process and may have sent a slip to the middle or inferior constrictors of the pharynx. The intermediate tendon was categorized as piercing the stylohyoid muscle (type I), passing superficial to the stylohyoid (type II), or passing deep to the stylohyoid (type III).

Prevalence

See digastricus anterior entry for prevalence information on the patterns described by De-Ary-Pires et al. (2003). Hallett (1848) found a third belly of the digastric muscle in about 1 in 15 subjects (6.7%). Macalister (1875) notes that Wood found a third belly in 1 out of 17 subjects (5.9%). Sato (1968b) found that the digastricus muscle was completely absent in 7 out of 324 sides (2.16%) in Kyushu-Japanese males and in 2 out of 232 sides (0.86%) in females.

Anomalies

Description

Bersu et al. (1976) describe a male infant with Hanhart syndrome in which the right mandible was represented by a small bone. On the right side, digastricus posterior had a normal origin and traveled laterally to hyoglossus and inserted by its intermediate tendon onto the body of the hyoid bone at the base of the greater cornu. The anterior digastricus originated from this bony attachment and traveled anterolaterally to attach along the inferior margin of the right mandible.

Colacino and Pettersen (1978), Pettersen (1979), and Pettersen et al. (1979) report anomalies of the posterior belly of the digastric in individuals with trisomy 13. In one neonate, the left posterior belly of the digastricus originated via two distinct bellies from the mastoid notch and from the styloid process and inserted with stylohyoid into the hyoid bone (Colacino and Pettersen 1978). The right posterior belly was split and sent a deep bundle to stylopharyngeus. In another neonate, the posterior belly of the digastric was doubled bilaterally, with the extra bellies inserting onto the hyoid bone (Pettersen et al. 1979). On the left side of the specimen, the extra posterior belly received a contribution from sternothyroid.

In a fetus with trisomy 13, the posterior bellies of the digastric were doubled bilaterally (Pettersen et al. 1979). On the left side, each posterior belly had a separate origin from the mastoid process and a separate insertion into the hyoid. On the right side, the superomedial belly inserted into the hyoid bone and the inferolateral belly inserted into the infrahyoid muscles. In another fetus, the left posterior belly of the digastric inserted into the hyoid bone without connecting to the anterior belly (Pettersen et al. 1979). The same condition was found on the right side, with an extension of the hyoid attachment of the posterior belly into the posterior aspect of hyoglossus. In a boy with trisomy 13q, the posterior belly on the left side of the body was small and blended with the stylohyoid (Pettersen 1979).

Digastricus posterior is also variable in some individuals with trisomy 18 (Bersu and Ramirez-Castro 1977; Aziz 1979; Smith et al. 2015). The intermediate tendon was absent bilaterally in all cases examined by Bersu and Ramirez-Castro (1977), and all posterior bellies of the digastric had an insertion into the hyoid when it was present. A tendinous inscription into the posterior belly was found on the left side of one infant (Bersu and Ramirez-Castro 1977). In another infant, the right posterior belly passed deep to the external and internal carotid arteries. In a third, the muscle was absent on the right side. Multiple infants exhibited slips extending from digastricus posterior to the styloid process and/or to the superior or middle pharyngeal constrictors (Bersu and Ramirez-Castro 1977). In the fetus with trisomy 18 and cyclopia dissected by Smith et al. (2015), the digastricus posterior bellies were broad on both sides of the body but had normal attachments.

Mieden (1982) describes an infant with median cleft lip, hypotelorism, and alobar holoprosencephaly (case I) and two male fetuses with cyclopia and alobar holoprosencephaly (cases II and III). In case I, there was an accessory muscle slip extending between the intermediate tendon of digastricus and the superior pharyngeal constrictor. In case III, an accessory muscle belly was present along the hyoid bone and extended between the right stylohyoid and left posterior digastric muscles (Mieden 1982). On both sides of the fetus with craniorachischisis, the posterior belly attached to the "temporo-occipital" bone (Alghamdi et al. 2017). On the left side, the intermediate tendon of the digastric sent a tendinous slip to the fascia over the left mylohyoid.

Prevalence

In their literature review, Smith et al. (2015) found that digastricus posterior was variable in 5 out of 20 individuals with trisomy 13 (25%). Digastricus posterior sent slips to either the styloid process and/or the superior or middle pharyngeal constrictors in 4 out of 17 individuals with trisomy 18 (23.5%). The intermediate tendon was absent in all eight infants (100%) with trisomy 18 described by Bersu and Ramirez-Castro (1977).

Clinical Implications

McMurtry and Yahr (1966) found that an accessory posterior belly of the digastric coursed diagonally across the origin of the internal and external carotid arteries and caused extracranial occlusion of the right internal carotid artery.

STYLOHYOIDEUS (STYLOHYOID) (FIGURE 2.10)

Synonyms

N/A

Typical Presentation

Description

Stylohyoid originates via a tendon from the posterior aspect of the styloid process (Standring 2016). It inserts onto the hyoid at the junction of the body and the greater horn (Standring 2016). The intermediate tendon of the digastric perforates stylohyoid near its insertion (Standring 2016).

Innervation

Stylohyoid is innervated by the stylohyoid branch of the facial nerve (Standring 2016).

Comparative Anatomy

Stylohyoideus has a similar typical presentation in most apes, extending from the styloid process to the hyoid with perforation at its insertion by the intermediate tendon of the digastric (Sonntag 1923; Raven 1950; Miller 1952; Gibbs 1999; Diogo et al. 2010, 2013a,b, 2017). As the styloid process is typically reduced or absent in gibbons, the stylohyoid muscle originates from the tympanic region (Diogo et al. 2012). It may originate from the temporal bone in gorillas (Dean 1984). Stylohyoideus is not perforated by the intermediate tendon in orangutans (Sonntag 1924).

Variations

Description

Stylohyoid may be absent (Macalister 1875; Knott 1880, 1883a; Bergman et al. 1988; Lee and Yang 2016; Standring 2016). In some cases, the muscle may pass medial to the

external carotid artery (Standring 2016). Its fibers may occasionally cover the anterior aspect of the hyoid bone (Ozgur et al. 2010) or end in either the suprahyoid or infrahyoid musculature (Standring 2016). The intermediate tendon of the digastric may pass in front of or behind stylohyoid instead of perforating it (Macalister 1875; Mori 1964; De-Ary-Pires et al. 2003; Harvey et al. 2015). In this case, the stylohyoid would have a single insertion onto the hyoid (Macalister 1875; Bergman et al. 1988; Lee and Yang 2016). Stylohyoid may also fuse with digastricus posterior or insert onto the intermediate tendon (Macalister 1875; Knott 1883a; Bergman et al. 1988; Lee and Yang 2016). Hallett (1848) reports a case in which stylohyoid split upon its insertion, with the lower part inserting onto the body of the hyoid and the upper part inserting onto the intermediate tendon.

Stylohyoid is associated with named accessory muscles and other accessory slips. Stylohyoid may send a slip to omohyoid, mylohyoid, or to the tongue (Macalister 1875). The stylohyoid may also insert into the outer border of mylohyoid (Macalister 1875). Stylohyoid may be doubled (Macalister 1875; Knott 1880; Standring 2016) with the second bundle sometimes referred to as stylohyoideus profundus (Bergman et al. 1988) or stylohyoideus nanus (Santorini) (Lee and Yang 2016). Stylohyoideus profundus may course parallel to the main bundle of stylohyoideus or replace the stylohyoid ligament (Macalister 1875; Bergman et al. 1988; Lee and Yang 2016). A second stylohyoid may have attachments to the base of the styloid process, the tip of the styloid process, and/or to the lesser horn of the hyoid (Macalister 1875; Knott 1880; Bergman et al. 1988; Lee and Yang 2016). Macalister (1875) notes that Petsche found a second slip of stylohyoid that inserted onto the cartilago triticea. A doubled stylohyoid may also send one slip over the intermediate tendon and another slip under the intermediate tendon (Macalister 1875). Stylohyoid may also be tripled (Macalister 1875).

Stylochondrohyoideus refers to a supernumerary muscle that extends from the styloid process to the lesser horn of the hyoid (Lambert et al. 2010; Lee and Yang 2016) It may replace, envelop, or have an attachment into, the stylohyoid ligament (Joshi et al. 2007; Lambert et al. 2010; Lee and Yang 2016). Stylochondrohyoideus may be used interchangeably or confused with stylohyoideus profundus in the literature (Lambert et al. 2010). A second head for an otherwise normal stylohyoid muscle may originate from the angle of the mandible (Macalister 1875). When this head is completely distinct from the stylohyoid, it forms the hyoangularis muscle (Macalister 1875). Stylomandibularis refers to a bundle that extends from the tip of the styloid process to the angle of the mandible (Bergman et al. 1988; Lee and Yang 2016).

Prevalence

Macalister (1875) notes that Hallett claims that stylohyoid is absent in 1 out of 200 cases (0.5%). From a sample of Japanese cadavers, Mori (1964) found that the stylohyoid passed medial to the intermediate tendon of the digastric in 178 sides out of 254 sides (70.1%), passed lateral to the intermediate tendon on five sides (2%), and was perforated by the intermediate tendon on 71 sides (27.9%). In a sample of 56 sides from 28 Anatolian cadavers, Ozgur et al. (2010) found that the stylohyoid muscle inserted into the body of the hyoid at its junction with the greater horn on 34 sides (60.7%). In the remaining 22 sides (39.3%), fibers from stylohyoid elongated in front of the hyoid and formed an arch or circle in front of it, having the appearance of covering the hyoid bone as a collar.

Anomalies

Description

On the right side of one neonate with trisomy 13, stylohyoid did not bifurcate around the intermediate tendon of the digastric (Colacino and Pettersen 1978). On the left side, stylohyoid inserted with some fibers of the posterior belly of the digastric into the hyoid. On the left side of another neonate, stylohyoid was hypoplastic and inserted into the intermediate tendon of the digastric (Pettersen et al. 1979). This morphology was present on the right, but a slip was present from the stylohyoid muscle to the hyoid. Stylohyoid was absent bilaterally in a neonate with trisomy 13 (Aziz 1980). In one fetus with trisomy 13, stylohyoid was absent on the left side (Pettersen et al. 1979). On the left side of another fetus, the stylohyoid inserted into the hyoid and continued into the anterior belly of the digastric (Pettersen et al. 1979). In a boy with trisomy 13q, the posterior belly of the digastric on the left side of the body was small and blended with the stylohyoid (Pettersen 1979).

Stylohyoid was absent either bilaterally or unilaterally in nearly all the infants with trisomy 18 studied by Bersu and Ramirez-Castro (1977). In two cases, stylohyoid muscles were doubled unilaterally. When present, the stylohyoid was not perforated by the digastric tendon, except for in the following case. On the right side of one infant, an accessory stylohyoid muscle originated from the temporal bone (Bersu and Ramirez-Castro 1977). This muscle gave origin to a tendon that split around digastricus and then attached to the body of the hyoid near its junction with the greater horn. The accessory stylohyoid muscle blended with the normal stylohyoid muscle. On the left side of this specimen, stylohyoid was absent. In the female fetus with trisomy 18 dissected by Alghamdi et al. (2018), stylohyoid was absent bilaterally.

Mieden (1982) describes an infant with median cleft lip, hypotelorism, and alobar holoprosencephaly (case I) and two male fetuses with cyclopia and alobar holoprosencephaly (cases II and III). Stylohyoideus was absent bilaterally in case I and absent on the left side in case III. In case III, an accessory belly was present along the hyoid bone and extended between the right stylohyoid and left posterior digastric muscles (Mieden 1982). In an infant with mandibulofacial dysostosis, stylohyoid received a slip from digastricus posterior (Herring et al. 1979).

Prevalence

In their literature review, Smith et al. (2015) found that stylohyoideus was absent in 5 out of 20 individuals with trisomy 13 (25%) and 7 out of 17 individuals with trisomy 18 (41.2%). Stylohyoideus blended with the digastric in 2 out of 20 individuals with trisomy 13 (10%) and was anomalous in 5 out of 17 individuals with trisomy 18 (29.4%).

Clinical Implications

A variant stylohyoid muscle can be confused with some pathological conditions and may compress surrounding neurovascular structures, inducing stylohyoid syndrome (Ozgur et al. 2010).

EXTRAOCULAR MUSCLES

LEVATOR PALPEBRAE SUPERIORIS (FIGURE 2.11)

See also: Tensor trochleae

Synonyms

N/A

Typical Presentation

Description

Levator palpebrae superioris originates via a tendon from the lesser wing of the sphenoid (Standring 2016). It ends in an aponeurosis that attaches to the superior tarsus, with some fibers inserting into the skin of the upper eyelid (Standring 2016). Anteriorly, the fascia between levator palpebrae superioris and the superior rectus attaches to the superior conjunctival fornix, which may be considered a third attachment of this muscle (Standring 2016).

Innervation

Levator palpebrae superioris is innervated by a branch from the superior division of the oculomotor nerve (Standring 2016).

Comparative Anatomy

In common chimpanzees, levator palpebrae superioris has attachments only into the superior tarsus and superior conjunctival fornix, lacking an insertion into the skin of the eyelid (Sonntag 1923). All three attachments are present in orangutans and the muscle also gives off a lateral band and medial band (Sonntag 1924). The lateral band splits the lacrimal gland and attaches to the deep surface of the malar bone. The medial band divides into two slips that surround the lacrimal sac and insert into the lacrimal bone. Some fibers of levator palpebrae superioris fused with superior rectus (Sonntag 1924).

Variations

Description

Levator palpebrae superioris may be fused with rectus superior at its origin (Macalister 1875). It may originate from the posterior margin of the frontal part of the roof of the orbit (Macalister 1875). Macalister (1875) observed a case in which

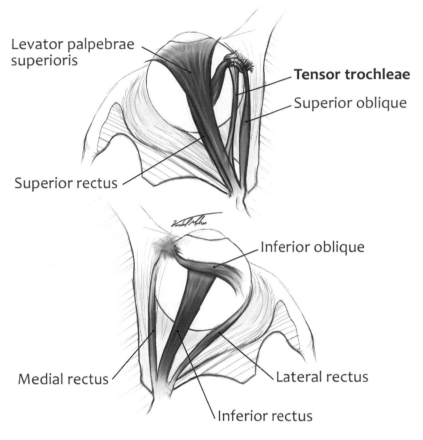

Levator palpebrae
superioris

Tensor trochleae

Superior oblique

Superior rectus

Inferior oblique

Medial rectus

Lateral rectus

Inferior rectus

FIGURE 2.11 Superior view (above) and inferior view (below) of the extraocular muscles.

levator palpebrae superioris only exhibited an insertion into the superior conjunctival fornix. Levator palpebrae superioris may be absent (Macalister 1875; Bergman et al. 1988). Levator palpebrae superioris may also be split, doubled, or associated with accessory slips (Macalister 1875; Knott 1883a; Whitnall 1921; Bergman et al. 1988; Amonoo-Kuofi and Darwish 1998; von Lüdinghausen et al. 1999; Plock et al. 2005; Yalçin et al. 2009; Kocabiyik 2016; Haładaj et al. 2020a). It may have a bipartite origin (Haładaj et al. 2020a).

Amonoo-Kuofi and Darwish (1998) describe a bilateral supernumerary muscle situated between the superior oblique and levator palpebrae superioris. These 'levator palpebrae superioris accessorius' muscles originated from the lesser wing of the sphenoid and inserted into the medial portion of the skin of the eyelid (Amonoo-Kuofi and Darwish 1998). The three accessory slips described by Yalçin et al. (2009) include a lateral slip divided anteriorly into superior and inferior parts, a medial fibromuscular slip, and slip situated between the levator and superior rectus that ended in a wide aponeurosis. This aponeurosis attached to the medial orbital septum, palpebral part of orbicularis oculi, and the medial skin of the upper eyelid (Yalçin et al. 2009).

A slip of levator palpebrae superioris may extend to the lacrimal gland and may be referred to as retractor glandulae lacrimalis (Whitnall 1921; Bergman et al. 1988; von Lüdinghausen et al. 1999; Haładaj et al. 2020a). An accessory muscle of levator palpebrae superioris that attaches to the superior oblique may also be referred to as obliquus accessorius, obliqui superioris (Albinus), gracillimus orbitis (Bochdalek), or gracillimus oculi (Macalister 1875; Knott 1883a; Bergman et al. 1988). A variant of this slip, tensor trochleae, may insert into the trochlea of superior oblique (see the entry for this muscle). Levator palpebrae superioris may also be connected with transversus orbitis, which extends from the os planum of the ethmoid bone to the lateral wall of the orbit, coursing across the superior surface of the eyeball (Bochdalek 1868; Macalister 1875; Whitnall 1921; Bergman et al. 1988; Kocabiyik 2016). Haładaj et al. (2020a) describe a slip attaching to the lateral wall of the orbit that resembles a partially developed transversus orbitis muscle.

Prevalence

In a sample of 20 sides of 10 fetuses, Plock et al. (2005) found medial accessory bellies of levator palpebrae superioris on seven sides (35%), and singular muscle fibers within medial fibrous bands on five sides (25%). Out of 35 cadavers, Amonoo-Kuofi and Darwish (1998) found bilateral levator palpebrae superioris accessorius muscles in one cadaver (2.9%). Yalçin et al. (2009) found accessory slips of levator palpebrae superioris in 3 out of 60 orbits (5%).

In a sample of 70 orbits, Haładaj et al. (2020a) found a typical presentation of levator palpebrae superioris in 58 orbits (82.8%). Lateral slips of levator palpebrae superioris that inserted into the lacrimal gland were present in seven specimens (10%). In one case (1.4%), the muscle sent a slip to the lateral wall of the orbit. In another case (1.4%), levator palpebrae superioris had a bipartite origin.

Anomalies

Description

In a fetus with 18p-, levator palpebrae superioris was absent on the left side and reduced in size on the right side (Urban and Bersu 1987). In a fetus with prosencephaly, von Lüdinghausen et al. (1999) found a bipartite levator palpebrae superioris that formed a retrobulbar arch. Levator palpebrae superioris was absent bilaterally in a fetus with occipital meningocele (Plock et al. 2007). In anencephalic fetuses, levator palpebrae superioris may be reduced, absent, or have insertions into the lacrimal gland and periorbita (Plock et al. 2007).

Prevalence

In a sample of 15 anencephalic fetuses, levator palpebrae superioris was absent bilaterally in six fetuses (40%) and absent on one side in one fetus (6.7%) (Plock et al. 2007).

Clinical Implications

Variations of levator palpebrae superioris (including absence, deficiency, or accessory slips) may cause ptosis or congenital eyelid retraction (Urban and Bersu 1987; Wylen et al. 2001; Plock et al. 2005; Yalçin et al. 2009).

TENSOR TROCHLEAE (FIGURE 2.11)

See also: Levator palpebrae superioris

Synonyms

This muscle may also be referred to as rectus quintus (Molinetti) (Knott 1883a) or the levator-trochlear muscle (Sacks 1985). Tensor trochleae is a variant of the accessory muscle referred to as comes obliquus accessorius, obliqui superioris (Albinus), gracillimus orbitis (Bochdalek), or gracillimus oculi (Macalister 1875; Knott 1883a; Whitnall 1921).

Typical Presentation

This muscle is only present as a variation or anomaly.

Comparative Anatomy

von Lüdinghausen (1998) states that tensor trochleae and similar muscles are remnants of the membrana nictitans (third eyelid) of amniotes.

Variations

Description

Tensor trochleae presents as a medial bundle of levator palpebrae superioris that inserts into the trochlea of the superior oblique (Budge 1859; Macalister 1875; Knott 1883a; Haładaj et al. 2020a). It may also have attachments into the sclera and fascia near the trochlea, the supratrochlear artery, or the medial rectus muscle (Whitnall 1921; Isomura 1977; Sacks 1985; Bergman et al. 1988; von Lüdinghausen 1998; von Lüdinghausen et al. 1999; Kocabiyik 2016). Tensor trochleae may be distinct from levator palpebrae superioris only at its insertion, or for most of its length (Macalister 1875).

Tensor trochleae may be split into two bundles (Whitnall 1921; von Lüdinghausen 1998). In a case observed by Whitnall (1921), tensor trochleae consisted of two bundles, one that inserted into the fascia bulbi near the superior oblique and one that inserted beneath the trochlea. In the case described by von Lüdinghausen (1998), the muscle split at its midpoint, with a medial portion that became ligamentous and inserted into the tissue between the trochlea and the eyeball, and a lateral portion that rejoined levator palpebrae superioris.

Innervation

Tensor trochleae is innervated by a branch from the superior division of the oculomotor nerve (Isomura 1977; Sacks 1985).

Prevalence

Isomura (1977) found tensor trochleae in five orbits from 85 subjects (5.9%). Sacks (1985) found tensor trochleae in 7 out of 98 cadaver orbits (7.1%). Haładaj et al. (2020a) found tensor trochleae in 3 out of 70 orbits (4.3%), and Haładaj et al. (2020c) found tensor trochleae in 2 out of 78 orbits (2.6%).

Anomalies

Description

Macalister (1875) notes that in 1724, Kulmus found a muscle corresponding to tensor trochleae in an abnormal fetus.

Prevalence

N/A

Clinical Implications

Sacks (1985) argued that it may be possible for tensor trochleae to be a cause of some hypertropias or unexplained ocular deviations.

RECTUS SUPERIOR (SUPERIOR RECTUS) (FIGURE 2.11)

Synonyms

N/A

Typical Presentation

Description

Superior rectus originates from the common tendinous ring and the dural sheath surrounding the optic nerve and inserts into the upper surface of the sclera (Standring 2016).

Innervation

Superior rectus is innervated by the superior division of the oculomotor nerve (Standring 2016).

Comparative Anatomy

In common chimpanzees, orangutans, and gibbons, superior rectus has a similar typical presentation to that of humans (Sonntag 1923, 1924; Diogo et al. 2012). In orangutans, some fibers fuse with levator palpebrae superioris (Sonntag 1924).

Variations

Description

Superior rectus may be fused with levator palpebrae superioris at its origin (Macalister 1875). Drummond and Keech (1989) describe a case in which superior rectus and superior oblique were absent in the right eye and variant in the left eye. Nayak et al. (2019) describe a double-bellied superior rectus. The muscle had two bellies with separate origins from the common tendinous ring that joined prior to insertion (Nayak et al. 2019).

Accessory slips that originate from the tendinous ring may connect the superior rectus with inferior rectus (Whitnall 1921; Bergman et al. 1988; von Lüdinghausen 1998; von Lüdinghausen et al. 1999; Kakizaki et al. 2006; Kocabiyik 2016; Haładaj et al. 2018; 2020b). These muscles may divide into two heads, one that inserts into superior rectus and one that inserts into inferior rectus (Kakizaki et al. 2006; Haładaj et al. 2018).

Superior rectus is associated with retractor bulbi, which has numerous presentations (Bergman et al. 1988; Kocabiyik 2016). It may present as a slip from the common tendinous ring to the posterior globe, a slip between the superior rectus and lateral rectus, four slips that attach to the back of the globe, or four slips that insert into the deep surfaces of the recti (Whitnall 1911; Bergman et al. 1988; Valmaggia et al. 1996; Krasny et al. 2011; Kocabiyik 2016).

Prevalence

In a sample of 70 hemiheads, Haładaj et al. (2020b) found slips that connected superior rectus and inferior rectus in two cases (2.9%).

Anomalies

Description

Superior rectus may be absent in individuals with Apert syndrome, craniofacial dysostosis, or anencephaly (Weinstock and Hardesty 1965; Cuttone et al. 1979; Diamond et al. 1980; Plock et al. 2007). In a patient with oculocutaneous albinism, superior rectus had a bifid insertion bilaterally (Verma and Hertle 2014).

In two fetuses with triploidy, the attachments of the recti onto the sclera were shifted posteriorly (Moen et al. 1984). In a fetus with occipital meningocele, the left superior rectus was very thin (Plock et al. 2007). In fetuses with anencephaly, there was hypoplasia of superior rectus (Plock et al. 2007). In a fetus with trisomy 18 and cyclopia, superior rectus was doubled bilaterally (Smith et al. 2015).

Prevalence

Diamond et al. (1980) found superior rectus absent in three out of five patients (60%) with craniofacial dysostosis. In a sample of 15 anencephalic fetuses, superior rectus was absent on the left side in one fetus (6.7%) (Plock et al. 2007).

Clinical Implications

The absence of superior rectus may cause ptosis (Posey 1923).

RECTUS INFERIOR (INFERIOR RECTUS) (FIGURE 2.11)

Synonyms

N/A

Typical Presentation

Description

Inferior rectus originates from the common tendinous ring and inserts into the sclera below the cornea (Standring 2016).

Innervation

Inferior rectus is innervated by a branch from the inferior division of the oculomotor nerve (Standring 2016).

Comparative Anatomy

In common chimpanzees and gibbons, inferior rectus has a similar typical presentation to that of humans (Sonntag 1923; Diogo et al. 2012). In orangutans, inferior rectus is cylindrical and has a more intimate attachment to the globe than the other extraocular muscles (Sonntag 1924).

Variations

Description

Inferior rectus may be absent (Ingham et al. 1986; Muñoz 1996; Taylor and Kraft 1997; Astle et al. 2003; Matsuo et al. 2009). Accessory slips that originate from the tendinous ring may connect the inferior rectus with superior rectus (Whitnall 1921; Bergman et al. 1988; von Lüdinghausen 1998; von Lüdinghausen et al. 1999; Kakizaki et al. 2006; Kocabiyik 2016; Haładaj et al. 2018; 2020b). These muscles may divide into two heads: one that inserts into superior rectus and one that inserts into inferior rectus (Kakizaki et al. 2006; Haładaj et al. 2018). Inferior rectus may also receive a fascicle from lateral rectus (Whitnall 1921; Bergman et al. 1988; Kocabiyik 2016). Macalister (1875) observed the partial fusion of inferior rectus and medial rectus in the posterior third of the orbit. There may be a muscular bridge between the inferior rectus and inferior oblique (Yalçin et al. 2004). It may also receive a slip from an accessory inferior oblique (Whitnall 1921). Inferior rectus may be attached to retractor bulbi, which has numerous presentations (Bergman et al. 1988; Kocabiyik 2016; see the entry for superior rectus for more information).

Prevalence

In a sample of 60 orbits, Yalçin et al. (2004) found a muscular bridge between inferior rectus and inferior oblique in four orbits (6.7%). In a sample of 70 hemiheads, Haładaj et al. (2020b) found slips that connect superior rectus and inferior rectus in two cases (2.9%).

Anomalies

Description

Inferior rectus muscles were thinner than normal in fetuses with anencephaly (Plock et al. 2007) and in a fetus with trisomy 18 and cyclopia (Smith et al. 2015). In a fetus with prosencephaly, there was a tripartite inferior rectus (von Lüdinghausen et al. 1999). Its lateral belly blended with the posterior tendon of inferior oblique and its medial belly attached medial to the main belly of inferior rectus (von Lüdinghausen et al. 1999). In two fetuses with triploidy, the attachments of the recti onto the sclera were shifted posteriorly (Moen et al. 1984). Diamond et al. (1980) noted the absence of the right inferior rectus in a child with craniofacial dysostosis. In a child with Axenfeld-Rieger syndrome, there was hypoplasia of inferior rectus on the right side (Bhate and Martin 2012).

Prevalence

Diamond et al. (1980) found inferior rectus absent in one out of five patients (20%) with craniofacial dysostosis.

Clinical Implications

The absence of inferior rectus may mimic inferior rectus paresis and cause strabismus and compensatory head posture (Muñoz 1996; Taylor and Kraft 1997; Astle et al. 2003). The absence of inferior rectus may also be associated with microphthalmos, microcornea, or coloboma (Matsuo et al. 2009).

RECTUS MEDIALIS (MEDIAL RECTUS) (FIGURE 2.11)

Synonyms

This muscle may also be referred to as rectus internus (Macalister 1875).

Typical Presentation

Description

Medial rectus originates from the common tendinous ring and the dural sheath surrounding the optic nerve and inserts into the medial surface of the sclera (Standring 2016).

Innervation

Medial rectus is innervated by a branch from the inferior division of the oculomotor nerve (Standring 2016).

Comparative Anatomy

In common chimpanzees, orangutans, and gibbons, medial rectus has a similar typical presentation to that of humans (Sonntag 1923, 1924; Diogo et al. 2012).

Variations

Description

Medial rectus may be bifurcated at its insertion (Bergman et al. 1988; Sundaram et al. 2005). Its insertion may also be shifted inferiorly (Matsuo et al. 2009). Medial rectus may

be absent (Bergman et al. 1988; Lee et al. 2013; Kocabiyik 2016). Macalister (1875) observed the partial fusion of inferior rectus and medial rectus in the posterior third of the orbit. A fascicle of lateral rectus may join with medial rectus (Whitnall 1921; Bergman et al. 1988; Kocabiyik 2016). An accessory medial rectus may be present superior and posterior to the insertion of medial rectus (Lee and Kim 2009). Tensor trochleae may send a slip to medial rectus (Sacks 1985).

Prevalence

In a sample of 16 patients with aplasia of the inferior rectus muscle, the insertion of medial rectus was shifted inferiorly in five patients (31.3%) (Matsuo et al. 2009).

Anomalies

Description

In a child with craniosynostosis, the left medial rectus was bifurcated at its insertion (Coats and Ou 2001). In fetuses with anencephaly, there was hypoplasia of medial rectus (Plock et al. 2007). Medial rectus was absent bilaterally in a fetus with trisomy 18 and cyclopia (Smith et al. 2015). In an individual with trisomy 21, medial rectus was doubled on the right side (Fernández-de-Luna et al. 2020). In two fetuses with triploidy, the attachments of the recti onto the sclera were shifted posteriorly (Moen et al. 1984).

Prevalence

N/A

Clinical Implications

The absence of medial rectus may be associated with divergent strabismus (Macalister 1875; Le Double 1897; Lee et al. 2013). A bifid insertion of medial rectus may contribute to intermittent distance exotropia (Sundaram et al. 2005). An accessory medial rectus muscle may be present in cases of strabismus fixus convergens (Lee and Kim 2009). An inferiorly shifted insertion of medial rectus may be associated with microcornea and iris coloboma (Matsuo et al. 2009).

RECTUS LATERALIS (LATERAL RECTUS) (FIGURE 2.11)

Synonyms

This muscle may also be referred to as rectus externus (Macalister 1875).

Typical Presentation

Description

Lateral rectus originates from the common tendinous ring and greater wing of the sphenoid and inserts into the lateral surface of the sclera (Standring 2016).

Innervation

Lateral rectus is innervated by the abducens nerve (Standring 2016).

Comparative Anatomy

In common chimpanzees, orangutans, and gibbons, lateral rectus has a similar typical presentation to that of humans (Sonntag 1923, 1924; Diogo et al. 2012). An accessory lateral rectus is often present in macaque monkeys and considered a remnant of retractor bulbi (Schnyder 1984; Boothe et al. 1990; Liao and Hwang 2014).

Variations

Description

Some authors may describe lateral rectus as having two heads, as it arises via two tendinous bands (Haładaj 2019). It may be bifurcated at its insertion (Duranoğlu and Gözkaya 2005). Its insertion may also be shifted superiorly (Matsuo et al. 2009). Lateral rectus may be absent (Bergman et al. 1988; Zöller et al. 2001; Kocabiyik 2016).

Lateral rectus may send a fascicle to inferior rectus, medial rectus, or the lateral wall of the orbit (Whitnall 1921; Bergman et al. 1988; Kocabiyik 2016). An accessory lateral rectus may be present (Macalister 1875; Bergman et al. 1988; Park and Oh 2003; Liao and Hwang 2014). Lateral rectus is associated with retractor bulbi, which may present as a slip between the superior rectus and lateral rectus (Bergman et al. 1988; Kocabiyik 2016). Nussbaum (1893) described an accessory muscle that originated with lateral rectus and split into three heads that united with the superior, inferior, and lateral recti.

Prevalence

In a sample of 16 patients with aplasia of the inferior rectus muscle, the insertion of lateral rectus was shifted superiorly in one patient (6.3%) (Matsuo et al. 2009).

Anomalies

Description

In fetuses with anencephaly, there was hypoplasia of lateral rectus (Plock et al. 2007). In a fetus with trisomy 18 and cyclopia, lateral rectus received one slip from inferior oblique on the left side, and two slips from inferior oblique on the right side (Smith et al. 2015). In two fetuses with triploidy, the attachments of the recti onto the sclera were shifted posteriorly (Moen et al. 1984). In a child with Axenfeld-Rieger syndrome, the left lateral rectus was absent (Sandall and Morrison 1979).

Prevalence

N/A

Clinical Implications

The absence of lateral rectus may be associated with convergent strabismus (Macalister 1875; Whitnall 1921; Sandall and Morrison 1979; Zöller et al. 2001). Park and Oh (2003) found that an accessory lateral rectus was associated with exotropia, ptosis, pupil dilation, and limited eye movement. Symptoms associated with accessory lateral rectus muscles may be diagnosed as exotropic Duane syndrome (Pineles and Velez 2015; Neves and Curi 2019).

OBLIQUUS OCULI SUPERIOR (SUPERIOR OBLIQUE) (FIGURE 2.11)

See also: Tensor trochleae

Synonyms

N/A

Typical Presentation

Description

Superior oblique originates from the body of the sphenoid (Standring 2016). The muscle ends in a tendon that courses through a trochlea (a cartilaginous loop or pulley) that is attached to the frontal bone (Standring 2016). The tendon inserts into the sclera deep to superior rectus (Standring 2016).

Innervation

Superior oblique is innervated by the trochlear nerve (Standring 2016).

Comparative Anatomy

In common chimpanzees and gibbons, superior oblique has a similar typical presentation to that found in humans (Sonntag 1923; Diogo et al. 2012). In orangutans, the superior oblique runs closely along the medial wall of the orbit and its tendon is connected via fascia to the superior rectus (Sonntag 1924). The tendon does not expand toward the globe (Sonntag 1924).

Variations

Description

The position and length of the tendinous insertion of superior oblique are variable (Whitnall 1921; Howe 1923; Kocabiyik 2016; Haładaj et al. 2020c). The insertion may also be bifurcated (Park et al. 2009a). Superior oblique or its tendon may be absent (Helveston et al. 1981; Matsuo et al. 1988; Drummond and Keech 1989; Wallace and von Noorden 1994; Chan and Demer 1999). There may be a muscular band that connects the insertion of superior oblique with that of inferior oblique (Macalister 1875).

Summarizing Le Double, Whitnall (1921) states that there may be accessory fasciculi associated with the tendon of the superior oblique. In another case, the belly of superior oblique was absent, and the tendon was replaced by muscular fibers that originated from the trochlea (Whitnall 1921). An accessory muscle of levator palpebrae superioris that attaches to the superior oblique may also be referred to as comes obliquus accessorius, obliqui superioris (Albinus), gracillimus orbitis (Bochdalek), or gracillimus oculi (Macalister 1875; Knott 1883a; Bergman et al. 1988). A variant of this slip, tensor trochleae, may insert into the trochlea of superior oblique (see the entry for this muscle).

Prevalence

In a sample of 34 patients diagnosed with congenital superior oblique palsy, Helveston et al. (1981) found the superior oblique tendon absent on at least one side of the body in six patients (17.6%). In a sample of 127 patients with strabismus, Chan and Demer (1999) found superior oblique absent in six patients (4.7%).

Anomalies

Description

The tendon of superior oblique may be absent in individuals with anencephaly, trisomy 21, craniofacial dysostosis, or neurofibromatosis (Barnes and Boniuk 1972; Diamond et al. 1980; Pinchoff and Sandall 1985; Pollard 1988; Newman and Cogen 1997). In a child with Axenfeld-Rieger syndrome, Park et al. (2009b) found that superior oblique inserted more posteriorly than normal.

In two fetuses with triploidy, the attachments of the superior oblique and inferior oblique were shifted anterior to those of the recti (Moen et al. 1984). Superior oblique was absent bilaterally in a fetus with trisomy 18 and cyclopia (Smith et al. 2015). In fetuses with anencephaly, the belly of superior oblique was markedly reduced, and the insertion of the tendon was variable (Plock et al. 2007). In a fetus with occipital meningocele, the superior oblique muscles were very thin (Plock et al. 2007).

Prevalence

Diamond et al. (1980) found the tendon of superior oblique absent bilaterally in one out of five patients (20%) with craniofacial dysostosis. Out of seven patients with Apert syndrome and bilateral superior oblique palsy, Pollard (1988) found that the tendon of superior oblique was absent bilaterally in five patients (71.4%) and superior oblique was replaced by a small fibrous band bilaterally in two patients (28.6).

Clinical Implications

The absence of superior oblique or its tendon may mimic superior oblique palsy and be associated with vertical deviations, horizontal strabismus, or amblyopia (Helveston et al. 1981; Matsuo et al. 1988; Pollard 1988; Wallace and von Noorden 1994; Chan and Demer 1999). A bifid insertion of the superior oblique may cause congenital Brown syndrome (Park et al. 2009a).

Obliquus oculi inferior (Inferior oblique) (Figure 2.11)

Synonyms

N/A

Typical Presentation

Description

Inferior oblique originates from the orbital surface of the maxilla and inserts into the inferolateral surface of the sclera (Standring 2016).

Innervation

Inferior oblique is innervated by a branch from the inferior division of the oculomotor nerve (Standring 2016).

Comparative Anatomy

Inferior oblique has a tendinous insertion in common chimpanzees, but the muscle is entirely fleshy in orangutans (Sonntag 1923, 1924). In common chimpanzees and orangutans, it inserts more posteriorly onto the sclera than in humans (Sonntag 1923, 1924). Diogo et al. (2012) found that inferior oblique in gibbons is similar to that of humans.

Variations

Description

The origin of inferior oblique may be laterally displaced (Whitnall 1921). Some fibers of inferior oblique may originate from the periosteal covering of the lacrimal sac (Whitnall 1921). The size and position of the insertion are variable (Whitnall 1921; Howe 1923; Prakash et al. 1983; Paik and Shin 2009). Inferior oblique may have two bellies (Wilson and Landers 1982; Bergman et al. 1988; DeAngelis et al. 1999; DeAngelis and Kraft 2001; Yalçin and Ozan 2005a). Inferior oblique may also be divided into three or more slips at its insertion (DeAngelis et al. 1999; Yalçin and Ozan 2005a; Paik and Shin 2009).

There may be a muscular band that connects the insertion of superior oblique with that of inferior oblique (Macalister 1875). There may also be a muscular bridge between the inferior rectus and inferior oblique (Yalçin et al. 2004). An accessory inferior oblique, or obliquus accessorius inferior, extends between the apex of the orbit and inferior oblique and may send a slip to inferior rectus (Rex 1887; Whitnall 1921; Bergman et al. 1988; Kocabiyik 2016; Richardson et al. 2017). The case described by Richardson et al. (2017) inserted into the inferior oblique and the lower eyelid.

Prevalence

In a sample of 100 orbits, Whitnall (1921) found that the origin of inferior oblique was adjacent (<1 mm away) to the nasolacrimal fossa in 45 cases (45%), 2 mm away from the edge of the nasolacrimal fossa in 14 cases (14%), 3 mm away in 19 cases (19%), 4 mm away in eight cases (8%), 5 mm away in six cases (6%), 6 mm away in four cases (4%), and 7 mm away in four cases (4%).

In a sample of 100 orbits, DeAngelis et al. (1999) found that 17 inferior oblique muscles (17%) had multiple divisions upon insertion. Eight inferior oblique muscles (8%) had two bellies. In four of these cases, the two bellies shared an insertion and in the other four cases, the two bellies had separate insertions (DeAngelis et al. 1999). DeAngelis and Kraft (2001) found 27 doubled-bellied inferior oblique muscles out of a sample of 247 muscles (10.9%).

In a sample of 60 orbits, Yalçin et al. (2004) found a muscular bridge between inferior rectus and inferior oblique in four orbits (6.7%). In a sample of 60 orbits, Yalçin and Ozan (2005a) studied how many bellies of inferior oblique were present at insertion. There was a single belly in five cases (8.3%), two bellies in 30 cases (50%), three bellies in 16 cases (26.7%), and more than three bellies in nine cases (15%). Paik and Shin (2009) studied how many bellies of inferior oblique were present at insertion in 62 orbits.

Inferior oblique had a single belly in 44 cases (71%), two bellies in 14 cases (22.5%), three bellies in two cases (3.2%), and four bellies in two cases (3.2%).

Anomalies

Description

Inferior oblique may be absent in individuals with anencephaly or craniofacial dysostosis (Diamond et al. 1980; Plock et al. 2007). In fetuses with anencephaly that had inferior oblique muscles, Diamond et al. (1980) found they were reduced in size. In two fetuses with triploidy, the attachments of the superior oblique and inferior oblique were shifted anterior to those of the recti (Moen et al. 1984). In a fetus with trisomy 18 and cyclopia, both inferior oblique muscles sent a slip to lateral rectus and had another slip that fused with its counterpart on the other side (Smith et al. 2015). On the right side, an additional slip inserted into lateral rectus, and on the left side, a slip passed to an accessory band of muscle parallel to the limbus of the eye (Smith et al. 2015). In an infant with mandibulofacial dysostosis, inferior oblique originated from an enlarged and poorly ossified fossa for the lacrimal sac (Herring et al. 1979).

Prevalence

Diamond et al. (1980) found the inferior oblique absent bilaterally in one out of five patients (20%) with craniofacial dysostosis. Plock et al. (2007) found inferior oblique absent unilaterally in 2 out of 15 anencephalic fetuses (13.3%).

Clinical Implications

The absence of inferior oblique may cause ptosis (Poscy 1923). DeAngelis and Kraft (2001) found that eyes with double-bellied inferior oblique muscles had a higher incidence of fundus excyclotropia. A band from the apex of the orbit to the inferior oblique and lower eyelid may cause congenital paradoxical lower eyelid retraction (Richardson et al. 2017). A variant insertion of inferior oblique may be associated with divergent strabismus (Prakash et al. 1983).

SCALENE, PREVERTEBRAL, AND SUBOCCIPITAL MUSCLES

SCALENUS ANTERIOR (ANTERIOR SCALENE) (FIGURE 2.12)

See also: Roos band, scalenus minimus

Synonyms

This muscle may also be referred to as scalenus anticus (Macalister 1875).

Typical Presentation

Description

Scalenus anterior originates from the anterior tubercles of the transverse processes of the third through sixth cervical vertebrae (Standring 2016). It inserts onto the scalene tubercle and superior margin of the first rib (Standring 2016).

Innervation

Scalenus anterior is innervated by the ventral rami of the fourth through sixth cervical spinal nerves (Standring 2016).

Comparative Anatomy

Scalenus anterior has a similar typical presentation in the apes, extending from the transverse processes of various cervical vertebrae to the first rib (Stewart 1936; Sonntag 1923, 1924; Miller 1952; Gibbs 1999; Diogo et al. 2010, 2012, 2013a,b, 2017). The origin is typically from the third through fifth or fourth through sixth cervical vertebrae (Stewart 1936; Sonntag 1923, 1924; Miller 1952; Gibbs 1999). It may originate from only the fifth and sixth cervical vertebrae in gorillas (Raven 1950). There may be an attachment to the seventh cervical vertebra in common chimpanzees (Champneys 1872).

Variations

Description

The origin of scalenus anterior may vary in terms of which vertebrae contribute fascicles to the muscle (Macalister 1875; Knott 1883a; Mori 1964; Rusnak-Smith et al. 2001; Bergman et al. 1988; Sakamoto 2012, 2016b). Its costal attachment may also vary (Bergman et al. 1988; Wayman et al. 1993; Sakamoto 2016b). Width of the anterior scalene varies among individuals (Rusnak-Smith et al. 2001). The lower third of the muscle may be tendinous (Macalister 1875). The muscle may be divided into two bellies (Macalister 1875; Goubran et al. 2010; Sakamoto 2016b; Perumal et al. 2018).

Scalenus anterior may exchange fibers with scalenus medius or scalenus minimus (Wood 1867b; Macalister 1875; Rajanigandha et al. 2008; Sakamoto 2012, 2016b). Its fibers may be continuous with longus capitis or the intertransverse muscles (Macalister 1875; Rusnak-Smith et al. 2001; Sakamoto 2016b). Scalenus anterior may be absent (Macalister 1875; Murakami et al. 2003; Collins et al. 2014). In the case reported by Murakami et al. (2003), scalenus anterior was replaced by aberrant muscle slips that originated from the lower cervical vertebrae and joined with scalenus medius.

An accessory anterior scalene muscle may be present (Bergman et al. 1988; Sakamoto 2016b). Scalenus anterior may be associated with transversalis cervicis medius (Krause), which originates from the second and fourth cervical vertebrae and inserts into the seventh and eighth cervical vertebrae (Knott 1883a; Bergman et al. 1988). A Roos band may extend from anterior scalene to subclavius and the costal cartilage (see the entry for this muscle).

Prevalence

In a sample of 240 sides (120 cadavers), Mori (1964) found that scalenus anterior arose from the second through fifth cervical vertebrae on eight sides (3.3%), from the third through fifth cervical vertebrae on 108 sides (45%), and from the fourth through sixth cervical vertebrae on 124 sides (51.7%). In a sample of ten cadavers, Rusnak-Smith et al. (2001) found that scalenus anterior arose from the third through sixth cervical vertebrae in two cases (20%), from the third through seventh cervical vertebrae in three cases (30%), from the fourth and fifth cervical vertebrae in two cases (20%), and from the fourth through sixth cervical vertebrae in three cases (30%). Tendinous fibers of scalenus anterior blended with longus capitis in one case (10%).

In a sample of 52 cadaveric sides, Sakamoto (2012) found that scalenus anterior originated from the fifth and sixth cervical vertebrae on three sides (5.8%), from the fourth through sixth cervical vertebrae on 26 sides (50%), and from the third through sixth cervical vertebrae on 23 sides (44.2%). Scalenus anterior sent fibers to scalenus minimus on one side (1.9%). Scalenus anterior and the ventral part of scalenus medius exchanged fibers on seven sides (13.5%).

Anomalies

Description

The right anterior scalene muscle was absent in a fetus with craniorachischisis (Alghamdi et al. 2017).

Prevalence

N/A

Clinical Implications

An anteriorly shifted insertion of scalenus anterior may cause venous compression syndromes in the root of the neck (Wayman et al. 1993). Blending of some anterior scalene fibers with longus capitis may cause tension and headaches in the occipital region (Rusnak-Smith et al. 2001). A relatively wide scalenus anterior muscle may impinge the surrounding structures, leading to vascular compromise causing symptoms of coldness and pallor (Rusnak-Smith et al. 2001). Compression of the subclavian artery between the two bellies of a divided scalenus anterior may lead to the development of vascular thoracic outlet syndrome (Goubran et al. 2010). The absence of scalenus anterior may present with the symptoms of thoracic outlet syndrome (Collins et al. 2014). A Roos band that arises from scalenus anterior and attaches to subclavius and the costal cartilage may cause subclavian vein compression (Spears et al. 2011).

SCALENUS MEDIUS (MIDDLE SCALENE) (FIGURE 2.12)

See also: Roos band

Synonyms

N/A

Typical Presentation

Description

Scalenus medius originates from the transverse processes of the second through seventh cervical vertebrae (Standring 2016). It inserts into the superior margin of the first rib (Standring 2016).

Innervation

Scalenus medius is innervated by the ventral rami of the third through eighth cervical spinal nerves (Standring 2016).

Comparative Anatomy

In the apes, scalenus medius and scalenus posterior are fused, and the combined muscle complex typically originates from the second through sixth or seventh cervical vertebrae and inserts onto the first rib (Sonntag 1923, 1924; Stewart 1936; Miller 1952; Jouffroy 1971; Gibbs 1999; Diogo et al. 2010, 2012, 2013a,b, 2017). In common chimpanzees, there may be an insertion onto the second rib (Macalister 1871). In one common chimpanzee, Sonntag (1923) found that the scalenus medius-posterior muscle sheet attached to the first five ribs.

Variations

Description

The origin of scalenus medius may vary in terms of which vertebrae contribute fascicles to the muscle (Macalister 1875; Knott 1883a; Cave 1933; Bergman et al. 1988; Rusnak-Smith et al. 2001; Sakamoto 2012, 2016b; Standring 2016). It often has an origin from the transverse process of the first cervical vertebra (Wood 1867b; Macalister 1875; Cave 1933; Bergman et al. 1988; Rusnak-Smith et al. 2001; Sakamoto 2016b; Standring 2016). Fibers of scalenus medius may originate from a cervical rib when this structure is present (Tokat et al. 2011). The insertion of scalenus medius onto the first rib may be shifted anteriorly to just behind the anterior scalene (Thomas et al. 1983). It may also insert partially or entirely into the second rib (Macalister 1875; Knott 1883a; Sakamoto 2012, 2016b). Width of the middle scalene varies among individuals (Rusnak-Smith et al. 2001). Scalenus medius may be absent (Macalister 1875).

Scalenus medius may exchange fibers with scalenus anterior (Wood 1867b; Macalister 1875; Rajanigandha et al. 2008; Sakamoto 2012, 2016b). Paraskevas et al. (2007) found an accessory middle scalene that arose from the middle portion of scalenus medius and inserted with scalenus anterior onto the first rib. Scalenus medius may be fused with scalenus posterior (Macalister 1875; Knott 1883a; Cave 1933; Rusnak-Smith et al. 2001; Sakamoto 2016b; Standring 2016). It may also join with multifidus or semispinalis cervicis (Macalister 1875). It may send a slip to levator scapulae (Macalister 1875; Wood 1867b, 1868). A Roos band may originate from the middle scalene and attach to the first rib or its cartilage (see the entry for this muscle).

Prevalence

Out of 60 subjects, Cave (1933) found that scalenus medius originated from all cervical vertebrae in 37 subjects (61.7%), from the second through seventh cervical vertebrae in nine cases (15%), from the third through seventh cervical vertebrae in six cases (10%), and from the third through sixth cervical vertebrae in six cases (10%). The origins could not be determined in two cases (3.3%). In a sample of 29 arms, Thomas et al. (1983) found that scalenus medius inserted anteriorly and behind anterior scalene in 14 arms (483%). In a sample of ten cadavers, Rusnak-Smith et al. (2001) found that scalenus medius originated from all cervical vertebrae in five cases (50%), from the second through seventh cervical vertebrae in one case (10%), and from the second through sixth cervical vertebrae in four cases (40%). Scalenus medius was fused with scalenus posterior in three cases (30%).

In a sample of 52 cadaveric sides, Sakamoto (2012) found that the ventral part of scalenus medius originated from the fourth through seventh cervical vertebrae on 42 sides (80.8%) and from the third through seventh cervical vertebrae on ten sides (19.2%). The ventral part of scalenus medius inserted onto the first rib on 42 sides (80.8%) and onto both the first and second ribs on ten sides (19.2%). Scalenus anterior and the ventral part of scalenus medius exchanged fibers on seven sides (13.5%). The dorsal part of scalenus medius originated from the third through seventh cervical vertebrae on two sides (3.8%), from the second through seventh cervical vertebrae on seven sides (13.5%), and from all cervical vertebrae on 43 sides (82.7%).

Anomalies

Description

In a boy with trisomy 13q, scalenus medius inserted onto the first and second ribs on the right side and to the first rib only on the left side (Pettersen 1979). In a fetus with craniorachischisis, levator scapulae fused with the distal portion of scalenus medius on the left side (Alghamdi et al. 2017).

Prevalence

N/A

Clinical Implications

An anterior insertion of scalenus medius (Thomas et al. 1983) or the presence of an accessory middle scalene (Paraskevas et al. 2007) may cause thoracic outlet syndrome. Fusion of scalenus medius and scalenus posterior may compromise the long thoracic and dorsal scapular nerves, leading to shoulder pain and weakness of levator scapulae, serratus anterior, and the rhomboid muscles (Rusnak-Smith et al. 2001).

SCALENUS POSTERIOR (POSTERIOR SCALENE) (FIGURE 2.12)

Synonyms

This muscle may also be referred to as scalenus posticus (Macalister 1875).

Typical Presentation

Description

Scalenus posterior originates from the posterior tubercles of the transverse processes of the fourth through sixth cervical vertebrae (Standring 2016). It inserts onto the outer aspect of the second rib (Standring 2016).

Innervation

Scalenus posterior is innervated by the ventral rami of the sixth through eighth cervical spinal nerves (Standring 2016).

Comparative Anatomy

In the apes, scalenus medius and scalenus posterior are fused, and the combined muscle complex typically originates from the second through sixth or seventh cervical vertebrae and inserts onto the first rib (Sonntag 1923, 1924; Stewart 1936; Miller 1952; Jouffroy 1971; Gibbs 1999; Diogo et al. 2010, 2012, 2013a,b, 2017). In common chimpanzees, there may be an insertion onto the second rib (Macalister 1871). In one common chimpanzee, Sonntag (1923) found that the scalenus medius-posterior muscle sheet attached to the first five ribs.

Variations

Description

The origin of scalenus posterior may vary in terms of which vertebrae contribute fascicles to the muscle (Mori 1964; Bergman et al. 1988; Rusnak-Smith et al. 2001; Sakamoto 2012, 2016b). It inserts variously into the first three ribs (Macalister 1875; Knott 1883a; Mori 1964; Bergman et al. 1988; Rusnak-Smith et al. 2001; Sakamoto 2012, 2016b). The muscle may be divided into three separate portions, one portion inserting onto each of the first three ribs (Macalister 1875). Width of the posterior scalene varies among individuals (Rusnak-Smith et al. 2001). Scalenus posterior may be absent (Macalister 1875; Knott 1883a; Rusnak-Smith et al. 2001; Sakamoto 2012, 2016b).

Scalenus posterior may be fused with scalenus medius (Macalister 1875; Knott 1883a; Cave 1933; Rusnak-Smith et al. 2001; Standring 2016). It may also be fused with the first external intercostal muscle (Bergman et al. 1988). Scalenus posterior may also connect with serratus anterior, levator scapulae, or the first levator costae (Wood 1868; Macalister 1875; Rickenbacher et al. 1985; Smith et al. 2003; Bakkum and Miller 2016).

Prevalence

In a sample of 102 cadaveric sides, Mori (1964) found that scalenus posterior inserted into the first rib on 21 sides (20.6%), the first and second ribs on 71 sides (69.6%), and the first three ribs on nine sides (8.8%). In a sample of ten cadavers, Rusnak-Smith et al. (2001) found that scalenus posterior originated from the fourth through sixth cervical vertebrae in two cases (20%), from the fourth and fifth cervical vertebrae in two cases (20%), and from the fifth and sixth cervical vertebrae in four cases (40%). Scalenus posterior inserted into the third rib in one case (10%). The muscle was absent in two cases (20%). Scalenus medius was fused with scalenus posterior in three cases (30%).

In a sample of 52 cadaveric sides, Sakamoto (2012) found that scalenus posterior originated from the fifth cervical vertebra only on 25 sides (61%), from the fifth and sixth cervical vertebrae on nine sides (21.9%), from the fourth through sixth cervical vertebrae on four sides (9.8%), from the fourth and fifth cervical vertebrae on two sides (4.9%), and from the third and fourth cervical vertebrae on one side (2.4%). Scalenus posterior inserted onto the first rib on two sides (4.9%), onto the second rib on 28 sides (68.3%), onto

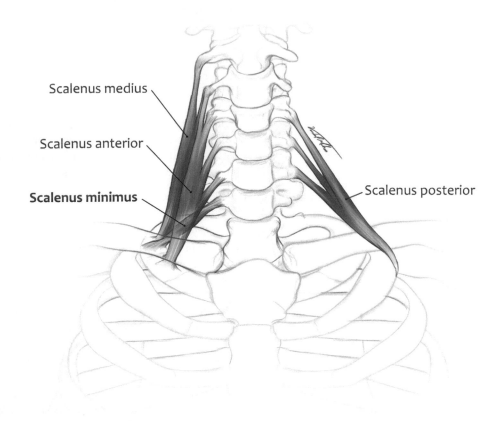

FIGURE 2.12   Lateral vertebral muscles in anterior view.

the first and second ribs on eight sides (19.5%), and onto the second and third ribs on three sides (7.3%). Scalenus posterior was absent on 11 sides (21.2%).

Anomalies

Description
The origin of scalenus posterior may blend with levator scapulae in individuals with trisomy 18 (Smith et al. 2015).

Prevalence
In their literature review, Smith et al. (2015) found that the origin of scalenus posterior was blended with levator scapulae in 1 out of 26 individuals with trisomy 18 (3.8%).

Clinical Implications
A relatively wide scalenus posterior muscle may affect the long thoracic nerve and dorsal scapular nerve, causing pain and tension in serratus anterior and levator scapulae (Rusnak-Smith et al. 2001). Fusion of scalenus medius and scalenus posterior may also compromise the long thoracic and dorsal scapular nerves, leading to shoulder pain and weakness of levator scapulae, serratus anterior, and the rhomboid muscles (Rusnak-Smith et al. 2001).

SCALENUS MINIMUS (FIGURE 2.12)

See also: Roos band

Synonyms
This muscle may also be referred to as scalenus pleuralis (Sibson) or scalenus intermedius (Testut) (Bergman et al. 1988; Standring 2016).

Typical Presentation
This muscle is present only as a variation.

Comparative Anatomy
In a gorilla, Stewart (1936) reported a slip that extended from the transverse processes of the sixth and seventh cervical vertebrae to the first rib, which may correspond to scalenus minimus. Diogo et al. (2017) found scalenus minimus in one bonobo extending between the transverse process of the seventh cervical vertebra and the first rib.

Variations

Description
Scalenus minimus originates from the transverse process of the seventh cervical vertebra and inserts onto the first rib just behind the groove for the subclavian artery, and into the cervical pleura (Fawcett 1896; Shore 1926; Stott 1928;

Boyd 1934; Rickenbacher et al. 1985; Bergman et al. 1988; Rusnak-Smith et al. 2001; Natsis et al. 2013; Sakamoto 2012, 2016b; Standring 2016).

It may sometimes have an origin from the sixth cervical vertebra (Bergman et al. 1988; Rusnak-Smith et al. 2001; Sakamoto 2012, 2016b). Some early accounts report that scalenus minimus extends from the fifth through seventh cervical vertebrae to the second rib (Macalister 1875; Knott 1883a). Under the Roos band classification scheme, a type 5 band is the scalenus minimus muscle attached to the first rib between the subclavian artery and the brachial plexus, and a type 6 band is the scalenus minimus muscle attached only to the cervical pleura (Roos 1976; entry for this muscle).

Scalenus minimus may exchange fibers with scalenus anterior (Sakamoto 2012). If scalenus minimus is not present, a fibrous band often referred to as the scalenus medius band may take its place (Shore 1926; Bonney 1965; Thomas et al. 1983; Bergman et al. 1988; Sakamoto 2016b).

Innervation

Scalenus minimus is innervated by the seventh and eighth cervical spinal nerves (Sakamoto 2012).

Prevalence

Knott (1883a) found scalenus minimus in 5 out of 23 bodies (21.7%). Stott (1928) found scalenus minimus on 39 out of 100 cadaveric sides (39%). In a sample of 30 cadaveric sides, Boyd (1934) found scalenus minimus on ten sides (33.3%). In a sample of 29 arms, Thomas et al. (1983) found scalenus minimus in one case (3%). In a sample of 102 cadaveric sides, Harry et al. (1997) found scalenus minimus in 46% of sides. In a sample of 10 cadavers, Rusnak-Smith et al. (2001) found scalenus minimus definitively present in one cadaver (10%) and potentially present in two other cadavers (20%). Natsis et al. (2013) found scalenus minimus in 3 out of 73 cadavers (4.1%).

Out of 241 patients that underwent surgery for thoracic outlet syndrome, Roos (1976) found type 5 bands in 40 cases (16.6%) and type 6 bands in five cases (2.1%). Out of 58 thoracic outlet dissections in 29 cadavers, Roos (1976) found type 5 bands present in eight cases (13.8%). Out of 100 cases, Spears et al. (2011) found type 5 bands in 11 cases (11%).

In a sample of 52 cadaveric sides, Sakamoto (2012) found that scalenus minimus was present on 25 sides (48.1%). Out of these 25 cases, it originated from the sixth cervical vertebra on two sides (8%), from the seventh cervical vertebra on 14 sides (56%), and from both the sixth and seventh cervical vertebrae on nine sides (36%). Scalenus anterior sent fibers to scalenus minimus on one side (1.9%).

Anomalies
N/A

Clinical Implications

Scalenus minimus may compress the brachial plexus and/or subclavian artery and cause thoracic outlet syndrome (Levi 1948; Harry et al. 1997; Rusnak-Smith et al. 2001; Natsis et al. 2013).

LONGUS COLLI (FIGURE 2.13)

Synonyms

This muscle may also be referred to as rectus colli (Luschka) or longus cervicis (Macalister 1875; Rusnak-Smith et al. 2001).

Typical Presentation

Description

Longus colli is divided into inferior oblique, vertical (intermediate), and superior oblique parts (Standring 2016). The inferior oblique part originates from the bodies of the first three thoracic vertebrae and inserts onto the transverse processes of the fifth and sixth cervical vertebrae (Standring 2016). The vertical part originates from the bodies of the fifth cervical through third thoracic vertebrae and inserts onto the bodies of the second through fourth cervical vertebrae (Standring 2016). The superior oblique part originates from the transverse processes of the third through fifth cervical vertebrae and inserts onto the anterior tubercle of the first cervical vertebra (Standring 2016).

Innervation

Longus colli is innervated by the ventral rami of the second through sixth cervical spinal nerves (Standring 2016).

Comparative Anatomy

There is no information available for gibbons. In orangutans, the superior oblique part is typically absent, while the inferior oblique and vertical parts originate from the seventh cervical through the fifth thoracic vertebrae and insert onto the first cervical vertebra (Sonntag 1924). In gorillas, there is no origin from the thoracic vertebrae (Gibbs 1999; Raven 1950; Diogo et al. 2010). The presentation in common chimpanzees and bonobos is most like that of humans, with similar origins and insertions (Gibbs 1999; Sonntag 1923; Miller 1952; Diogo et al. 2013a, 2017).

Variations

Description

Longus colli may vary in terms of which structures it arises from and inserts into (Macalister 1875; Rickenbacher et al. 1985; Bergman et al. 1988; Sakamoto 2012, 2016b). It may have an origin from the body of the fourth thoracic vertebra (Eisler 1912; Rickenbacher et al. 1985; Sakamoto 2016b). It may also originate from the heads of the first, second, or third rib (Eisler 1912; Rickenbacher et al. 1985; Sakamoto 2016b). The origins from the bodies of the thoracic vertebrae or lower cervical vertebrae may be absent (Rickenbacher et al. 1985). The most superior bundles of the muscle may insert into the base of the skull (Rickenbacher et al. 1985).

Longus colli may be thin or absent (Macalister 1875). Longus colli may fuse with or send bundles to longus capitis (Macalister 1875; Rickenbacher et al. 1985; Bergman et al. 1988; Sakamoto 2012, 2016b). It may be associated with an accessory intertransverse muscle referred to as transversalis cervicis anticus (Retzius), which extends from the fourth through sixth cervical vertebrae to the first three cervical vertebrae (Macalister 1875; Knott 1883a; Bakkum and Miller 2016; Sakamoto 2016b).

Prevalence

In a sample of 52 cadaveric sides, Sakamoto (2012) found that the vertical and inferior oblique parts were fused at their origins, with their lowermost origin from the third thoracic vertebra on 15 sides (28.9%), from the second thoracic vertebra on 36 sides (69.2%), and from the first thoracic vertebra on one side (1.9%). The inferior oblique part inserted onto the fifth and sixth cervical vertebrae on 44 sides (84.7%), the sixth cervical vertebra on two sides (3.8%), the fourth and fifth cervical vertebrae on two sides (3.8%), and the fourth through sixth cervical vertebrae on four sides (7.7%). The vertical part originated from the fifth cervical vertebra on one side (1.9%), from the fourth and fifth cervical vertebrae on three sides (5.8%), from the fifth and sixth cervical vertebrae on 18 sides (34.6%), from the fourth through sixth cervical vertebrae on 24 sides (46.2%), and from the third through sixth cervical vertebrae on six sides (11.5%). The superior oblique part originated from the third through fifth cervical vertebrae on 26 sides (50%), the third and fourth cervical vertebrae on 17 sides (32.7%), from the second through fourth cervical vertebrae on one side (1.9%), from the second through fifth cervical vertebrae on four sides (7.7%), and from the third through sixth cervical vertebrae on four sides (7.7%). Longus capitis and the inferior oblique part connected via tendinous fibers on 43 sides (82.7%).

Anomalies
N/A

Clinical Implications
N/A

LONGUS CAPITIS (FIGURE 2.13)

Synonyms
This muscle may also be referred to as rectus capitis anticus major (Macalister 1875).

Typical Presentation

Description
Longus capitis originates from the anterior tubercles of the transverse processes of the third through sixth cervical vertebrae and inserts into the basilar part of the occipital bone (Standring 2016).

Innervation
Longus capitis is innervated by the ventral rami of the first through third cervical spinal nerves (Standring 2016).

Comparative Anatomy
There is no information available for gibbons. The muscle has a similar typical presentation to that of humans in the other apes, extending from the transverses processes of the cervical vertebrae to the basiocciput (Sonntag 1923, 1924; Raven 1950; Miller 1952; Dean 1985; Gibbs 1999; Diogo et al. 2010, 2013a,b, 2017). It may originate from the second through sixth cervical vertebrae in gorillas (Raven 1950) and from the second through fifth (Diogo et al. 2017) or fourth through seventh cervical vertebrae (Miller 1952) in bonobos. It may receive a slip from the anterior scalene in common chimpanzees (Sonntag 1923).

Variations

Description
Longus capitis may vary in terms of which structures it arises from and inserts into (Macalister 1875; Rickenbacher et al. 1985; Bergman et al. 1988; Sakamoto 2012, 2016b). It may have additional origins from the first and/or second cervical vertebrae (Macalister 1875; Rickenbacher et al. 1985; Sakamoto 2012, 2016b). The origin from the fifth or sixth cervical vertebrae may be absent (Macalister 1875; Rickenbacher et al. 1985; Sakamoto 2016b). At its insertion, fibers may decussate with those of the contralateral muscle (Rickenbacher et al. 1985). Longus capitis may split into two muscles or multiple fascicles (Macalister 1875; Knott 1883a; Rickenbacher et al. 1985). It may also be bilaminar (Macalister 1875). Longus capitis may fuse with longus colli (Macalister 1875; Rickenbacher et al. 1985; Bergman et al. 1988; Sakamoto 2012, 2016b). It may also connect with the anterior scalene, rectus capitis anterior, or intertransverse muscles (Macalister 1875; Bergman et al. 1988; Sakamoto 2016b).

Longus capitis is associated with atlantobasilaris internus (Gruber), which originates from the anterior tubercle of the first cervical vertebra, courses along the medial margin of longus capitis, and inserts near longus capitis into the base of the skull (Rickenbacher et al. 1985; Bergman et al. 1988; Sakamoto 2016b). If the insertion of this accessory muscle is shifted onto the anterior longitudinal ligament, it is referred to as axobasilaris or axiobasilaris (Rickenbacher et al. 1985). If it originates from the second cervical vertebra, it is referred to as epistropheobasilaris (Gruber) (Bergman et al. 1988; Sakamoto 2016b).

Prevalence
Likely summarizing the work of Gruber, Rickenbacher at al. (1985) states that atlantobasilaris internus is present in about 4% of subjects and axobasilaris is present in about 2% of subjects. In a sample of 52 cadaveric sides, Sakamoto (2012) found that longus capitis originated from the third through sixth cervical vertebrae on 32 sides (61.5%) and from the second through sixth cervical vertebrae on 20 sides (38.5%). Longus capitis and the inferior oblique part of longus colli connected via tendinous fibers on 43 sides (82.7%).

Anomalies

N/A

Clinical Implications

N/A

RECTUS CAPITIS ANTERIOR (FIGURE 2.13)

Synonyms

This muscle may also be referred to as rectus capitis anticus minor (Macalister 1875).

Typical Presentation

Description

Rectus capitis anterior originates on the first cervical vertebra from the lateral mass and base of the transverse process (Standring 2016). It inserts into the basilar part of the occipital bone (Standring 2016).

Innervation

Rectus capitis anterior is innervated by the ventral rami of the first and second cervical spinal nerves (Standring 2016).

Comparative Anatomy

Rectus capitis anterior has a similar typical presentation in apes, extending from the first cervical vertebra to the basilar part of the occipital bone (Sonntag 1923, 1924; Raven 1950; Dean 1985; Gibbs 1999; Diogo et al. 2010, 2012, 2013a,b, 2017).

Variations

Description

Rectus capitis anterior may be reduced or absent (Macalister 1875; Rickenbacher et al. 1985; Bergman et al. 1988; Sakamoto 2016b). It may insert exclusively into the anterior atlanto-occipital ligament (Macalister 1875; Rickenbacher et al. 1985; Bergman et al. 1988; Sakamoto 2016b). It may receive a slip from the second cervical vertebra (Macalister 1875). It may connect with longus capitis (Macalister 1875). Rectus capitis anterior may be doubled (Macalister 1875; Knott 1883a; Rickenbacher et al. 1985). There may be a separate bundle along its medial border, rectus capitis minimus, that originates from the anterior arch of the first cervical vertebra (Macalister 1875; Rickenbacher et al. 1985; Bergman et al. 1988; Sakamoto 2016b). If the origin of this bundle is shifted inferiorly over the lateral atlantoaxial joint, it may be referred to as rectus capitis anterior medius (Eisler) (Rickenbacher et al. 1985).

Prevalence

Rickenbacher et al. (1985) state that rectus capitis anterior is reduced or absent in 4% of cases and rectus capitis anterior medius is present in 10%–12% of cases.

Anomalies

N/A

Clinical Implications

N/A

RECTUS CAPITIS LATERALIS (FIGURE 2.13)

Synonyms

N/A

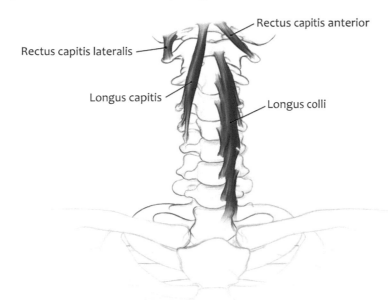

FIGURE 2.13   Anterior vertebral muscles in anterior view.

Typical Presentation

Description

Rectus capitis lateralis originates from the transverse process of the first cervical vertebra and inserts into the jugular process of the occipital bone (Standring 2016).

Innervation

Rectus capitis lateralis is innervated by the ventral rami of the first and second cervical spinal nerves (Standring 2016).

Comparative Anatomy

Rectus capitis lateralis has a similar typical presentation in apes, inserting from the transverse process of the first cervical vertebra to the jugular process of the occipital bone (Sonntag 1923; Raven 1950; Dean 1984; Gibbs 1999; Diogo et al. 2010, 2012, 2013a,b, 2017). Rectus capitis lateralis may be absent in some orangutans (Gibbs 1999; Sonntag 1924).

Variations

Description

Rectus capitis lateralis may be deficient (Macalister 1875). The muscle may be fan-shaped (Macalister 1875; Rickenbacher et al. 1985). Levator scapulae may fuse with the inferior attachment of rectus capitis lateralis (Gonzales et al. 2017). Rectus capitis lateralis may be doubled (Macalister 1875; Rickenbacher et al. 1985). The accessory belly may be referred to as rectus capitis lateralis accessorius (Winslow) (Macalister 1875; Knott 1883a). A rectus capitis lateralis longus (Otto) may be present, extending from the transverse process of the second cervical vertebra to the occipital bone (Macalister 1875; Rickenbacher et al. 1985; Bergman et al. 1988; Sakamoto 2016b).

Prevalence

Knott (1883a) found rectus capitis lateralis accessorius in 3 out of 33 subjects (9.1%).

Anomalies

Description

Rectus capitis lateralis may be absent in individuals with atlas assimilation, or in individuals with a well-developed paracondylar process that articulates with the transverse process of the atlas (Rickenbacher et al. 1985).

Prevalence

N/A

Clinical Implications

Fusion of levator scapulae with the origin of rectus capitis lateralis may cause greater flexion of the craniocervical junction (Gonzales et al. 2017).

RECTUS CAPITIS POSTERIOR MAJOR (FIGURE 2.14)

Synonyms

This muscle may also be referred to as rectus capitis posticus major or rectus capitis posterior superficialis (Macalister 1875; Bakkum and Miller 2016).

Typical Presentation

Description

Rectus capitis posterior major originates from the spinous process of the second cervical vertebra (Standring 2016). It inserts onto the occipital bone along the lateral half of the inferior nuchal line and onto the bone just below the line (Standring 2016).

Innervation

Rectus capitis posterior major is innervated by the suboccipital nerve (Standring 2016).

Comparative Anatomy

Rectus capitis posterior major has a similar typical presentation in the apes, extending from the spinous process of the second cervical vertebra to the occipital bone (Sonntag 1923, 1924; Raven 1950; Miller 1952; Gibbs 1999; Diogo et al. 2010, 2012, 2013a,b, 2017). Sonntag (1923) notes that the rectus capitis posterior major muscles mostly conceal the rectus capitis posterior minor muscles in common chimpanzees. The rectus capitis posterior minor muscles are concealed to a lesser extent in orangutans (Sonntag 1924). Grider-Potter (2017) found an accessory suboccipital muscle in one gibbon. It had the same origin and insertion as rectus capitis posterior major but was situated lateral and deep to that muscle and deep to obliquus capitis superior. This location is similar to that of the rectus capitis posterior medius muscle found in cats.

Variations

Description

Rectus capitis posterior major may contact its counterpart at the midline such that the rectus capitis posterior minor muscles are not visible (Mori 1964). Rectus capitis posterior major may receive accessory slips from the spine of the third cervical vertebra or the ligamentum nuchae (Rickenbacher et al. 1985). It may also receive slips from the spinalis or semispinalis (Macalister 1875), or from rectus capitis posterior minor or obliquus capitis inferior (Mori 1964). There may be a soft-tissue connection (myodural bridge) between rectus capitis posterior major and the dura mater in the atlanto-axial interspace (Scali et al. 2011, 2013; Bakkum and Miller 2016).

Rectus capitis posterior major may be doubled (Wood 1867b; Macalister 1875; Mori 1964; Rickenbacher et al. 1985; Tagil et al. 2005; Nayak et al. 2011; Bakkum and Miller 2016). When doubled, the more lateral belly may extend to near rectus capitis lateralis (Rickenbacher et al. 1985). Loukas and Tubbs (2007) describe an accessory

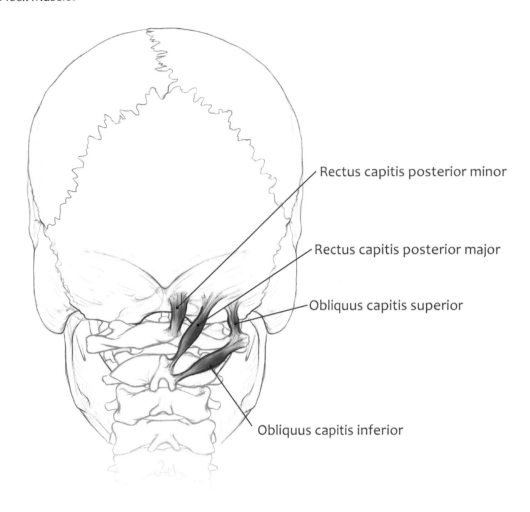

Rectus capitis posterior minor

Rectus capitis posterior major

Obliquus capitis superior

Obliquus capitis inferior

FIGURE 2.14 Suboccipital muscles in posterior view.

suboccipital muscle that originated from the spinous process of the second cervical vertebra inferior to rectus capitis posterior major and inserted into the inferior nuchal line lateral and posterior to the insertion of rectus capitis posterior major.

Prevalence

In a sample of 13 cadavers, 11 cadavers (84.6%) had connections between rectus capitis posterior major and the dura mater in the atlanto-axial interspace (Scali et al. 2011). In a sample of 112 cadavers, Mori (1964) found rectus capitis posterior major with a typical presentation bilaterally in 84 cadavers (75%), on the right side only in seven cadavers (6.3%), and on the left side only in six cadavers (5.4%). The muscle was longitudinally split into two parts bilaterally in three cadavers (2.7%), on the right side only in one cadaver (0.9%), and on the left side only in two cadavers (1.8%). Rectus capitis posterior major received accessory slips from rectus capitis posterior

minor bilaterally in three cadavers (2.7%), on the right side only in two cadavers (1.8%), and on the left side only in nine cadavers (8%). The left rectus capitis posterior major muscle received a slip from obliquus capitis inferior in one cadaver (0.9%).

Anomalies

Description

When the spinous process of the second cervical vertebra is absent, rectus capitis posterior major may originate from the spinous process of the third cervical vertebra (Asakawa et al. 1999). In an individual with atlas assimilation, the right rectus capitis posterior major muscle was comprised of two fan-shaped bellies, and the left muscle was reduced in size (Ciołkowski et al. 2014).

Prevalence

N/A

Clinical Implications

The myodural communication between rectus capitis posterior major and the dura mater may monitor dural tension or be involved in some cervicogenic pathologies (Scali et al. 2011, 2013). A doubled rectus capitis posterior major may strain the spine of the second cervical vertebra or contribute to cervicogenic headaches (Nayak et al. 2011). Accessory muscles like the one described by Loukas and Tubbs (2007) may compress the vertebral artery.

RECTUS CAPITIS POSTERIOR MINOR (FIGURE 2.14)

Synonyms

This muscle may also be referred to as rectus capitis posticus minor, rectus posticus minor, or rectus capitis posterior profundus (Macalister 1875; Bakkum and Miller 2016).

Typical Presentation

Description

Rectus capitis posterior minor originates from the posterior tubercle of the first cervical vertebra and inserts onto the occipital bone along the medial half of the inferior nuchal line and onto the bone just below the line (Standring 2016).

Innervation

Rectus capitis posterior minor is innervated by the suboccipital nerve (Standring 2016).

Comparative Anatomy

Rectus capitis posterior minor has a similar typical presentation in the apes, extending from the posterior tubercle of the first cervical vertebra to the occipital bone (Sonntag 1923, 1924; Raven 1950; Miller 1952; Gibbs 1999; Diogo et al. 2010, 2012, 2013a,b, 2017). Sonntag (1923) notes that the rectus capitis posterior major muscles mostly conceal the rectus capitis posterior minor muscles in common chimpanzees. The rectus capitis posterior minor muscles are concealed to a lesser extent in orangutans (Sonntag 1924).

Variations

Description

Rectus capitis posterior minor may be reduced or absent (Mori 1964; Rickenbacher et al. 1985; Zumpano et al. 2006; Nayak et al. 2011). It may be separated from its counterpart at the midline (Mori 1964). Rectus capitis posterior minor may receive accessory slips from the second cervical vertebra or the ligamentum nuchae (Mori 1964; Rickenbacher et al. 1985). It may send a slip to rectus capitis posterior major (Mori 1964). It may fuse with spinalis capitis at its insertion (Martin 1994; Bakkum and Miller 2016). Rectus capitis posterior minor often has a soft-tissue connection to the posterior atlanto-occipital membrane and the dura mater in the atlanto-occipital interspace (Hack et al. 1995; Hack and Hallgren 2004; Zumpano et al. 2006; Scali et al. 2011; Bakkum and Miller 2016; Standring 2016; Yuan

et al. 2016). Yuan et al. (2016) also found that rectus capitis posterior minor may connect to the dura via the posterior atlanto-axial interspace.

Rectus capitis posterior minor may be doubled (Macalister 1875; Mori 1964; Rickenbacher et al. 1985; Tagil et al. 2005; Bakkum and Miller 2016; Standring 2016). It may also be divided into three parts (Mori 1964; Bakkum and Miller 2016). When doubled or divided, the second muscle is often smaller and situated lateral to the normal muscle and deep to rectus capitis posterior major (Mori 1964; Rickenbacher et al. 1985).

Prevalence

In a sample of 112 cadavers, Mori (1964) found rectus capitis posterior minor with a typical presentation bilaterally in 54 cadavers (48.2%), on the right side only in 16 cadavers (14.3%), and on the left side only in ten cadavers (8.9%). Rectus capitis posterior minor was absent bilaterally in two cadavers (1.8%), on the right side only in one cadaver (0.9%), and on the left side only in three cadavers (2.7%). The muscle was longitudinally split into two parts bilaterally in 17 cadavers (15.2%), on the right side only in 11 cadavers (9.8%), and on the left side only in 12 cadavers (10.7%). Rectus capitis posterior minor received an accessory slip that originated from the spine of the second cervical vertebra or the ligamentum nuchae bilaterally in seven cadavers (6.3%) and on the left side only in one cadaver (0.9%). Rectus capitis posterior minor sent accessory slips to rectus capitis posterior major bilaterally in three cadavers (2.7%), on the right side only in two cadavers (1.8%), and on the left side only in nine cadavers (8%).

In a sample of 75 cadavers, Zumpano et al. (2006) found that rectus capitis posterior minor was absent bilaterally in five cadavers (6.7%). A soft tissue bridge between rectus capitis posterior minor and the posterior atlanto-occipital membrane was found on the right side in 53 cadavers (70.7%) and on the left side in 55 cadavers (73.3%). Out of 11 cases, Hack et al. (1995) found a connection between rectus capitis posterior minor and the dorsal spinal dura at the atlanto-occipital junction in all cases (100%). In a sample of 13 cadavers, all of them (100%) had connection between rectus capitis posterior minor and the dura mater (Scali et al. 2011).

Yuan et al. (2016) studied the origin of rectus capitis posterior minor in 14 specimens using P45 sheet plastination and in five cadavers via dissection. Out of the sample of 14 specimens, the tendon of rectus capitis posterior minor attached only to the posterior arch of the atlas in one case (type I, 7.1%). The tendon terminated in both the posterior arch of the atlas and the posterior atlanto-occipital interspace in six cases (type II, 42.9%) and in both the posterior arch of the atlas and the posterior atlanto-axial interspace in one case (type III, 7.1%). The tendon terminated in all three locations in six cases (type IV, 42.9%). Among the five cadavers, a type I attachment was found in two cases (40%), a type II attachment was found in one case (20%), and a type III attachment was found in two cases (40%).

Anomalies

Description

When the posterior tubercle of the first cervical vertebra is absent, rectus capitis posterior minor may originate from an unusual prominence on the spinous process of the second cervical vertebra (Brown 1941). In an individual with atlas assimilation, the right rectus capitis posterior minor muscle was vestigial, and the left muscle was replaced by a band of connective tissue (Ciołkowski et al. 2014).

Prevalence

N/A

Clinical Implications

The absence of rectus capitis posterior minor may lead to a lack of coordination among the suboccipital muscles while balancing the head or contribute to cervicogenic headaches (Nayak et al. 2011). The myodural communication between rectus capitis posterior minor and the dorsal spinal dura may help resist dural infolding (Hack et al. 1995). Surgical separation of this myodural connection can provide relief from chronic headache (Hack and Hallgren 2004). The rectus capitis posterior minor myodural bridge may influence the circulation of cerebrospinal fluid (Yuan et al. 2016).

OBLIQUUS CAPITIS SUPERIOR (FIGURE 2.14)

See also: Atlantomastoideus

Synonyms

This muscle may be referred to as obliquus superior or obliquus capitis major (Macalister 1875; Bakkum and Miller 2016).

Typical Presentation

Description

Obliquus capitis superior originates from the transverse process of the first cervical vertebra and inserts onto the occipital bone between the inferior and superior nuchal lines (Standring 2016).

Innervation

Obliquus capitis superior is innervated by the suboccipital nerve (Standring 2016).

Comparative Anatomy

Obliquus capitis superior has a similar typical presentation in the apes, extending from the transverse process of the first cervical vertebra to the occipital bone (Sonntag 1923, 1924; Raven 1950; Miller 1952; Gibbs 1999; Diogo et al. 2010, 2012, 2013a,b, 2017).

Variations

Description

Obliquus capitis superior may be bilaminar (Flower and Murie 1867; Macalister 1875; Rickenbacher et al. 1985). Its origin may receive bundles from obliquus capitis inferior (Rickenbacher et al. 1985). It is associated with atlantomastoideus, which extends from the transverse process of the first cervical vertebra to the mastoid process (see the entry for this muscle).

Prevalence

N/A

Anomalies

Description

In a fetus with trisomy 13, the left obliquus capitis superior had an extra belly (Pettersen et al. 1979). In an individual with atlas assimilation, the left obliquus capitis superior muscle was replaced by a bundle of connective tissue (Ciołkowski et al. 2014).

Prevalence

In their literature review, Smith et al. (2015) found that an extra belly of obliquus capitis superior was present in only 1 out of 20 individuals with trisomy 13 (5%).

Clinical Implications

N/A

OBLIQUUS CAPITIS INFERIOR (FIGURE 2.14)

Synonyms

This muscle may be referred to as obliquus inferior or obliquus capitis minimus (Macalister 1875; Bakkum and Miller 2016).

Typical Presentation

Description

Obliquus capitis inferior originates from the spinous process of the second cervical vertebra and inserts onto the transverse process of the first cervical vertebra (Standring 2016).

Innervation

Obliquus capitis inferior is innervated by the suboccipital nerve (Standring 2016).

Comparative Anatomy

Obliquus capitis inferior has a similar typical presentation in the apes, extending from the spinous process of the second cervical vertebra to the transverse process of the first cervical vertebra (Sonntag 1923, 1924; Raven 1950; Miller 1952; Gibbs 1999; Diogo et al. 2010, 2012, 2013a,b, 2017).

Variations

Description

Obliquus capitis inferior may overlap rectus capitis posterior major (Macalister 1875). It may send a slip to rectus capitis posterior major (Mori 1964) or bundles to the origin of obliquus capitis superior (Rickenbacher et al. 1985). It may also send bundles to the transverse processes of the second or third cervical vertebrae (Rickenbacher et al. 1985). There may be a myodural bridge connecting obliquus capitis inferior with the dura mater (Scali et al. 2011; Pontell et al. 2013; Bakkum and Miller 2016). Obliquus capitis inferior may be doubled (Macalister 1875; Rickenbacher et al. 1985).

Prevalence

In a sample of 112 cadavers, Mori (1964) found that the left rectus capitis posterior major muscle received a slip from obliquus capitis inferior in one cadaver (0.9%). In a sample of 14 obliquus capitis inferior muscles, Pontell et al. (2013) found that all of the muscles (100%) were connected with the dura mater.

Anomalies

Description

On the right side of one male neonate with trisomy 13, obliquus capitis inferior sent an accessory slip to semispinalis cervicis (Pettersen et al. 1979). On the left side, obliquus capitis inferior had an extra belly. In an individual with atlas assimilation, the left obliquus capitis inferior muscle was thinner than the right muscle (Ciołkowski et al. 2014).

Prevalence

In their literature review, Smith et al. (2015) found that accessory muscles associated with obliquus capitis inferior were found only in 1 out of 20 individuals with trisomy 13 (5%).

Clinical Implications

The obliquus capitis inferior myodural bridge may be involved in monitoring dural tension or resisting dural infolding (Pontell et al. 2013).

POSTEROLATERAL NECK MUSCLES

STERNOCLEIDOMASTOIDEUS (STERNOCLEIDOMASTOID) (FIGURES 2.3 AND 3.3)

See also: Cleido-occipitalis cervicalis, Platysma cervicale, Levator claviculae, Supraclavicularis proprius, Sternalis

Synonyms
N/A

Typical Presentation

Description

Sternocleidomastoid has two heads. The sternal (medial) head originates from the manubrium, and the clavicular (lateral) head originates from the medial third of the clavicle (Standring 2016). The two heads join and insert into the mastoid process and the superior nuchal line (Standring 2016).

Innervation

Sternocleidomastoid is innervated by the accessory nerve (Standring 2016).

Comparative Anatomy

Sternocleidomastoid has a similar typical presentation in the apes, with a sternomastoid head that extends from the sternum to the mastoid and nuchal crest and a cleidomastoid head that extends from the medial clavicle to the mastoid (Gratiolet and Alix 1866; Primrose 1899, 1900; Sonntag 1923, 1924; Miller 1952; Gibbs 1999; Diogo et al. 2010, 2012, 2013a,b, 2017). Accessory heads may be found in gibbons or bonobos (Schück 1913; Miller 1952). Schück (1913) found that the muscle may fuse with trapezius in gibbons. In bonobos, the clavicular attachment may be absent (Diogo et al. 2017). An insertion of the cleidomastoid head into the axis has been observed in orangutans (Owen 1868; Diogo et al. 2013b) while an insertion into the atlas has been observed in common chimpanzees (Sutton 1883; Diogo et al. 2013a).

Variations

Description

The sternal head (sternomastoid) and the clavicular head (cleidomastoid) may be completely separated (Hallett 1848; Macalister 1875; Knott 1880, 1883a; Mori 1964; Lee and Yang 2016). They may also be completely fused (Hallett 1848; Macalister 1875). The sternal head (Macalister 1875) or the entire sternocleidomastoid muscle may be absent (McKinley and Hamilton 1976; Vajramani et al. 2010). The sternal head may be doubled (Macalister 1875; Nayak et al. 2006; Raikos et al. 2012). The clavicular origin may be doubled or tripled (Wood 1868; Macalister 1875; Ramesh Rao et al. 2007; Raikos et al. 2012; Heo et al. 2020). The clavicular head may also be divided into multiple fascicles, or into superficial and deep sheets (Macalister 1875; Knott 1880, 1883a; Mori 1964). There are reports of sternocleidomastoid with six heads, comprised of a doubled sternal head and quadrupled clavicular head (Natsis et al. 2009; Kaur et al. 2013). Surendran et al. (2016) report a sternocleidomastoid with 13 tendons of origin and five fleshy bellies (four clavicular bellies, one sternal belly). The insertion of sternocleidomastoid may also be doubled or divided (Macalister 1875; Mori 1964). The entire sternocleidomastoid muscle may be doubled (Lee and Yang 2016).

The extent of the origin along the clavicle may vary (Hallett 1848; Macalister 1875; Lee and Yang 2016). The clavicular head may be narrow and tendinous (Macalister 1875). Sato (1968b) found that sternocleidomastoid formed a thick band anteriorly and a thin band posteriorly. Sternocleidomastoid may blend with the clavicular attachment of trapezius (Hallett 1848; Macalister 1875;

Rickenbacher et al. 1985; Bakkum and Miller 2016; Standring 2016). It may send accessory slips to the mastoid process, tympanic ring, parotid fascia, stylomandibular ligament, thyroid cartilage, hyoid, angle of the mandible, or clavicle on the opposite side of the body (Macalister 1875; Lee and Yang 2016).

Sternocleidomastoid is associated with multiple named accessory muscles. Coskun et al. (2002) report a case in which sternomastoid and cleidomastoid were accompanied by a "sternocleidooccipital" muscle, which had a single origin from the occiput and a split attachment onto the clavicle and the manubrium. This accessory muscle sent an additional bundle to sternomastoid. Platysma cervicale (transversus nuchae, occipital platysma) runs from the occipital region to the mouth or posterior ear region and may insert into the anterior border of sternocleidomastoid (see the entry for this muscle). Levator claviculae originates from the transverse processes of some cervical vertebrae and inserts onto the clavicle, sometimes inserting into sternocleidomastoid (see the entry for this muscle). Supraclavicularis proprius originates from the cervical fascia overlying the clavicular head of sternocleidomastoid and the sternoclavicular joint and inserts onto the distal end of the clavicle or the fascial sheath of trapezius (see the entry for this muscle). Sternalis, a variable accessory muscle that extends from the sternal/infraclavicular area to the upper abdominal wall or costal cartilages, may originate from or blend with sternocleidomastoid (see the entry for this muscle). Cleido-occipitalis cervicalis is situated near the posterior border of sternocleidomastoid, extending between the occiput and the clavicle (see the entry for this muscle).

Prevalence

Hallett (1848) found a lengthened attachment of the clavicular head toward the middle of the clavicle in one out of eight cases (12.5%). Wood (1868) found that sternocleidomastoid had a doubled or divided clavicular origin in 7 out of 36 subjects (19.4%). Mori (1964) found complete separation of the sternal and clavicular heads in 450 out of 510 cases (88.2%). Mori (1964) also found sternocleidomastoid separated into superficial and deep layers in 10 out of 1020 sides (1%). The occipital insertion was separated from the rest of the muscle in 102 out of 1020 sides (10%). The variant described by Sato (1968b, see above) was present on 12 out of 354 sides (3.39%) in Kyushu-Japanese males and on 10 out of 216 sides (4.63%) in females.

Anomalies

Description

Sternocleidomastoid was absent on the right side in a male infant with triploidy studied by Moen et al. (1984). Sternocleidomastoid had three bellies on both sides of an infant with trisomy 13 (Pettersen et al. 1979). The lateral belly attached to the clavicle, the medial belly attached to the manubrium, and the middle belly attached to the sternoclavicular junction. On the left side, the medial belly sent slips

to platysma. In a neonate with trisomy 18, the left sternocleidomastoid was divided into two distinct parts (Aziz 1979). In a fetus with trisomy 18 and cyclopia, sternocleidomastoid was split into fascicles; had a broad attachment to the skull, a strong fascial connection to platysma; and formed a complex with rhomboideus occipitalis and trapezius (Smith et al. 2015). In a fetus with craniorachischisis, the left sternocleidomastoid had a small clavicular head and a large sternal head, attached to the "temporo-occipital bone," and fused with trapezius (Alghamdi et al. 2017). The right sternocleidomastoid had three heads: a lateral head attached to the "temporo-occipital bone," a middle head attached to the skull inferior to the ear, and a small head attached to the mandibular ramus.

Prevalence

In their literature review, Smith et al. (2015) found that sternocleidomastoid was divided into three bellies in 1 out of 20 individuals with trisomy 13 (5%). The muscle was divided into sternomastoid and cleidomastoid portions in 2 out of 17 individuals with trisomy 18 (11.8%).

Clinical Implications

The absence of sternocleidomastoid may be associated with torticollis (McKinley and Hamilton 1976; Vajramani et al. 2010). Accessory heads may lead to stenosis of the supraclavicular fossa (Natsis et al. 2009; Raikos et al. 2012; Lee and Yang 2016).

CLEIDO-OCCIPITALIS CERVICALIS (FIGURE 2.3)

See also: Sternocleidomastoideus, Trapezius

Synonyms

This muscle may be referred to as the cleido-occipital muscle (Wood 1866, 1867b, 1870; Macalister 1875), cleido-occipitalis (Rickenbacher et al. 1985; Rahman and Yamadori 1994), or accessory cleido-occipital muscle of trapezius (Paraskevas et al. 2013; note: these authors consider the cleido-occipital muscle of Wood to be separate muscle that is a variant of sternocleidomastoid).

Typical Presentation

This muscle is present only as a variation or anomaly.

Comparative Anatomy

A cleido-occipital head of sternocleidomastoid (but not trapezius) has been observed in a few orangutans and common chimpanzees (Sonntag 1923, 1924; Miller 1952; Diogo et al. 2013a,b).

Variations

Description

When present, cleido-occipitalis cervicalis (Kwak et al. 2003) presents as a separate slip that courses along the anterior border of trapezius, originating from the occiput and inserting into the clavicle (Hallett 1848; Wood 1866, 1867b, 1870; Macalister 1867b, 1875; Mori 1964; Rickenbacher et al. 1985; Rahman and Yamadori 1994; Kwak et al. 2003; Ravindra et al. 2012; Paraskevas et al. 2013; Bakkum and Miller 2016). It likely forms as an isolated muscle during the separation of trapezius and sternocleidomastoid from the common muscle anlage (Rahman and Yamadori 1994; Kwak et al. 2003; Paraskevas et al. 2013; Bakkum and Miller 2016).

It may join with trapezius or sternocleidomastoid at its origin or insertion (Wood 1867b, 1870; Macalister 1875; Rahman and Yamadori 1994; Kwak et al. 2003). It may be split into separate fascicles (Wood 1870; Macalister 1875). It may be doubled (Wood 1870; Macalister 1875). It may be comprised of tendinous or muscular fibers (Mori 1964). The external jugular vein may pass through the space created between cleido-occipitalis cervicalis and the clavicle (Mori 1964; Ravindra et al. 2012). Paraskevas et al. (2013) observed a fibrous arch at the clavicular insertion of cleido-occipitalis, through which the main trunk of the supraclavicular nerves passed. Rickenbacher et al. (1985) report that cleido-occipitalis cervicalis may take the form of cleido-occipitalis totalis, which connects trapezius to sternocleidomastoid, filling the posterior triangle of the neck.

Innervation

The cleido-occipitalis cervicalis is likely innervated by the accessory nerve.

Prevalence

Wood (1867b) found the cleido-occipital muscle in 12 out of 34 subjects (35.3%). Wood (1870) states that the muscle was found in 37 out of 102 subjects (36.3%). Mori (1964) found a bundle along the anterior margin of trapezius that inserted into the clavicle bilaterally in 16 out of 130 cadavers (12.3%) and unilaterally in 11 cadavers (8.5%).

Anomalies

Description

In an infant with median cleft lip, hypotelorism, and alobar holoprosencephaly, Mieden (1982) found cleido-occipitalis present on the right side, extending between the superior nuchal line and the clavicle.

Prevalence

Mieden (1982) found cleido-occipitalis in one out of three specimens with alobar holoprosencephaly (33%).

Clinical Implications

The external jugular vein may become entrapped between cleido-occipitalis cervicalis and trapezius (Ravindra et al. 2012). The supraclavicular nerve trunk may be entrapped by a fibrous arch at the insertion of the cleido-occipital muscle (Paraskevas et al. 2013).

TRAPEZIUS (FIGURES 2.3 AND 3.3)

See also: Cleido-occipitalis cervicalis, Platysma cervicale, Levator claviculae, Supraclavicularis proprius

Synonyms

This muscle may also be referred to as cucullaris (Henle) (Bakkum and Miller 2016).

Typical Presentation

Description

Trapezius originates from the superior nuchal line, external occipital protuberance, nuchal ligament, and the spinous processes and supraspinous ligaments of the seventh cervical through the twelfth thoracic vertebrae (Standring 2016). It inserts onto the lateral third of the clavicle, the acromion, and the scapular spine (Standring 2016). The muscle can therefore be divided into three parts: the superior part (descending fibers with occipital and clavicular attachments), middle part (transverse fibers with vertebral, acromial, and scapular spine attachments), and inferior part (ascending fibers with vertebral and scapular spine attachments) (Rickenbacher et al. 1985; Bakkum and Miller 2016; Standring 2016).

Innervation

Trapezius is innervated by the accessory nerve (Standring 2016).

Comparative Anatomy

Trapezius has a similar typical presentation in the great apes, differentiated into three parts with origins from the cranium and vertebral column and insertions into the acromion, scapular spine, and lateral third of the clavicle (Diogo et. 2010, 2013a,b, 2017). As in humans, the extent of the attachment along the clavicle may vary (Hepburn 1892; Diogo et. 2010, 2013a,b). The clavicular attachment was reported absent in one orangutan (Schück 1913). The lowest attachment of trapezius in common chimpanzees varies between the eighth and thirteenth thoracic vertebrae (Gratiolet and Alix 1866; Macalister 1871; Sonntag 1923; Stewart 1936; Swindler and Wood 1973). The lowest attachment of trapezius in bonobos is either onto the ninth or tenth thoracic vertebrae (Miller 1952; Diogo et al. 2017). The occipital origin is absent in most gibbons (Deniker 1885; Kohlbrügge 1890–1892; Gibbs 1999; Michilsens et al. 2009; Diogo et al. 2012).

Variations

Description

Trapezius may be partially or entirely absent (Hallett 1848; Wood 1864; Macalister 1875; Testut 1884; Le Double 1897; Bing 1902; Rickenbacher et al. 1985; Emsley and Davis 2001; Garbelotti et al. 2001; Allouh et al. 2004; Vajramani et al. 2010; Bakkum and Miller 2016; Standring 2016). The occipital attachment may be missing (Hallett 1848; Macalister 1875; Testut 1884; Le Double 1897; Rickenbacher et al. 1985; Standring 2016). The inferior part may be reduced or absent (Hallett 1848; Wood 1867b; Macalister 1875; Mori 1964; Rickenbacher et al. 1985; Bakkum and Miller 2016; Standring 2016). Isolated absence of the middle part can also occur (Macalister 1875; Rickenbacher et al. 1985). The clavicular insertion may also be reduced or absent (Hallett 1848; Macalister 1875; Rickenbacher et al. 1985). Reduction or absence of the scapular insertion is rare (Macalister 1875; Rickenbacher et al. 1985). Due to these variations, there may be asymmetry in development of the left and right muscles (Macalister 1875; Hallett 1848; Wood 1867b; Mori 1964; Rickenbacher et al. 1985; Emsley and Davis 2001; Bakkum and Miller 2016).

Hallett (1848) reports a case in which trapezius was partially absent on the left side, with muscle fibers ending at the level of the third thoracic vertebra and a thin fascial layer replacing the inferior part of the muscle. Similarly, Garbelotti et al. (2001) and Valtanen et al. (2017) report cases in which an aponeurosis completely replaced the ascending fibers and partially replaced transverse fibers of left trapezius muscles.

Its origin from the occiput or its insertion into the clavicle may occur via a tendinous arch that also connects to sternocleidomastoid (Macalister 1875; Rickenbacher et al. 1985). The origin of the inferior part may extend to the lumbar vertebrae (Mori 1964). When the occipital origin is missing, it may originate from the posterior border of sternocleidomastoid (Macalister 1875). The extent of the insertion along the clavicle may vary (Hallett 1848; Macalister 1875; Rickenbacher et al. 1985; Bakkum and Miller 2016; Standring 2016). The occipital and cervical parts may be divided into multiple fasciculi (Macalister 1875). The dorsal and cervical parts of the trapezius muscles can be partially separated (Macalister 1875; Mori 1964; Rickenbacher et al. 1985; Standring 2016; Ferreli et al. 2019). A cleft may also be found separating the inferior part of the muscle (Macalister 1875; Rickenbacher et al. 1985). The entire muscle may be partially or entirely split into superficial and deep layers (Rickenbacher et al. 1985).

Trapezius may blend with sternocleidomastoid at its clavicular attachment (Hallett 1848; Macalister 1875; Rickenbacher et al. 1985; Bakkum and Miller 2016; Standring 2016). It may send slips to latissimus dorsi, sternocleidomastoid, levator claviculae, deltoideus, the fascia of the neck, the lower angle or medial margin of the scapula, or the sternum (Wood 1867b; Macalister 1875; Rickenbacher et al. 1985; Bakkum and Miller 2016).

Trapezius is also associated with multiple named accessory muscles. Platysma cervicale (transversus nuchae, occipital platysma) may extend from near the occipital attachment of trapezius to the region of auricularis posterior or to the mouth near the parotid fascia (see the entry for this muscle). Levator claviculae (cleidocervical muscle) originates from the transverse processes of some cervical vertebrae and inserts onto the clavicle near trapezius (see the entry for this muscle). Supraclavicularis proprius originates from the cervical fascia overlying the clavicular head of sternocleidomastoid and the sternoclavicular joint and inserts onto the distal end of the clavicle or the fascial sheath of trapezius (see the entry for this muscle). Cleido-occipitalis cervicalis courses along the anterior margin of

trapezius, extending between the occiput and the clavicle (see the entry for this muscle).

Prevalence

In a review of 186 cases of congenital muscle absences, Bing (1902) reported that trapezius was absent in 18 cases. Macalister (1875) states that Wood found that the inferior part of trapezius extended only to the eighth and ninth, or tenth, thoracic vertebrae in about 4 out of 70 subjects (5.7%). In a sample of 216 sides, Mori (1964) found that the lower limit of trapezius was the eighth thoracic vertebra on two sides (0.9%), the ninth thoracic vertebra on seven sides (3.2%), the tenth thoracic vertebra on 49 sides (22.7%), the eleventh thoracic vertebra on 79 sides (36.6%), the twelfth thoracic vertebra on 65 sides (30%), the first lumbar vertebra on 12 sides (5.6%), and the second lumbar vertebra on two sides (0.9%). Mori (1964) also found the cervical and occipital parts separated on 15 sides (6.9%).

Anomalies

Description

On the right side of a fetus with cyclopia and alobar holoprosencephaly, an "occipito-trapezius" muscle was present, extending from the superior nuchal line to the deep surface of trapezius (Mieden 1982). In cases of triploidy, the middle part of trapezius may be absent and replaced with connective tissue (Moen et al. 1984). In a trisomy 18 cyclopic fetus, trapezius had a broad origin from the skull and was part of a complex with rhomboideus occipitalis and sternocleidomastoid (Smith et al. 2015). Trapezius was also closely associated with splenius capitis at the midline origin on both sides (Smith et al. 2015). In a fetus with craniorachischisis, the left trapezius presented as a small muscle on top of supraspinatus, with attachments to the clavicle, acromion, scapular spine, and temporo-occipital bone (Alghamdi et al. 2017). On the right side, trapezius presented as undifferentiated tissue between the right eye and scapular spine and was fused with sternocleidomastoid (Alghamdi et al. 2017). Poland syndrome, a rare congenital anomaly, can cause the partial or complete absence of trapezius (Debeer et al. 2002; Yiyit et al. 2014). Bilateral absence of trapezius was observed in male fetus with CHARGE syndrome (Beger et al. 2019).

Prevalence

Moen et al. (1984) found that the middle fibers of trapezius were absent bilaterally and replaced with a sheet of connective tissue in three specimens with triploidy (100%). Mieden (1982) found occipito-trapezius in one out of three specimens with alobar holoprosencephaly (33%).

Clinical Implications

The absence of trapezius may be associated with torticollis (Vajramani et al. 2010). Stevenson et al. (2014) describe a cadaver with a severe case of congenital scoliosis and found significant asymmetry in the trapezius muscles. Valtanen et al. (2017) report a partial unilateral absence of a left trapezius associated with 5-degree thoracic scoliosis toward the right side.

3 Upper Limb Muscles

Eve K. Boyle
Howard University College of Medicine

Vondel S. E. Mahon
University of Maryland Medical Center

Rui Diogo
Howard University College of Medicine

CONTENTS

DOI: 10.1201/9781003083535-3

AXIAL PECTORAL GIRDLE MUSCLES

SERRATUS ANTERIOR (FIGURE 3.1)

Synonyms

Serratus anterior may also be referred to as serratus anticus, serratus magnus, or serratus anticus major (Macalister 1875; Bakkum and Miller 2016).

Typical Presentation

Description

Serratus anterior originates from ribs one through eight and inserts onto the medial border of the scapula (Standring 2016).

Innervation

Serratus anterior is innervated by the long thoracic nerve (Standring 2016).

Comparative Anatomy

Serratus anterior has a similar typical presentation in the apes, extending from the ribs to the medial side of the scapula (Gratiolet and Alix 1866; Macalister 1871, 1873; Champneys 1872; Deniker 1885; Kohlbrügge 1890–1892; Hepburn 1892; Beddard 1893; Primrose 1899, 1900; Schück 1913; Sonntag 1923; Sullivan and Osgood 1927; Stewart 1936; Raven 1950; Miller 1952; Gibbs 1999; Diogo et al. 2010, 2012, 2013a,b, 2017). In the apes, serratus anterior tends to have origins more often from the inferior-most ribs (Gibbs 1999; Diogo et al. 2010, 2012, 2013a,b, 2017).

In a bonobo fetus, serratus anterior was fused with the insertion of levator scapulae (Diogo et al. 2017).

Variations

Description

The superior part of serratus anterior may be split into two layers or it may be absent (Macalister 1875). The middle portion of the muscle may also be absent, or it may be reduced and replaced with connective tissue (Macalister 1875; Bergman et al. 1988; Bakkum and Miller 2016; Standring 2016). Slips to the first or eighth rib may be absent (Macalister 1875; Mori 1964; Bergman et al. 1988; Smith et al. 2003; Standring 2016). Serratus anterior may have origins from ribs nine and ten (Macalister 1875; Mori 1964; Bergman et al. 1988; Bakkum and Miller 2016; Standring 2016). Every slip beyond the first two may be absent (Macalister 1875). There may be connections to coracobrachialis, pectoralis minor, or scalenus posterior (Smith et al. 2003; Bakkum and Miller 2016). Serratus anterior may also be continuous with the external oblique, intercostal muscles, supracostalis anterior, or levator scapulae (Macalister 1875; Bergman et al. 1988; Bakkum and Miller 2016; Standring 2016).

Prevalence

In a study cited by Bergman et al. (1988) and Bakkum and Miller (2016), the inferior most attachment of serratus anterior was to rib seven in 1% of cases, rib eight in 40% of cases, rib nine in 38% of cases, rib ten in 10% of cases, and

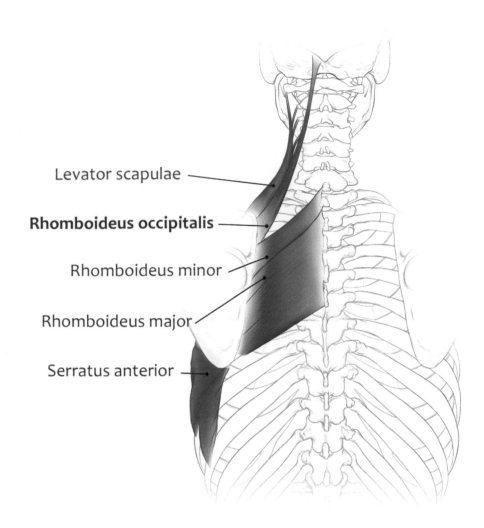

Levator scapulae

Rhomboideus occipitalis

Rhomboideus minor

Rhomboideus major

Serratus anterior

FIGURE 3.1　Thoracoscapular muscles in posterior view.

rib 11 in 0.5% of cases. The superior most attachment of the muscle was to rib one in 75% of cases, to the fascia of the rib one in 21% of cases, and to rib two in 3% of cases (Bergman et al. 1988). Based on a study of 204 sides, Mori (1964) reported that the inferior most attachment of serratus anterior was to rib seven on 14 sides (6.8%), rib eight on 26 sides (12.7%), rib nine on 152 sides (74.5%), and rib ten on 12 sides (5.8%). The superior most attachment was to rib one on 182 sides (89.2%) and to rib two on 22 sides (10.7%) of cases. In a study of 13 sides, Smith et al. (2003) observed that the superior most attachment was to both ribs one and two on six sides (46%), to rib one only on two sides (15%), to rib two only on four sides (31%), and to ribs two and three on one side (8%).

Anomalies

Description

Poland syndrome, a rare congenital anomaly, can lead to the absence of serratus anterior (Cingel et al. 2013). In a male fetus with triploidy, the upper half of serratus anterior was absent bilaterally (Moen et al. 1984).

Prevalence

N/A

Clinical Implications

The absence of serratus anterior can cause winged scapula (Levin and Trummer 1973).

RHOMBOIDEUS MAJOR (RHOMBOID MAJOR) (FIGURE 3.1)

See also: Rhomboideus minor

Synonyms

Rhomboideus major may also be referred to as rhomboideus inferior (Bakkum and Miller 2016).

Typical Presentation

Description

Rhomboideus major originates from the spines of the second through fifth thoracic vertebrae (Standring 2016). It attaches to the medial border of the scapula inferior to the spine (Standring 2016).

Innervation

Rhomboideus major is innervated by the dorsal scapular nerve (Standring 2016).

Comparative Anatomy

In the apes, the rhomboid muscles are typically fused and extend between the cervical and thoracic vertebrae and the scapula (Macalister 1873; Deniker 1885; Kohlbrügge 1890–1892; Schück 1913; Sonntag 1923, 1924; Stewart 1936; Raven 1950; Miller 1952; Preuschoft 1965; Swindler and Wood 1973; Gibbs 1999; Diogo et al. 2010, 2012, 2013a,b, 2017). In a bonobo fetus, rhomboideus was fused with its counterpart on the other side of the body and partially fused with levator scapulae and serratus anterior (Diogo et al. 2017).

Variations

Description

The rhomboid major muscle may vary in its vertebral attachments, with the inferior most attachments varying anywhere between the third and sixth thoracic vertebrae (Macalister 1875; Mori 1964; Bakkum and Miller 2016). Rhomboideus major can also be divided into many discrete bundles (Macalister 1875; Bergman et al. 1988; Bakkum and Miller 2016). When fasciculated, it may connect with serratus anterior (Macalister 1875). The lower part of the muscle may be bilaminar (Macalister 1875). The rhomboid muscles may be fused (Macalister 1875; Mori 1964; Bergman et al. 1988). Together, the rhomboids can send slips to infraspinatus, latissimus dorsi, or teres major (Macalister 1875; Rickenbacher et al. 1985; Bergman et al. 1988; Bakkum and Miller 2016). Rhomboideus minimus, or rhomboid minus, refers to a slip that extends between the upper thoracic or lower cervical vertebral spines and the scapula and/or teres major fascia (Mori 1964; Bergman et al. 1988; Bakkum and Miller 2016).

Prevalence

Based on a study of 60 sides, Mori (1964) found that the inferior most vertebral attachment was T3 on two sides (3.3%), T4 on 20 sides, (33.3%), T5 on 28 sides (46.7%), and T6 on 10 sides (16.7%). Mori (1964) also observed that the rhomboids were fused on 70 out of 500 sides (14%). Mori (1964) reports the presence of rhomboideus minimus in 56 out of 505 sides (11.1%) and states that Nishi found this muscle in 16% of cases.

Anomalies

Description

In both a neonate with trisomy 18 (Aziz 1979) and a fetus with craniorachischisis (Alghamdi et al. 2017), the rhomboid muscles were present as a continuous sheet of muscle. Rhomboideus major and minor were also fused in a trisomy 18 cyclopic fetus dissected by Smith et al. (2015), and these muscles attached higher onto the scapula than is normally observed. Furthermore, the composition of the rhomboid muscles in this specimen was about one-third fibrous and two-thirds tendinous (Smith et al. 2015). In a male fetus with triploidy, rhomboid major had an extra muscle slip on the right side (Moen et al. 1984). In a cadaver with a severe case of congenital scoliosis, Stevenson et al. (2014) found significant asymmetry in the rhomboid muscles.

Prevalence

In their literature review, Smith et al. (2015) found that rhomboideus major and minor were fused in 2 out of 26 individuals with trisomy 18 (7.7%).

Clinical Implications

N/A

RHOMBOIDEUS MINOR (RHOMBOID MINOR) (FIGURE 3.1)

See also: Rhomboideus major

Synonyms

Rhomboideus minor may also be referred to as rhomboideus superior or kleiner Rautenmuskel (Bakkum and Miller 2016).

Typical Presentation

Description

Rhomboid minor originates from the inferior end of the ligamentum nuchae and spines of the seventh cervical and first thoracic vertebrae (Standring 2016). It attaches to the medial border of the scapula at the root of the scapular spine (Standring 2016).

Innervation

Rhomboideus minor is innervated by the dorsal scapular nerve (Standring 2016).

Comparative Anatomy

In the apes, the rhomboid muscles are typically fused and extend between the cervical and thoracic vertebrae and the scapula (Macalister 1873; Deniker 1885; Kohlbrügge 1890–1892; Schück 1913; Sonntag 1923, 1924; Stewart 1936; Raven 1950; Miller 1952; Preuschoft 1965; Swindler and Wood 1973; Gibbs 1999; Diogo et al. 2010, 2012, 2013a,b, 2017). In a bonobo fetus, rhomboideus was fused with its counterpart on the other side of the body and partially fused with levator scapulae and serratus anterior (Diogo et al. 2017).

Variations

Description

The rhomboid minor muscle may vary in its vertebral attachments, with the superior most attachments varying anywhere between the fourth and sixth cervical vertebrae (Macalister 1875; Mori 1964; Rickenbacher et al. 1985; Bakkum and Miller 2016). Rhomboideus minor can also be divided into many discrete bundles (Bergman et al. 1988; Bakkum and Miller 2016). It may also be bilaminar (Macalister 1875). The rhomboid muscles may be fused (Macalister 1875; Mori 1964; Bergman et al. 1988). Together, the rhomboids can send slips to infraspinatus, latissimus dorsi, or teres major (Macalister 1875; Rickenbacher et al. 1985; Bergman et al. 1988; Bakkum and Miller 2016). Rhomboideus minimus, or rhomboid minus, refers to a slip that extends between the upper thoracic or lower cervical vertebral spines and the scapula and/or teres major fascia (Mori 1964; Bergman et al. 1988; Bakkum and Miller 2016).

Prevalence

Based on a study of 60 sides, Mori (1964) found that the superior most vertebral attachment was C4 on 10 sides (~16.7%), C5 on 36 sides (60%), and C6 on 14 sides (~23.3%). Mori (1964) also observed that the rhomboids were fused on 70 out of 500 sides (14%). Mori (1964) reports the presence of rhomboideus minimus in 56 out of 505 sides (~11.1%) and states that Nishi found this muscle in 16% of cases.

Anomalies

Description

In both a neonate with trisomy 18 (Aziz 1979) and a fetus with craniorachischisis (Alghamdi et al. 2017), the rhomboid muscles were present as a continuous sheet of muscle. Rhomboideus major and minor were also fused in a trisomy 18 cyclopic fetus dissected by Smith et al. (2015), and these muscles attached higher onto the scapula than is normally observed. Furthermore, the composition of the rhomboid muscles in this specimen was about one-third fibrous and two-thirds tendinous (Smith et al. 2015). The bilateral presence of a bipartite rhomboid minor with superficial and deep parts was observed in a 26-week-old male fetus with CHARGE syndrome (Beger et al. 2019). Stevenson et al. (2014) describe a cadaver with a severe case of congenital scoliosis and found significant asymmetry in the rhomboid muscles.

Prevalence

In the literature review completed by Smith et al. (2015), they found that rhomboideus major and minor were fused in 2 out of 26 individuals with trisomy 18 (7.7%).

Clinical Implications
N/A

RHOMBOIDEUS OCCIPITALIS (FIGURE 3.1)

Entry adapted by permission from Springer Nature Customer Service Centre GmbH: Springer Current Molecular Biology Reports, Muscles Lost in Our Adult Primate Ancestors Still Imprint in Us: on Muscle Evolution, Development, Variations, and Pathologies. E. Boyle, V. Mahon, R. Diogo, 2020.

See also: Rhomboideus major, Rhomboideus minor

Synonyms

Rhomboideus occipitalis may also be referred to as occipito-scapularis (Wood), omo-occipitalis, rhomboideus cervicis, rhomboideus capitis, levator scapulae minor vel posterior, or levator anguli scapulae minor (Wood 1867a,b; Macalister 1875; Knott 1883a; Patten 1935; Aziz 1981; Sullivan and Osgood 1927; Jouffroy 1971; Bakkum and Miller 2016).

Typical Presentation

This muscle is only present as a variation or anomaly.

Comparative Anatomy

Among the apes, rhomboideus occipitalis seems to only be present in orangutans as a variation and extends from the medial border of the scapula to the cranium (Diogo et al. 2013b). In orangutans, this muscle is innervated by C4 and C5 (Kallner 1956).

Variations

Description

Rhomboideus occipitalis is present in karyotypically normal humans as an extremely rare variation (Rogawski 1990; Smith et al. 2015). It is not known whether this muscle appears during normal muscle formation and then disappears before birth. However, Jelev and Landzhov (2012–2013) suggest that variation in the rhomboid muscles may happen in the embryo when the rhomboid mass migrates to its usual position after its formation at CR14 mm (crown-rump length of 14 mm).

When present, rhomboideus occipitalis passes from the superior nuchal line on the occipital bone to attach to the medial border of the scapula at the level of the scapular spine (Wood 1867a,b; Knott 1883a; Bakkum and Miller 2016). As noted by Patten (1935), Zağyapan et al. (2008), and Stanchev et al. (2017), this muscle can also originate from the superior angle of the scapula between the origins of rhomboideus minor and levator scapulae.

In the case described by Patten (1935), rhomboideus occipitalis sent slips to the fascia of serratus posterior superior. This muscle can also send slips to levator scapulae, splenius, and serratus anterior (Wood 1870; Bakkum and Miller 2016). It may also be connected to trapezius (Macalister 1875). In the cadaver examined by Rogawski (1990), there were three other muscular variations on the left side of the body, including a third head of biceps brachii, absence of plantaris, and insertion of the tertius onto the distal phalanx of the fifth digit. Stanchev et al. (2017) describe a bilateral presentation of rhomboideus occipitalis that appeared to be comprised of an inferior oblique and superior oblique part on the left side, and an inferior oblique, middle straight, and superior oblique part on the right side.

Innervation

Zağyapan et al. (2008) and Stanchev et al. (2017) observed innervation of rhomboideus occipitalis by the dorsal scapular nerve.

Prevalence

N/A

Anomalies

Description

Mieden (1982) describes two male fetuses with cyclopia and alobar holoprosencephaly. Rhomboideus occipitalis was present on the right side of one specimen and on the left side of the other specimen. In both cases, the muscle extended between the superior nuchal line and the scapular attachment of rhomboid minor (Mieden 1982). In an otocephalic fetus examined by Lawrence and Bersu (1984), rhomboideus occipitalis extended from the spinous processes of the fourth and fifth cervical vertebrae to the medial border of the scapula, just above the level of the scapular spine.

Aziz (1979) found rhomboideus occipitalis present bilaterally in a neonate with trisomy 18. It arose deep to trapezius near the superior nuchal line and attached to the scapula. In a fetus with trisomy 18 and cyclopia, rhomboideus occipitalis was part of a complex with trapezius and a broad sternocleidomastoid (Smith et al. 2015). Rhomboideus occipitalis was also present in a fetus with craniorachischisis (Alghamdi et al. 2017). On the left sides of one adult and one fetus with trisomy 21, Bersu (1980) found an "occipitoscapular" muscle that extended between the superior nuchal line and serratus anterior.

Prevalence

In the literature review conducted by Smith et al. (2015), they found that rhomboideus occipitalis was present in 1 out of 24 individuals with trisomy 13 (4.2%) and 8 out of 26 individuals with trisomy 18 (30.8%). The "occipitoscapular" muscle described by Bersu (1980) was found in two out of five individuals with trisomy 21 (40%).

Clinical Implications

N/A

RHOMBOIDEUS TERTIUS (NOT ILLUSTRATED)

See also: Rhomboideus major, Rhomboideus minor

Synonyms

It is possible that rhomboideus tertius may be synonymous with rhomboideus minimus (rhomboideus minus), as it is in a similar location to this muscle (Jelev and Landzhov 2012–2013).

Typical Presentation

This muscle is only present as a variation.

Comparative Anatomy

In the apes, the rhomboid muscles are typically fused, and there is no portion that has been designated as a "rhomboideus tertius" (Diogo et al. 2010, 2012, 2013a,b, 2017).

Variations

Description

Rhomboideus tertius is a rare variation of the rhomboid muscles. Jelev and Landzhov (2012–2013) document a case in which rhomboideus tertius is present bilaterally, originating from the spinous processes of the sixth, seventh, and (on the left side) eighth thoracic vertebrae and attaching to the inferior most part of the medial border of the scapula. The muscle was nearly 1.5 times as wide (40 mm) on the left side than on the right side (27 mm). Lee and Jung (2015) describe a similar case in which this muscle originates from the spinous processes of the fourth and fifth thoracic vertebrae on the left side and the spinous processes of the second through fifth thoracic vertebrae on the right side. This case also presented with asymmetry, as the right muscle was about 3.5 times as wide at origin (90.50 mm) than the left muscle (25.13 mm).

Innervation

Rhomboideus tertius is innervated by the dorsal scapular nerve (Jelev and Landzhov 2012–2013).

Prevalence

N/A

Anomalies

N/A

Clinical Implications

Jelev and Landzhov (2012–2013) suggest that when present, rhomboideus tertius may be used with rhomboid major and rhomboid minor for intrathoracic muscle flap transfer, or for muscle transfer for the paralysis of trapezius.

LEVATOR SCAPULAE (FIGURE 3.1)

Synonyms

Levator scapulae may also be referred to as levator anguli scapulae (Macalister 1875).

Typical Presentation

Description

Levator scapulae originates from the transverse processes of the first four cervical vertebrae and inserts onto the medial border of the scapula (Standring 2016).

Innervation

Levator scapulae is innervated C3 and C4, and by the dorsal scapular nerve (C5) (Standring 2016).

Comparative Anatomy

Levator scapulae has a similar typical presentation in the apes, extending between various cervical vertebrae and the scapula (Gratiolet and Alix 1866; Champneys 1872; Deniker 1885; Kohlbrügge 1890–1892; Hepburn 1892; Primrose 1899, 1900; Pira 1913; Schück 1913; Sonntag 1923, 1924;

Sullivan and Osgood 1927; Stewart 1936; Raven 1950; Miller 1952; Preuschoft 1965; Swindler and Wood 1973; Gibbs 1999; Michilsens et al. 2009; Diogo et al. 2010, 2012, 2013a,b, 2017).

Variations

Description

Levator scapulae may be completely absent (Rickenbacher et al. 1985). Levator scapulae may vary in its vertebral attachments (Mori 1964; Macalister 1875; Rickenbacher et al. 1985; Standring 2016; Bakkum and Miller 2016). Levator scapulae can separate into multiple slips and may have additional attachments to the temporal bone/mastoid process, occipital bone, first or second rib, upper thoracic vertebrae, ligamentum nuchae, scalene muscles, longissimus cervicis, subclavius, subscapularis, trapezius, splenius capitis, rhomboideus muscles, or serratus muscles (Wood 1870; Curnow 1873; Flower and Murie 1867; Macalister 1875; Humphry 1873; Mori 1964; Rickenbacher et al. 1985; Bergman et al. 1988; Loukas et al. 2006a, Lima et al. 2012; Standring 2016; Bakkum and Miller 2016; Au et al. 2017). Gonzales et al. (2017) describe a variable presentation of this muscle on the right side of a cadaver in which the upper fibers of levator scapulae fused with the inferior attachment of rectus capitis lateralis. Au et al. (2017) suggest that the frequent connections between levator scapulae, serratus anterior, and serratus posterior superior may be due to the shared somitic cell origin of these muscles. A slip of levator scapulae that extends from some of the cervical vertebrae to the lateral end of the clavicle and the acromion has been identified as levator claviculae (see the entry for this muscle) (Bergman et al. 1988).

Prevalence

Based on observations from 60 sides, Mori (1964) reported that levator scapulae arose from cervical vertebrae one through four on 40 sides (66.7% of cases), from the first three cervical vertebrae on 16 sides (26.7%), from the first two cervical vertebrae on two sides (3.3%), and from the first five cervical vertebrae on two sides (3.3%). This author also found two types of anomalous slips. One type ran from the medial margin of levator scapulae to the spinous process of the second thoracic vertebra, to the dorsal surface of serratus posterior superior, or to the lumbodorsalis fascia in 9 out of 100 sides (9%) (Mori 1964). The other ran from the medial margin of levator scapulae to the ventral surface of subscapularis in 22 out of 100 sides (22%) (Mori 1964).

Au et al. (2017) studied variations of levator scapulae using MRI and found that this muscle had caudal accessory attachments in 16 out of 37 subjects (43.2%). Ten subjects exhibited unilateral attachments to serratus anterior, serratus posterior superior, or the first or second rib. Four subjects exhibited bilateral attachments to serratus anterior. One subject exhibited bilateral attachments to serratus posterior superior and a unilateral attachment to serratus anterior. One subject had bilateral attachments to both serratus anterior and serratus posterior superior.

Anomalies

Description

In a fetus with craniorachischisis, levator scapulae was absent on the right side and fused with the distal portion of the middle scalene and rhomboideus occipitalis on the left side (Alghamdi et al. 2017). In a male fetus with triploidy, Moen et al. (1984) found that the muscle bellies of levator scapulae were replaced by tendons on both sides of the body. Levator scapulae may blend with the origin of scalenus posterior in cases of trisomy 18 (Smith et al. 2015).

Mieden (1982) describes two male fetuses with cyclopia and alobar holoprosencephaly. On the right side of one specimen, levator scapulae was divided into superficial and deep heads, with the former attaching to the first and second cervical vertebrae and the latter to the third and fourth cervical vertebrae. A supernumerary slip of the superficial head originated from the third rib just posterior to serratus anterior (Mieden 1982).

Prevalence

In their literature review, Smith et al. (2015) found that the origin of scalenus posterior was blended with levator scapulae in 1 out of 26 individuals with trisomy 18 (3.8%).

Clinical Implications

Shpizner and Holliday (1993) suggest that asymmetry of levator scapulae may present as a palpable muscle mass in the posterior triangle and may be confused with disease. Loukas et al. (2006a) suggest that variable slips and insertions of levator scapulae may contribute to myofascial pain syndrome.

SUBCLAVIUS (FIGURE 3.2)

See also: Sternoscapularis, Pectoralis intermedius, Subclavius posticus

Synonyms

N/A

Typical Presentation

Description

Subclavius originates from the first rib and its costal cartilage and inserts onto the inferior aspect of the middle third of the clavicle (Standring 2016).

Innervation

Subclavius is innervated by the subclavian nerve (Standring 2016).

Comparative Anatomy

Subclavius has a similar typical presentation in the apes, extending from the first rib to the clavicle (Primrose 1899, 1900; Sullivan and Osgood 1927; Stewart 1936; Kallner 1956; Gibbs 1999; Diogo et al. 2010, 2012, 2013a,b, 2017). There may be an origin from the second rib in

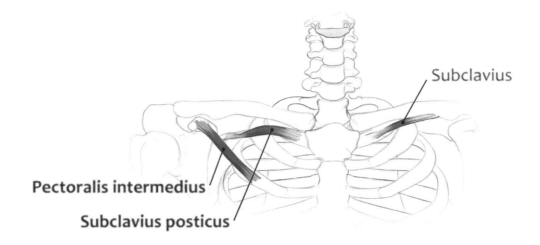

Subclavius

Pectoralis intermedius

Subclavius posticus

FIGURE 3.2 Thoracoclavicular muscles in anterior view.

orangutans, and from the second and/or third ribs in gibbons (Kohlbrügge 1890–1892; Hepburn 1892; Sonntag 1924; Gibbs 1999; Michilsens et al. 2009).

Variations

Description

Subclavius may also arise from the second rib (Bergman et al. 1988). Subclavius may insert onto the coracoclavicular ligament, transverse ligament of the scapula, acromion process, coracoid process, the superior border of the scapula, or the humerus (Macalister 1875; Bergman et al. 1988; Standring 2016). Subclavius may be doubled or divided into two parts (Macalister 1875). This muscle may also be completely absent and in some cases can be replaced by a fibrous band (Macalister 1875; Knott 1883a; Crerar 1892; Georgiev and Jelev 2009; Snosek and Loukas 2016; Yun et al. 2018).

Mori (1964) observed that subclavius could have a lateral end that divides into two portions: one inserting on the inferior surface of the clavicle and the other inserting onto the base of the coracoid process (type I variation). Alternatively, the lateral end of the muscle may insert into the inferior surface of the clavicle, but then courses on to insert onto the base of the coracoid or the superior border of the scapula (type II variation).

Subclavius is associated with scapuloclavicularis, which passes from the base of the coracoid and transverse scapular ligament to the posterior side of the clavicle (Figure 3.3) (Macalister 1875; Bergman et al. 1988). It may be connected to omohyoid at its origin and subclavius at its insertion (Macalister 1875). A variant of scapuloclavicularis is scapulocostoclavicularis, which originates from the upper border of the scapula and inserts onto the clavicle and first costal cartilage (Bergman et al. 1988). Other variations of subclavius include sternoscapularis, pectoralis intermedius, and subclavius posticus (see the entries for these muscles).

Prevalence

Out of 72 cases, Mori (1964) noted that 12 out of 72 sides (16.7%) exhibited type I variation (see above), while 6 out of 72 sides (8.3%) exhibited type II variation.

Anomalies

Description

Subclavius was absent bilaterally in a neonate with trisomy 18 (Aziz 1979) and a neonate with trisomy 13 (Aziz 1980).

Prevalence

In their literature review, Smith et al. (2015) found that subclavius was absent in 10 out of 20 individuals with trisomy 13 (50%) and in 11 out of 17 individuals with trisomy 18 (64.7%).

Clinical Implications

Georgiev and Jelev (2009) found that the fibrous band that may replace subclavius in cases of its absence can reduce the costoclavicular space and possibly lead to entrapment of the brachial plexus and the subclavian/axillary vessels and could thus contribute to the development of thoracic outlet syndrome.

Pectoralis Intermedius (Figure 3.2)

See also: Subclavius, Pectoralis major, Pectoralis minor

Synonyms

N/A

Typical Presentation

This muscle is only present as a variation.

Comparative Anatomy

Pectoralis intermedius was not present in the common chimpanzees or bonobos dissected by Potau et al. (2018), and there is little information about this muscle for other species.

Variations

Description

Pectoralis intermedius is a variant of subclavius (Bergman et al. 1988). It originates from the third and fourth ribs, in between pectoralis major and minor, and inserts onto the coracoid process (Bergman et al. 1988). Mori (1964) describes pectoralis intermedius as the deep layer of pectoralis major that arises from ribs three through six and is fused with the lateral insertion of pectoralis major. Sawada et al. (1991) observed that pectoralis intermedius can arise from the fourth and fifth ribs. Arican et al. (2006) found that this muscle originated from the third and fourth ribs and joined the tendon of the short head of biceps brachii upon insertion, just below the coracoid process.

Innervation

Pectoralis intermedius is innervated by the lateral pectoral nerve (Arican et al. 2006).

Prevalence

Mori (1964) states that pectoralis intermedius was found in 112 out of 351 cases (31.9%).

Anomalies

N/A

Clinical Implications

Potau et al. (2018) suggest that pectoralis intermedius could be mistaken for masses or tumors in medical imaging or interfere with the surgical use of pectoralis major flaps.

SUBCLAVIUS POSTICUS (FIGURE 3.2)

See also: Subclavius

Synonyms

This muscle is also referred to as scapulo-costalis (Knott 1883a), scapulocostalis minor (Gruber) (Macalister 1875), or chondroscapularis (Shetty et al. 2006).

Typical Presentation

This muscle is only present as a variation or anomaly.

Comparative Anatomy

N/A

Variations

Description

This muscle is a variant of subclavius (Bergman et al. 1988). Subclavius posticus (Rosenmüller) extends from the first rib or the first costal cartilage and inserts onto the superior margin of the scapula (Knott 1883a; Mori 1964; Bergman et al. 1988; Snosek and Loukas 2016). Moyano et al. (2018) report the presence of subclavius posticus in an adult male cadaver that originated from the cranial surface of the first costal cartilage near the insertion of subclavius, coursed laterally over the brachial plexus and subclavian vessels, and ended on the fascia of serratus anterior between its first two digitations near the superior border of the scapula.

Innervation

Innervation to subclavius posticus is variable (Cogar et al. 2015). This muscle can be innervated by the subclavian branch of the brachial plexus, the nerve to the omohyoid from the ansa cervicalis, or the suprascapular nerve (Cogar et al. 2015).

Prevalence

Macalister (1875) states that subclavius posticus is present in about 1 out of 15 subjects (6.7%). Mori (1964) found this muscle in five out of 500 sides from 250 cadavers (1%) and states that Nishi found this muscle in 2 out of 12 cadavers (16.7%). Akita et al. (2000) recorded the presence of this muscle in 11 out of 124 cadavers (8.9%).

Anomalies

Description

In individuals with trisomy 13 and trisomy 18, subclavius posticus extends from the upper margin of the scapula, and sometimes the transverse scapular ligament, to the first rib (Ramirez-Castro and Bersu 1978; Aziz 1979; Smith et al. 2015).

Prevalence

In the literature review conducted by Smith et al. (2015), they found that subclavius posticus was present in 3 out of 20 individuals with trisomy 13 (15%) and 5 out of 17 individuals with trisomy 18 (29.4%).

Clinical Implications

The presence of subclavius posticus can contribute to thoracic outlet syndrome and its consequences, including Paget-von-Schroetter syndrome (Akita et al. 2000; Forcada et al. 2001; Cogar et al. 2015). Kolpattil et al. (2009) report that the presence of the muscle could be confused with a pathological mass on a mammogram.

LEVATOR CLAVICULAE (FIGURE 3.3)

Entry adapted by permission from Springer Nature Customer Service Centre GmbH: Springer Current Molecular Biology Reports, Muscles Lost in Our Adult Primate Ancestors Still Imprint in Us: on Muscle Evolution, Development, Variations, and Pathologies. E. Boyle, V. Mahon, R. Diogo, 2020.
See also: Levator scapulae

Synonyms

Levator claviculae is also referred to as omocervicalis, levator scapulae anticus, or levator scapulae ventralis (Diogo et al. 2018), trachelo-clavicularis superior (Knott 1883a), cleido-cervicalis superior (Knott 1883a) or the cleidocervical muscle (Leon et al. 1995), cleidoatlanticus (Rodríguez-Vázquez et al. 2009), cleidotrachelian (Newell et al. 1991), or musculus trachleo-acromialis (Kuiper et al. 2014).

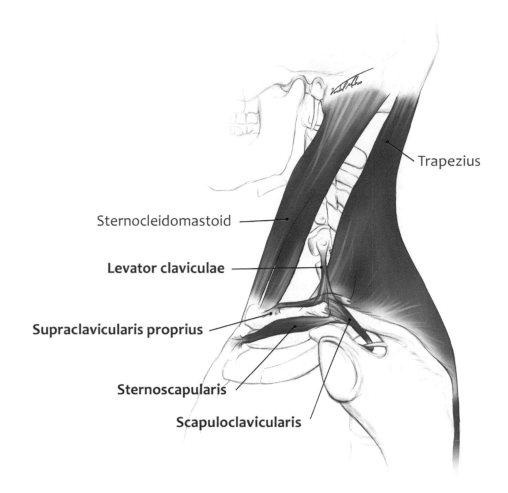

Trapezius

Sternocleidomastoid

Levator claviculae

Supraclavicularis proprius

Sternoscapularis

Scapuloclavicularis

FIGURE 3.3 Lateral view of additional thoracoclavicular variations, shown relative to trapezius and sternocleidomastoid.

Typical Presentation

This muscle is only present as a variation or anomaly.

Comparative Anatomy

Levator claviculae is normally present as a distinct muscle in the apes (Diogo et al. 2010, 2012, 2013a,b, 2017). In the apes, levator claviculae typically passes deep to trapezius, originating from the atlas and inserting onto the lateral end of the clavicle (Gratiolet and Alix 1866; Champneys 1872; Deniker 1885; Kohlbrügge 1890–1892; Chapman 1900; Schück 1913; Sullivan and Osgood 1927; Stewart 1936; Raven 1950; Miller 1952; Kallner 1956; Preuschoft 1965; Jouffroy 1971; Gibbs 1999; Diogo et al. 2010, 2012, 2013a,b, 2017). It may have an additional attachment onto the scapula in gorillas (Preuschoft 1965).

Variations

Description

Early in development, specifically between CR9 mm (crown-rump length of 9 mm) to CR 10.5 mm, the axial pectoral muscles resemble those of adult humans as subclavius is present but levator claviculae is absent (Diogo and Abdala 2010). Though closely associated with and

considered a variant of levator scapulae (Loukas et al. 2008b; Odate et al. 2012), levator claviculae has been argued to have embryological origins from scalenus anterior (Gruber 1876), sternocleidomastoid (Wood 1870), trapezius (Parsons 1898a), longus colli (Tomo et al. 1994), or the ventrolateral muscle primordia of the neck (Leon et al. 1995). In their review, Odate et al. (2012) arrive at the conclusion that levator scapulae shares a common embryological origin with levator scapulae (i.e., arise from the same myotome), based on the work of McKenzie (1955) and shared characteristics between these two muscles, including similar innervation and origin/insertion. This idea is reinforced by a detailed study of the comparative myology of tetrapods (Diogo et al. 2018).

When present, levator claviculae seems to be found more often on the left side than on the right side of the body (Rubinstein et al. 1999; Loukas et al. 2008b; Odate et al. 2012; Ferreli et al. 2019). Levator claviculae extends from the transverse processes of various cervical vertebrae (rarely from the first, but often from the second and third, or third and fourth) and attaches onto the middle third or lateral end of the clavicle, and the acromion (Wood 1864, Macalister 1875; Macdonald Brown 1880; Knott 1883a; Rickenbacher et al. 1985; Bergman et al. 1988; Leon et al.

1995; Ginsberg and Eicher 1999; Loukas et al. 2008b; Odate et al. 2012; Raikos et al. 2012; Bakkum and Miller 2016). It may also originate from the fifth or sixth cervical vertebrae (Macalister 1875; Knott 1883a; Billings and Sherrill 2015). Levator claviculae may insert onto the sternocleidomastoid or serratus anterior muscles (Flower and Murie 1867; Feigl and Pixner 2011) or blend with trapezius (Macalister 1875; Knott 1883a).

Innervation

This muscle can be innervated by cervical spinal nerve 3, 4, 5, or 6 (Leon et al. 1995; Loukas et al. 2008b; Odate et al. 2012)

Prevalence

Wood (1870) observed that levator claviculae is present in only 4 out of 202 humans (2%). Loukas et al. (2008b) observed levator claviculae in only 2 out of 2000 cadavers (0.1%). Based on CT scans of 300 individuals, Rubinstein et al. (1999) noted seven instances of the muscle (one bilateral case, five unilateral cases) in six individuals (2%). Review articles (e.g., Leon et al. 1995; Ginsberg et al. 1999; Rubinstein et al. 1999; Odate et al. 2012) report a prevalence of 2%–3%.

Anomalies

Description

Levator claviculae was present bilaterally in an adult with trisomy 21, extending from the basilar portion of the occipital bone to the clavicle (Bersu 1980).

Prevalence

In the literature review conducted by Smith et al. (2015), they found that levator claviculae was present in one out of five individuals with trisomy 21 (20%).

Clinical Implications

Levator claviculae can be misidentified as various pathologies. It can resemble a neck mass, cyst, lymphadenopathy or cervical adenopathy, metastasis, neurofibroma, arterial aneurysm, or thrombosed vein, and can present as an abnormal levator scapulae or sternocleidomastoid (Rüdisüli 1995; Ginsberg et al. 1999; Rubinstein et al. 1999; Santiago et al. 2001; Feigl and Pixner 2011; Odate et al. 2012). This muscle may also compress the supraclavicular nerve (Billings and Sherrill 2015) or contribute to thoracic outlet syndrome (Aydoğ et al. 2007).

Sternoscapularis (Figure 3.3)

See also: Subclavius

Synonyms

Sternoscapularis also known as sternoacromialis (Snosek and Loukas 2016).

Typical Presentation

This muscle is only present as a variation.

Comparative Anatomy

N/A

Variations

Description

This muscle is a variant of subclavius (Bergman et al. 1988). It arises from the sternum, courses between the clavicle and the coracoid process, and then attaches to the medial border of the acromion (Huntington 1904; Snosek and Loukas 2016).

Innervation

This muscle is innervated by the lateral pectoral nerves (Snosek and Loukas 2016).

Prevalence

N/A

Anomalies

N/A

Clinical Implications

N/A

Supraclavicularis proprius (Figure 3.3)

Synonyms

This muscle is also referred to as tensor fascia colli (Gruber) (Laidlaw 1902) or anomalus claviculae (Knott 1883a).

Typical Presentation

This muscle is only present as a variation.

Comparative Anatomy

N/A

Variations

Description

Supraclavicularis proprius courses from the sternal end of the clavicle to the acromial end and is sheathed in cervical fascia (Macalister 1875; Bergman et al. 1988; Snosek and Loukas 2016). It may have origins from the sternoclavicular joint and the fascia over sternocleidomastoid (Macalister 1875; Bergman et al. 1988; Ottone and Medan 2009; Snosek and Loukas 2016). It inserts onto the distal portion of the clavicle or the trapezius fascia (Macalister 1875; Laidlaw 1902; Bergman et al. 1988; Ottone and Medan 2009; Raikos et al. 2014; Snosek and Loukas 2016). Raikos et al. (2014) describe a case in which this muscle arose posteriorly from the medial surface of the clavicle, formed a muscular arch over the supraclavicular nerve, and split into three slips that inserted onto the trapezius, acromion, and the distal end of the clavicle.

Innervation

This muscle is innervated by the supraclavicular nerve (Laidlaw 1902).

Prevalence

Ottone and Medan (2009) observed the presence of this muscle on the left side of 1 out of 156 sides from 78 cadavers (0.64%).

Anomalies

N/A

Clinical Implications

Ottone and Medan (2009) and Raikos et al. (2014) suggest that the presence of supraclavicularis proprius could be a potential cause of supraclavicular nerve entrapment syndrome.

PECTORAL GIRDLE AND ARM MUSCLES

STERNALIS (FIGURE 3.4)

Synonyms

This muscle may also be referred to as episternalis, japonicas, parasternalis, presternalis, rectus sternalis, rectus sterni, rectus thoracis, rectus thoracicus superficialis, sternalis brutorum, superficial rectus abdominis, and thoracicus (Macalister 1875; Jelev et al. 2001; Snosek and Loukas 2016).

Typical Presentation

This muscle is only present as a variation or anomaly.

Comparative Anatomy

Sternalis is normally absent in nonhuman primates (Diogo and Wood 2012a). According to the literature reviews and dissections done by Diogo et al. (2010, 2012, 2013a,b, 2017), this muscle is absent in orangutans, gorillas, common chimpanzees, and bonobos, and its presence is variable in gibbons.

Variations

Description

Sternalis has several presentations and varies widely in width, length, and attachments (Macalister 1875; Snosek and Loukas 2016; Standring 2016). When present, sternalis is a vertical slip of fibers in the anterior thoracic wall that lies close to the sternum and runs on top of pectoralis major, extending from the sternal/infraclavicular area to the upper abdominal wall or costal cartilages (Mori 1964; Jouffroy 1971; Jelev et al. 2001; Snosek and Loukas 2016; Standring 2016). It may originate from the manubrium, sternum, clavicle, upper ribs, upper costal cartilages, pectoralis fascia, pectoralis major and/or sternocleidomastoid and its fascia (Macalister 1875; Mori 1964; Jelev et al. 2001; Hung et al. 2012; Poveda et al. 2013; Snosek and Loukas 2016;

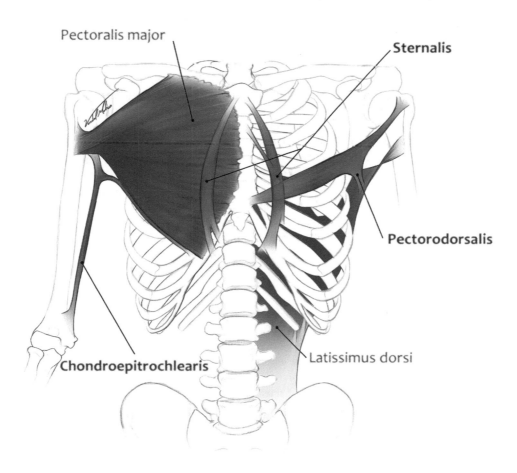

FIGURE 3.4 Thoracohumeral muscles in anterior view.

Standring 2016; Duque-Parra et al. 2019). It may insert into the lower ribs and costal cartilages, pectoral fascia, pectoralis major, external oblique aponeurosis, and/or the rectus sheath (Macalister 1875; Mori 1964; Jelev et al. 2001; Hung et al. 2012; Poveda et al. 2013; Snosek and Loukas 2016; Standring 2016; Duque-Parra et al. 2019). Duque-Parra et al. (2019) found that sternalis fibers extended between sternocleidomastoid to the fascia of the seventh intercostal muscle. In this case, the muscle had two bellies.

Sternalis can be partially or completely absent and also can have unilateral or bilateral presentations (Young Lee et al. 2006; Duque-Parra et al. 2019), though a unilateral presence is more frequent (Snosek and Loukas 2016; Standring 2016). When muscles are present on both sides, they may fuse across the sternum (Mori 1964; Snosek and Loukas 2016). Kalpana and Usha (2010) and Dudgeon et al. (2017) report sternalis muscles with three bellies. Macalister (1875) states that tendinous intersections in the muscle have been observed by some researchers.

Snosek and Loukas (2016) provide a comprehensive review of this muscle, including speculation on its homology and embryological origin. The authors review the four common arguments for origin of sternalis—that it is a remnant of panniculus carnosus, a downward extension of sternocleidomastoid, an upward extension of rectus abdominis, or a derivative of pectoralis major—and appear to favor this last hypothesis, suggesting that sternalis should be classified as one of the many muscular variations caused by abnormal pectoral muscle development (Snosek and Loukas 2016). Standring (2016) also considers sternalis a variant of pectoralis major.

Snosek and Loukas (2016) also note that other supernumerary muscles found on the anterior thoracic wall may be described as novel muscle variants but are more likely variants of sternalis. Examples include oblique pectoralis anterior, which passes from the sternum to the lower ribs and the rectus sheath (Huber et al. 2012), rectus thoracis bifurcalis, which extends between the aponeurosis of external oblique and the manubrium and sends two diverging aponeurotic bands to sternocleidomastoid (Mehta et al. 2010), and sternomastalis, which passes from the pectoral fascia and sternocostal junction to the tissue of the breast and nipple-areola complex (Kale et al. 2006).

Innervation

Musculus sternalis is innervated by the medial or lateral pectoral nerve in most cases (Mori 1964; O'Neill and Folan-Curran 1998; Kida et al. 2000; Kumar et al. 2003; Hung et al. 2012; Snosek and Loukas 2016; Duque-Parra et al. 2019). It may also be innervated the anterior cutaneous branches of the intercostal nerves, or both of these nerves in rare cases (Mori 1964; O'Neill and Folan-Curran 1998; Jelev et al. 2001; Motabagani et al. 2004; Snosek and Loukas 2016; Duque-Parra et al. 2019). It may be the case that sternalis is not supplied by the intercostal nerves, but that they may pass near to or through sternalis on their way to innervate other structures (Snosek and Loukas 2016).

Prevalence

Sternalis is estimated to be present in 3%–8% of the world population (Pérez et al. 2008). Snosek and Loukas (2016) provide a comprehensive list of prevalence rates from cadaveric studies and clinical investigations and state that the overall prevalence in the general population is about 7.8%. Macalister (1875) states that Gruber found sternalis in 5 out of 95 cases (5.3%) and that Turner found it in 21 out of 650 subjects (3.2%). Macalister (1875) himself found sternalis present in 11 out of 350 subjects (3.1%) and connected to the sternal head of sternocleidomastoid in 2 out of 600 subjects (0.3%).

Prevalence can be anywhere from ~1%, as observed in a Chilean population (Molina et al. 2017) and a Taiwanese population, to 23.5% as observed in a Chinese population (Jelev et al. 2001; Raikos et al. 2011; Vishal et al. 2013; Snosek and Loukas 2016). Sato (1968c) reported that sternalis was present in 61 out of 426 sides (14.3%) in Kyushu-Japanese males and present in 42 of 266 sides (15.79%) in females. Mehta et al. (2010) found sternalis in 1 out of 88 cadavers of Asian origin (1.1%).

Mori (1964) searched for sternalis in 350 Japanese male cadavers and 25 Japanese female cadavers. This author found sternalis in 36 male cadavers (10.3%) and 3 female cadavers (12%). Among males, 12 presented the muscle bilaterally and 24 presented the muscle unilaterally, while two females presented the muscle bilaterally and one presented the muscle unilaterally. Therefore, sternalis was present in 53 out of 750 sides (7.1%). Mori (1964) also classified the 53 instances of sternalis into six types and noted that on seven sides (1%) both ends of the muscle attached to the pectoral fascia, on seven sides (1%) the muscle extended from the sternum superiorly to the pectoral fascia inferiorly, on 12 sides (1.7%) the muscle extended from the sternum superiorly to the rectus sheath inferiorly, on eight sides (1.1%) the muscle extended from the pectoral fascia superiorly to the rectus sheath inferiorly, on two sides (0.3%) the muscle extended from the tendon of sternocleidomastoid superiorly to the pectoral fascia inferiorly, and on 17 sides (2.4%) the muscle extended from the tendon of sternocleidomastoid superiorly to the rectus sheath inferiorly.

Duque-Parra et al. (2019) found this muscle in 2 out of 68 Colombian cadavers (2.94%). Saeed et al. (2002) found a prevalence of 4% in the Kingdom of Saudi Arabia. In Europeans, prevalence is estimated at 4.4%, while prevalence is estimated at 8.4% in Africans (Loukas et al. 2004). Jelev et al. (2001) found sternalis in 3 out of 102 Bulgarian cadavers (2.9%). Krishnan et al. (2017) observed the presence of sternalis in 3 out of 18 cadavers from Wales (16.7%). Sonne (2020) found a bilateral presentation of sternalis in 2 out of 36 cadavers from the United States (5.5%). This muscle may be more prevalent in women than in men (Snosek and Loukas 2016; Aguado-Henche et al. 2018).

Anomalies

Description

Anomalous presentations are similar to the above, extending from the infraclavicular region near the sternum to the lower ribs or rectus abdominis (Smith et al. 2015). Macalister (1875) states that Barkow (1828) found sternalis in an abnormal individual extending between the second and seventh ribs.

Prevalence

Windle (1893) conducted dissections on ten anencephalic fetuses and noted the presence of sternalis on the left side in two females and one male, and on both sides in one female, yielding a prevalence of 5 out of 20 sides (25%). Abraham (1883) found sternalis in 6 out of 11 anencephalic fetuses (54.5%). In their literature review, Smith et al. (2015) found that sternalis was reported in 1 out of 17 (5.8%) trisomy 18 individuals.

Clinical Implications

Sternalis can be mistaken for pathology, especially mammary cancer, when evaluating mammograms, CT scans, or MRI scans (Bradley et al. 1996; Goktan et al. 2006; Marques et al. 2009; Mehta et al. 2010; Standring 2016; Molina et al. 2017). Standring (2016) and Snosek and Loukas (2016) note that sternalis may be as useful as a muscular flap in reconstructive surgeries.

DORSOEPITROCHLEARIS (FIGURE 3.11)

Entry adapted by permission from Springer Nature Customer Service Centre GmbH: Springer Current Molecular Biology Reports, Muscles Lost in Our Adult Primate Ancestors Still Imprint in Us: on Muscle Evolution, Development, Variations, and Pathologies. E. Boyle, V. Mahon, R. Diogo, 2020.

See also: Latissimus dorsi, Triceps brachii

Synonyms

Alternative names for this muscle include latissimo-condylus or latissimo-epitrochlearis (Barnard 1875), latissimo-condyloideus (Kohlbrügge 1890–1892; Chapman 1878, 1879; 1880, 1900; Hepburn 1892; Primrose 1899, 1900; Grönroos 1903; Sommer 1907; MacDowell 1910; Pira 1913; Sullivan and Osgood 1927; Loth 1931), latissimo-tricipitalis (Schück 1913; Fick 1925; Kallner 1956; Preuschoft 1965), appendix of latissimus dorsi (Tyson 1699), accessorium tricipitis (Bergman et al. 1988) or tricipiti accessorius (Macalister 1875), and tensor fasciae antebrachii, anconeus accessorius, accessorius latissimus dorsi, dorso-antebrachialis, anconeus quintus, anconeus longus, or extensor cubiti sensu Jouffroy (1971).

Typical Presentation

This muscle is only present as a variation or anomaly.

Comparative Anatomy

While typically absent in adult humans, dorsoepitrochlearis is present in nonhuman primates (Diogo and Wood 2011, 2012a). This muscle is present in all apes, typically extending from latissimus dorsi to the medial epicondyle of the humerus (Tyson 1699; Gratiolet and Alix 1866; Barnard 1875; Chapman 1880, 1900; Kohlbrügge 1890–1892; Beddard 1893; Dwight 1895; Primrose 1899, 1900; Michaelis 1903; MacDowell 1910; Schück 1913; Sonntag 1923, 1924; Sullivan and Osgood 1927; Raven 1950; Miller 1952; Swindler and Wood 1973; Michilsens et al. 2009; Gibbs 1999; Diogo et al. 2010, 2012, 2013a,b, 2017). Dorsoepitrochlearis is innervated by the radial nerve in the apes (Gibbs 1999; Diogo et al. 2010, 2012, 2013a,b, 2017).

In gibbons, it is often blended with the short head of the biceps (Howell and Straus 1932; Michilsens et al. 2009; Diogo et al. 2012). MacDowell (1910) observed a slip from coracobrachialis to dorsoepitrochlearis in one common chimpanzee. There may be an additional origin from the coracoid process in common chimpanzees (Gratiolet and Alix 1866; Diogo et al. 2013a). It may attach to the intermuscular septum in orangutans (Barnard 1875; Hepburn 1982; Diogo et al. 2013b). In orangutans and common chimpanzees, there may be an insertion onto the olecranon process (Grönroos 1903; Ziegler 1964; Diogo et al. 2013a,b).

Variations

Description

Dorsoepitrochlearis is typically only present in the early stages of human development, usually appearing in human embryos at CR15 mm (crump-round length of 15 mm) and disappearing in embryos at CR18 mm (Haninec et al. 2009). However, Diogo et al. (2019) state that since all other arm muscles are differentiated earlier (CR10.5 mm), further research is needed to reveal if dorsoepitrochlearis is differentiated earlier than CR15 mm.

When present in adults, dorsoepitrochlearis originates from latissimus dorsi near to or on the tendon of insertion, passes through the axilla, and inserts onto the medial epicondyle of the humerus (Haninec et al. 2009; Bakkum and Miller 2016). It may also insert into the brachial and forearm fascia, the humerus, the lateral epicondyle and olecranon, or the long head of triceps (Bergman et al. 1988; Bakkum and Miller 2016). When the dorsoepitrochlearis inserts onto the medial epicondyle of the humerus, its distal part is similar to that of the chondroepitrochlearis (Figure 3.4), the main difference being that proximally the former is often linked to the latissimus dorsi, while the latter is often linked to the pectoral muscles. Farfán et al. (2019) report a case in which dorsoepitrochlearis originated via three fascicles.

Innervation

In three of the cases described by Haninec et al. (2009), dorsoepitrochlearis was innervated by the thoracodorsal nerve. This differs from the innervation observed in other primates (see above).

Prevalence

Haninec et al. (2009) observe the presence of this muscle in 4 out of 209 adults (1.9%). Bergman et al. (1988) and Bakkum and Miller (2016) note this muscle is present in 5% of bodies.

Anomalies

Description

An anomalous dorsoepitrochlearis muscle connects latissimus dorsi to pectoralis major or to the long head of the triceps (Windle 1893; Aziz 1979; Smith et al. 2015; Alghamdi et al. 2017). Alghamdi et al. (2017) note that in a fetus with craniorachischisis, dorsoepitrochlearis was fused to the inner side of the inferior band (costohumeralis) of pectoralis major. Alghamdi et al. (2017) note that this muscle is similar in presentation to dorsoepitrochlearis found on the right side of one female fetus with anencephaly by Windle (1893).

Prevalence

Testut (1884) and Aziz (1981) suggest that this muscle is present in about 5% of anomalous humans. Barash et al. (1970) state that this muscle is present in an infant with trisomy 18, and Aziz (1980, 1981) notes the presence of dorsoepitrochlearis in two trisomy 18 neonates, but not in three trisomy 13 neonates. In the literature review conducted by Smith et al. (2015), they noted the presence of this muscle in 4 out of 26 individuals with trisomy 18 (15.4%).

Clinical Implications

Haninec et al. (2009) note that the presence of dorsoepitrochlearis can compress nerves in the axilla and lead to symptoms such as paresthesia, pain, and muscle weakness.

PANNICULUS CARNOSUS (NOT ILLUSTRATED)

Entry adapted by permission from Springer Nature Customer Service Centre GmbH: Springer Current Molecular Biology Reports, Muscles Lost in Our Adult Primate Ancestors Still Imprint in Us: on Muscle Evolution, Development, Variations, and Pathologies. E. Boyle, V. Mahon, R. Diogo, 2020.

Synonyms

According to the summary by Naldaiz-Gastesi et al. (2018), alternative names for this muscle include cutaneous trunci, musculus cutaneous, cutaneous maximus muscle, subcutaneous muscle, and superficial fascia system.

Typical Presentation

Remnants of panniculus carnosus are present only as variations, and the entire muscle is present as a rare anomaly.

Comparative Anatomy

This muscle is present in basal primates and several species of monkeys and can be vestigial in gorillas (Jouffroy 1971;

Diogo and Wood 2011; Diogo et al. 2018), although dissections by Sommer (1907), Raven (1950), and Diogo et al. (2010) did not find this muscle.

Variations

Description

Panniculus carnosus is a cutaneous muscle sheet arising from the pectoral muscle mass and covering various trunk regions (Smith et al. 2015). It is present in many mammals and derives from the pectoralis muscle of amphibians and reptiles (Diogo et al. 2018). Bergman et al. (1988) state that panniculus carnosus is represented only by vestigial remnants in humans, which may present as extra muscular slips in the pectoral region. These slips may have attachments to the abdominal aponeurosis, rectus sheath, serratus anterior fascia, axillary fascia, the fascia between coracobrachialis and pectoralis minor, the humerus, or the coracoid process (Bergman et al. 1988). Several muscles in adult humans are considered to be remnants of panniculus carnosus, including some craniofacial muscles, platysma, pectorodorsalis, sternalis, abdominal external oblique, palmaris brevis, and potentially several other striated muscles in the upper limb, pectoral region, and trunk (Naldaiz-Gastesi et al. 2018).

Innervation

Panniculus carnosus is innervated by various nerves in different species, depending on where in the body the panniculus carnosus fibers are located (Naldaiz-Gastesi et al. 2018).

Prevalence

N/A

Anomalies

Description

Dunlap et al. (1986) describe panniculus carnosus in a fetus with trisomy 18 and a fetus with trisomy 21. On the left side of the fetus with trisomy 18, panniculus carnosus arose from the level of the tenth rib in the midaxillary line and inserted onto the humerus and onto the deep aspect of pectoralis major. It had a third tendinous insertion into the tendon of latissimus dorsi, which Dunlap et al. (1986) state is pectorodorsalis. On the right side, it arose from the level of the seventh rib in the midaxillary line and inserted onto the humerus. In the fetus with trisomy 21, panniculus carnosus was adjacent to the axillary border of latissimus dorsi and inserted onto the humerus.

Prevalence

In their literature review, Smith et al. (2015) found that panniculus carnosus was reported in 1 out of 26 trisomy 18 individuals (3.8%) and 1 out of 7 individuals with trisomy 21 (14.3%).

Clinical Implications

N/A

PECTORALIS MAJOR (FIGURES 3.4 AND 3.5)

See also: Sternalis, Sternoclavicularis, Pectoralis quartus, Pectorodorsalis, Chondroepitrochlearis, Dorsoepitrochlearis, Pectoralis abdominis

Synonyms

This muscle may also be referred to as the great pectoral (Macalister 1875).

Typical Presentation

Description

Pectoralis major has three heads. The clavicular head originates from the medial half of the clavicle (Standring 2016). The sternocostal head originates from the body of the sternum and the second through sixth costal cartilages (Standring 2016). The abdominal or rectus head originates from the external oblique aponeurosis (Standring 2016). The muscle inserts via a tendon onto the humerus at the lateral lip of the intertubercular sulcus (Standring 2016).

Innervation

Pectoralis major is innervated by the medial and lateral pectoral nerves (Standring 2016).

Comparative Anatomy

Pectoralis major has a similar typical presentation in the apes, with clavicular, sternocostal, and abdominal heads (Gibbs 1999; Diogo et al. 2010, 2012, 2013a,b, 2017). In gibbons and gorillas, pectoralis major is often blended with biceps brachii (Deniker 1885; Kohlbrügge 1890–1892; Howell and Straus 1932; Stewart 1936; Raven 1950; Preuschoft 1965; Michilsens et al. 2009; Diogo et al. 2012).

In bonobos, pectoralis major can be fused with deltoid, sternocleidomastoid, and/or pectoralis minor (Diogo et al. 2017). In orangutans, the clavicular head originates from the sternum and does not have an attachment to the clavicle (Chapman 1880; Hepburn 1892; Beddard 1893; Primrose 1899, 1900; Michaelis 1903; Sullivan and Osgood 1927; Stewart 1936; Kallner 1956; Diogo et al. 2013b).

Variations

Description

The three heads of pectoralis major may be completely distinct from one another (Macalister 1875; Knott 1883a). Absence or reduction of one or more heads has been observed (Macalister 1875; Bing 1902; Bergman et al. 1988; Snosek and Loukas 2016; Standring 2016; Haładaj et al. 2019). The clavicular head may be divided (Macalister 1875). It can also extend laterally on the clavicle as far as deltoideus (Bergman et al. 1988; Snosek and Loukas 2016; Haładaj et al. 2019). The sternocostal head may extend laterally to latissimus dorsi (Bergman et al. 1988). It may also be bilaminar (Macalister 1875). There may also be variation in the number of costal attachments of this head, with inclusion of the first, seventh, and/or eighth costal cartilages (Macalister 1875; Snosek and Loukas 2016; Standring 2016).

Pectoralis major may be continuous with deltoid, external oblique, or rectus abdominis (Macalister 1875; Bergman et al. 1988). It may send an accessory slip to biceps brachii or latissimus dorsi (Macalister 1875; Knott 1883a; Mori 1964). An accessory head of pectoralis major has been observed originating from serratus anterior (Loukas et al. 2006b). Hammad and Mohamed (2006) observed an accessory tendon originating from the lateral portion of pectoralis

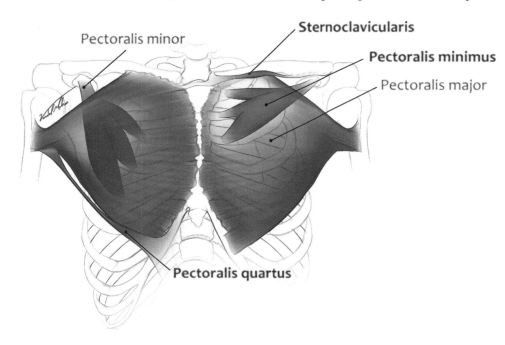

FIGURE 3.5 Anterior view of the pectoralis muscles and pectoral region variations.

major that had an attachment to the shoulder joint capsule. Tubbs et al. (2008a) also note an insertion of pectoralis major onto the shoulder joint capsule.

The fibers of the left and right pectoralis major muscles may fuse over the sternum (Macalister 1875; Snosek and Loukas 2016; Standring 2016). In rare cases, the entire pectoralis major muscle may be absent or even doubled (Macalister 1867a, 1875; Bergman et al. 1988; Upasna et al. 2015; Snosek and Loukas 2016). Pectoralis major is associated with supernumerary muscles including sternalis, pectoralis quartus, pectorodorsalis, and chondroepitrochlearis (see these entries).

Prevalence

In a study of 40 cadavers, Haładaj et al. (2019) observe the fusion of the clavicular head of pectoralis major with deltoideus in two male cadavers (5%), and hypotrophy of the clavicular head in one female (2.5%). In a literature review of 186 cases of congenital muscle absences, Bing (1902) reported that the sternocostal part of pectoralis major is defective or absent more than any other muscle (deficient in 102 cases). Upasna et al. (2015) report the absence of the pectoralis major in 1 out of 50 cases (2%), and Lee and Chun (1991) report its absence in one case. Upasna et al. (2015) cite notes from Bergman and colleagues that suggest that this muscle was absent in 3 of 15,000 cases in one study, the muscle was absent in 5 of 54,000 cases in another study. Mori (1964) reports a slip connecting pectoralis major to biceps brachii in 15 out of 320 arms from 160 Japanese individuals (4.7%). Mori (1964) also reports a slip connecting pectoralis major to latissimus dorsi in 12 out of 320 arms from 160 Japanese individuals (3.75%), but this slip is not designated as an axillary arch, simply an "abnormous slip."

Anomalies

Description

Poland syndrome, a rare congenital anomaly, can lead to the absence of the sternocostal head, deficiencies of the clavicular head, or the absence of the entire pectoralis major muscle (Cingel et al. 2013; Snosek and Loukas 2016).

In a fetus with craniorachischisis, dorsoepitrochlearis was fused to the inner side of the inferior band (costohumeralis) of pectoralis major on the right side of the body (Alghamdi et al. 2017). On the left side of the body, pectoralis major was fused with deltoideus, and an additional bundle was present on the inner side of this muscle. This bundle originated from the anterior capsule of the shoulder joint and attached distally to the crest of the greater tubercle of the humerus (Alghamdi et al. 2017). Mieden (1982) describes an infant with median cleft lip, hypotelorism, and alobar holoprosencephaly. On the right side, pectoralis major split into superficial and deep layers at the costal cartilages (Mieden 1982).

In a neonate with trisomy 13, the right pectoralis major was divided into clavicular, sternal, and costal portions (Aziz 1980). In two neonates with trisomy 18 (Aziz 1979, 1981) and in a female fetus with trisomy 18 (Alghamdi et al.

2018), deltoid was fused with pectoralis major bilaterally, forming the deltopectoral complex. In the neonate, the pectoral portion did not insert directly onto the humerus but instead was continuous with biceps brachii (Aziz 1979). In the fetus, the abdominal portion of pectoralis major on the left side was absent (Alghamdi et al. 2018). The fascia on the deep surface of pectoralis major was fused with the fascia of the short head of biceps brachii bilaterally.

Prevalence

In their literature review, Smith et al. (2015) found that pectoralis major was fused with deltoideus in 21 out of 26 individuals with trisomy 18 (80.8%).

Clinical Implications

Haładaj et al. (2019) state that knowledge of the numerous anatomical variations of pectoralis major is important for planning and conducting surgeries in this region.

Pectoralis minor (Figure 3.5)

See also: Pectoralis minimus, Costocoracoideus, Sternoclavicularis, Tensor semivaginae articulationis humeroscapularis

Synonyms

N/A

Typical Presentation

Description

Pectoralis minor lies deep to pectoralis major (Standring 2016). It originates from the third, fourth, and fifth ribs and from the intercostal fascia and has a tendinous insertion into the coracoid process (Standring 2016).

Innervation

Pectoralis minor is innervated by the medial and lateral pectoral nerves (Standring 2016).

Comparative Anatomy

Pectoralis minor has a similar typical presentation in the apes, extending from the ribs to the coracoid process, with similar variability in costal origins (Gratiolet and Alix 1866; Deniker 1885; Kohlbrügge 1890–1892; Hepburn 1892; Beddard 1893; Primrose 1899, 1900; Sonntag 1923, 1924; Sullivan and Osgood 1927; Stewart 1936; Miller 1952; Kallner 1956; Gibbs 1999; Michilsens et al. 2009; Gibbs 1999; Diogo et al. 2010, 2012, 2013a,b, 2017).

The costal attachments may include the first rib in gibbons, common chimpanzees, and bonobos (Hepburn 1892; Michilsens et al. 2009; MacDowell 1910, Diogo et al. 2012, 2013a, 2017). In common chimpanzees, the insertion into the coracoid may be absent (Champneys 1872; Chapman 1879; Sutton 1883; Hepburn 1892; MacDowell 1910; Ziegler 1964; Swindler and Wood 1973; Diogo et al. 2013a, 2017). It may have an insertion into the clavicle in gibbons (Hepburn 1892; Sonntag 1924, Stewart 1936; Gibbs 1999;

Michilsens et al. 2009; Gibbs 1999; Diogo et al. 2012). It may have additional attachments to the proximal humerus or glenohumeral joint capsule in orangutans and common chimpanzees (Diogo et al. 2013a,b).

Variations

Description

Pectoralis minor may arise from the second to fourth ribs (Macalister 1875; Standring 2016). Other origin patterns include the second to fifth ribs, second to fourth ribs, third to fourth ribs, or third to fifth ribs (Macalister 1875; Mori 1964; Standring 2016), or only from the fifth rib in a rare case (Turan-Özdemir and Cankur 2004). An origin from the sixth rib has been observed (Macalister 1875; Bergman et al. 1988). The tendon may cross the coracoid process into the coraco-acromial ligament, or even extend beyond the ligament and attach to shoulder joint capsule or the humerus (Macalister 1875; Knott 1883a; Bergman et al. 1988, Tubbs et al. 2005a; Uzel et al. 2008; Snosek and Loukas 2016; Standring 2016). Other potential attachments include the clavicle, costocoracoid membrane, costohumeral ligament, or the supraspinatus tendon (Macalister 1875; Uzel et al. 2008; Snosek and Loukas 2016).

Pectoralis minor may be connected with subclavius, pectoralis major, biceps brachii, latissimus dorsi, or coracobrachialis (Macalister 1875; Bergman et al. 1988; Snosek and Loukas 2016). Pectoralis minor may be absent unilaterally or bilaterally, especially when pectoralis major is absent (Macalister 1875; Bergman et al. 1988, Snosek and Loukas 2016; Standring 2016). It may also be doubled when pectoralis major is doubled (Macalister 1875). Variations of this muscle also include slips that are defined as discrete muscles including pectoralis minimus, costocoracoideus, sternoclavicularis, and tensor semivaginae articulationis humeroscapularis (see these entries).

Prevalence

Macalister (1875) notes that the tendon of pectoralis minor was prolonged over the coracoid process in 17 out of 106 subjects (16.04%). Upasna et al. (2015) report the absence of the pectoralis minor in 1 out of 50 cases (2%). Mori (1964) found that pectoralis minor originated from the first three ribs in 2 out of 326 cases (0.6%), ribs two through four in 46 cases (14.1%), ribs two through five in 115 cases (35.3%), ribs three and four in nine cases (2.8%), ribs three through five in 153 cases (46.9%), and ribs three through six in one case (0.3%). The superior most attachment was to rib one in two cases (0.6%), rib two in 161 cases (49.4%), and rib three in 163 cases (50%). The inferior most attachment was to rib three in two cases (0.6%), rib four in 55 cases (16.9%), rib five in 268 cases (82.2%), and rib six in one case (0.3%).

Anomalies

Description

Poland syndrome, a rare congenital anomaly, can cause the underdevelopment or absence of pectoralis minor (Snosek and Loukas 2016; Standring 2016; Petleshkova et al. 2019).

Alghamdi et al. (2017) note that on the left side of the body of a fetus with craniorachischisis, pectoralis minor had a normal insertion but sent an abnormal slip connecting it to pectoralis major. On the right side of the body, pectoralis minor originated from ribs two through four and inserted onto the lesser tubercle of the humerus (Alghamdi et al. 2017).

In a neonate with trisomy 13, pectoralis minor was absent on the left side (Aziz 1980). In a neonate with trisomy 18, the left pectoralis minor was divided into two fascicles (Aziz 1979). One extended from the fifth rib to the coracoid process and the other extended from the fourth rib to the coracoid process. In a female fetus with trisomy 18, the insertion of pectoralis minor on the right side extended inferiorly to the fascia of coracobrachialis (Alghamdi et al. 2018).

Prevalence

In their literature review, Smith et al. (2015) found that pectoralis minor was absent in 3 out of 24 individuals with trisomy 13 (12.5%) and in 1 out of 26 trisomy 18 individuals (3.8%).

Clinical Implications

Aberrant lateral insertions (ectopic insertions) of the pectoralis minor tendon beyond the coracoid process may lead to pain, clicking, or restricted range of motion (Moineau et al. 2008; Low and Tan 2010; Pandey et al. 2016; Snosek and Loukas 2016; Ruiz Santiago et al. 2019).

CHONDROEPITROCHLEARIS (FIGURE 3.4)

See also: Pectoralis major, Pectoralis quartus

Synonyms

This muscle may also be referred to as costoepitrochlearis, chondrohumeralis (Bergman et al. 1988), thoracoepicondylaris, chondrofascialis, chondrobrachialis, costohumeralis (Snosek and Loukas 2016), and chondroepicondylaris sensu (Palagama et al. 2016).

Typical Presentation

This muscle is only present as a variation or anomaly.

Comparative Anatomy

Chondroepitrochlearis is present in rare cases in common chimpanzees and bonobos, originating from the ribs and inserting onto the proximal humerus at the crest of the greater tubercle (MacDowell 1910; Diogo et al. 2013a, 2017). Palagama et al. (2016) suggest that chondroepitrochlearis, acting as an insertion point for pectoralis major on the medial epicondyle, would impede shoulder extension in suspensory primates, likely contributing to why it is rare in humans and our closest relatives.

Variations

Description

Chondroepitrochlearis is considered a variant of pectoralis major. It originates from one or more ribs, the chondrocostal junction of pectoralis major, or the external oblique aponeurosis (Macalister 1875; Knott 1880, 1883a; Bergman et al. 1988; Snosek and Loukas 2016). It courses through the axilla to insert onto the medial intermuscular septum or medial epicondyle of the humerus (Macalister 1875; Knott 1880, 1883a; Bergman et al. 1988; Snosek and Loukas 2016). Macalister (1875) found an insertion into the brachial aponeurosis. Standring (2016) describes chondroepitrochlearis as an extra head of pectoralis major that originates deep to the sternal and abdominal heads from the fifth through seventh ribs and their associated costal cartilages. It can be present unilaterally or bilaterally (Lin 1988; Snosek and Loukas 2016). It may have two bellies (Macalister 1875). It frequently occurs with pectorodorsalis (Macalister 1875; Chiba et al. 1983; Lin 1988; Spinner et al. 1991; Snosek and Loukas 2016; Palagama et al. 2016).

Macalister (1875) suggests that chondroepitrochlearis may be a variant of pectoralis quartus (see the entry for this muscle). In a cadaver examined by Carroll et al. (2019), chondroepitrochlearis was present along with a third head of biceps brachii. These authors suggest that chondroepitrochlearis may be a remnant of panniculus carnosus (Carroll et al. 2019). Barcia and Genovés (2009) consider chondrofascialis to be a separate muscle from, not a synonym of, chondroepitrochlearis, as they argue that chondrofascialis inserts into the fascia of the arm without direct connections to pectoralis major or the humerus and should thus be considered intermediate in form between pectoralis quartus and chondroepitrochlearis.

Innervation

Chondroepitrochlearis is innervated by the medial pectoral nerve (Barcia and Genovés 2009; Palagama et al. 2016).

Prevalence

Flaherty et al. (1999) observed chondroepitrochlearis in only 1 out of 200 cadavers over the course of 20 years (0.5%). Natsis et al. (2012) report a prevalence of this muscle in 1 out of 119 cadavers (0.84%), based on dissections done by them and Natsis et al. (2010).

Anomalies

Description

In a neonate with trisomy 13, Aziz (1980) describes chondroepitrochlearis as a derivative of the sternal portion of pectoralis major that became aponeurotic near its humeral insertion. The aponeurosis was divided into superficial and deep flaps. The superficial flap attached to the lateral crest of the bicipital groove, and then became muscular along the humeral shaft. This muscle, chondroepitrochlearis, inserted onto the medial epicondyle.

Prevalence

In their literature review, Smith et al. (2015) found that chondroepitrochlearis was present in 5 out of 24 individuals with trisomy 13 (20.8%).

Clinical Implications

Due to its position in the axilla, the presence of chondroepitrochlearis may interfere with axillary lymphadenectomy (Natsis et al. 2010, 2012; Palagama et al. 2016). Furthermore, its presence can limit abduction at the shoulder joint (Lin 1988; Redler et al. 2012; Palagama et al. 2016) or lead to entrapment of the ulnar nerve (Spinner et al. 1991).

STERNOCLAVICULARIS (FIGURE 3.5)

See also: Pectoralis major, Pectoralis minor

Synonyms

Sternoclavicularis is also referred to as preclavicularis medialis, sternoclavicularis anterior, sternoclavicularis anticus, or supraclavicularis (Gruber 1860; Macalister 1875; Knott 1883a; Eisler 1912; Snosek and Loukas 2016).

Typical Presentation

This muscle is only present as a variation or anomaly.

Comparative Anatomy

Sternoclavicularis has been observed in one orangutan (Michaelis 1903) but has not been recorded in any other orangutan dissections, nor in dissections of the other apes (Diogo et al. 2010, 2012, 2013a,b, 2017).

Variations

Description

Sternoclavicularis is considered a variant of pectoralis major and pectoralis minor. It may be present when pectoralis major is deficient (Macalister 1875; Snosek and Loukas 2016). It can originate from the manubrium, the capsule of the sternoclavicular joint, the anterior sternoclavicular ligament, or the first or second costal cartilage (Macalister 1875; Knott 1883a; Mori 1964; Bergman et al. 1988; Sakuma et al. 2007; Sontakke et al. 2013; Snosek and Loukas 2016). It may insert into the middle or distal portions of the clavicle (Macalister 1875; Knott 1883a; Mori 1964; Smith et al. 2015; Bergman et al. 1988; Snosek and Loukas 2016). When sternoclavicularis is present bilaterally, a tendinous band can connect the muscles, which is referred to as musculus interclavicularis (Knott 1883a) or interclavicularis anticus digastricus (Sakuma et al. 2007; Snosek and Loukas 2016). It attaches onto the manubrium via a tendinous intersection and connects the two clavicles (Bergman et al. 1988). If sternoclavicularis inserts into the coracoid process, it may be referred to as coraco-clavicularis anticus (Knott 1883a).

Innervation

Sternoclavicularis is innervated by the lateral pectoral nerve (Sakuma et al. 2007; Sontakke et al. 2013).

Gruber (1860) suggests it is present in about 3% of bodies. Mori (1964) found this muscle in 2 out of 1050 cadavers (0.2%).

Anomalies

Description

As in karyotypically normal humans, sternoclavicularis originates from the anterior surface of the manubrium and capsule of the sternoclavicular joint and inserts onto the anterior surface of the clavicle (Smith et al. 2015). Barash et al. (1970) report the unilateral presence of sternoclavicularis in a trisomy-18 infant.

Prevalence

In their literature review, Smith et al. (2015) found that sternoclavicularis was present in 1 out of 17 individuals with trisomy 18 (5.9%).

Clinical Implications

Sontakke et al. (2013) note that sternoclavicularis muscle could be mistaken for a mass or tumor in medical imaging, and Sakuma et al. (2007) suggest that it could interfere with subclavian-vein catheter insertion.

PECTORALIS QUARTUS (FIGURE 3.5)

See also: Pectoralis major

Synonyms

This muscle is also referred to as pectoralis abdominis (Potau et al. 2018) or pectoralis abdominalis (Dunlap et al. 1986).

Typical Presentation

This muscle is only present as a variation or anomaly.

Comparative Anatomy

In one gibbon, pectoralis quartus originated from between the abdominal head of pectoralis major and the rectus sheath and inserted into the humerus (Van den Broek 1909; Diogo et al. 2012). Pectoralis quartus (pectoralis abdominis) has been described in gorillas, but Diogo et al. (2010) argue that these structures correspond to the abdominal head of pectoralis major.

Variations

Description

Pectoralis quartus is a variant of pectoralis major, extending laterally along the inferior border of this muscle (Bergman et al. 1988; Arican et al. 2006; Snosek and Loukas 2016). It usually arises near the costochondral junction of ribs five and six, crosses the axilla, and inserts on the tendon of pectoralis major (Macalister 1875; Knott 1883a; Birmingham 1889; Bergman et al. 1988; Arican et al. 2006; Cardoso

Souza et al. 2019). This muscle can also arise from the rectus sheath (Bascho 1906; Bonastre et al. 2002; Snosek and Loukas 2016). Pectoralis quartus can also insert onto the fascia of the arm, the short head of the biceps, the bicipital groove of the humerus, or the coracoid process (Birmingham 1889; Arican et al. 2006; Snosek and Loukas 2016; Potau et al. 2018). Hunt (2017) reports a case in which a conjoined tendon of pectoralis major and pectoralis quartus passed superiorly through the intertubercular groove to insert over the glenohumeral joint capsule. Pectoralis quartus can be connected to the axillary arch or sternalis when these muscles are present (Knott 1883a; Bergman et al. 1988; Bonastre et al. 2002; Snosek and Loukas 2016).

Pectoralis quartus is similar in presentation to a muscle that some refer to as pectoralis tertius, which runs between the lower ribs and the humerus or coracoid process (Snosek and Loukas 2016). This muscle appears to be equivalent to the xiphihumeralis muscle that runs between the xiphoid and coracoid process in rodents (Snosek and Loukas 2016; Diogo et al. 2018). Pectoralis quartus is also similar in presentation to costocoracoideus (see the entry for this muscle).

Innervation

Pectoralis quartus is innervated by the medial pectoral nerve (Birmingham 1889; Snosek and Loukas 2016). Arican et al. (2006) observe that this muscle is innervated by the fourth intercostal nerve in one specimen.

Prevalence

Pectoralis quartus has been reported to have a prevalence between 2.8% and 11%–16% (Diogo and Wood 2012a; Testut 1884; Wagenseil 1937; Bonastre et al. 2002; Snosek and Loukas 2016; Hunt 2017; Cardoso Souza et al. 2019).

Anomalies

Description

As in karyotypically normal humans, pectoralis quartus may arise below pectoralis major and extend to the humerus (Howell and Straus 1933; Dunlap et al. 1986).

Prevalence

In their literature review, Smith et al. (2015) found that pectoralis quartus ("pectoralis abdominalis") was present in one out of seven individuals with trisomy 21 (14.3%).

Clinical Implications

Hunt (2017) suggests that the presence of pectoralis quartus could obscure the long head of the biceps during imaging studies, leading to the misdiagnosis of pathology to this structure. Furthermore, Hunt (2017) notes that pain attributed to the long head of the biceps could actually be due to pectoralis quartus. Bonastre et al. (2002) state that pectoralis quartus can contribute to axillary thrombosis and may complicate the removal of lymph nodes during axillary lymphadenectomy.

Pectorodorsalis (Figure 3.4)

See also: Pectoralis major, Latissimus dorsi

Synonyms

Pectorodorsalis is also referred to as the axillary arch, achselbogen, Langer's arch, Langer's muscle, axillopectoral muscle, and arcus axillans (Langer 1846; Bergman et al. 1988; Bakkum and Miller 2016; Rai et al. 2018).

Typical Presentation

This muscle is only present as a variation or anomaly.

Comparative Anatomy

Dorsoepitrochlearis is considered to be the manifestation of axillary arch muscles in the apes. Pectorodorsalis is therefore not present in the apes (Diogo et al. 2010, 2012, 2013a,b, 2017).

Variations

Description

Pectorodorsalis is present as a slip of muscle that crosses the axilla and connects latissimus dorsi to pectoralis major or its tendon (Macalister 1875; Mori 1964; Bergman et al. 1988; Chavan and Wabale 2014; Bakkum and Miller 2016; Standring 2016). It can also attach to the axillary fascia, biceps brachii or its fascia, coracobrachialis or its fascia, pectoralis minor, teres major, or the coracoid process (Ramsay 1812; Macalister 1875; Mori 1964; Bergman et al. 1988; Bakkum and Miller 2016; Standring 2016). It may be present bilaterally (Chavan and Wabale 2014).

Innervation

Pectorodorsalis may be innervated by the medial pectoral nerve or the thoracodorsal nerve (Chavan and Wabale 2014; Bakkum and Miller 2016).

Prevalence

Ramsay (1812) observed the presence of this muscle in 1 out of 30 cadavers (3.3%). Macalister (1875) notes that it has been found by Struthers in 8 out of 105 cases (7.6%) and by Wood in 6 out of 106 cases (5.7%). In a review by Khan et al. (2008) they list a prevalence ranging as low as 0.2% (Serpell and Baum 1991) to as high as 10% (Clarys et al. 1996). Wagenseil (1927) reports a prevalence of 43.8% in a Chinese population. Mori (1964) reports an axillary arch in 52 out of 1050 sides from Japanese cadavers (5%). Mori (1964) also reports a slip from pectoralis major to coracobrachialis in 3 out of 50 arms (6%) and suggests it is a type of axillary arch. Kasai and Chiba (1977) suggest a prevalence of 9.1% in a Japanese population. Miguel et al. (2001) observe a presence of 3% in Spain. Turgut et al. (2005) provide a prevalence of 1.9% in a Turkish population. A prevalence of 3.6% in a Bulgarian population is provided by Georgiev et al. (2007). Turki and Adds (2017) found only three axillary arch muscles from the examination of 280 Caucasian cadavers spanning 14 years of dissection (1%).

Anomalies

Description

Aziz (1980, 1981) reports the presence of pectorodorsalis, a muscle bundle connecting latissimus dorsi to pectoralis major, in three trisomy 13 neonates. In a female fetus with trisomy 18, Langer's axillary arch was present on the left side, extending from the lateral side of latissimus dorsi to the inferior aspect of pectoralis major near its insertion onto the humerus (Alghamdi et al. 2018). In a fetus with trisomy 18, Dunlap et al. (1986) describe a pectorodorsalis that presents as a tendinous insertion of panniculus carnosus into the latissimus dorsi tendon. However, they do not include this as a case of pectorodorsalis in their summary tables.

Prevalence

In their literature review, Smith et al. (2015) found that pectorodorsalis was present in 16 out of 24 individuals with trisomy 13 (66.7%).

Clinical Implications

Ucerler et al. (2005) note that the presence of pectorodorsalis can lead to entrapment of the axillary vein or median nerve, difficulty staging lymph nodes in malignancy cases, problems with axillary surgery, and shoulder instability (Chavan and Wabale 2014). Chavan and Wabale (2014) also suggest that the presence of this muscle can lead to neurovascular symptoms in the upper limb or the development of upper limb lymph edema after breast surgery. Regarding neurovascular compression, Rai et al. (2018) state that pectorodorsalis can lead to brachial plexus compression, thoracic outlet syndrome, and hyperabduction syndrome.

Pectoralis minimus (Figure 3.5)

See also: Pectoralis minor

Synonyms

Pectoralis minimus is also referred to as chondrocoracoideus ventralis, sternocostocoracoidian, sternochondrocoracoideus, or sternochondrocoracoideus ventralis (Snosek and Loukas 2016). Sternochondroscapularis is potentially another synonym (Aziz 1980).

Typical Presentation

This muscle is only present as a variation or anomaly.

Comparative Anatomy

N/A

Variations

Description

Pectoralis minimus (Gruber) originates from the cartilage of the first, second, or potentially the third rib, and inserts onto the coracoid process (Macalister 1875; Knott 1883a; Bergman et al. 1988; Turgut et al. 2000; Rai et al. 2008; Soni et al. 2008; Ebenezer and Rathinam 2013;

Khizer Hussain Afroze et al. 2015; Snosek and Loukas 2016). It may also have origins from the manubrium or costoclavicular ligament (Macalister 1875; Knott 1883a). Turgut et al. (2000) observed insertions into the shoulder joint capsule, the lateral clavicle, and fascia of subclavius. It may be present bilaterally (Turgut et al. 2000).

Innervation

Pectoralis minimus is innervated by the lateral pectoral nerve (Soni et al. 2008; Khizer Hussain Afroze et al. 2015).

Prevalence

Khizer Hussain Afroze et al. (2015) observed the presence of this muscle in 3 out of 56 cadavers in India (5.4%).

Anomalies

Description

Pectoralis minimus arises from the first rib, superior to pectoralis minor, and inserts onto the coracoid process (Smith et al. 2015). Barash et al. (1970) report the unilateral presence of pectoralis minimus in a trisomy-18 infant. Aziz (1980) reports a "sternochondroscapularis" on the right side of a neonate with trisomy 13 that originated from the manubrium and first rib and inserted onto the coracoid process and humeral head.

Prevalence

In their literature review, Smith et al. (2015) found that pectoralis minimus was present in 9 out of 26 individuals with trisomy 18 (34.6%).

Clinical Implications

The presence of pectoralis minimus can cause impingement or compression of nearby thoracoacromial vessels (Turgut et al. 2000; Rai et al. 2008; Ebenezer and Rathinam 2013; Khizer Hussain Afroze et al. 2015; Snosek and Loukas 2016).

COSTOCORACOIDEUS (FIGURE 3.6)

See also: Pectoralis minor

Synonyms

This muscle is also known as chondrocoracoideus (Bergman et al. 1988).

Typical Presentation

This muscle is only present as a variation.

Comparative Anatomy

Although Jouffroy (1971) states that costocoracoideus may be present in some primates, dissections and literature reviews by Diogo et al. (2010, 2012, 2013a,b, 2017) do not find costocoracoideus present as a distinct muscle in the apes. Rather, all these species present a costocoracoid ligament, as in humans, which corresponds to the costocoracoid muscle of monotremes (Diogo et al. 2013a). A distinct costocoracoideus muscle may be present in common chimpanzees as a variant, similar to the condition in humans (Diogo et al. 2013a).

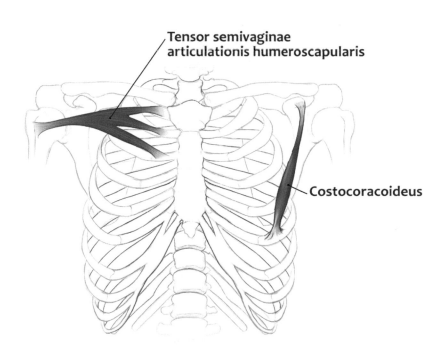

FIGURE 3.6 Thoracoscapular variations in anterior view.

Variations

Description

Humans typically only have a costocoracoid ligament. When present as a distinct muscle, costocoracoideus typically originates via one or more slips from ribs six to eight or the rectus sheath and inserts onto the coracoid process (Macalister 1875; Bergman et al. 1988; Snosek and Loukas 2016). It thus has a similar origin and insertion to pectoralis quartus (see the entry for this muscle). It may also originate from ribs five through seven (Macalister 1875). Wood (1864) reports a "chondro-coracoid muscle" that arose from latissimus dorsi at the tenth rib and inserted into the apex of the coracoid process. Venieratos et al. (2017) report a "chondrocoracoideus" arising via three slips from ribs six, seven, and eight and from the aponeurosis of the external oblique, fusing with the sternocostal head of pectoralis major at the level of rib five and six, and fusing with the tendon of the short head of biceps brachii before insertion onto the coracoid process. Sonne (2020) reports a "chondrocoracoideus" muscle originating from the costal cartilage of the sixth rib.

Innervation

Costocoracoideus is innervated by the medial pectoral nerve (Venieratos et al. 2017; Sonne 2020).

Prevalence

Sonne (2020) found this muscle in 1 out of 36 cadavers (2.8%).

Anomalies

N/A

Clinical Implications

Venieratos et al. (2017) suggest that "chondrocoracoideus" can potentially compress the axillary artery and branches of the brachial plexus, contributing to thoracic outlet syndrome.

TENSOR SEMIVAGINAE ARTICULATIONIS HUMEROSCAPULARIS (FIGURE 3.6)

See also: Pectoralis minor

Synonyms

Alternative names for this muscle include sternohumeralis and sternochondrohumeralis (Snosek and Loukas 2016), and tensor semivaginae scapulohumeralis (Ramirez-Castro and Bersu, 1978; Smith et al. 2015).

Typical Presentation

This muscle is only present as a variation or anomaly.

Comparative Anatomy

Macalister (1871) found tensor semivaginae articulationis humeroscapularis on the left side of a female chimpanzee. In this specimen, it originated from the sternum and cartilage of the first and second ribs.

Variations

Description

Tensor semivaginae articulationis humeroscapularis (Gruber) originates from one or two of the upper rib cartilages and from the sternum (Macalister 1875; Knott 1883a; Bergman et al. 1988; Snosek and Loukas 2016). It inserts into the shoulder joint capsule, the fascia deep to deltoid, or the subacromial bursa (Macalister 1875; Huntington 1904; Knott 1883a; Bergman et al. 1988; Snosek and Loukas 2016). Snosek and Loukas (2016) note that this muscle may be a displaced portion of pectoralis major, and it is often present when pectoralis major is deficient.

Innervation

Tensor semivaginae articulationis humeroscapularis is innervated by the lateral pectoral nerve (Huntington 1904).

Prevalence

N/A

Anomalies

Description

Smith et al. (2015) state that "tensor semivaginae scapulohumeralis" passes from the manubrium to the humeral head and/or the scapula. This is based on the description from Ramirez-Castro and Bersu (1978), who describe this muscle as passing from the first sternochondral joint to the tendinous attachments over the glenohumeral joint capsule. In a neonate with trisomy 18, tensor semivaginae articulationis humeroscapularis arose from the costal surfaces of ribs one and two, coursed below the clavicle, and ended as an aponeurosis over the glenohumeral joint that inserted into the scapula (Aziz 1979).

Prevalence

In their literature review, Smith et al. (2015) found that "tensor semivaginae scapulohumeralis" was present in 1 out of 24 individuals with trisomy 13 (4.2%) and 10 out of 26 individuals with trisomy 18 (38.5%).

Clinical Implications

N/A

INFRACLAVICULARIS (FIGURE 3.7)

Synonyms

N/A

Typical Presentation

This muscle is only present as a variation.

Comparative Anatomy

N/A

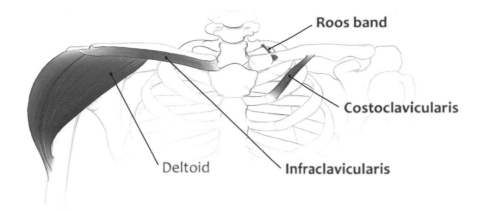

FIGURE 3.7 Deltoideus and clavicular region variations in anterior view.

Variations

Description

Infraclavicularis (Bardeleben) is a rare muscle situated inferior to the clavicle (Knott 1883a; Snosek and Loukas 2016). It arises from the middle third of the clavicle or the anterior sternoclavicular ligament and inserts onto the lateral end of the clavicle and deltopectoral fascia (Knott 1883a; Ingalls 1913; Snosek and Loukas 2016; Wehrli et al. 2017). Snosek and Loukas (2016) note that this muscle may be a displaced portion of the clavicular head of pectoralis major. It may be present bilaterally (Wehrli et al. 2017).

Innervation

Infraclavicularis is innervated by the lateral pectoral nerve (Snosek and Loukas 2016).

Prevalence

N/A

Anomalies

N/A

Clinical Implications

N/A

COSTOCLAVICULARIS (FIGURE 3.7)

Synonyms

N/A

Typical Presentation

This muscle is only present as a variation.

Comparative Anatomy

N/A

Variations

Description

Costoclavicularis is situated deep to the upper part of pectoralis minor and inferior to subclavius (Mori 1964; Snosek and Loukas 2016). It arises from the second rib and attaches to the inferior aspect of the middle portion of the clavicle (Mori 1964; Snosek and Loukas 2016).

Innervation

Mori (1964) states that Nishi reports this muscle may be innervated by a branch of the anterior thoracic nerve (either a branch of the medial or lateral pectoral nerve).

Prevalence

Mori (1964) observed costoclavicularis in 3 out of 367 cases (0.8%) and reports that Nishi found this muscle in 1 out of 12 cadavers (8.3%).

Anomalies

N/A

Clinical Implications

N/A

ROOS BANDS/MUSCLES (FIGURE 3.7)

See also: Scalenus minimus

Synonyms

N/A

Typical Presentation

This muscle is only present as a variation.

Comparative Anatomy

To our knowledge, most Roos bands have not been described in the apes (Diogo et al. 2010, 2012, 2013a,b,

2017). Scalenus minimus muscles corresponding to a type 5 band have been found in gorillas and bonobos (see the entry for this muscle).

Variations

Description

Roos bands or muscles are fibro-muscular structures that originate in the neck, anterior to the T1 root, and insert onto the first rib (Roos 1976; Spears et al. 2011; Snosek and Loukas 2016). Roos (1976) classifies seven types of presentations for these bands and recorded their prevalence in 241 patients that underwent operations for thoracic outlet syndrome and in 58 thoracic outlet dissections from 29 cadavers. A type 1 band is classified as a tough fibrous ligament extending from the top of an incomplete cervical rib to the midsection of the first rib. A type 2 band extends from an elongated seventh cervical rib vertebra to the first rib. A type 3 band is the smallest and deepest and presents as a muscular band extending between the neck of the first rib to the inner surface of the posterior curve of this rib. A type 4 band is a muscle connection between the anterior and middle scalene muscles that attach to the first rib. A type 5 band is the scalenus minimus muscle attaching onto the first rib between the subclavian artery and the brachial plexus. A type 6 band is the scalenus minimus muscle attaching to the cupula of the pleura beneath the first rib. A type 7 band extends between the middle scalene muscle to the costal cartilage of the first rib. Spears et al. (2011) list three other band types, including a band extending from the anterior scalene muscle to subclavius and the costal cartilage (type 8), a band running along the posterior inner surface of the first rib (type 9), and a double fibrous band that extends over the cupula of the lung (type 10).

Innervation

N/A

Prevalence

Out of 241 patients that underwent surgery for thoracic outlet syndrome, Roos (1976) found type 1 bands in 18 cases (7.5%), type 2 bands in 10 cases (4.1%), type 3 bands in 146 cases (60.6%), type 4 bands in 13 cases (5.4%), type 5 bands in 40 cases (16.6%), type 6 bands in five cases (2.1%), type 7 bands in two cases (0.8%), and no bands were present in seven cases (2.9%). Out of 58 thoracic outlet dissections in 29 cadavers, Roos (1976) found type 3 bands present in 10 cases (17.2%), a type 4 band present in one case (1.7%), type 5 bands present in eight cases (13.8%), and no bands were present in 39 cases (67.2%). Spears et al. (2011) found type 3 bands in 29 out 70 cadavers (41.4%) and in 35 out of 100 (35%) first ribs from these cadavers. Type 5 bands were found in 11 ribs (11%).

Anomalies

N/A

Clinical Implications

The presence of these bands creates a tunnel through which the T1 nerve root passes, which also compresses the T1 nerve root against the first rib, therefore predisposing individuals with these muscles to thoracic outlet syndrome (Roos 1976; Spears et al. 2011).

DELTOIDEUS (DELTOID) (FIGURE 3.7)

Synonyms

N/A

Typical Presentation

Description

Deltoid originates from the lateral third of the clavicle, the acromion, and the crest of the scapular spine (Standring 2016). It inserts via a tendon onto the deltoid tubercle on the humeral midshaft (Standring 2016).

Innervation

Deltoid is innervated by the axillary nerve (Standring 2016).

Comparative Anatomy

Deltoid has a similar typical presentation in the apes, with clavicular, acromial, and spinal portions that converge to insert into the humerus (Gratiolet and Alix 1866; Primrose 1899, 1900; Sonntag 1923, 1924; Sullivan and Osgood 1927; Miller 1952; Kallner 1956; Swindler and Wood 1973; Gibbs 1999; Diogo et al. 2010, 2012, 2013a,b, 2017). The insertion of deltoid into the humerus in gibbons is more distal than in the other apes (Diogo et al. 2012). In bonobos, deltoid may be fused with pectoralis major or infraspinatus (Diogo et al. 2017).

Variations

Description

Each part of the deltoid, or the entire muscle, can be reduced or absent (Otto 1830; Gruber 1872; Macalister 1875; Bing 1902; Bergman et al. 1988; Lamb 2016). The muscle sheet of the deltoid can split into multiple parts (Bergman et al. 1988), including a variation in which the posterior-most fibers are separated from the rest of the muscle sheet by a layer of fascia (Kayikçioglu et al. 1993; Kamburoğlu et al. 2008; Lamb 2016). The muscle may also split into numerous fascicles (Macalister 1875; Lamb 2016). The completeness of the division between the clavicular, acromial, and spinous portions can vary (Macalister 1875; Mori 1964; Lamb 2016).

Deltoid can fuse with pectoralis major (deltopectoral complex, see anomalous description below), or may have connections to trapezius, infraspinatus, supraspinatus, latissimus dorsi, teres major, biceps brachii, brachialis, brachioradialis, the infraspinous fascia, or the lateral scapular border (Macalister 1875; Mori 1964; Bergman et al. 1988; Lamb 2016; Standring 2016). Acromioclavicularis or prae-clavicularis lateralis extends between the acromion and the clavicular portion of the deltoid (Gruber 1865; Macalister 1875; Knott 1883a; Lamb 2016). Basiodeltoideus or fasciculus infraspinata deltoideus (Gruber) extends from the infraspinatus fascia or axillary border of the scapula to the lower fibers of the deltoid (Knott 1883a; Lamb 2016). Costodeltoideus (Calori) refers to a slip that originates from the scapula between teres minor and infraspinatus, or between teres minor and teres major, that connects deltoid to the clavicle or to the acromion process (Macalister 1875; Knott 1883a; Bergman et al. 1988; Lamb 2016). Fraser et al. (2014) report an accessory slip connecting deltoid with teres minor that they do not believe corresponds to costodeltoideus. Infraspinatohumeralis is a slip that originates from the scapula and ends in the fascia of the arm (Calori 1867; Bergman et al. 1988; Lamb 2016).

Prevalence

Mori (1964) studied the deltoid in 50 arms. The acromial portion was fully separated from the rest of the muscle in 12 arms (24%), partially separated from the rest of the muscle in 19 arms (38%), and not separated from the rest of the muscle in 19 arms (38%). The clavicular portion was fully separated from the rest of the muscle in two arms (4%), partially separated from the rest of the muscle in two arms (4%), and not separated from the rest of the muscle in 46 arms (92%). The spinous portion originated from only the scapular spine in 16 arms (32%), from the spine and the infraspinous fascia in 31 arms (62%), and from only the infraspinous fascia in three arms (6%).

Anomalies

Description

Macalister (1875) states that Haller found deltoid with an insertion into brachialis into an abnormal individual. In two neonates with trisomy 18 (Aziz 1979, 1981) and in a female fetus with trisomy 18 (Alghamdi et al. 2018), deltoid was fused with pectoralis major bilaterally, forming the deltopectoral complex. Alghamdi et al. (2017) note that in a fetus with craniorachischisis, a deltopectoral complex was present bilaterally. In a neonate with trisomy 13, deltoid was divided into clavicular, acromial, and spinous portions (Aziz 1980).

Prevalence

In their literature review, Smith et al. (2015) found a bilateral deltopectoral complex, in which there was a complete fusion of deltoid and pectoralis major, in 21 out of 26 fetuses/neonates with trisomy 18 (80.8%). The deltoid was divided into three distinct parts in 1 out of 24 individuals with trisomy 13 (4.2%).

Clinical Implications

Understanding variations in deltoid anatomy and insertions is important for successful shoulder surgery (Kamburoğlu et al. 2008; Fraser et al. 2014).

INFRASPINATUS (FIGURE 3.8)

Synonyms
N/A

Typical Presentation

Description

Infraspinatus originates from the infraspinous fossa and infraspinous fascia and has a tendinous insertion onto the greater tubercle of the humerus (Standring 2016).

Innervation

Infraspinatus is innervated by the suprascapular nerve (Standring 2016).

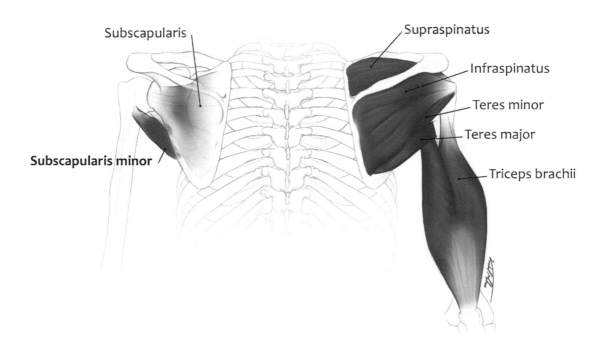

FIGURE 3.8 Scapulohumeral muscles in posterior view.

Comparative Anatomy

Infraspinatus has a similar typical presentation in the apes, extending from the infraspinous fossa and fascia to the greater tubercle of the humerus and often also to the capsule of the glenohumeral joint (Beddard 1893; Miller 1952; Gibbs 1999; Diogo et al. 2010, 2012, 2013a,b, 2017).

Variations

Description

Infraspinatus can be completely absent as a rare variation (Bing 1902; Lamb 2016). Infraspinatus can be fused with teres minor (Macalister 1875; Knott 1883a; Aasar 1947; Mori 1964; Bergman et al. 1988; Lamb 2016; Standring 2016). It may also fuse with the insertion of supraspinatus or connect with deltoid (Macalister 1875; Knott 1883a; Lamb 2016; Standring 2016). Infraspinatus may be bilaminar (Macalister 1875). Scapulohumeralis digastricus singularis of Gruber refers to an accessory muscle that originates from the acromion and scapular spine, courses between deltoid and infraspinatus, and inserts into the humerus (Macalister 1875; Lamb 2016).

Two other accessory fascicles have been named; infraspinatus minor (see below) and infraspinatus superficialis extends from the scapular spine to the greater tubercle of the humerus (Knott 1883a; Aasar 1947; Bergman et al. 1988; Lamb 2016). Ashaolu et al. (2015) report the presence of infraspinatus minor together with a teres minor that partially divided into three bundles upon insertion onto the humerus on the left side of a Nigerian male cadaver. The authors' description of infraspinatus minor—arising inferior to infraspinatus "major" and extending between the lateral aspect of the infraspinous fossa and the greater tubercle of the humerus—seems to correspond to the definition of infraspinatus superficialis provided by Bergman et al. (1988). Typically, infraspinatus minor is defined as the superior or upper part of a divided infraspinatus (Aasar 1947; Knott 1883a; Bergman et al. 1988; Lamb 2016).

Prevalence

Mori (1964) found infraspinatus fused with teres minor in 10 out of 50 arms (20%).

Anomalies

Description

Poland syndrome can cause the underdevelopment or absence of infraspinatus (Kutluk and Metin 2017). In a fetus with craniorachischisis, infraspinatus was fused with teres minor on both the left and right sides (Alghamdi et al. 2017). This fusion was also observed bilaterally in a fetus with trisomy 18 (Alghamdi et al. 2018).

Prevalence

N/A

Clinical Implications

Variant bundles of infraspinatus may interfere with successful posterior portal placement for shoulder arthroscopy (Ashaolu et al. 2015).

SUPRASPINATUS (FIGURE 3.8)

Synonyms

N/A

Typical Presentation

Description

Supraspinatus originates from the supraspinous fossa and the supraspinous fascia and has a tendinous insertion into the greater tubercle of the humerus (Standring 2016).

Innervation

Supraspinatus is innervated by the suprascapular nerve (Standring 2016).

Comparative Anatomy

Supraspinatus has a similar typical presentation in the apes, extending from the supraspinous fossa and fascia to the greater tubercle of the humerus and often also to the capsule of the glenohumeral joint (Gibbs 1999; Diogo et al. 2010, 2012, 2013a,b, 2017). In orangutans, supraspinatus may have additional origins from the scapular spine and/or acromion and may also be fused with infraspinatus (Gibbs 1999; Diogo et al. 2013b). In common chimpanzees, it may have an additional insertion into the acromioclavicular ligaments (Gratiolet and Alix 1866).

Variations

Description

Macalister (1875), Bergman et al. (1988), and Lamb (2016) note that the presentation of supraspinatus is largely similar among humans. Supraspinatus may be absent in rare cases (Bing 1902). Other rare variations of supraspinatus include a division of the muscle belly into two portions, connections to the tendons of pectoralis minor, pectoralis major, or subscapularis, and an attachment to a tendinous lamella below pectoralis major (Macalister 1875; Le Double 1897; Bergman et al. 1988; Uzel et al. 2008; Lamb 2016). It may also receive a slip from the suprascapular ligament (Macalister 1875). Supraspinatus can also blend with the insertion of infraspinatus (Lamb 2016).

Prevalence

N/A

Anomalies

Description

Poland syndrome can cause the underdevelopment or absence of supraspinatus (Kutluk and Metin 2017).

Teres minor (Figure 3.8)

Synonyms

N/A

Typical Presentation

Description

Teres minor originates from the lateral margin of the scapula and inserts via a tendon onto the greater tubercle of the humerus (Standring 2016). Its insertion blends with the capsule of the shoulder joint (Standring 2016).

Innervation

Teres minor is innervated by the axillary nerve (Standring 2016).

Comparative Anatomy

Teres minor has a similar typical presentation in the apes, extending from the lateral border of the scapula to the greater tubercle of the humerus (Gibbs 1999; Diogo et al. 2010, 2012, 2013a,b, 2017). The insertion often extends to the shaft of the humerus in all apes except orangutans (Gratiolet and Alix 1866; Sonntag 1924; Raven 1950; Swindler and Wood 1973; Gibbs 1999; Diogo et al. 2010, 2012, 2013a,b, 2017). Teres minor may be blended with infraspinatus in gibbons, gorillas, and orangutans (Gibbs 1999; Diogo et al. 2012). It may have an additional insertion into the shoulder joint capsule in bonobos (Miller 1952; Gibbs 1999; Diogo et al. 2017).

Variations

Description

Teres minor may be absent entirely (Macalister 1875; Knott 1883a; Mori 1964; Sato 1968c; Bergman et al. 1988; Lamb 2016). A common variation of teres minor is fusion with infraspinatus (Macalister 1875; Knott 1883a; Mori 1964; Sato 1968c; Bergman et al. 1988; Lamb 2016; Standring 2016). Teres minor may send a slip to deltoideus (Aasar 1947; Lamb 2016). There may be an insertion onto the surgical neck of the humerus (Jain et al. 2012; Lamb 2016). Ashaolu et al. (2015) report the presence of a teres minor that partially divided into three bundles upon insertion onto the humerus on the left side of a Nigerian male cadaver. The superior portion inserted onto the posterior facet of the greater tubercle, the middle portion inserted onto the inferior facet of the greater tubercle, and the inferior portion inserted onto the antero-inferior surface of the greater tubercle (Ashaolu et al. 2015).

Prevalence

Mori (1964) found teres minor fused with infraspinatus in 10 out of 50 arms (20%) and absent in 2 arms (4%). Sato (1968c) found teres minor absent in 33 out of 346 sides (9.5%) in Kyushu-Japanese males and absent in 27 of 214 sides (12.6%) in females. Teres minor was partially fused with infraspinatus in 74 out of 268 sides in males (27.6%) and in 54 out of 166 sides in females (32.5%).

Anomalies

Description

Teres minor was fused bilaterally with infraspinatus in both a fetus with craniorachischisis (Alghamdi et al. 2017) and a fetus with trisomy 18 (Alghamdi et al. 2018).

Prevalence

N/A

Clinical Implications

Variable slips of teres minor may be surrounded by vascular structures (Ashaolu et al. 2015). In their case, a branch of the posterior circumflex artery lied between the superior and middle bundles of the teres minor insertion, thus having the potential to complicate surgery in that region (Ashaolu et al. 2015).

Teres major (Figure 3.8)

Synonyms

N/A

Typical Presentation

Description

Teres major originates from the inferior scapular angle and inserts via a tendon onto the intertubercular sulcus of the humerus (Standring 2016).

Innervation

Teres major is innervated by the lower subscapular nerve (Standring 2016).

Comparative Anatomy

Teres major has a similar typical presentation in the apes, extending from the lateral border and inferior angle of the scapula to the proximal humerus (Gibbs 1999; Diogo et al. 2010, 2012, 2013a,b, 2017). Fusion with the tendon of latissimus dorsi is observed as a common variant in all apes (Gratiolet and Alix 1866; Champneys 1872; Barnard 1875; Kohlbrügge 1890–1892; Hepburn 1892; Beddard 1893; Primrose 1899, 1900; Sonntag 1923, 1924; Sullivan and Osgood 1927; Stewart 1936; Miller 1952; Kallner 1956; Gibbs 1999; Michilsens et al. 2009; Diogo et al. 2010, 2012, 2013a,b, 2017). In one bonobo fetus, teres major was fused with triceps brachii and subscapularis (Diogo et al. 2017).

Variations

Description

Teres major may be absent (Macalister 1867a, 1875; Bergman et al. 1988; Lamb 2016). Teres major can fuse with latissimus dorsi or its tendon, send a slip to the long head of the triceps or the brachial fascia, or fuse with rhomboid major (Macalister 1875; Le Double 1897; Aasar 1947; Bergman et al. 1988; Iamsaard et al. 2012; Standring 2016; Lamb 2016). Slips connecting teres major to biceps brachii or coracobrachialis have also been observed (Macalister 1875; Aggarwal et al. 2009; Lamb 2016). It may connect with the shoulder joint capsule (Macalister 1875).

Prevalence

In a sample of 52 arms, Mori (1964) found that the tendon of teres major was fused with the tendon of latissimus dorsi in 28 arms (53.8%), the insertions of teres major and latissimus dorsi were parallel on the humerus in 13 arms (25%), the insertions of teres major and latissimus dorsi made a v shape on the humerus in 10 arms (19.2%), and a slip passed from the infraglenoid tubercle of the scapula to the tendon of teres major in one arm (1.9%).

Anomalies

Description

On the left side of a fetus with craniorachischisis, a muscular slip connected teres major to triceps brachii (Alghamdi et al. 2017). In a fetus with trisomy 18 and cyclopia, teres major fused with latissimus dorsi near their humeral insertion at the intertubercular sulcus (Smith et al. 2015). In a male fetus with triploidy, teres major was doubled on the right side (Moen et al. 1984).

Prevalence
N/A

Clinical Implications

Iamsaard et al. (2012) suggest that variations in teres major insertions (such as the insertion these authors observed onto the tendon of latissimus dorsi) may cause unusual movement of the arm, and knowledge of such variations is important when planning tendon transfer to treat rotator cuff tears.

SUBSCAPULARIS (FIGURE 3.8)

See also: Subscapularis minor

Synonyms
N/A

Typical Presentation

Description

Subscapularis occupies the subscapular fossa. It primarily originates from the costal surface of the scapula and inserts via a tendon onto the lesser tubercle of the humerus (Standring 2016).

Innervation

Subscapularis is innervated by the upper and lower subscapular nerves (Standring 2016).

Comparative Anatomy

Subscapularis has a similar typical presentation in the apes, extending from the subscapular fossa to the lesser tubercle of the humerus (Gibbs 1999; Diogo et al. 2010, 2012, 2013a,b, 2017). The insertion can sometimes extend to the shaft of the humerus as a variant in all apes except gibbons (Beddard 1893; Sonntag 1923; Gibbs 1999; Diogo et al. 2010, 2012, 2013a,b, 2017). It may insert onto the shoulder joint capsule in bonobos (Miller 1952; Diogo et al. 2017).

Variations

Description

Standring (2016) reports that variation in subscapularis is not common, while Lamb (2016) states that this muscle has the most reported variations of any of the rotator cuff muscles. In addition to the lesser tubercle, its tendon can insert into the bicipital groove or greater tubercle (MacDonald et al. 2007; Cash et al. 2009; Lamb 2016). Subscapularis can divide into two discrete parts or numerous slips (Macalister 1867a, 1875; Lamb 2016). Subscapularis may connect with biceps brachii, pectoralis major, or triceps brachii (Macalister 1875; Le Double 1897; Bergman et al. 1988; Lamb 2016). Mori (1964) found an abnormal slip that extended from levator scapulae to subscapularis. Coracobrachialis profundus may insert into subscapularis or its tendon (Macalister 1875; Knott 1883a). Le Double (1897) describes a slip that originated from the subscapular tendon and attached to the axillary fascia or skin. An accessory slip may extend from the shoulder joint capsule and lesser tubercle and insert onto latissimus dorsi (Namking et al. 2013).

Subscapularis is associated with several named variations. Glenobrachialis (Gruber) refers to a slip that originates with the long head of biceps brachii and attaches onto the surgical neck of the humerus (Macalister 1875; Knott 1883a; Bergman et al. 1988). Subscapulo-capsularis may insert into the bicipital groove, shoulder joint capsule, or neck of the humerus (Macalister 1867a, 1875; Lamb 2016). Subscapularis-teres-latissimus is an accessory muscle that has three different presentations and fuses with the subscapularis insertion (Kameda 1976; Lamb 2016). Depressor tendinis subscapularis majoris (also referred to as deltoidius profundus, tensor capsulae humeralis, or retinaculum musculare tendinis subscapularis majoris (Gruber) originates from the subscapularis tendon and inserts into the surgical neck of the humerus (Macalister 1875; Knott 1883a). Subscapularis minor may also be present as a variation (see the entry for this muscle).

Prevalence

Mori (1964) found a slip from the medial margin of levator scapulae to the ventral surface of subscapularis in 22 out of 100 sides (22%). Kameda (1976) observed the presence of subscapularis-teres-latissimus in 3.8% of cases. In an MRI study of 50 individuals, Cash et al. (2009) found that subscapularis primarily inserted onto the lesser tubercle in ten cases (20%), the bicipital groove in 33 cases (66%), and the greater tubercle in seven cases (14%).

Anomalies

Description

An anomalous presentation of subscapularis includes the insertion splitting the plane of muscle (Smith et al. 2015).

Prevalence

In the literature review conducted by Smith et al. (2015), they found that subscapularis with insertion splitting the plane of muscle was present in 1 out of 26 individuals with trisomy 18 (3.8%).

Clinical Implications

N/A

Subscapularis Minor (Figure 3.8)

See also: Subscapularis

Synonyms

This muscle is also referred to as scapularis secundus or accessory subscapularis (Gruber 1859; Le Double 1897; Bergman et al. 1988), infraspinatus secundus, subscapulo-humeralis, subglenoidalis (Knott 1883a), and potentially the infraglenoid muscle (Lee et al. 2019a).

Typical Presentation

This muscle is only present as a variation.

Comparative Anatomy

In a common chimpanzee dissected by Ziegler (1964), an accessory head arose from the superior-most part of the axillary border of subscapularis. A few fibers of this head inserted onto the capsular ligament while the rest attached to the humerus distal to the lesser tubercle. In an orangutan dissected by Sullivan and Osgood (1927), there was an upper bundle of subscapularis that was distinct from the rest of the muscle.

Variations

Description

This muscle is a variation of subscapularis. When present, subscapularis minor originates from the upper axillary border of the scapula (Knott 1883a; Bergman et al. 1988) or the anterior and lateral surface of subscapularis (Breisch 1986; Pires et al. 2017). Its insertion is variable, with possible attachments to the shoulder joint capsule, the crest of the lesser tubercle of the humerus, the intertubercular sulcus,

or just below the lesser tubercle (Knott 1883a; Aasar 1947; Bergman et al. 1988; Standring 2016; Pires et al. 2017). Although Staniek and Brenner (2012) suggested that the infraglenoid muscle described by them (and by Lee et al. 2019a) should be distinguished from subscapularis minor, this muscle is similar in morphology, origin, and insertion.

Innervation

The infraglenoid muscles described by Staniek and Brenner (2012) were innervated by the axillary nerve.

Prevalence

Gruber (1859) noted the presence of subscapularis minor in ten out of 200 limbs (5%). Knott (1883a) found this muscle in four out of 39 subjects (10.3%). Le Double (1897) reports that Krause found this muscle in 3 out of 35 specimens (8.6%) and Testut found this muscle in 3 out of 18 specimens (16.7%).

Anomalies

N/A

Clinical Implications

Breisch (1986) states that an accessory subscapularis muscle can create a myotendinous tunnel through which the axillary and subscapular nerves pass, which may lead to nerve entrapment and its associated neurological symptoms. Pires et al. (2017) similarly state that an accessory subscapularis passing over the axillary nerve can contribute to quadrangular space compression syndrome.

Latissimus dorsi (Figures 3.4, 3.9, and 3.11)

See also: Pectorodorsalis, Dorsoepitrochlearis, Levator tendinis musculi latissimus dorsi

Synonyms

Latissimus dorsi is also referred to as the grand dorsal (Bakkum and Miller 2016).

Typical Presentation

Description

Latissimus dorsi originates from the spines of the lower six thoracic vertebrae, the thoracolumbar fascia and therefore the spines of the lumbar and sacral vertebrae, the posterior portion of the iliac crest, and the lower three or four ribs (Standring 2016). Its fibers converge into a tendon that inserts onto the intertubercular sulcus of the humerus (Standring 2016).

Innervation

Latissimus dorsi is innervated by the thoracodorsal nerve (Standring 2016).

Comparative Anatomy

Latissimus dorsi has a similar typical presentation in the apes, extending from the vertebrae, ribs, pelvis, and

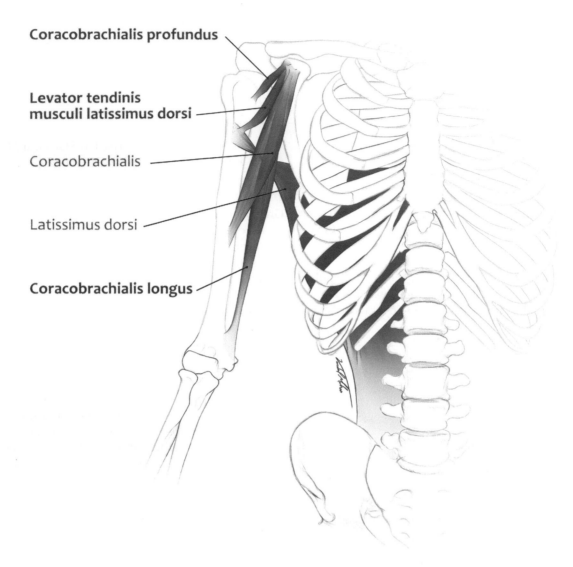

Coracobrachialis profundus

Levator tendinis musculi latissimus dorsi

Coracobrachialis

Latissimus dorsi

Coracobrachialis longus

FIGURE 3.9   Coracobrachialis and associated variations in anterior view.

thoracolumbar fascia to the intertubercular sulcus of the humerus (Gibbs 1999; Michilsens et al. 2009; Diogo et al. 2010, 2012, 2013a,b, 2017). Fusion of the latissimus dorsi tendon with teres major is observed as a common variant in all apes (see the entry for teres major). In orangutans, latissimus dorsi is often divided into two or more bundles or sends accessory slips to other structures (Beddard 1893; Primrose 1899, 1900; Schück 1913; Stewart 1936; Diogo et al. 2013b). In gorillas, latissimus dorsi often blends with trapezius (Raven 1950; Preuschoft 1965; Gibbs 1999; Diogo et al. 2010). Latissimus dorsi was also partially blended with trapezius in a fetal bonobo (Diogo et al. 2017). An additional origin from the inferior angle of the scapula has been observed in an adult bonobo (Miller 1952).

Variations

Description

Latissimus dorsi may be absent on one or both sides of the body (Bergman et al. 1988; Bakkum and Miller 2016).

It can vary in the number of costal attachments (Wood 1868; Macalister 1875; Mori 1964; Bakkum and Miller 2016; Standring 2016). It may originate only from the lumbar vertebrae (Rickenbacher et al. 1985). It can also originate only from the ribs, instead of a more extensive attachment, or it can be divided into multiple fascicles (Macalister 1875; Bergman et al. 1988; Bakkum and Miller 2016). Common variations include additional attachments to the inferior angle of the scapula; the presence of pectorodorsalis (axillary arch), which connects latissimus dorsi to pectoralis major or other nearby muscles; and the presence of dorsoepitrochlearis, which connects latissimus dorsi the upper arm (see the entries for these muscles) (Macalister 1875; Mori 1964; Bergman et al. 1988; Standring 2016; Bakkum and Miller 2016). Latissimus dorsi or its tendon may be continuous with, or send a slip to, teres major (Macalister 1875; Mori 1964; Aasar 1947; Bergman et al. 1988; Iamsaard et al. 2012; Bhatt et al. 2013; Bakkum and Miller 2016; Lamb 2016; Standring 2016). A slip can also pass to the long head of the triceps (Macalister 1875;

Standring 2016; Bakkum and Miller 2016) or to the first rib (Miyauchi 1982a). It may overlap with the external oblique (Macalister 1875).

Prevalence

Mori (1964) studied the attachments of latissimus dorsi on 100 sides from 50 cadavers. This author found that the upper limit of the aponeurosis from the vertebral column was the spinous process of the fifth thoracic vertebra on two sides (2%), sixth thoracic vertebra on 16 sides (16%), seventh thoracic vertebra on 44 sides (44%), eighth thoracic vertebra on 30 sides (30%), and ninth thoracic vertebra on eight sides (8%). Mori (1964) studied the costal origins of this muscle on 60 sides and found that latissimus dorsi had origins from ribs 9–12 on 25 sides (41.7%) and ribs 10–12 on 35 sides (58.3%). This author also observed an attachment to the inferior angle of the scapula in 53.3% of cases.

Anomalies

Description

In a cadaver with a severe case of congenital scoliosis, Stevenson et al. (2014) found significant asymmetry in the latissimus dorsi muscles. In a fetus with craniorachischisis, the right latissimus dorsi was reduced compared to the left side (Alghamdi et al. 2017). Smith et al. (2015) observed the fusion of teres major with latissimus dorsi near their humeral insertion at the intertubercular sulcus in one fetus with trisomy 18 and cyclopia. On both sides of a male infant with triploidy, latissimus dorsi was divided into scapular and humeral heads (Moen et al. 1984).

Prevalence

N/A

Clinical Implications

Understanding variations in latissimus dorsi is important for the planning and execution of the numerous reconstructive and cosmetic surgeries that utilize parts of this muscle (Bhatt et al. 2013).

LEVATOR TENDINIS MUSCULI LATISSIMUS DORSI (FIGURE 3.9)

See also: Coracobrachialis longus, Latissimus dorsi

Synonyms

This muscle is also referred to as coracobrachialis accessorius, coracobrachialis superior, coracobrachialis minor or secundus, le court coracobrachialis (Bergman et al. 1988; Del Sol and Olave 2005; Akita and Nimura 2016a), or coracobrachialis brevis s. rotator humeri (Wood 1864).

Typical Presentation

This muscle is only present as a variation or anomaly.

Comparative Anatomy

N/A

Variations

Description

Levator tendinis musculi latissimus dorsi (Gruber) originates from the coracoid process and shoulder joint capsule and has a tendinous insertion onto the tendon of latissimus dorsi (Gruber 1844; Wood 1868; Macalister 1875; Knott 1883a; Le Double 1897; Bergman et al. 1988; Del Sol and Olave 2005; Moore and Rice 2018). Moore and Rice (2018) suggest that the presence of this muscle may represent a failed migration of a coracobrachialis longus variant.

Innervation

Innervation of levator tendinis musculi latissimus dorsi has not been described, but it is found in close proximity to the nerves passing through the axilla (Del Sol and Olave 2005).

Prevalence

Del Sol and Olave (2005) observed the presence of this muscle in 1 out of 108 adult male cadavers (0.9%).

Anomalies

Description

On the left side of a neonate with trisomy 13, levator tendinis musculi latissimus dorsi originated just beneath the coracoid from the fascia covering the shoulder joint capsule and inserted into the latissimus dorsi tendon (Pettersen et al. 1979).

Prevalence

In their literature review, Smith et al. (2015) found that this muscle was present in 1 out of 24 individuals with trisomy 13 (4.2%).

Clinical Implications

Del Sol and Olave (2005) suggest that the presence of this muscle may lead to compression of branches of the brachial plexus or axillary vessels.

CORACOBRACHIALIS (FIGURE 3.9)

See also: Coracobrachialis profundus, Coracobrachialis longus

Synonyms

N/A

Typical Presentation

Description

Coracobrachialis originates from the coracoid process along with the tendon of the short head of the biceps and inserts onto the shaft of the humerus (Standring 2016).

Innervation

Coracobrachialis is innervated by the musculocutaneous nerve (Standring 2016).

Comparative Anatomy

Coracobrachialis has a similar typical presentation in the apes, extending from the coracoid process to the proximal humerus (Gibbs 1999; Diogo et al. 2010, 2012, 2013a,b, 2017).

Variations

Description

Coracobrachialis is comprised of three parts: the proximal (deep) portion, the middle portion (corresponding to cora-cobrachialis proprius/medius), and the distal (superficial) portion, and only in some cases do the parts appear distinct from one another (Mori 1964; Bergman et al. 1988; Akita and Nimura 2016a). The proximal portion occasionally presents as a muscle referred to as coracobrachialis profundus, and the distal portion occasionally presents in the form of coracobrachialis longus (see the entries for these muscles) (Bergman et al. 1988; Akita and Nimura 2016a). Georgiev et al. (2017a) report a coracobrachialis muscle in a male cadaver in which coracobrachialis brevis, coracobrachialis, and a variant of coracobrachialis longus (their "coracoepi-trochlearis") are distinct from each other and well-developed.

Coracobrachialis can send additional slips to the lesser tubercle, medial epicondyle, supracondylar process of the humerus, brachialis, triceps brachii, or the medial inter-muscular septum (Macalister 1875; Bergman et al. 1988; Standring 2016; Akita and Nimura 2016a). Its origin may connect with the insertion of pectoralis minor (Macalister 1875). Its tendon may receive slips from the tendons of latissimus dorsi or teres major (Macalister 1875). Garbelotti et al. (2017) report a slip of coracobrachialis that inserted into the intermuscular septum in the proximal humerus, trapping the lateral cord of the brachial plexus against it and coracobrachialis. Coracobrachialis can also be absent as a variation (Bergman et al. 1988; Akita and Nimura 2016a).

Several authors report variations in coracobrachialis associated with variations in biceps brachii. El-Naggar and Zahir (2001) reported a coracobrachialis with two bellies that formed inferior to its origin on the coracoid, the first inserting onto the middle of the humerus and the second onto the medial head of the triceps, with the musculocutaneous nerve passing in between them. This muscle was associated with a "three-headed" biceps, with the third head originat-ing mostly from the humerus and partly from the tendinous origin of the medial head of the triceps to insert onto the common tendon for the biceps (El-Naggar and Zahir 2001). Catli et al. (2012) observed the presence of a coracobrachi-alis with a superficial and deep head that both originated from the coracoid process and inserted onto the middle third of the humerus, and a "capsular" head that originated from the articular capsule of the glenohumeral joint. This muscle was associated with a "four-headed" biceps brachii that had two supernumerary heads (Catli et al. 2012). The first super-numerary head arose from the insertion of coracobrachialis as a united tendon and inserted onto the medial aspect of the short head of biceps brachii (Catli et al. 2012). The second arose from the upper third of the humerus and was fused

along the medial border of the long head of the biceps (Catli et al. 2012). Piagkou et al. (2019) report a coracobrachialis with a superficial and deep head that was connected with an accessory muscle bundle. This muscle was associated with a "three-headed" biceps, with the third head originating from the tendon of the short head and the coracobrachialis to insert onto the radial tuberosity (Piagkou et al. 2019).

Prevalence

In a study of 50 arms, Mori (1964) found that coracobra-chialis was completely separated into superficial and deep layers in eight arms (16%), partially separated into super-ficial and deep layers in four arms (8%), and not separated into layers in 38 arms (76%).

Anomalies

Description

Macalister (1875) notes that Barkow observed the absence of coracobrachialis in an anomalous individual. In a fetus with craniorachischisis dissected by Alghamdi et al. (2017), they found that coracobrachialis on the right side of the body was fused with the short head of biceps brachii at its proximal end and fused with dorsoepitrochlearis at its distal end. The fusion of the proximal end of this muscle with the short head of biceps brachii was also observed on the left side of the body. Alghamdi et al. (2017) note that coracobrachialis was associated with the median nerve in this specimen.

In the female fetus with trisomy 18 dissected by Alghamdi et al. (2018), the insertion of pectoralis minor on the right side extended inferiorly to the fascia of cora-cobrachialis. The proximal end of coracobrachialis was completely fused with the proximal end of the short head of biceps brachii (side not indicated). In a dissection of a trisomy 18 and cyclopic fetus completed by Smith et al. (2015), they observed that coracobrachialis on the right side of the body was fused with the short head of the biceps and inserted through its entire length along the anteromedial proximal humerus.

Bersu et al. (1976) describe a male infant with Hanhart syndrome. On the left side of this specimen, the upper limb was absent below the elbow, and rudiments of the radius and ulna were present. Coracobrachialis bifurcated and had a deep medial portion that represented the usual muscle and a superficial portion that attached to the capsule of the elbow joint, the latter of which sent a slip to the biceps tendon. On the left arm of a male neonate with Meckel syndrome, cor-acobrachialis had two heads and the superficial head was encircled by the two roots of the median nerve (Pettersen 1984). A partial fusion of coracobrachialis with the short head of biceps brachii has been observed in infants with Neu-Laxova syndrome (Shved et al. 1985).

Prevalence

In their literature review, Smith et al. (2015) found that coracobrachialis was split into proximal and middle por-tions in 1 out of 24 individuals with trisomy 13 (4.2%).

Coracobrachialis had otherwise anomalous presentations in 3 out of 26 individuals with trisomy 18 (11.5%); in two female neonates, coracobrachialis was represented by small bellies in addition to the short head of the biceps, and in another female neonate, coracobrachialis was fused with the short head of the biceps (Smith et al. 2015). In a study of six upper limbs from three infants with Neu-Laxova syndrome, Shved et al. (1985) found that coracobrachialis was partially fused with the short head of biceps brachii in all six upper limbs (100%).

Clinical Implications

Division of coracobrachialis into distinct parts can lead to the compression of the musculocutaneous nerve as the nerve passes between the parts (El-Naggar and Zahir 2001).

CORACOBRACHIALIS PROFUNDUS (FIGURE 3.9)

See also: Coracobrachialis

Synonyms

This muscle is also referred to as coracocapsularis, coracobrachialis superior, or coracobrachialis brevis (Macalister 1875; Bergman et al. 1988; Smith et al. 2015; Akita and Nimura 2016a).

Typical Presentation

This muscle is only present as a variation or anomaly.

Comparative Anatomy

Coracobrachialis profundus is typically not present as a distinct structure in the apes (Diogo et al. 2010, 2012, 2013a,b, 2017). Kallner (1956) reports the presence of this muscle in one orangutan, and Hepburn (1892) reports the presence of some fibers corresponding to this muscle in one gorilla. Coracobrachialis profundus may be present as a variation in common chimpanzees (Parsons 1898a,b; Howell and Straus 1932).

Variations

Description

Coracobrachialis profundus refers to a deep accessory bundle near the proximal part of coracobrachialis that originates from the coracoid process and inserts into the shoulder joint capsule or into the surgical neck of the humerus below the lesser tubercle (Macalister 1875; Knott 1883a; Bergman et al. 1988; Akita and Nimura 2016a). It may also insert into the tendon of subscapularis, fibers of subscapularis, or the capsular ligament of the shoulder (Macalister 1875; Knott 1883a). Macalister (1875) notes that coracobrachialis profundus may be a variation of the deltoid or subscapularis.

Innervation

This muscle is likely innervated by the musculocutaneous nerve.

Prevalence

Howell and Straus (1932) observed the presence of coracobrachialis profundus in 3 out of 39 arms that they dissected (7.7%).

Anomalies

Description

In a fetus with trisomy 18 and cyclopia, Smith et al. (2015) found coracobrachialis profundus on the left side of the body. This muscle was also present on the left side of a neonate with trisomy 13 (Aziz 1980).

Prevalence

In their literature review, Smith et al. (2015) found that this muscle was present in 2 out of 24 individuals with trisomy 13 (8.3%).

Clinical Implications

N/A

CORACOBRACHIALIS LONGUS (FIGURE 3.9)

See also: Coracobrachialis

Synonyms

This muscle is also referred to as coracobrachialis inferior or coracobrachialis superficialis (Wood 1864; Bergman et al. 1988; Smith et al. 2015).

Typical Presentation

This muscle is only present as a variation or anomaly.

Comparative Anatomy

Coracobrachialis longus is typically not present as a distinct structure in the apes (Diogo et al. 2010, 2012, 2013a,b, 2017). Kallner (1956) describes a coracobrachialis longus in one orangutan, but the presence of this muscle is not corroborated by the illustrations provided by the author (Diogo et al. 2013b). In one gorilla, Hepburn (1892) reports the presence of some fibers potentially corresponding to this muscle inserting onto the intermuscular septum of the arm, but Howell and Straus (1932) suggest that this is just an extension of the coracobrachialis proprius. Coracobrachialis longus may be present as a rare variation in common chimpanzees (Howell and Straus 1932; Oishi et al. 2009).

Variations

Description

Coracobrachialis longus is a superficial and distal bundle of coracobrachialis and extends from coracoid process to the distal humerus, potentially inserting onto the medial epicondyle or medial intermuscular septum of the arm (Wood 1864; Macalister 1875; Knott 1883a; Akita and Nimura 2016a; Paraskevas et al. 2016). It may be continuous with brachialis (Macalister 1875). Georgiev et al. (2017a) use coracoepitrochlearis to refer to a variant of coracobrachialis longus that originates from the coracoid process to insert onto the medial epicondyle. Georgiev et al. (2018a) use humero-epitrochlearis to refer to a variant of coracobrachialis longus that originates from the medial surface of the middle part of the humerus to insert onto the medial epicondyle.

Innervation

Coracobrachialis longus is innervated by the musculocutaneous nerve (Georgiev et al. 2017a, 2018a).

Prevalence

N/A

Anomalies

Description

Bersu et al. (1976) describe a male infant with Hanhart syndrome. On the left side of this specimen, the upper limb was absent below the elbow, and rudiments of the radius and ulna were present. Coracobrachialis bifurcated and had a deep medial portion that represented the usual muscle and a superficial portion that attached to the capsule of the elbow joint, the latter of which sent a slip to the biceps tendon. In a neonate with trisomy 18, coracobrachialis longus extended from the coracoid process to the medial epicondyle of the humerus (Aziz 1979).

Prevalence

In the literature review conducted by Smith et al. (2015), they found that this muscle was present in 2 out of 26 individuals with trisomy 18 (7.7%).

Clinical Implications

El-Naggar and Al-Saggaf (2004) noted that the presence of coracobrachialis longus can contribute to compression of the median nerve and brachial artery, as well as palsy hypoxia of the forearm and hand. Paraskevas et al. (2016) suggest that the presence of this muscle could induce symptoms of median, ulnar, or medial antebrachial cutaneous neuropathy. Georgiev et al. (2017a) note that an accessory belly of coracobrachialis inserting onto the medial epicondyle of the humerus may be a good candidate to be used as a graft for surgery, but its presence may lead to confusion during medical imaging of the arm.

BRACHIALIS (FIGURE 3.10)

Synonyms

Other names for brachialis include brachialis anticus and flexor brachii brevis (Hepburn 1892; Parsons 1898b).

Typical Presentation

Description

Brachialis originates from the lower half of the humeral shaft and the associated intermuscular septa and inserts via a tendon onto the coronoid process and the tuberosity of the ulna (Standring 2016).

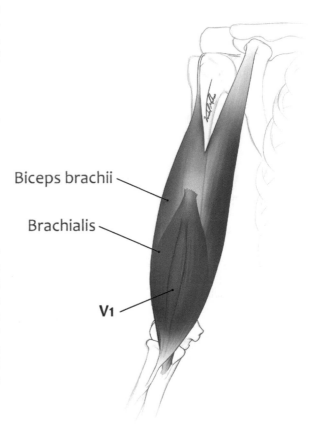

FIGURE 3.10 Brachialis and biceps brachii in anterior view. V1 indicates an additional bundle of biceps brachii that originates from brachialis and joins the biceps insertion tendon.

Innervation

Brachialis is typically innervated by the musculocutaneous nerve and radial nerve (Standring 2016). It may sometimes be supplied by the median nerve (Machida 1961; Akita and Nimura 2016a).

Comparative Anatomy

Brachialis has a similar typical presentation in the apes, extending from the humeral shaft to the ulnar tuberosity, and sometimes the coronoid process (Raven 1950; Miller 1952; Gibbs 1999; Diogo et al. 2010, 2012, 2013a,b, 2017). Many of the same variations are also present in the apes, including division into multiple parts, the presence of accessory slips, or fusion with other muscles (Sonntag 1924; Sullivan and Osgood 1927; Howell and Straus 1932; Ziegler 1964; Gibbs 1999; Diogo et al. 2010, 2012, 2013a,b, 2017).

Variations

Description

Brachialis may send slips or otherwise have connections to the radius near the tuberosity, both the radius and ulna, the bicipital aponeurosis, the forearm fascia, or the semilunar fascia (Macalister 1875; Mori 1964; Bergman et al. 1988;

Standring 2016; Akita and Nimura 2016a). Other common variations include division into multiple parts, complete absence, and fusion with biceps brachii, brachioradialis, coracobrachialis, extensor carpi radialis, or pronator teres (Wood 1864, 1866, 1867a, 1868; Macalister 1875; Machida 1961; Mori 1964; Bergman et al. 1988; Standring 2016; Akita and Nimura 2016a). Brachialis may have three or four heads (Wood 1864; Macalister 1875; Akita and Nimura 2016a). Macalister (1875) notes that in rare cases, brachialis may send a slip to flexor digitorum superficialis.

Brachialis lateralis minor is a supernumerary muscle associated with brachialis that inserts into the ulnar tuberosity, while brachialis internus minor is medially situated and also inserts into the ulna (Macalister 1875; Knott 1883a). Capsularis sub-brachialis (Portal) or artecularis cubiti anterior refers to one or two deep bundles of brachialis that attach to the capsule of the elbow joint (Macalister 1875; Nishi 1966; Bergman et al. 1988; Akita and Nimura 2016a). Supinator radii brevis accessorius extends from brachialis to the radial tuberosity (Knott 1883a). Pai et al. (2008a) report an accessory brachialis that originated from the lateral part of brachialis and the lateral intermuscular septum and split into two slips, the medial slip inserting onto the deep fascia of pronator teres and the lateral slip inserting onto the fascia of supinator. Vadgaonkar et al. (2008) report an accessory brachialis that inserted on the shaft of the radius and formed a fibro-muscular tunnel above the cubital fossa containing the median nerve, brachial artery, and other structures.

Prevalence

Knott (1883a) found an accessory slip between brachialis and biceps brachii in 3 out of 49 subjects (6.1%). Knott (1883a) also found brachialis internus minor in 3 out of 49 subjects (6.1%). Mori (1964) found that in 12 out of 50 arms (24%), brachialis was divided into two distinct heads. In one arm (2%), an accessory slip originated from brachialis to insert onto the radial tuberosity (Mori 1964).

Anomalies

Description

In a neonate with trisomy 13, brachialis sent two accessory slips to biceps brachii on the right side (Aziz 1980). In a neonate with trisomy 18, the right brachialis was divided into a thick part that originated below the deltoid tuberosity and a deep, thin sheet that originated from the distal humerus (Aziz 1979). In a fetus with craniorachischisis, Alghamdi et al. (2017) observed that brachialis on the right upper limb was absent, while the left brachialis was connected to an extra head of triceps brachii. In this specimen, Alghamdi et al. (2017) note that brachialis was associated with the median nerve.

Bersu et al. (1976) describe a male infant with Hanhart syndrome. On the left side of this specimen, the upper limb was absent below the elbow, and rudiments of the radius and ulna were present. Brachialis was absent. Mieden (1982) describes an infant with median cleft lip, hypotelorism, and

alobar holoprosencephaly. On the right side, brachialis was divided into a superficial and deep head. A low origin of brachialis was observed in infants with Neu-Laxova syndrome (Shved et al. 1985).

Prevalence

In their literature review, Smith et al. (2015) found that brachialis had two accessory slips joining biceps in 2 out of 24 individuals with trisomy 13 (8.3%). Brachialis was otherwise anomalous (high origin, divided into two portions) in 3 out of 26 individuals with trisomy 18 (11.5%). An accessory brachialis was present in 1 out of 26 individuals with trisomy 18 (3.8%). In a study of six upper limbs from three infants with Neu-Laxova syndrome, Shved et al. (1985) found that a low origin of brachialis was present in two upper limbs (33%).

Clinical Implications

Loukas et al. (2006c) suggest that an accessory brachialis can contribute to median nerve palsy. Pai et al. (2008a) state that an accessory brachialis may contribute to radial-tunnel syndrome. Vadgaonkar et al. (2008) suggest that an accessory brachialis can lead to various compression syndromes involving the median nerve or the brachial artery.

Biceps brachii (Figure 3.10)

Synonyms

This muscle is also referred to as biceps flexor cubiti (Owen 1868; Hepburn 1892).

Typical Presentation

Description

The short head of biceps brachii originates via a tendon from the coracoid process (Standring 2016). The long head of biceps brachii originates within the shoulder joint capsule via a tendon from the supraglenoid tubercle of the scapula (Standring 2016). Both bellies converge into a tendon to insert onto the radial tuberosity (Standring 2016). The tendon has a medial expansion, termed the bicipital aponeurosis (Standring 2016).

Innervation

Biceps brachii is innervated by the musculocutaneous nerve (Standring 2016).

Comparative Anatomy

Biceps brachii has a similar typical presentation in the apes, arising from the coracoid process or proximal humerus and the supraglenoid tubercle and inserting into the radial tuberosity (Gibbs 1999; Diogo et al. 2010, 2012, 2013a,b, 2017). Accessory heads are occasionally present in common chimpanzees (Howell and Straus 1932; Diogo et al. 2013a). The bicipital aponeurosis is usually absent in bonobos and orangutans (Diogo et al. 2013b, 2017). In gibbons, the distal portion of biceps brachii is blended with flexor digitorum superficialis (Kohlbrügge 1890–1892; Howell and Straus 1932; Gibbs 1999; Michilsens et al. 2009; Diogo et al. 2012).

Variations

Description

The short head and the long head can sometimes be fused or one of them could be absent (Macalister 1875; Knott 1883a; Bergman et al. 1988; Akita and Nimura 2016a). When the long head is deficient or absent, it may be replaced by a singular or doubled tendon that originates from the proximal humerus, shoulder joint capsule, or the pectoralis major tendon (Bergman et al. 1988; Akita and Nimura 2016a; Katsuki et al. 2018). Cutler et al. (2018) report a long head of the biceps tendon with a trifurcate origin. Collett et al. (2018) report a short head of biceps brachii with an origin from an aponeurotic sheet that extended over the coracoid process, coracoacromial ligament, the inferior surface of the acromion, and the greater tubercle of the humerus. Biceps brachii may be entirely absent (Macalister 1875; Bergman et al. 1988). Several authors report variations in biceps brachii associated with variations in coracobrachialis (see coracobrachialis entry for more details). Other variations of biceps brachii recorded by Macalister (1875) include information on absence, variable origins and insertions, supernumerary heads, and accessory slips.

A third or humeral head may be present, which typically arises from brachialis (Macalister 1875; Mori 1964; Sato 1969; Bergman et al. 1988; Akita and Nimura 2016a; Standring 2016; Ravi et al. 2020). Moore and Rice (2018) report a "four-headed" biceps with both an inferomedial and inferolateral humeral head. Accessory slips may also be present and give biceps brachii the appearance of having up to five heads (Macalister 1875; Bergman et al. 1988; Akita and Nimura 2016a). An accessory slip may originate from the humerus at the insertion of coracobrachialis, extend to brachialis, and connect with the short head of biceps brachii and the semilunar fascia (Bergman et al. 1988). Other accessory slips can arise from the neck of the humerus and connect to the short and long head, or from the intertubercular sulcus, lesser tubercle, deltoid tuberosity, lower end of the humerus, shoulder joint capsule, tendon of pectoralis major, ulna, radius, or antebrachial fascia (Macalister 1875; Mori 1964; Bergman et al. 1988; Akita and Nimura 2016a; Standring 2016). Muscular slips can connect biceps brachii to other muscles including the deltoid, brachialis, brachioradialis, pronator teres, flexor carpi radialis, or flexor digitorum profundus (Macalister 1875; Knott 1883a; Bergman et al. 1988; Akita and Nimura 2016a). Brachiofascialis (Struthers), also referred to as brachialis accessorius or supinator brevis accessorius, is a slip extending between biceps brachii and fascia over pronator teres (Wood 1864; Macalister 1875; Knott 1883a; Akita and Nimura 2016a).

Prevalence

Macalister (1875) found a third head present in about one in ten subjects (10%) and reports that a third head was found by Theile in one in nine subjects (11.1%), by Hallett in 1 out of 15 subjects (6.7%), and by Wood in 18 out of 175 subjects (10.3%). In a sample of 49 subjects, Knott (1883a) found an accessory slip between brachialis and biceps brachii in three subjects (6.1%) and an additional head between biceps and coracobrachialis in five subjects (10.2%). Sato (1969) found a third head in 35 out of 286 limbs from Kyushu-Japanese males (9.07%) and in 17 out of 250 limbs (6.8%) from females.

Mori (1964) found the third head of the biceps in 10 out of 50 arms (20%). The third head originated from the distal aspect of the deltoid tuberosity in four arms (8%), the distal aspect of the insert site of coracobrachialis in three arms (6%), the tendon of pectoralis major in two arms (4%), and the lesser tubercle in one arm (2%). Ravi et al. (2020) reported supernumerary heads of the biceps in 5 out of 50 arms (10%). The biceps in one of the specimens had four heads, and the muscle in the other specimens had three heads (Ravi et al. 2020).

Anomalies

Description

In a fetus with craniorachischisis, Alghamdi et al. (2017) observed that biceps brachii on the left upper limb demonstrated a fusion between the short head and coracobrachialis. There was also an abnormal slip connecting teres major to the long head. A fusion of the short head and coracobrachialis was also observed on the right side. The short head of the right biceps brachii also had an abnormal origin at the lesser tubercle of the humerus, and an abnormal insertion onto the lateral condyle and medial supracondylar ridge of the humerus. The long head of the right biceps brachii was missing. In this specimen, Alghamdi et al. (2017) note that biceps brachii was associated with the median nerve.

In a neonate with trisomy 13, the right biceps brachii had two accessory heads (Aziz 1980). One arose from the medial crest of the bicipital groove, and the other arose from the distal half of the humerus. Biceps brachii on this side also received two slips from brachialis. On the left side, the short head of the biceps was absent, but there were also two accessory heads. One arose from the lesser tubercle, and the other arose from the proximal humerus.

In a neonate with trisomy 18, the superior portion of biceps brachii was divided into a long head, short head, and a fascicle that was continuous with the deltopectoral complex (Aziz 1979). In a female fetus with trisomy 18, the proximal end of coracobrachialis was completely fused with the proximal end of the short head of biceps brachii (side not indicated) (Alghamdi et al. 2018). In a fetus with trisomy 18 and cyclopia, Smith et al. (2015) observed the presence of a tendon connecting biceps brachii to pectoralis major, as well as the bilateral absence of the bicipital aponeurosis. The short head of the left biceps brachii was missing, and the short head of the right biceps brachii was fused with coracobrachialis. In an adult with trisomy 21, the long head of biceps brachii was absent bilaterally (Bersu 1980).

Bersu et al. (1976) describe a male infant with Hanhart syndrome. On the left side of this specimen, the upper limb was absent below the elbow, and rudiments of the radius and ulna were present. The insertion tendon of biceps brachii inserted onto the radial rudiment and the long head was deficient in fibers. In a male fetus with triploidy, Moen et al. (1984) found an extra muscle belly between the short head of biceps and the supraglenoid tubercle on the right side. In a female fetus with triploidy, the long head of biceps brachii was absent bilaterally (Moen et al. 1984). Doubling of the short head of biceps brachii has been observed in infants with Neu-Laxova syndrome (Shved et al. 1985).

Mieden (1982) describes an infant with median cleft lip, hypotelorism, and alobar holoprosencephaly (case I) and two male fetuses with cyclopia and alobar holoprosencephaly (cases II and III). On the right side of case I, an accessory muscle belly originated from the biceps tendon and inserted onto the radius proximal to the attachment of supinator. In case III, an accessory muscle belly was associated with biceps brachii on both sides of the body. On the right side, it originated from the coracoid process and attached to the humerus proximal to brachialis. On the left, it originated from the humerus lateral to coracobrachialis and fused with biceps brachii at its distal insertion (Mieden 1982).

Prevalence

In a study of six upper limbs from three infants with Neu-Laxova syndrome, Shved et al. (1985) found that the short head of biceps brachii was doubled in two upper limbs (33%). In their literature review, Smith et al. (2015) found that biceps brachii muscle was variable (with accessory heads, abnormal connections to other muscles, extra tendons, and variable origins and insertions) in 12 out of 24 individuals with trisomy 13 (50%), 15 out of 26 individuals with trisomy 18 (57.7%), and 1 out of 7 individuals with trisomy 21 (14.3%). These authors also found that an extra biceps brachii tendon inserting into pectoralis major was present in 9 out of 26 individuals with trisomy 18 (34.6%). A muscle belly extending between the biceps and the pectoralis major tendon was present in 4 out of 26 individuals with trisomy 18 (15.4%). The short head of biceps brachii was absent in 2 out of 24 specimens with trisomy 13 (8.3%). Fusion of the short head with coracobrachialis was observed in 3 out of 26 individuals with trisomy 18 (11.5%) and in one out of seven individuals with trisomy 21 (14.3%). The long head of biceps brachii was absent in 1 out of 26 individuals with trisomy 18 (3.8%) and in one 1 of 7 individuals with trisomy 21 (14.3%) (Smith et al. 2015).

Clinical Implications

Nakatani et al. (1998) suggest that a biceps brachii with four heads can contribute to median nerve palsy or brachial artery compression. El-Naggar and Zahir (2001) state that the presence of a third head could lead to musculocutaneous nerve compression. Ravi et al. (2020) state that supernumerary heads of the biceps may be useful for muscle transfer surgeries.

Triceps brachii (Figure 3.8)

Synonyms

Triceps brachii is also referred to as multiceps extensor cubiti (Barnard 1875) or triceps extensor cubiti (Hepburn 1892).

Typical Presentation

Description

The long head of triceps brachii originates via a tendon from the infraglenoid tubercle of the scapula, the lateral head originates via a tendon the posterior humeral shaft and the lateral intermuscular septum, and the medial head originates from the entire posterior surface of the humeral shaft and the medial and lateral intermuscular septa (Standring 2016). The heads converge into a tendon that inserts onto the olecranon process of the ulna (Standring 2016).

Innervation

Triceps brachii is innervated by the radial nerve (Standring 2016).

Comparative Anatomy

Triceps brachii has a similar typical presentation in the apes, but the long head has a more extensive origin along the axillary border of the scapula in all apes (Diogo et al. 2010, 2012, 2013a,b, 2017). Articularis cubiti (subanconeus) is present in some common chimpanzees (Champneys 1872; Sonntag 1923; Diogo et al. 2013a).

Variations

Description

Fibers of the long head of triceps brachii may extend to the capsule of the shoulder joint or to the axillary border of the scapula, and the medial head may sometimes extend to form an arch across the ulnar groove (Macalister 1875; Mori 1964; Bergman et al. 1988; Akita and Nimura 2016a). Prabhu et al. (2012) report a muscular connection between the long head and the lateral head. There may be a tendinous connection between the tendon of the long head of the triceps and the latissimus dorsi tendon (Knott 1883a; Koizumi 1934; Ishimi 1950; Akita and Nimura 2016a). There may also be a fleshy slip connecting triceps brachii with latissimus dorsi or subscapularis (Macalister 1875; Knott 1883a). Triceps brachii may be fused with anconeus (Macalister 1875; Knott 1883a; Bergman et al. 1988; Akita and Nimura 2016a). It may also fuse with extensor carpi ulnaris (Macalister 1875). Subanconeus or articularis cubiti refers to the deep layer/medial head of triceps attaching to the joint capsule of the elbow (Tubbs et al. 2006a; Akita and Nimura 2016a; Standring 2016). An accessory or fourth head of the triceps can originate from the medial surface of the humerus, the axillary border of the scapula, the coracoid process, or the capsule of the shoulder joint (Macalister 1875; Sato 1969; Bergman et al. 1988).

Prevalence

Mori (1964) reports that the long head originated from the capsule of the shoulder joint and the axillary border of the scapula in 49 out of 50 arms (98%), while in one arm (2%) the long head originated only from the axillary border of the scapula. The medial head was proximal to the lateral head in 36 arms (72%) while the two heads originated at an equal level in 14 arms (28%). In one arm (2%), a slip originated between the medial and lateral heads and travelled distally to fuse with the lateral head. In another arm (2%), a slip originated from the capsule of the shoulder joint and traveled distally to fuse with the medial head of the triceps. Sato (1969) found a fourth head of triceps brachii present in 9 out of 364 limbs from Kyushu-Japanese males (2.47%) and present in 9 out of 438 limbs (2.05%) from females.

Anomalies

Description

In a fetus with craniorachischisis, Alghamdi et al. (2017) observed that both the left and right triceps brachii had four heads, with the fourth head originating from the lateral aspect of the humerus inferior to the deltoid, with fibers extending to the medial condyle and the olecranon process of the ulna on the right side. These authors also observed slips between triceps brachii and teres major and latissimus dorsi on the left side.

In a male fetus with triploidy, Moen et al. (1984) found that the long head of triceps brachii was doubled on the right side. Triceps brachii has been observed to have a low origin of the medial head in infants with Neu-Laxova syndrome (Shved et al. 1985). In a study of six upper limbs from three infants with Neu-Laxova syndrome, Shved et al. (1985) found that triceps had a low origin of the medial head in all six upper limbs (100%).

Prevalence

In their literature review, Smith et al. (2015) found that triceps brachii had a more proximal origin than usual in 2 out of 24 individuals with trisomy 13 (8.3%). Triceps brachii was also variable (with extensive and/or variable origins, or accessory slips) in 18 out of 26 individuals with trisomy 18 (69.2%). In a study of six upper limbs from three infants with Neu-Laxova syndrome, Shved et al. (1985) found that triceps had a low origin of the medial head in all six upper limbs (100%).

Clinical Implications

The presence of a fourth head of triceps brachii can contribute to radial nerve palsy, vascular compromise due to the compression of the deep radial artery, profunda brachii artery compression, and snapping elbow (Fabrizio and Clemente 1997; Tubbs et al. 2006b). A muscular fascicle connecting the long head and the lateral head may lead to radial nerve entrapment (Prabhu et al. 2012).

EPITROCHLEOANCONEUS (FIGURE 3.11)

Entry adapted by permission from Springer Nature Customer Service Centre GmbH: Springer Current Molecular Biology Reports, Muscles Lost in Our Adult Primate Ancestors Still Imprint in Us: on Muscle Evolution, Development, Variations, and Pathologies. E. Boyle, V. Mahon, R. Diogo, 2020.

Synonyms

Alternative names for this muscle include anconeus quintus, anconeus minimus, anconeus epitrochlearis muscle (Wood) (Knott 1883a); flexor antebrachii ulnaris (Kallner 1956), epitrochleo-olecranonis, accessory anconeus, ulnaris internis, cubital anterieur (Wilson et al. 2016), anconeus quartus, anconeus medialis, anconeus sextus, anconeus parvus, and tensor fasciae antebrachii (Jouffroy 1971), epitrochleocubital or artecularis cubiti posterior (Nishi 1966).

Typical Presentation

This muscle is only present as a variation or anomaly.

Comparative Anatomy

While typically absent in adult humans, epitrochleoanconeus is present often in several primate species including common chimpanzees and bonobos (Gratiolet and Alix 1866; Macalister 1871, 1875; Miller 1952; Ziegler 1964; Swindler and Wood 1973; Diogo and Wood 2011, 2012a; Diogo et al. 2013a, 2017). The presentation and innervation in nonhuman primates are the same as in humans. It is usually not present as a distinct muscle in gibbons, orangutans, or gorillas (Diogo et al. 2010, 2012, 2013b).

Variations

Description

Epitrochleoanconeus (Gruber) is typically only present in the early stages of human development, appearing as a distinct muscle at CR25mm (crown-rump length of 25mm) and persisting until at least CR33.5mm (Diogo et al. 2019). When present as a distinct muscle in adults, epitrochleoanconeus extends from the medial epicondyle of the humerus to the medial side of the olecranon process of the ulna (Gruber 1867a; Galton 1874; Macalister 1875; Knott 1883a; Jouffroy 1971; Lewis 1989; Akita and Nimura 2016a,b). Its origin may present as narrow, wide and fleshy, or tendinous (Macalister 1875). It may sometimes be fused with anconeus (Bergman et al. 1988; Akita and Nimura 2016a). It may also be doubled (Macalister 1875).

Innervation

Epitrochleoanconeus is innervated by the ulnar nerve (Howell and Strauss 1932; Miller 1952; Kallner 1956; Ziegler 1964; Akita and Nimura 2016a,b).

Prevalence

Gruber (1867a) reports a prevalence of 34 out of 100 cadavers (34%). Galton (1874) suggests that the epitrochleoanconeus

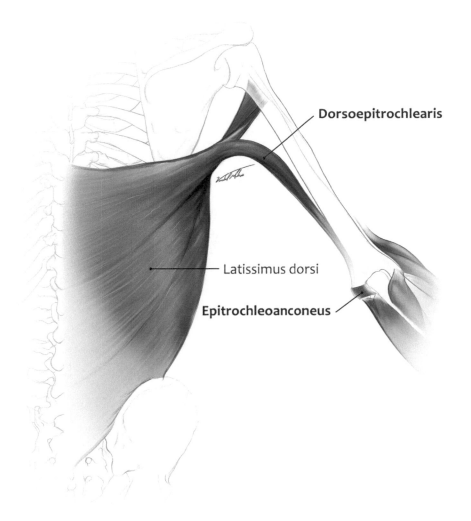

FIGURE 3.11 Posterior view of latissimus dorsi and posterior humeral variations. (Figure adapted by permission from Springer Nature Customer Service Centre GmbH: Springer Current Molecular Biology Reports, Muscles Lost in Our Adult Primate Ancestors Still Imprint in Us: on Muscle Evolution, Development, Variations, and Pathologies. E. Boyle, V. Mahon, R. Diogo, 2020.)

is found in about 53 out of 200 human upper limbs (26.5%). Macalister (1875) found this muscle in 16 out of 63 subjects (25.4%). Le Double (1897) reports its presence in 32 out of 102 cadavers (31%). Clemens (1957) found the muscle in 4 out of 100 cadavers (4%). From a sample of 96 arms, Mori (1964) reported a prevalence of 5%. In a study of 218 Brazilian adults, Nascimento and Ruiz (2018) found that this muscle was present in 29 cases (13.3%).

Anomalies

Description

Anomalous presentation is same as above, running from the back of the medial condyle to the medial side of the olecranon (Smith et al. 2015).

Prevalence

In their literature review, Smith et al. (2015) found that epitrochleoanconeus was reported in 2 out of 26 individuals with trisomy 18 (7.7%).

Clinical Implications

The presence of epitrochleoanconeus can lead to ulnar compression neuropathy at the elbow (Masear et al. 1988). Wilson et al. (2016) suggest that the presence of this muscle may protect against the development of cubital tunnel syndrome, as it may decrease the rigidity of the entrance into the cubital tunnel, replacing Osborne's ligament as the roof of this tunnel.

ANTERIOR FOREARM MUSCLES

FLEXOR POLLICIS LONGUS (FIGURE 3.12)

See also: Gantzer's muscle

Synonyms

This muscle is also referred to as flexor longus proprius pollicis (Todd 1839).

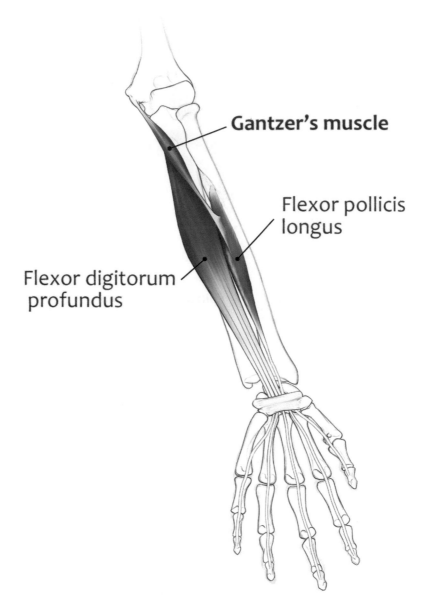

FIGURE 3.12   Deep anterior forearm muscles in anterior view.

Typical Presentation

Description

Flexor pollicis longus originates from the radius and the interosseous membrane and inserts via a tendon onto the base of the distal phalanx of the first digit (Standring 2016).

Innervation

Flexor pollicis longus is innervated by the anterior interosseous branch of the median nerve (Standring 2016).

Comparative Anatomy

Although it has been suggested that flexor pollicis longus is unique to humans (e.g., Bergman et al. 1988; Akita and Nimura 2016b), it is also present in gibbons as a distinct muscle separate from flexor digitorum profundus that extends from the radius and interosseous membrane to digit one and/or digit two (Diogo et al. 2012, 2017).

Variations

Description

Flexor pollicis longus can also arise via a variable accessory head from the coronoid process or from the medial epicondyle of the humerus (Macalister 1875; Knott 1883a; Sato 1969; Akita and Nimura 2016b; Standring 2016). Flexor pollicis longus may also originate from brachialis (Macalister 1875; Bergman et al. 1988). Other variations include connections to flexor digitorum superficialis, flexor digitorum profundus, pronator teres, and the synovial bursa (a slip termed tensor bursae mucosae tendinum) (Macalister 1875; Knott 1883a; Mori 1964; Bergman et al.

1988; Akita and Nimura 2016b). Flexor pollicis longus may send a tendon to the first lumbrical (Macalister 1875; Bergman et al. 1988). Flexor pollicis longus can be partially or completely absent (Macalister 1875; Akita and Nimura 2016b; Standring 2016). Other variations of flexor pollicis longus described by Macalister (1875) include the presence of accessory slips and doubling of the muscle or its tendon. Linburg-Comstock variation is described as a tendinous connection between flexor pollicis longus and the digit two slip of flexor digitorum profundus, or the tendons of these muscles (Linburg and Comstock 1979). Flexor pollicis longus is also associated with Gantzer's muscle (see the entry for this muscle).

Prevalence

In a sample of 34 subjects, Knott (1883a) found an accessory head from the medial epicondyle in two cases (5.9%). A head from the coronoid was present in some form in 18 cases (52.9%): arising separately in nine cases (26.5%), arising with the deep head of pronator teres in three cases (8.8%), closely associated with the flexor digitorum superficialis in four cases (11.8%), and via a slip common to all three muscles in two cases (5.9%).

Mori (1964) found that there was a muscular bundle from flexor pollicis longus inserting into flexor digitorum profundus in 12.5% of cases. These two muscles were connected with a muscular bundle in 4.5% of cases. The tendons of these muscles were fused upon insertion into digit two in 7.5% of cases. The origin of flexor pollicis longus from the interosseous membrane was absent in 7.5% of cases. Sato (1969) found an accessory head of flexor pollicis longus present in 83 out of 356 limbs (23.31%) from Kyushu-Japanese males and present in 68 out of 248 limbs (27.42%) from females.

Linburg and Comstock (1979) note that in a large sample of humans, only 69% of them had a flexor pollicis longus fully independent from the flexor digitorum profundus. Yurasakpong et al. (2018) studied 130 upper limbs and found that the tendons of flexor pollicis longus and flexor digitorum profundus were connected in 32 limbs (24.6%) and varied between fibrous, tendinous, and musculotendinous connections. Erić et al. (2019) clinically diagnosed Linburg-Comstock variation via two tests (inability to flex the thumb without simultaneous flexion of the index finger; pain during active flexion of the thumb while long fingers were fully extended, and the wrist was in supination) in 130 out of 215 subjects (60.5%).

Anomalies

Description

Bersu et al. (1976) describe a male infant with Hanhart syndrome. On the right side of this specimen, the wrist and hand were deficient. Flexor pollicis longus inserted onto the trapezium. In a fetus with craniorachischisis, Alghamdi et al. (2017) observed that flexor pollicis longus on the left upper limb had an insertion onto the proximal phalanx of the first digit, in addition to the normal attachment to the distal phalanx. This muscle was also connected to flexor digitorum profundus. In a trisomy 18 cyclopic fetus, flexor pollicis longus had a bifurcated tendon with insertions into the base of the proximal phalanx and the distal phalanx of digit one (Smith et al. (2015).

Mieden (1982) describes two male fetuses with cyclopia and alobar holoprosencephaly. On the left side of one specimen, an extra muscle belly originated from flexor pollicis longus and fused with the tendon of flexor digitorum profundus going to digit two. On the left arm of a male neonate with Meckel syndrome, Pettersen (1984) observed a small slip that extended between the tendon of brachioradialis and flexor pollicis longus at the wrist.

Prevalence

A presentation similar to that of the trisomy 18 cyclopic fetus examined by Smith et al. (2015, see above) was also recorded in 2 out of 24 individuals with trisomy 13 (8.3%) and 4 out of 26 individuals with trisomy 18 (15.4%). Flexor pollicis longus was otherwise variable (e.g., tendinous or aponeurotic attachments to the first metacarpal, split tendons, tendon to the second digit) in 2 out of 24 individuals with trisomy 13 (8.3%), in 13 out of 26 individuals with trisomy 18 (50%), and in 1 out of 7 individuals with trisomy 21 (14.3%). Flexor pollicis longus was also absent in 1 out of 26 individuals with trisomy 18 (3.8%).

Clinical Implications

Shrewsbury et al. (2003) explain that the clinical evidence of restrictive thumb/index tendosynovitis and pain in humans is associated with connections between the flexor pollicis longus and the flexor digitorum profundus (e.g., Linburg-Comstock variations).

GANTZER'S MUSCLE (FIGURE 3.12)

Synonyms

This muscle is also known as Gantzer's (also Gantzner's or Ganzer's) fasciculus, accesorius ad pollicem, flexor digitorum profundus accessorius, or accessorius ad flexorem profundus (Macalister 1875; Knott 1883a; Mori 1964; Bergman et al. 1988).

Typical Presentation

This muscle is only present as a variation or anomaly.

Comparative Anatomy

N/A

Variations

Description

Gantzer's muscle is associated with flexor pollicis longus, flexor digitorum profundus, and flexor digitorum superficialis. It is generally described as an accessory head of flexor pollicis longus. It can arise from the medial epicondyle, the coronoid process, from both of these structures, or from flexor digitorum superficialis (Macalister 1875;

Knott 1883a; Mori 1964; Bergman et al. 1988; Akita and Nimura 2016b). Zdilla et al. (2019) reported an origin from the brachialis fascia. It inserts onto the tendons or muscle bellies of flexor pollicis longus and/or flexor digitorum profundus (Macalister 1875; Knott 1883a; Mori 1964; Bergman et al. 1988; Caetano et al. 2015; Akita and Nimura 2016b).

Innervation

Gantzer's muscle is innervated by the anterior interosseous nerve (Kulkarni et al. 2014; Caetano et al. 2015; Zdilla et al. 2019).

Prevalence

Macalister (1875) reports that Gantzer's muscle can be found in about two out of five subjects (40%). Mori (1964) found this muscle in 50% of cases. In a study of 80 limbs from 40 cadavers, Caetano et al. (2015) observed that this muscle was present in 54 limbs (67% of limbs). Kulkarni et al. (2014) state that prevalence ranges from 39% to 90% in the literature, with an average of about 67%.

Mori (1964) found that Gantzer's muscle arose from the medial epicondyle in 24% of cases, from the coronoid process in 68% of cases, and from both these structures in 8% of cases. In a sample of 80 limbs, Caetano et al. (2015) observed that this muscle originated from the medial epicondyle in about 9% of limbs, from the coronoid process in 10% of limbs, and from the deep surface of flexor digitorum superficialis in about 53% of limbs.

Mori (1964) also observed variation in how the insertion tendon of flexor pollicis longus relates to Gantzer's muscle. The tendon arose from Gantzer's muscle in 40% of cases, arose from both flexor pollicis longus and Gantzer's muscle in 40% of cases, arose from the point of fusion of flexor pollicis longus and Gantzer's muscle in 16% of cases, and both muscles fused to form one tendon in 4% of cases. Caetano et al. (2015) observed that this muscle inserted into flexor pollicis longus in 26 out of 80 limbs (45%) and into flexor digitorum profundus in 21 out of 80 limbs (26.3%).

Anomalies

Description

Anomalous presentation is similar to the above, running from the medial epicondyle to flexor pollicis longus (Smith et al. 2015).

Prevalence

Smith et al. (2015) noted that flexor digitorum superficialis sent an accessory slip to flexor pollicis longus in 3 out of 24 individuals with trisomy 13 (12.5%), 8 out of 26 individuals with trisomy 18 (30.8%), and 1 out of 7 individuals with trisomy 21 (14.3%).

Clinical Implications

Gantzer's muscle can contribute to median nerve and/or anterior interosseous nerve palsy, entrapment, or pressure neuritis, as well as Kiloh-Nevin syndrome (Oh et al. 2000;

Pai et al. 2008b; Kulkarni et al. 2014; Caetano et al. 2015; Zdilla et al. 2019). It may also simulate a soft-tissue tumor or a ganglion (Kulkarni et al. 2014).

FLEXOR DIGITORUM PROFUNDUS (FIGURE 3.12)

See also: Gantzer's muscle

Synonyms

This muscle is also known as flexor digitorum perforans (Wood) (Macalister 1875), musculus perforans, cubito-phalangettien commun (Todd 1839).

Typical Presentation

Description

Flexor digitorum profundus originates from the anterior and medial surfaces of the ulna and the interosseous membrane (Standring 2016). The muscle converges into four tendons that pass through the tendons of flexor digitorum superficialis to insert onto the bases of the distal phalanges of digits two through five (Standring 2016).

Innervation

Innervation for this muscle is split; the portion that sends tendons to digits four and five is innervated by the ulnar nerve while the portion that sends tendons to digits two and three is innervated by the anterior interosseous branch of the median nerve (Standring 2016).

Comparative Anatomy

Flexor digitorum profundus has a similar typical presentation in the apes, extending from the radius, ulna, and interosseous membrane to digits two through five (Gibbs 1999; Diogo et al. 2010, 2012, 2013a,b, 2017). In some cases, a poorly developed tendon to digit one is present in common chimpanzees, orangutans, and gorillas (Gibbs 1999; Diogo et al. 2010, 2013a,b, 2017). In bonobos, the tendon to digit one was well-developed, stout and continuous with the main body of the muscle in two specimens, and absent entirely in another specimen (Diogo et al. 2017). Bergman et al. (1988) suggest that the distinct separation of the part of the muscle that acts on the second digit is unique to humans, relating to the functional specialization of the index finger.

Variations

Description

The part of the muscle that inserts onto the second digit is distinct from origin to insertion (Bergman et al. 1988; Standring 2016). When completely distinct, it forms flexor indicis profundus (Macalister 1875; Knott 1883a; Bergman et al. 1988). The tendon to the third digit may be absent (Bergman et al. 1988). Flexor digitorum profundus is frequently joined by slips from other structures including flexor digitorum superficialis, flexor pollicis longus, the medial epicondyle, the coronoid process, or the radius (Macalister 1875; Mori 1964; Akita and Nimura 2016b;

Standring 2016). Other variations of flexor digitorum profundus described by Macalister (1875) include the distinct separation of flexor indicis profundus, accessory slips to and from other structures, and cases in which other forearm or hand muscles arose from this muscle or its tendons. Linburg-Comstock variation is described as a tendinous connection between flexor pollicis longus and the digit two slip of flexor digitorum profundus, or the tendons of these muscles (Linburg and Comstock 1979). Flexor digitorum profundus is also associated with Gantzer's muscle (see the entry for this muscle).

Prevalence

See flexor pollicis longus entry for prevalence information about Linburg-Comstock variation. Knott (1883a) found flexor indicis profundus in 2 out of 34 subjects (5.9%). Mori (1964) observed that flexor digitorum profundus had a radial origin in 84% of cases. Mori (1964) also noted that out of 205 arms, this muscle received a slip from the coronoid process in 40% of arms, from the medial epicondyle in one case (about 0.5%), from the flexor pollicis longus in 12.5% of arms, and its tendon was fused that of with flexor digitorum superficialis in 11% of arms. Flexor digitorum profundus and flexor pollicis longus were connected with a muscular bundle in 4.5% of cases. The tendons of these muscles were fused upon insertion into digit two in 7.5% of cases. Furnas (1965) found that the muscle belly and tendon going to digit two was doubled in 4 out of 117 cadavers (3.4%).

Anomalies

Description

In a fetus with craniorachischisis, Alghamdi et al. (2017) observed that the tendon of the left flexor digitorum profundus that attached to the distal phalanx of the fifth digit also sent a small tendon to the middle phalanx of this digit. Also, a slip connected this muscle to flexor pollicis longus. On the right side of the body, flexor digitorum profundus only sent tendons to digits four and five. There were two deeper bundles of flexor digitorum profundus deep to this main belly. The first bundle sent one tendon to the forearm fascia and a second tendon that joined the tendons of the second bundle and flexor digitorum superficialis going to digit three. Windle (1893) described a slip running from the inner condyle of the humerus to flexor digitorum profundus in two female fetuses with anencephaly.

In a neonate with trisomy 13, the left flexor digitorum profundus was divided into three fascicles (Aziz 1980). In a female fetus with trisomy 18, the tendons of flexor digitorum profundus on the left side split more proximally than is normal (Alghamdi et al. 2018). On the right side, flexor digitorum profundus had two bellies that were fused proximally. The lateral belly sent one tendon to digit two and the medial belly sent three tendons to the three medial digits. The lateral belly was fused proximally to flexor pollicis longus.

Bersu et al. (1976) describe a male infant with Hanhart syndrome. On the right side of this specimen, the wrist and hand were deficient. Flexor digitorum profundus inserted via a single tendon onto the capsule of the fused carpal mass with the single anomalous tendon of flexor digitorum superficialis. The fifth tendon of flexor digitorum profundus arising from the fourth tendon has been observed in infants with Neu-Laxova syndrome (Shved et al. 1985). On the right hand of a male neonate with Meckel syndrome, Pettersen (1984) observed that flexor digitorum profundus sent tendons to all six digits.

Prevalence

According to the literature review conducted by Smith et al. (2015), flexor digitorum profundus was variable (e.g., diminutive or missing tendons, fusion with flexor digitorum superficialis, tendon to sixth digit when present, and variable presentation in how and which tendons insert onto each digit) in 5 out of 24 individuals with trisomy 13 (20.8%) and 6 out of 26 individuals with trisomy 18 (23.1%). In a study of six upper limbs from three infants with Neu-Laxova syndrome, Shved et al. (1985) found that the tendon of flexor digitorum profundus going to the fifth finger arose from the tendon to the fourth finger in two upper limbs (33%).

Clinical Implications

Shrewsbury et al. (2003) explain that the clinical evidence of restrictive thumb/index tendosynovitis and pain in humans is associated with connections between the flexor pollicis longus and the flexor digitorum profundus (e.g., Linburg-Comstock variations).

FLEXOR DIGITORUM SUPERFICIALIS (FIGURE 3.13)

See also: Gantzer's muscle

Synonyms

This muscle is also referred to as flexor digitorum sublimis (Standring 2016), musculus perforates, or epi-trochlophalanginien commun (Todd 1839).

Typical Presentation

Description

The humero-ulnar head of flexor digitorum superficialis originates from the medial epicondyle of the humerus, the coronoid process, the anterior band of the ulnar collateral ligament, and the intermuscular septa (Standring 2016). The radial head originates from the middle third of the radius (Standring 2016). The heads converge into a muscle with two layers; the superficial layer sends tendons to the third and fourth digits, while the deep layer sends tendons to the second and fifth digits (Standring 2016). The tendons for each digit enter the flexor sheaths, split to course around the tendons of flexor digitorum profundus, and insert onto the intermediate phalanx of each digit (Standring 2016).

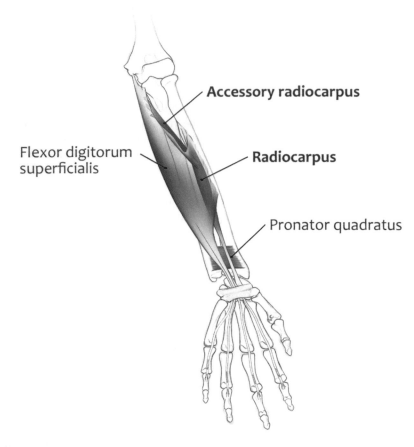

FIGURE 3.13 Flexor digitorum superficialis, pronator quadratus, radiocarpus, and accessory radiocarpus in anterior view.

Innervation

Flexor digitorum superficialis is innervated by the median nerve (Standring 2016).

Comparative Anatomy

Flexor digitorum superficialis has a similar typical presentation in the apes, extending from the radius, ulna, and medial epicondyle to the intermediate phalanges of digits two through five (Gibbs 1999; Diogo et al. 2010, 2012, 2013a,b, 2017). In all apes, the ulnar origin may be occasionally absent (Macalister 1873; Deniker 1885; Beddard 1893; Loth 1931; Kallner 1956; Gibbs 1999; Diogo et al. 2010, 2012, 2013a,b, 2017). The radial origin may be absent in gibbons, orangutans, and common chimpanzees (Gratiolet and Alix 1866; Deniker 1885; Michaelis 1903; Diogo et al. 2012, 2013b).

Variations

Description

The radial head of flexor digitorum superficialis and the insertions onto the third or fifth digit may be absent (Macalister 1875; Knott 1883a; Mori 1964; Furnas 1965; Shrewsbury and Kuczynski 1974; Bergman et al. 1988; Akita and Nimura 2016b; Standring 2016; Yammine and Erić 2018). Occasionally, the flexor digitorum superficialis tendons may be replaced by slips from other structures (Macalister 1875; Bergman et al. 1988; Akita and Nimura 2016b; Standring 2016). There is also frequent variation in how the tendons supply each digit (Macalister 1875; Furnas 1965; Kaplan 1969; Shrewsbury and Kuczynski 1974; Bergman et al. 1988; Akita and Nimura 2016b). Flexor digitorum superficialis can be connected via slips to flexor pollicis longus, palmaris longus, the brachioradialis tendon, or the ulnar tuberosity, or be fused with flexor pollicis longus, flexor digitorum profundus and its tendons, or pronator teres (Macalister 1875; Mori 1964; Bergman et al. 1988; Akita and Nimura 2016b). Other variations of flexor digitorum profundus described by Macalister (1875) include variation in tendon insertion, tendon doubling or absence, the presence of accessory slips, and presentation as a digastric muscle.

Flexor digitorum superficialis is associated with three supernumerary muscles. Radiopalmaris originates from the radius and attaches to the palmar aponeurosis and digital flexor sheath (Bergman et al. 1988; Akita and Nimura 2016b). Palmar flexor digitorum superficialis accessorius originates from the palmar fascia and transverse carpal ligament and ends in a tendon that joins the flexor tendon going to digit two (Bergman et al. 1988; Akita and Nimura 2016b). Flexor digitorum superficialis is also associated with Gantzer's muscle (see the entry for this muscle).

Prevalence

Mori (1964) noted that the radial head of flexor digitorum superficialis was absent in 7.5% of his subjects and diminutive in 12.5%. Mori (1964) also observed that this muscle was fused with pronator teres in 2.5% of the individuals examined by him, while it was fused with flexor digitorum profundus in 8%, and with flexor pollicis longus in 45%.

Furnas (1965) found that the tendon and muscle belly of flexor digitorum superficialis going to digit five was absent in 6 out of 117 arms (5.1%). Kaplan (1969) found that in 21 out of 68 hands the flexor superficialis tendons to digit five were connected with the tendon going to digit two (30.8%), while in 23 hands the flexor superficialis tendons to digit five were connected with the tendon going to digit four (33.8%). Shrewsbury and Kuczynski (1974) found that the tendon to digit five was absent in seven of 23 hands (30%) from 15 cadavers.

A meta-analysis of 34 studies with a total sample of 12,213 forearms by Yammine and Erić (2018) reveals that the clinical prevalence of functional absence of the flexor digitorum superficialis tendon to digit five is 7.45%, the clinical prevalence of the "common type" of the flexor digitorum superficialis tendon to digit five is 37.5%, and the cadaveric prevalence of muscle belly absence for flexor digitorum superficialis to digit five is 2.5%.

Anomalies

Description

In a neonate with trisomy 13, flexor digitorum superficialis was divided into four fascicles bilaterally, and the tendon to the fifth digit was absent on both sides (Aziz 1980). In a trisomy 18 cyclopic fetus dissected by Smith et al. (2015), the authors observed that the left flexor digitorum superficialis lacked both its radial origin and its insertion onto the fifth digit. On the right side of this individual, flexor digitorum superficialis sent a slip to flexor digitorum profundus (Smith et al. 2015). In a female fetus with trisomy 18, the tendon of flexor digitorum superficialis to the fifth digit was absent bilaterally (Alghamdi et al. 2018). The proximal end of this muscle was also fused with that of flexor carpi radialis on both sides of the body. Among individuals with trisomy 21, the tendon to the fifth digit was absent on the left side in one fetus, both sides of another fetus, and on the right side of an adult (Bersu 1980). There was a double belly of flexor digitorum superficialis to the fifth digit in a child with trisomy 21 (Bersu 1980).

In one anencephalic fetus, Windle (1893) observed that flexor digitorum superficialis did not send a tendon to the fifth digit. In a fetus with craniorachischisis, the right flexor digitorum superficialis was diminutive and only sent tendons to digits three and four (Alghamdi et al. 2017). On the left side of the body, this muscle only inserted onto digits two, three, and four, and its proximal end was fused with pronator teres and flexor carpi ulnaris.

Bersu et al. (1976) describe a male infant with Hanhart syndrome. On the right side of this specimen, the wrist and hand were deficient. Flexor digitorum superficialis inserted via a single tendon associated with palmaris longus onto the connective tissue capsule of the fused carpal mass. Mieden (1982) describes an infant with median cleft lip, hypotelorism, and alobar holoprosencephaly. The tendon of flexor digitorum superficialis to the fifth digit was absent on the right side (Mieden 1982). On the left side of a male neonate with Meckel syndrome, Pettersen (1984) observed that the flexor digitorum superficialis tendon to the fifth digit was absent. An accessory muscle associated with flexor digitorum superficialis and fifth tendon arising from the fourth tendon has been observed in infants with Neu-Laxova syndrome (Shved et al. 1985).

Prevalence

Overall, flexor digitorum superficialis was anomalous in many individuals included in the literature review conducted by Smith et al. (2015). This muscle was variable (e.g., diminutive radial head, doubled muscle bellies or tendons, variation in presentation or absence of tendons, tendons replaced by other structures) in 6 out of 24 individuals with trisomy 13 (25%), 11 out of 26 individuals with trisomy 18 (42.3%), and in 2 out of 7 individuals with trisomy 21 (28.6%). An absent radial head of this muscle was noted in 4 out of 24 individuals with trisomy 13 (16.7%) and 2 out of 26 individuals with trisomy 18 (7.7%). Flexor digitorum superficialis sent a slip to flexor digitorum profundus in 3 out of 24 individuals with trisomy 13 (12.5%), 7 out of 26 individuals with trisomy 18 (26.9%), and 2 out of 7 individuals with trisomy 21 (28.6%). These authors also noted that flexor digitorum superficialis sent an accessory slip to flexor pollicis longus in 3 out of 24 individuals with trisomy 13 (12.5%), 8 out of 26 individuals with trisomy 18 (30.8%), and 1 out of 7 individuals with trisomy 21 (14.3%). An accessory slip from flexor digitorum superficialis to radiocarpus was present in 1 out of 24 individuals with trisomy 13 (4.2%) and 1 out of 26 individuals with trisomy 18 (3.8%).

In a study of six upper limbs from three infants with Neu-Laxova syndrome, Shved et al. (1985) found that an accessory muscle associated with flexor digitorum superficialis was present in two upper limbs (33%) and the tendon going to the fifth finger arose from the tendon to the fourth finger in two upper limbs (33%).

Clinical Implications

A diminutive or absent flexor superficialis tendon may impair grip strength and can also functionally present as a tendon rupture, which can be assessed by clinical tests (Bowman et al. 2003; Yammine and Erić 2018; Belbl et al. 2020).

PRONATOR QUADRATUS (FIGURE 3.13)

Synonyms

This muscle is also referred to as pronator radii quadratus (Knott 1883a) or cubito-radial (Todd 1839).

Typical Presentation

Description

Pronator quadratus extends from the distal portion of the ulnar shaft to the distal portion of the radial shaft (Standring 2016).

Innervation

Pronator quadratus is innervated by the median nerve (Standring 2016).

Comparative Anatomy

Pronator quadratus has a similar typical presentation in the apes but appears to have a more oblique orientation in gibbons and orangutans (Gibbs 1999; Diogo et al. 2010, 2012, 2013a,b, 2017). Dwight (1895) observed that pronator quadratus can be separated into multiple layers as a variation in common chimpanzees.

Variations

Description

Pronator quadratus can be split into two or more parts or layers, and its fibers may run in different directions (Macalister 1875; Knott 1883a; Inoue 1934; Mori 1964; Johnson and Shrewsbury 1976; Sakamoto et al. 2015; Akita and Nimura 2016b; Das et al. 2008). Pronator quadratus may distally expand into the wrist or metacarpal region (Bergman et al. 1988; Akita and Nimura 2016b). It may also expand proximally to connect with pronator teres or flexor carpi radialis (Macalister 1875; Bergman et al. 1988; Akita and Nimura 2016b). Its fibers can insert into the thenar eminence and act as an accessory adductor of the first digit (Bergman et al. 1988; Akita and Nimura 2016b). Pronator quadratus can also be absent as a rare variation (Macalister 1875; Bergman et al. 1988; Akita and Nimura 2016b).

Pronator quadratus is in close proximity to several supernumerary muscles. Radiocubitocarpien (radialis internus brevis biceps) has an ulnar head and radial head and ends on the wrist (Calori 1870; Bergman et al. 1988; Akita and Nimura 2016b). Tensor capsulae radiocubitalis (inferioris) originates from the distal radius and courses over the anterior surface of pronator quadratus to insert onto the radioulnar capsule (Bergman et al. 1988; Akita and Nimura 2016b). Ulnocarpus brevis (flexor carpi ulnaris brevis or cubitocarpeus) originates from the distal end of the ulna and inserts onto the pisiform, hamate, fourth metacarpal, fifth metacarpal, capsule of carpal articulations, or abductor digiti minimi (Knott 1883a; Mori 1964; Bergman et al. 1988; Akita and Nimura 2016b).

Prevalence

Knott (1883a) found that pronator quadratus was split completely into two parts in 2 out of 34 subjects (5.9%). Mori (1964) recorded the presence of supernumerary muscle "flexor carpi ulnaris brevis" in 4 out of 205 arms (1.9%). Mori (1964) also classified pronator quadratus into eight types and found that the typical presentation of this muscle was only present in 39% of cases.

Anomalies

Description

In a fetus with craniorachischisis, Alghamdi et al. (2017) noted that pronator quadratus was absent on the right side. In a neonate with trisomy 18, "flexor carpi ulnaris brevis" was present on the left side, extending from the distal ulna to the hamate (Aziz 1979).

Prevalence

In their literature review, Smith et al. (2015) found that pronator quadratus was absent in 1 out of 26 individuals with trisomy 18 (3.8%).

Clinical Implications

N/A

RADIOCARPUS (FIGURE 3.13)

See also: Pronator quadratus, Flexor carpi radialis brevis

Synonyms

This muscle is also referred to as radiocarpeus, radiocarpien (Fano), or court radial anterieur (Le Double) (Bergman et al. 1988; Akita and Nimura 2016b). Though Knott (1883a) and Akita and Nimura (2016b) list flexor carpi radialis brevis as a synonym of radiocarpus, we treat these muscles as separate structures due to (1) the described tendinous and muscular connections between flexor carpus radialis brevis and flexor carpi radialis and (2) the possibility of radiocarpus extending proximally to the ulna or medial epicondyle.

Typical Presentation

This muscle is only present as a variation or anomaly.

Comparative Anatomy

N/A

Variations

Description

Radiocarpus is a supernumerary muscle that originates from the radius proximal to pronator quadratus and may extend proximally to the ulna or medial epicondyle of the humerus (Macalister 1875; Bergman et al. 1988; Akita and Nimura 2016b). It inserts onto one or more carpal or metacarpal bones, or bones from both regions (Macalister 1875; Bergman et al. 1988; Akita and Nimura 2016b). It may be divided into slips (Macalister 1875).

Innervation

N/A

Prevalence

Macalister (1875) notes that Wood has reported radiocarpus present in 4 out of 34 subjects in one study (11.8%) and in 2 out of 36 subjects (5.6%) in two studies. Over the course of three studies, Macalister (1875) found radiocarpus in 2 out of 53 subjects (3.8%), 1 out of 60 subjects (1.7%), and 4 out of 64 subjects (6.3%).

Anomalies

Description

In a neonate with trisomy 18, radiocarpus was present on the right side, extending from the proximal radius to the flexor retinaculum (Aziz 1979). Radiocarpus was present bilaterally in a neonate with trisomy 13 and extended from just below the radial tuberosity to the trapezium (Aziz 1980). Some anomalous cases exhibit an accessory radiocarpus that originates from the underside of flexor digitorum superficialis and inserts onto the belly of the radiocarpus (Figure 3.13) (Smith et al. 2015).

Prevalence

In their literature review, Smith et al. (2015) found that radiocarpus was present in 5 out of 24 individuals with trisomy 13 (20.8%) and in 5 out of 26 individuals with trisomy 18 (19.2%). The accessory radiocarpus was present in 2 out of 24 individuals with trisomy 13 (8.3%). An accessory slip from flexor digitorum superficialis to radiocarpus was present in 1 out of 24 individuals with trisomy 13 (4.2%) and 1 out of 26 individuals with trisomy 18 (3.8%).

Clinical Implications

N/A

PALMARIS LONGUS (FIGURE 3.14)

Synonyms

This muscle corresponds to palmaris longus externus sensu (Jouffroy 1971) and is also referred to as epitrochlo-palmaire (Todd 1839).

Typical Presentation

Description

Palmaris longus originates from the medial epicondyle of the humerus (Standring 2016). Some fibers attach onto the flexor retinaculum as its tendon of insertion passes into the hand to join with the palmar aponeurosis (Standring 2016).

Innervation

Palmaris longus is innervated by the median nerve (Standring 2016).

Comparative Anatomy

Palmaris longus is typically present in gibbons and orangutans, extending from the medial epicondyle of the humerus to the palmar aponeurosis (Chapman 1880; Kohlbrügge 1890–1892; Hepburn 1892; Beddard 1893; Primrose 1899, 1900; Grönroos 1903; Michaelis 1903; Sonntag 1924; Loth 1931; Kallner 1956; Michilsens et al. 2009; Oishi et al. 2009; Diogo et al. 2012, 2013b). It is sometimes absent in common chimpanzees and bonobos and typically absent in gorillas (Chapman 1878; Bischoff 1880; Deniker 1885; Hepburn

1892; Sommer 1907; Pira 1913; Sonntag 1923; Preuschoft 1965; Gibbs 1999; Diogo et al. 2010, 2013a, 2017).

Variations

Description

Macalister (1875), Knott (1883a), Bergman et al. (1988), and Akita and Nimura (2016b) note that palmaris longus is likely the most variable muscle in the human body. It can be absent bilaterally or unilaterally, is more often absent in females, and is more often absent on the left side of the body (Macalister 1875; Knott 1883a; Le Double 1897; Reimann et al. 1944; George 1953; Sato 1969; Hall 1984; Bergman et al. 1988; Akita and Nimura 2016b; Standring 2016; Georgiev et al. 2017b). Wilde et al. (2021) suggest that the absence of palmaris longus in adults is the result of the muscle failing to form early in development.

Both its origin and insertion are variable. Palmaris longus can originate from the medial intermuscular septum, biceps, brachialis, the fascia of the forearm, the coronoid process, or the radius (Macalister 1875; Knott 1883a; Bergman et al. 1988; Akita and Nimura 2016b). It can insert onto the interosseous membrane, forearm fascia, the flexor carpi ulnaris tendon, abductor pollicis brevis, the hypothenar eminence, any one of the flexor tendons, the pisiform, scaphoid, or digit four (Macalister 1875; Knott 1883a; Bergman et al. 1988; Akita and Nimura 2016b). The proportion of fleshy muscle belly to tendon in palmaris longus is variable (Macalister 1875; Knott 1883a; Bergman et al. 1988; Akita and Nimura 2016b). The tendon and muscle can be inverted so that palmaris longus is fleshy distally and the tendon is proximal, in which the muscle would be termed palmaris longus inversus (Macalister 1875; Mori 1964; Bergman et al. 1988; Akita and Nimura 2016b; Georgiev et al. 2017b).

Palmaris longus can be doubled or tripled (accessory palmaris longus), or either the muscle belly or tendon can be split (Macalister 1875; Reimann et al. 1944; Bergman et al. 1988; Akita and Nimura 2016b; Georgiev et al. 2017b). It is also associated with two supernumerary muscles. Palmaris profundus originates from the middle third of the radius and courses beneath the flexor retinaculum to insert with the palmar aponeurosis (Bergman et al. 1988; Akita and Nimura 2016b). Accessorius ad flexorem digiti minimi refers to a muscle that arises from the palmaris longus tendon to insert onto the fifth metacarpal (Bergman et al. 1988).

Prevalence

Macalister (1875) notes that palmaris longus deviates from the typical presentation in about every one out of four cases (25%). The rate of absence of palmaris longus has been reported to be anywhere between about 2%–25% (Hall 1984; Bergman et al. 1988). Bergman et al. report an absence of 11.2% across all bodies and cite a study of 800 subjects in which it was absent on both sides in 7.7% of cases, absent on the right side in 4.5% of cases, and absent

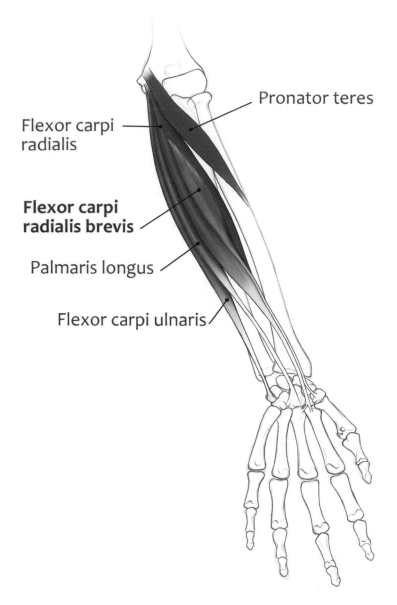

FIGURE 3.14 Superficial anterior forearm muscles in anterior view. This figure displays the anomalous presentation of flexor carpi radialis brevis as described by Smith et al. (2015).

on the left side in 5.2% of cases. Bergman et al. (1988) also note that prevalence of absence is lower in Asian populations, as it is absent in 3.4% of Japanese individuals (30 out of 884 arms; Adachi 1909) and 2.2% of Chinese individuals (two out of 95 arms; Nakano 1923). Knott (1883a) found the muscle absent in 4 out of 34 subjects (11.8%) and found an accessory head from the coronoid process in two subjects (5.9%). Le Double (1897) reports an absence in 91 out of 520 cases (17.5%). In a study of 276 cadavers by George (1953), palmaris longus was absent in 15.2% of the 552 limbs examined. Sato (1969) found palmaris longus absent in 33 out of 406 limbs from Kyushu-Japanese males (8.13%) and absent in 6 out of 262 limbs (2.29%) from females.

Reimann et al. (1944) conducted an extensive examination of palmaris longus in 1,600 arms. They found that this

muscle was absent in 205 arms (12.8%), which is close to the prevalence of 12.7% (178 out of 1,400 cases) reported by Gruber (Reimann et al. 1944). These authors also found that palmaris longus showed variations other than absence in 46 out of 530 arms (9%). Palmaris longus was doubled in 4 out of 530 arms (0.8%). Mori (1964) noted that an inverted palmaris longus was present in 3 out of 360 arms (0.8%), the tendon of insertion ended in the forearm fascia in 3 out of 205 arms (1.5%), the tendon of insertion was split into two fascicles in three or 4 out of 40 arms (10%), and the tendon of insertion was divided into three fascicles in 1 out of 40 arms (2.5%).

Through clinical testing of 7,000 teenagers in Turkey, Ceyhan and Mavt (1997) report an absence of 63.9%. Clinical testing of 300 Caucasian subjects revealed that palmaris longus was absent unilaterally in 49 subjects (16.3%) and absent bilaterally in 26 subjects (8.6%) (Thompson et al. 2001). Through clinical testing of 800 subjects in Serbia, Erić et al. (2010) determined that palmaris longus was absent unilaterally in 173 subjects (21.6%) and absent bilaterally in 127 subjects (15.9%). Clinical testing of 200 subjects in Marathwada, India, found that this muscle was absent unilaterally in 20 individuals (10%) and absent bilaterally in 11 individuals (6%) (Hussaini and Deshmukh 2018).

Georgiev et al. (2017b) studied palmaris longus anatomy in 112 limbs from 56 cadavers. They found that this muscle was only variable in nine cases (8%). Palmaris longus was absent in three cases (2.7%), doubled in two cases (1.8%), had an intermediate muscle belly in two cases (1.8%), was digastric in one case (0.9%), and was reversed and associated with an accessory abductor digiti minimi in one case (0.9%) (Georgiev et al. 2017b).

Anomalies

Description

Palmaris longus was absent bilaterally in two neonates with trisomy 18 and three neonates with trisomy 13 (Aziz 1979, 1980, 1981). In a female fetus with trisomy 18, palmaris longus was absent on the right side (Alghamdi et al. 2018). In a trisomy 18 cyclopic fetus, palmaris longus was absent on one side (Smith et al. (2015). Palmaris longus was absent bilaterally in four individuals with trisomy 21 described by Bersu (1980). In a fifth case (a fetus), the muscle belly was situated at the wrist in the right forearm and at the middle of the forearm in the left forearm.

In a male fetus with triploidy, Moen et al. (1984) found that palmaris longus was absent on the left side. The absence or "anomalous structure" of palmaris longus has been observed in infants with Neu-Laxova syndrome (Shved et al. 1985). In a fetus with craniorachischisis, Alghamdi et al. (2017) observed that the palmaris longus was absent on the left side. On the right side of the body, palmaris longus was fused with flexor carpi ulnaris at its proximal end.

Bersu et al. (1976) describe a male infant with Hanhart syndrome. On the right side of this specimen, the wrist and hand were deficient. Palmaris longus inserted onto the radial side of the reduced flexor digitorum superficialis tendon just proximal to the flexor retinaculum. Mieden (1982) describes an infant with median cleft lip, hypotelorism, and alobar holoprosencephaly (case I) and two male fetuses with cyclopia and alobar holoprosencephaly (cases II and III). In cases I and II, palmaris longus was absent bilaterally (Mieden 1982).

Prevalence

Among the limbs of ten anencephalic fetuses, Windle (1893) noted that palmaris longus was absent unilaterally in two males and missing bilaterally in one male (30%), while this muscle was doubled in one female (10%). In a study of six

upper limbs from three infants with Neu-Laxova syndrome, Shved et al. (1985) found that palmaris longus was absent in four upper limbs (66%) and an "anomalous structure" was present in two upper limbs (33%).

According to Smith et al. (2015), palmaris longus was absent in 20 out of 24 individuals with trisomy 13 (83.3%), 23 out of 26 individuals with trisomy 18 (88.5%), and in 6 out of 7 individuals with trisomy 21 (85.7%). This muscle was also variable (diminutive in one specimen and variable insertion onto metacarpal five in another) in 2 out of 26 individuals with trisomy 18 (7.7%) and was variable (diminutive in one specimen and distally located belly in another) in 2 out of 7 individuals with trisomy 21 (28.6%) (Smith et al. 2015).

Clinical Implications

Palmaris longus inversus can lead to forearm pain and swelling, compression and paresthesia of the median or ulnar nerve, and carpal tunnel syndrome (Backhouse and Churchill-Davidson 1975; Still and Kleinert 1973; Depuydt et al. 1998; Bhashyam 2017). Tiengo et al. (2006) note that the presence of an accessory palmaris longus can emulate a tumor in medical images and also contribute to median nerve compression or carpal tunnel syndrome. Palmaris profundus can cause compressive neuropathy of the anterior interosseous nerve and the median nerve (Akita and Nimura 2016b).

FLEXOR CARPI ULNARIS (FIGURE 3.14)

Synonyms

This muscle is also referred to as ulnaris internus, cubital interne, or cubito-carpien (Todd 1839).

Typical Presentation

Description

The humeral head of flexor carpi ulnaris originates from the medial epicondyle, and the ulnar head originates the proximal portion of the posterior ulna, including the olecranon (Standring 2016). It has insertions into the pisiform, hamate, and fifth metacarpal (Standring 2016).

Innervation

Flexor carpi ulnaris is innervated by the ulnar nerve (Standring 2016).

Comparative Anatomy

The insertion of flexor carpi ulnaris is confined to the pisiform in gibbons, orangutans, and gorillas (Diogo et al. 2010, 2012, 2013a,b, 2017). The presentation of flexor carpi ulnaris in common chimpanzees and bonobos is more similar to that of humans, as it can have attachments to structures beyond that of the pisiform including the fifth metacarpal and the hamate (Gratiolet and Alix 1866; Miller 1952; Diogo et al. 2013a, 2017).

Variations

Description

A slip may connect flexor carpi ulnaris to the coronoid process (Bergman et al. 1988; Akita and Nimura 2016b; Standring 2016). Flexor carpi ulnaris can also exhibit attachments to the flexor retinaculum, the third or fourth metacarpals, the metacarpophalangeal joint capsule of the fifth digit, or the abductor digiti minimi (Macalister 1875; Knott 1883a; Bergman et al. 1988; al-Qattan and Duerksen 1992; Akita and Nimura 2016b; Standring 2016). It may originate from triceps brachii (Macalister 1875). Bergman et al. (1988) describe a rare variation in which an accessory belly is present inferior to the main belly of this muscle and is innervated by the median nerve. Both Sakthivel and Verma (2017) and Kunc et al. (2019) report an accessory flexor carpi ulnaris associated with an absent palmaris longus, though in the former study the accessory muscle was innervated by the ulnar nerve and no innervation information was provided in the latter study.

Prevalence

Mori (1964) did not find any variation in origin or insertion of flexor carpi ulnaris but noted that in 6% of cases the muscular part extended distally past the radiocarpal joint.

Anomalies

Description

Macalister (1875) notes that Koster observed an insertion of flexor carpi ulnaris into the interosseous membrane in an individual with a congenital deformity and that Friedlowsky found a slip from flexor carpi ulnaris to the annular ligament in a hand that had only a thumb and two fingers. Bersu et al. (1976) describe a male infant with Hanhart syndrome. On the right side of this specimen, the wrist and hand were deficient. Flexor carpi ulnaris inserted onto the ulnar aspect of the fused carpal mass. In a fetus with craniorachischisis dissected by Alghamdi et al. (2017), the authors observed that the left flexor carpi ulnaris had two heads like the normal condition, but the ulnar nerve separated abnormally between the two heads. Additionally, the proximal end of flexor carpi ulnaris was fused with pronator teres and flexor digitorum superficialis. On the right side of the body, flexor carpi ulnaris was abnormally fused with palmaris longus near where these muscles arise from the medial epicondyle. Smith et al. (2015) noted the presence of an accessory belly, termed flexor carpi ulnaris accessorius, which originated from the middle of the ulna and inserted with flexor digiti minimi onto the fifth digit in a fetus with trisomy 18 and cyclopia.

Prevalence

Flexor carpi ulnaris accessorius was present in 9 out of 26 individuals with trisomy 18 (34.6%).

Clinical Implications

Variations of flexor carpi ulnaris and its tendon of insertion can cause ulnar nerve compression (O'Hara and Stone 1988; al-Qattan and Duerksen 1992).

FLEXOR CARPI RADIALIS (FIGURE 3.14)

Synonyms

This muscle is also referred to as flexor carpi radialis longus (Mori 1964), radialis internus, grand palmaire, or radial anterieur (Todd 1839).

Typical Presentation

Description

Flexor carpi radialis originates from the medial epicondyle of the humerus (Standring 2016). It inserts via a long tendon onto the base of the second metacarpal and sends a slip to the third metacarpal (Standring 2016).

Innervation

Flexor carpi radialis is innervated by the median nerve (Standring 2016).

Comparative Anatomy

An origin from the radius is frequently present in all apes (Gibbs 1999; Diogo et al. 2010, 2012, 2013a,b, 2017). Some individuals may lack an attachment to the third metacarpal (Gratiolet and Alix 1866; Kohlbrügge 1890–1892; Beddard 1893; Dwight 1895; Primrose 1899, 1900; Sullivan and Osgood 1927; Gibbs 1999; Miller 1952; Michilsens et al. 2009; Diogo et al. 2010, 2012, 2013a,b, 2017). An insertion into the trapezium may be found in gorillas (Preuschoft 1965; Diogo et al. 2010). In bonobos, flexor carpi radialis may fuse with pronator teres (Miller 1952) or the flexor digitorum superficialis tendon to digit four (Diogo et al. 2017).

Variations

Description

Flexor carpi radialis may be completely absent (Mori 1964; Bergman et al. 1988; Akita and Nimura 2016b; Standring 2016). It may be doubled (Mori 1964; Akita and Nimura 2016b). Accessory slips or accessory heads may connect this muscle to brachialis, the biceps tendon, the bicipital aponeurosis, coronoid process, or radius (Macalister 1875; Knott 1883a; Mori 1964; Bergman et al 1988; Akita and Nimura 2016b; Standring 2016). It may have insertions into the flexor retinaculum, scaphoid, trapezium, or fourth metacarpal (Macalister 1875; Knott 1883a; Bergman et al 1988; Akita and Nimura 2016b; Standring 2016).

Prevalence

In a sample of 34 specimens, Knott (1883a) found that flexor carpi radialis inserted into the second and third metacarpals in 19 cases (55.9%), into the trapezium in one case (2.9%), into the trapezium and second metacarpal in one case (2.9%), and into the third and fourth metacarpal in one case (2.9%). Mori (1964) noted that flexor carpi radialis had a radial origin in 7.5% of cases, received a slip from the coronoid process in 5% of cases, was doubled in 2% of cases, and was entirely absent in 2.5% of cases. Mori (1964) also observed that flexor carpi radialis inserted onto the second metacarpal in

90% of cases and sent a slip to the third metacarpal in 7.5% of cases. Mori (1964) noted a flexor carpi radialis accessorius inserting onto the scaphoid in 2.5% of cases (unclear if this is synonymous with flexor carpi radialis brevis).

Anomalies

Description

Macalister (1875) notes that Koster observed an insertion of flexor carpi radialis into the distal radius in an individual with a congenital deformity and that Friedlowsky found an insertion into the scapho-trapezium in a hand that had only a thumb and two fingers. In a trisomy 18 cyclopic fetus, Smith et al. (2015) observed that on both sides of the body, flexor carpi radialis was fused with pronator teres. In a fetus with craniorachischisis, Alghamdi et al. (2017) observed that the left flexor carpi ulnaris had an insertion onto the trapezoid. This muscle was absent on the right side. In a female fetus with trisomy 18, the proximal end of this muscle was fused with that of flexor digitorum superficialis on both sides of the body (Alghamdi et al. 2018). Absence or anomalous insertion of flexor carpi radialis has been observed in infants with Neu-Laxova syndrome (Shved et al. 1985). Bersu et al. (1976) describe a male infant with Hanhart syndrome. On the right side of this specimen, the wrist and hand were deficient. Flexor carpi radialis inserted onto the trapezoid.

Prevalence

In their literature review, Smith et al. (2015) found that flexor carpi radialis was absent in 3 out of 26 individuals with trisomy 18 (11.6%), and that this muscle had variable attachments (to the flexor retinaculum, to the base of metacarpal one) in 2 out of 26 individuals with trisomy 18 (7.7%). Fusion of pronator teres and flexor carpi radialis was noted in 2 out of 24 individuals with trisomy 13 (8.3%). In a study of six upper limbs from three infants with Neu-Laxova syndrome, Shved et al. (1985) found that flexor carpi radialis was absent in two upper limbs (33%) and an anomalous insertion was present in four upper limbs (66%).

Clinical Implications
N/A

Flexor carpi radialis brevis (Figure 3.14)

See also: Flexor carpi radialis, Pronator quadratus

Synonyms

This muscle is also referred to as flexor carpi radialis vel profundus (Wood) and the short radiocarpal flexor muscle (Hongsmatip et al. 2019). Though Knott (1883a) and Akita and Nimura (2016b) list flexor carpus radialis brevis as a synonym of radiocarpus, we treat these muscles as separate structures due to (1) the described tendinous and muscular connections between flexor carpus radialis brevis and flexor carpi radialis and (2) the possibility of radiocarpus extending proximally to the ulna or medial epicondyle.

Typical Presentation
This muscle is only present as a variation or anomaly.

Comparative Anatomy

According to Diogo and Wood (2012a), Lewis (1989) states that in chimpanzees (and humans), if flexor carpi radialis originates from the radius via two tendons, one is referred to as flexor carpi radialis brevis and the other is referred to flexor carpi radialis longus.

Variations

Description

Flexor carpi radialis brevis is a variant of flexor carpi radialis. It is a small muscle that originates from the radius and typically inserts onto the tendon of flexor carpi radialis, or with the flexor carpi radialis tendon onto the base of the second metacarpal (Knott 1883a; Nakahashi and Izumi 1987; Bergman et al. 1988). This muscle can also insert onto the retinacular septum, trapezium, capitate, or bases of the third or fourth metacarpals (Knott 1883a; Nakahashi and Izumi 1987; Hongsmatip et al. 2019).

Innervation

Flexor carpi radialis brevis is innervated by the anterior interosseous nerve (Dodds 2006; Hongsmatip et al. 2019).

Prevalence

Gruber observed flexor carpi radialis brevis in 1 out of 400 limbs (0.25%), and Wood (1867a) noted its presence in 6 out of 70 limbs (8.6%). Knott (1883a) found this muscle in 1 out of 34 subjects (2.9%).

Anomalies

Description

According to Smith et al. (2015), an anomalous flexor carpi radialis brevis can originate from the flexor carpi radialis belly and insert onto the trapezium.

Prevalence

In the literature review conducted by Smith et al. (2015), they found that this muscle was present in 1 out of 26 individuals with trisomy 18 (3.8%).

Clinical Implications

Hongsmatip et al. (2019) suggest that the interaction between the tendons of flexor carpi radialis and flexor carpi radialis brevis could lead to tendon intersection syndrome or tenosynovitis.

Pronator teres (Figure 3.14)

Synonyms

This muscle is also referred to as pronator radii teres (Knott 1883a).

Typical Presentation

Description

The humeral head of pronator teres originates from the medial supracondylar ridge of the humerus, the intermuscular septum it shares with flexor carpi radialis, and the antebrachial fascia (Standring 2016). The ulnar head originates from the coronoid process of the ulna (Standring 2016). The muscle inserts via a tendon onto the lateral radial shaft (Standring 2016).

Innervation

Pronator teres is innervated by the median nerve (Standring 2016).

Comparative Anatomy

Pronator teres has a similar typical presentation in the apes, but the ulnar head is frequently absent as a variation (Gratiolet and Alix 1866; Chapman 1878; Bischoff 1880; Deniker 1885; Hepburn 1892; Chapman 1900; Loth 1931; Preuschoft 1965; Jouffroy 1971; Lewis 1989; Gibbs 1999; Michilsens et al. 2009; Diogo et al. 2010, 2012, 2013a,b, 2017).

Variations

Description

The ulnar head can be reduced or absent (Macalister 1875; Mori 1964; Bergman et al. 1988; Nebot-Cegarra et al. 1991–1992; Vymazalová et al. 2015; Standring 2016; Olewnik et al. 2018a). The two heads may be partially or completely divided (Macalister 1875; Knott 1883a; Akita and Nimura 2016b). Both heads may also be doubled (Macalister 1875; Bergman et al. 1988). An accessory slip may originate from a supracondylar process of the humerus, or a ligament can connect pronator teres to the medial epicondyle (Bergman et al. 1988; Standring 2016; Akita and Nimura 2016b). A third head may arise from the ulna from below the coronoid process (Macalister 1875; Knott 1883a; Akita and Nimura 2016b). Slips can extend to the fascia of the arm, the medial intermuscular septum, or the humerus (Macalister 1875; Bergman et al. 1988; Akita and Nimura 2016b; Standring 2016). This muscle can also be connected to biceps, brachialis, flexor carpi radialis, flexor pollicis longus, or flexor digitorum superficialis (Macalister 1875; Mori 1964; Bergman et al. 1988; Akita and Nimura 2016b; Standring 2016).

Prevalence

In a sample of 80 arms, Mori (1964) found that pronator teres received a slip from brachialis in 15% of cases and a slip from biceps brachii in 17.5% of cases. The ulnar head was poorly developed in 10% of cases. The insertion was divided into two parts in 4% of cases. In a study of 50 limbs, Olewnik et al. (2018a) found that the humeral head of pronator teres originated from both the medial epicondyle and medial intermuscular septum in 36 cases (72%), but only from the medial epicondyle in 14 cases (28%). These frequencies are similar to the ones provided by Vymazalová et al. (2015), who studied pronator teres in 68 adults and 3 fetuses and noted an origin from both the medial epicondyle and medial intermuscular septum in 70.6% of cases and an origin from only the medial epicondyle in 29.4% of cases. Olewnik et al. (2018a) observed that the ulnar head was present in 43 limbs (86%), therefore yielding an absence prevalence of 14%. Vymazalová et al. (2015) found that the ulnar head was absent in 4.4% of cases. Nebot-Cegarra et al. (1991–1992) observed an absence of the ulnar head of pronator teres in 22% of cases.

Anomalies

Description

Macalister (1875) notes that Koster observed an insertion of pronator teres into the distal radius in an individual with a congenital deformity. In a fetus with craniorachischisis, Alghamdi et al. (2017) observed that the right pronator teres only had a humeral head, and some of its fibers had an abnormal insertion onto the fascia at the level of the hand. On the left side, the proximal end of pronator teres was fused with flexor carpi ulnaris and flexor digitorum superficialis. In a male infant with triploidy, Moen et al. (1984) found that pronator teres was absent bilaterally. Absence of the ulnar head and fusion of pronator teres with flexor carpi radialis has been observed in infants with Neu-Laxova syndrome (Shved et al. 1985).

In a neonate with trisomy 13, pronator teres partially originated from flexor carpi radialis (Aziz 1980). On the right side, it inserted into radiocarpus. In a trisomy 18 cyclopic fetus, Smith et al. (2015) observed that on both sides of the body, pronator teres was fused with flexor carpi radialis and there was a second deep belly of pronator teres that had an insertion that extended more distally onto the radius.

Prevalence

In their literature review, Smith et al. (2015) found that fusion of pronator teres and flexor carpi radialis, and pronator teres with two bellies, were both noted in 2 out of 24 individuals with trisomy 13 (both at a prevalence of 8.3%). Altogether, pronator teres was variant (accessory slips, doubled superficial head, variable origins and insertions) in 4 out of 24 individuals with trisomy 13 (16.7%). In 2 out of 26 individuals with trisomy 18, the ulnar head of pronator teres was missing (7.7%). In a study of six upper limbs from three infants with Neu-Laxova syndrome, Shved et al. (1985) found that both absence of the ulnar head and fusion of pronator teres with flexor carpi radialis occurred in four upper limbs (66%).

Clinical Implications

As variations of pronator teres may affect the course of the median nerve, variations can lead to median nerve compression neuropathy or "pronator teres syndrome" (Hartz et al. 1981; Nebot-Cegarra et al. 1991–1992; Olewnik et al. 2018a).

POSTERIOR FOREARM MUSCLES

BRACHIORADIALIS (FIGURE 3.15)

Synonyms

Brachioradialis is also referred to as supinator longus, supinator primus, or grand supinateur (Todd 1839; Barnard 1875; Parsons 1898b; Jouffroy 1971).

Typical Presentation

Description

Brachioradialis originates from the lateral supracondylar ridge of the humerus and lateral intermuscular septum and inserts via a tendon onto the distal radius proximal to the styloid process (Standring 2016).

Innervation

Brachioradialis is innervated by the radial nerve (Standring 2016).

Comparative Anatomy

Brachioradialis has a similar typical presentation in the apes, extending from the distal humerus to the radial shaft (Kohlbrügge 1890–1892; Hepburn 1892; Miller 1952; Gibbs 1999; Michilsens et al. 2009; Diogo et al. 2010, 2012, 2013a,b, 2017). The origin may extend to the level of the deltoid insertion in gorillas and common chimpanzees (Sonntag 1923; Swindler and Wood 1973; Diogo et al. 2010). The insertion usually reaches the styloid process of the radius in gorillas (Diogo et al. 2010). It sometimes reaches the styloid process in gibbons, common chimpanzees, bonobos, and orangutans (Hepburn 1892; Primrose 1899, 1900; Ziegler 1964; Swindler and Wood 1973; Michilsens et al. 2009; Diogo et al. 2012, 2013a,b, 2017). Brachioradialis may be fused with brachialis in gibbons, common chimpanzees, and bonobos (Hepburn 1892; Straus 1941; Miller 1952; Diogo et al. 2012, 2017).

Variations

Description

Brachioradialis may insert more proximally on the radius (Bergman et al. 1988; Akita and Nimura 2016b; Standring 2016). In other cases, the insertion can extend distally to attach onto the scaphoid, trapezium, or base of the third

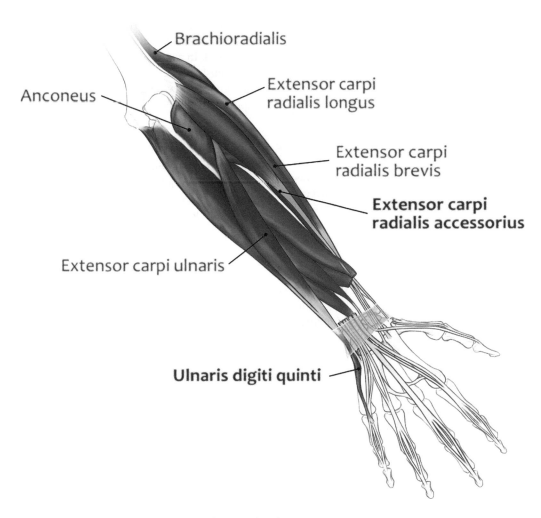

FIGURE 3.15 Superficial posterior forearm muscles in posterior view.

metacarpal (Macalister 1875; Bergman et al. 1988; Akita and Nimura 2016b). Its tendon may be bifurcated or trifurcated, or the entire muscle may be doubled (Macalister 1875; Mori 1964; Bergman et al. 1988; Turkof et al. 1994, 1995; Akita and Nimura 2016b; Standring 2016). Brachioradialis can be partially fused with or connected via slips to abductor pollicis longus, biceps brachii, brachialis, deltoid, extensor carpi radialis longus, supinator, or the forearm fascia (Macalister 1875; Inoue 1934; Mori 1964; Bergman et al. 1988; Akita and Nimura 2016b; Standring 2016). In rare cases, brachioradialis can be entirely absent (Macalister 1875; Bergman et al. 1988; Standring 2016).

An accessory brachioradialis may also be referred to as supinator radii longus accessorius, brachioradialis brevis, or brachioradialis minor (Knott 1883a). It originates next to or from brachioradialis and attaches to the radial tuberosity (Lauth 1830; Gruber 1867b; Knott 1883a; Le Double 1897; Bergman et al. 1988; Rodríguez-Niedenführ et al. 2001; Akita and Nimura 2016b). This muscle can also insert onto the supinator, pronator teres tendon, or the ulna (Bergman et al. 1988; Rodríguez-Niedenführ et al. 2001; Akita and Nimura 2016b).

Prevalence

Mori (1964) found that brachioradialis was connected (via muscular slips) with brachialis in 2.5% of cases, abductor pollicis longus in 12.5% of cases, extensor carpi radialis longus in 5% of cases, and biceps brachii in 2.5% of cases. The insertion tendon of brachioradialis attached to the dorsal radiocarpal ligament in 2.5% of cases (Mori 1964). In another 2.5% of cases, the insertion tendon was doubled, and the superficial branch of the radial nerve passed between the slips (Mori 1964).

In a study of 176 upper limbs from 88 cadavers, Rodríguez-Niedenführ et al. (2001) found an accessory brachioradialis present in five upper limbs (2.8%) from three cadavers. Turkof et al. (1994) found that the superficial branch of the radial nerve emerged between a split brachioradialis tendon in 5 out of 150 arms (3.3%) from 4 out of 75 cadavers. Turkof et al. (1995) found that in 143 patients with Wartenberg's syndrome (radial sensory nerve entrapment at the forearm), seven of them (4.9%) exhibited a superficial branch of the radial nerve passing between a split brachioradialis tendon.

Anomalies

Description

Windle (1893) observed a slip connecting brachioradialis and supinator on the right side of one male fetus with anencephaly. On the left side of the body of a fetus with craniorachischisis, Alghamdi et al. (2017) observed that brachioradialis had a normal origin but it had two tendons. The first attached to the distal end of the radius. The other attached to the base of the first metacarpal, exhibiting bifurcation as it surrounded the tendon of

abductor pollicis longus, and then rejoining as one tendon distally. Opponens pollicis had an abnormal attachment to this tendon near the base of the first metacarpal.

In a female fetus with trisomy 18, brachioradialis was thin on both sides of the body (Alghamdi et al. 2018). In a trisomy 18 cyclopic fetus, Smith et al. (2015) observed that brachialis was fused with extensor carpi radialis longus and extensor carpi radialis brevis at their proximal ends on the left side of the body. In a study of specimens with triploidy, Moen et al. (1984) found that brachioradialis was doubled on the right side of a male fetus and doubled bilaterally in a female fetus. Partial fusion of brachioradialis with brachialis has been observed in infants with Neu-Laxova syndrome (Shved et al. 1985).

On the left arm of a male neonate with Meckel syndrome, a small slip extended between the tendon of brachioradialis and flexor pollicis longus (Pettersen 1984). Bersu et al. (1976) describe a male infant with Hanhart syndrome. On the right side of this specimen, the wrist and hand were deficient. Brachioradialis inserted onto the radius proximal to the styloid process.

Prevalence

In their literature review, Smith et al. (2015) found that brachioradialis was variable (e.g., more distal attachment, diminutive muscle) in 3 out of 26 individuals with trisomy 18 (11.5%). In a study of six upper limbs from three infants with Neu-Laxova syndrome, Shved et al. (1985) found that brachioradialis was partially fused with brachialis in all six upper limbs (100%).

Clinical Implications

An accessory brachioradialis muscle or a split brachioradialis muscle/tendon can create possible entrapment sites for the radial nerve (Turkof et al. 1994, 1995; Spinner and Spinner 1996; Akita and Nimura 2016b).

SUPINATOR (FIGURE 3.16)

Synonyms

This muscle is also referred to as supinator brevis (Parsons 1898b) or epicondylo-radial (Todd 1839).

Typical Presentation

Description

Supinator has two heads/two layers of fibers (Standring 2016). The humeral (superficial) head and ulnar (deep) head originate together from the lateral epicondyle of the humerus, radial collateral ligament, annular ligament of the superior radioulnar joint, and from the supinator crest on the ulna (Standring 2016; Akita and Nimura 2016b). Supinator inserts onto the proximal third of the radius (Standring 2016).

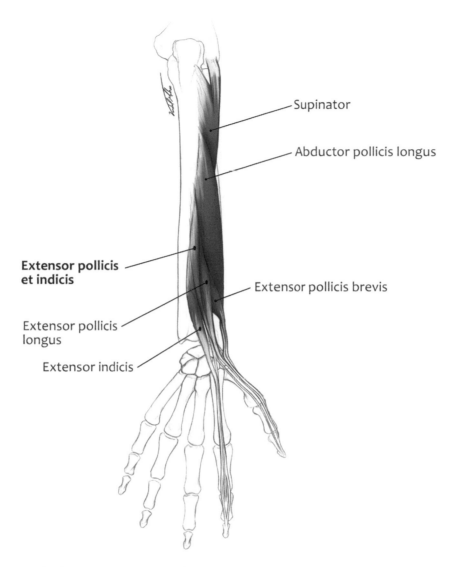

Supinator

Abductor pollicis longus

Extensor pollicis et indicis

Extensor pollicis brevis

Extensor pollicis longus

Extensor indicis

FIGURE 3.16 Deep posterior forearm muscles in posterior view.

Innervation

Supinator is innervated by the posterior interosseous nerve (Standring 2016).

Comparative Anatomy

Supinator has a similar typical presentation in the apes, extending from the lateral epicondyle of the humerus and from the proximal ulna to the proximal radius (Gibbs 1999; Diogo et al. 2010, 2012, 2013a,b, 2017). The humeral origin may be absent in some orangutans and bonobos (Barnard 1875; Straus 1941; Kallner 1956; Diogo et al. 2013b, 2017). The ulnar origin may be absent in gibbons (Michilsens et al. 2009; Diogo et al. 2012).

Variations

Description

The degree of division into two layers can vary (Bergman et al. 1988; Akita and Nimura 2016b). Its insertion may shift more distally along the radius (Mori 1964). Small

parts of supinator have been named as variations, including the lateral and medial tensors of the annular ligament (Macalister 1875; Standring 2016). Supinator may be doubled or divided (Macalister 1875). It may send accessory bundles to the biceps tendon, the bursa under the tendon, the radial tuberosity, or pronator teres (Clason 1869; Macalister 1875; Bergman et al. 1988; Akita and Nimura 2016b).

Prevalence

Mori (1964) found that the distal end of the supinator insertion was distal to the middle point of the radius in 16% of cases.

Anomalies

Description

Windle (1893) observed a slip connecting brachioradialis and supinator on the right side of one male fetus with anencephaly. On the left side of a fetus with craniorachischisis

(Alghamdi et al. 2017), supinator was fused with extensor carpi ulnaris.

Prevalence

N/A

Clinical Implications

If the most proximal portion of the humeral (superficial) head of supinator is tendinous and forms a fibrous arch (arcade of Frohse), this can cause paralysis of the posterior interosseous nerve (Spinner 1968).

ANCONEUS (FIGURE 3.15)

Synonyms

Alternative names for anconeus include extensor antebrachii ulnaris, epicondylo-cubitalis, anconeus brevis, anconeus parvus or anconeus quartus (Jouffroy 1971).

Typical Presentation

Description

Anconeus originates via a tendon from the lateral epicondyle of the humerus and inserts onto the lateral surface of the olecranon and the posterior surface of the proximal ulnar shaft (Standring 2016).

Innervation

Anconeus is innervated by the radial nerve (Standring 2016).

Comparative Anatomy

Anconeus has a similar typical presentation in the great apes, extending from the lateral epicondyle to the olecranon process and adjacent areas of the ulna (Miller 1952; Gibbs 1999; Diogo et al. 2010, 2013a,b, 2017). In gibbons, it is undifferentiated from extensor carpi ulnaris and does not appear as a distinct muscle (Kohlbrügge 1890–1892; Hepburn 1892; Gibbs 1999; Michilsens et al. 2009; Diogo et al. 2012).

Variations

Description

Anconeus can have connections to, or be partially fused with, epitrochleoanconeus, extensor carpi ulnaris, or triceps brachii (Macalister 1875; Bergman et al. 1988; Akita and Nimura 2016a; Standring 2016). This muscle may be divided into two portions (Macalister 1875). It can also be entirely absent (Bergman et al. 1988). Anconeus likely has developmental origins from the triceps brachii due to its position, propensity to be blended with this muscle, and the shared innervation between anconeus and the medial head of triceps (Bergman et al. 1988; Akita and Nimura 2016a).

Prevalence

N/A

Anomalies

Description

Anconeus had a normal presentation and innervation in a fetus with craniorachischisis dissected by Alghamdi et al. (2017).

Prevalence

N/A

Clinical Implications

N/A

EXTENSOR CARPI RADIALIS LONGUS (FIGURE 3.15)

See also: Extensor carpi radialis brevis, Extensor carpi radialis accessorius

Synonyms

This muscle is also referred to radialis externus longior or humero sus-metacarpien (Todd 1839).

Typical Presentation

Description

Extensor carpi radialis longus originates from the lateral supracondylar ridge of the humerus and the lateral intermuscular septum and inserts via a tendon onto the base of the second metacarpal (Standring 2016).

Innervation

Extensor carpi radialis longus is innervated by the radial nerve (Standring 2016).

Comparative Anatomy

Extensor carpi radialis longus has a similar typical presentation in the apes, sometimes with an additional attachment to the first metacarpal (Kohlbrügge 1890–1892; Hepburn 1892; Straus 1941; Bojsen-Møller 1978; Gibbs 1999; Michilsens et al. 2009; Diogo et al. 2010, 2012, 2013a,b, 2017). It may also attach to the third metacarpal in common chimpanzees and bonobos (Diogo et al. 2013a, 2017). It may be blended with extensor carpi radialis brevis in common chimpanzees, gibbons, and orangutans (Deniker 1885; Beddard 1893; Sonntag 1923; Gibbs 1999; Diogo et al. 2012, 2013b).

Variations

Description

Extensor carpi radialis longus shares a developmental origin with extensor carpi radialis brevis so these muscles may be completely or partially fused (Macalister 1875; Knott 1883a; Mori 1964; Albright and Linburg 1978; Bergman et al. 1988; Akita and Nimura 2016b; Standring 2016). The muscle belly or tendon of extensor carpi radialis longus can split into multiple slips prior to insertion (Macalister 1875; Knott 1883a; Mori 1964; Bergman et al. 1988; Tountas and Bergman 1993; Akita and Nimura 2016b; Standring 2016). This muscle may send a slip to the first metacarpal, third metacarpal, fourth metacarpal, or the trapezium (Macalister 1875; Knott 1883a; Albright and Linburg 1978; Bojsen-Møller 1978; Bergman et al. 1988; Lewis 1989; Akita and Nimura 2016b; Standring 2016). Its tendon may send a slip to brachioradialis (Macalister 1875). It may also have connections to abductor pollicis longus or to the interosseous muscles (Macalister 1875; Bergman et al. 1988; Akita and Nimura 2016b). Extensor carpi radialis longus may be trigastric and insert onto both the first and second metacarpals (Bergman et al. 1988; Akita and Nimura 2016b). Yang et al. (2018) report a similar case in which the lateral and intermediate heads of a trigastric extensor carpi radialis longus muscle fused and inserted onto the second metacarpal while the medial head merged with extensor carpi radialis brevis.

The radial extensor muscles are associated with two (potentially three) supernumerary muscles. Extensor carpi radialis intermedius originates from the lateral epicondyle between extensor carpi radialis longus and brevis, or directly from one of these muscles, and inserts onto the second and/or third metacarpals (Albright and Linburg 1978; Bergman et al. 1988; Tountas and Bergman 1993; Akita and Nimura 2016b; West et al. 2017). Nayak et al. (2007) and Bharambe et al. (2017) referred to an additional radial extensor they term extensor carpi radialis tertius. Nayak et al. (2007) suggest that extensor carpi radialis tertius originates from the lateral epicondyle between extensor carpi radialis longus and extensor digitorum and attaches to the second and third metacarpals via two tendons. Bharambe et al. (2017) use extensor carpi radialis tertius to refer to a muscle that originates from the posterolateral surface of the radius deep to extensor carpi radialis brevis and inserts onto the third metacarpal. Extensor carpi radialis tertius is likely synonymous with extensor carpi radialis intermedius. Extensor carpi radialis accessorius is the most radial of these supernumerary muscles, and its insertion is more closely associated with the thenar muscles (see the entry for this muscle).

Prevalence

Knott (1883a) found extensor carpi radialis longus fused with extensor carpi radialis brevis in 5 out of 34 subjects (14.7%). Bojsen-Møller (1978) found that extensor carpi radialis longus inserted onto both the first and second metacarpals in 2 out of 23 individuals (8.7%). In a study of 173 upper limbs, Albright and Linburg (1978) found that extensor carpi radialis longus and extensor carpi radialis brevis exhibited typical presentations (the former going to metacarpal two and the latter going to metacarpal three with no interconnections) in eight-six limbs (49.7%). Interconnections between the two muscles were observed in 61 limbs (35.3%). A tendon originating proximally from extensor carpi radialis longus inserted on the third metacarpal in front of the extensor carpi radialis brevis in 45 limbs (26%) (Albright and Linburg

1978). A tendon originating from extensor carpi radialis brevis and inserting onto the second metacarpal next to extensor carpi radialis longus was present in 37 limbs (21.4%). Extensor carpi radialis intermedius was present in 42 limbs (24.3%).

Mori (1964) describes several variations in extensor carpi radialis longus anatomy. In 2.5% of cases, the insertion tendon of this muscle was fused with that of extensor carpi radialis brevis, and this anatomy was associated with a two-headed flexor carpi radialis longus that was fused with flexor carpi radialis brevis. In another 2.5% of cases, the extensor carpi radialis longus arose from two heads that both fused with extensor carpi radialis brevis to some extent. The insertion tendon of extensor carpi radialis brevis was split into two, and the smaller one fused with the insertion tendon of extensor carpi radialis longus (Mori 1964). In another 2.5% of cases, extensor carpi radialis longus and extensor carpi radialis brevis were each divided into two bellies that each had their own insertion tendons, thus presenting as a group of four muscles that fused proximally to form extensor carpi radialis intermedius (Mori 1964). Lastly, 5.4% of the radial extensors showed overall variation in the separation of the tendon of insertion (Mori 1964).

Anomalies

Description

Extensor carpi radialis longus had a duplicate tendon on the right side of one anencephalic male studied by Windle (1893). Barash et al. (1970) found that extensor carpi radialis longus and extensor carpi radialis brevis were fused in a trisomy 18 infant. In a female neonate with trisomy 18 (Aziz 1979) and a female fetus with trisomy 18 (Alghamdi et al. 2018), the proximal ends of extensor carpi radialis longus and brevis were fused bilaterally. In a fetus with trisomy 18 and cyclopia, extensor carpi radialis longus was fused with extensor carpi radialis brevis and brachioradialis on the left side of the body (Smith et al. 2015), and both radial extensors were fused to each other on the right side. Extensor carpi radialis longus has been observed to share a common muscle belly with extensor carpi radialis brevis in infants with Neu-Laxova syndrome (Shved et al. 1985). Bersu et al. (1976) describe a male infant with Hanhart syndrome. On the right side of this specimen, the wrist and hand were deficient. Extensor carpi radialis longus inserted onto the trapezium.

Prevalence

In their literature review, Smith et al. (2015) found that the radial extensor muscles were fused in 1 out of 24 individuals with trisomy 13 (4.2%) and in 4 out of 26 individuals with trisomy 18 (15.4%). Smith et al. (2015) also found that extensor carpi radialis (both muscles) were variable (e.g., fusion of the two, variable origins and insertions, doubled tendon or muscle bellies) in 3 out of 24 individuals with trisomy 13 (12.5%) and in 10 out of 26 individuals with trisomy 18 (38.5%). In a study of six upper limbs from three infants with Neu-Laxova syndrome, Shved et al. (1985) found that extensor carpi radialis longus and extensor carpi radialis brevis shared a common muscular belly in all six upper limbs (100%).

Clinical Implications

The presence of extra tendons of extensor carpi radialis longus should be checked when planning for tendon transfer surgery (Albright and Linburg 1978).

Extensor carpi radialis brevis (Figure 3.15)

See also: Extensor carpi radialis longus, Extensor carpi radialis accessorius

Synonyms

This muscle is also referred to as radialis externus brevior or epicondylo sus-metacarpien (Todd 1839).

Typical Presentation

Description

Extensor carpi radialis brevis originates from the lateral epicondyle of the humerus and inserts via a tendon onto the base of the third metacarpal (Standring 2016).

Innervation

Extensor carpi radialis brevis is innervated by the radial nerve or the posterior interosseous nerve (Standring 2016).

Comparative Anatomy

Extensor carpi radialis brevis has a similar typical presentation in the apes, with an origin from the lateral epicondyle and frequent insertion onto both the second and third metacarpals (Kohlbrügge 1890–1892; Straus 1941; Raven 1950; Gibbs 1999; Michilsens et al. 2009; Diogo et al. 2010, 2013, 2013a,b, 2017). There may be an origin from extensor digitorum in gibbons (Michilsens et al. 2009; Diogo et al. 2012). There may be an origin from the lateral condyle of the humerus in gibbons and gorillas (Deniker 1885; Kohlbrügge 1890–1892; Diogo et al. 2010; 2012). It may be blended with extensor carpi radialis longus in common chimpanzees, gibbons, and orangutans (Deniker 1885; Beddard 1893; Sonntag 1923; Gibbs 1999; Diogo et al. 2012, 2013b).

Variations

Description

Extensor carpi radialis brevis shares a developmental origin with extensor carpi radialis longus so sometimes these muscles can be completely or partially fused (Macalister 1875; Knott 1883a; Mori 1964; Albright and Linburg 1978; Bergman et al. 1988; Akita and Nimura 2016b; Standring 2016). The muscle belly or tendon of extensor carpi radialis brevis can split into multiple slips prior to insertion (Macalister 1875; Knott 1883a; Mori 1964; Bergman

et al. 1988; Tountas and Bergman 1993; Akita and Nimura 2016b; Standring 2016). Slips may pass from this muscle to the second metacarpal, fourth metacarpal, trapezium, or dorsal interossei (Macalister 1875; Knott 1883a; Albright and Linburg 1978; Bergman et al. 1988; Lewis 1989; Akita and Nimura 2016b; Standring 2016). Reina-de la Torre et al. (1994) report a case in which extensor carpi radialis brevis was attached via a tendinous accessory slip to the insertion tendon of biceps brachii. Mitsuyasu et al. (2004) report a case in which extensor carpi radialis brevis had a normal insertion onto the base of the third metacarpal but originated from the fascia/tendon of extensor digitorum instead of the lateral epicondyle. Extensor carpi radialis brevis may be absent (Macalister 1875). It may also be doubled (Macalister 1875).

The radial extensor muscles are associated with two (potentially three) supernumerary muscles. See the entry for extensor carpi radialis longus for details on extensor carpi radialis intermedius and extensor carpi radialis tertius. Extensor carpi radialis accessorius is the most radial of these supernumerary muscles, and its insertion is more closely associated with the thenar muscles (see the entry for this muscle).

Prevalence

According to Macalister (1875), Wood observed extensor carpi radialis brevis sending tendons into both the second and third metacarpals in 4 out of 36 subjects (11%). Knott (1883a) found extensor carpi radialis longus fused with extensor carpi radialis brevis in 5 out of 34 subjects (14.7%). In a study of 173 upper limbs, Albright and Linburg (1978) found that extensor carpi radialis longus and extensor carpi radialis brevis exhibited typical presentations (the former going to metacarpal two and the latter going to metacarpal three with no interconnections) in eight-six limbs (49.7%). Interconnections between the two muscles were observed in 61 limbs (35.3%). A tendon originating proximally from extensor carpi radialis longus inserted on the third metacarpal in front of the extensor carpi radialis brevis in 45 limbs (26%) (Albright and Linburg 1978). A tendon originating from extensor carpi radialis brevis and inserting onto the second metacarpal next to extensor carpi radialis longus was present in 37 limbs (21.4%). Extensor carpi radialis intermedius was present in 42 limbs (24.3%).

Mori (1964) describes several variations in extensor carpi radialis brevis anatomy. In 2.5% of cases, the insertion tendon of this muscle was fused with that of extensor carpi radialis longus, and this anatomy was associated with a two-headed flexor carpi radialis longus that was fused with flexor carpi radialis brevis. In another 2.5% of cases, the extensor carpi radialis longus arose from two heads that both fused with extensor carpi radialis brevis to some extent. The insertion tendon of extensor carpi radialis brevis was split into two, and the smaller one fused with the insertion tendon of extensor carpi radialis longus (Mori 1964). In another 2.5% of cases, extensor carpi radialis longus and extensor carpi radialis brevis were each divided into two bellies that each had their own insertion tendons, thus presenting as a group of four muscles that fused proximally to form extensor carpi radialis intermedius (Mori 1964). Lastly, 5.4% of the radial extensors showed overall variation in the separation of the tendon of insertion (Mori 1964).

Anomalies

Description

Barash et al. (1970) found that extensor carpi radialis longus and extensor carpi radialis brevis were fused in a trisomy 18 infant. In a female neonate with trisomy 18 (Aziz 1979) and a female fetus with trisomy 18 (Alghamdi et al. 2018), the proximal ends of extensor carpi radialis longus and brevis were fused bilaterally. In a trisomy 18 cyclopic fetus, extensor carpi radialis brevis was fused with extensor carpi radialis longus and brachioradialis on the left side of the body (Smith et al. 2015), and both radial extensors were fused to each other on the right side. Extensor carpi radialis brevis has been observed to share a common muscle belly with extensor carpi radialis longus in infants with Neu-Laxova syndrome (Shved et al. 1985). Bersu et al. (1976) describe a male infant with Hanhart syndrome. On the right side of this specimen, the wrist and hand were deficient. Extensor carpi radialis brevis inserted onto the trapezoid.

Prevalence

In their literature review, Smith et al. (2015) found that the radial extensor muscles were fused in 1 out of 24 individuals with trisomy 13 (4.2%) and in 4 out of 26 individuals with trisomy 18 (15.4%). Smith et al. (2015) also found that extensor carpi radialis (both muscles) were variable (e.g., fusion of the two, variable origins and insertions, doubled tendon or muscle bellies) in 3 out of 24 individuals with trisomy 13 (12.5%) and in 10 out of 26 individuals with trisomy 18 (38.5%). Extensor carpi radialis brevis was absent in 2 out of 26 individuals with trisomy 18 (7.7%) (Smith et al. 2015). In a study of six upper limbs from three infants with Neu-Laxova syndrome, Shved et al. (1985) found that extensor carpi radialis longus and extensor carpi radialis brevis shared a common muscular belly in all six upper limbs (100%).

Clinical Implications

The presence of extra tendons of extensor carpi radialis brevis should be checked when planning for tendon transfer surgery (Albright and Linburg 1978). Mitsuyasu et al. (2004) suggest that a variant origin of the extensor carpi radialis brevis may affect the severity of, or ability to develop, lateral epicondylitis (tennis elbow).

EXTENSOR CARPI RADIALIS ACCESSORIUS (FIGURE 3.15)

See also: Extensor carpi radialis brevis, Extensor carpi radialis longus

Synonyms

N/A

Typical Presentation

This muscle is only present as a variation or anomaly.

Comparative Anatomy

N/A

Variations

Description

Extensor carpi radialis accessorius (Wood) originates from the humerus with, or from, extensor carpi radialis longus and inserts onto the first metacarpal (Wood 1867b; Macalister 1867b, 1875; Knott 1883a; Bergman et al. 1988; Hong and Hong 2005; Akita and Nimura 2016b; West et al. 2017). Macalister (1875) notes that other anatomists, including Wood and Cruveilhier, observed that this muscle arose from the fascia over the other radial extensors. West et al. (2017) note an origin in one case from extensor carpi radialis brevis.

Extensor carpi radialis accessorius may insert onto, or give origin to, abductor pollicis brevis (Macalister 1875; Knott 1883a; Frohse and Frankel 1908; Khaledpour and Schindelmeiser 1994; Hong and Hong 2005). It also may be continuous with the origin of flexor pollicis brevis (Macalister 1875; Knott 1883a). Knott (1883a) also observed an insertion into the scaphoid. This muscle can sometimes be represented by a slip that arises from the extensor carpi radialis longus tendon and inserts onto the first metacarpal and the first dorsal interosseous muscle (Wood 1867b; Macalister 1875; Bergman et al. 1988).

Hong and Hong (2005) suggest that extensor carpi radialis intermedius is an accessory head of extensor carpi radialis brevis, while extensor carpi radialis accessorius is an accessory head of extensor carpi radialis longus. These authors also note that the tendon of extensor carpi radialis accessorius can pass through its own dorsal tunnel under the extensor retinaculum as it enters the hand (Hong and Hong 2005), a feature that has been noted by others (Frohse and Frankel 1908; Claassen and Wree 2002; West et al. 2017).

Innervation

Extensor carpi radialis accessorius is innervated by the deep branch of the radial nerve (Khaledpour and Schindelmeiser 1994).

Prevalence

In a study of 82 forearms from 41 cadavers, West et al. (2017) found that additional wrist extensors were present in seven forearms (8.5%) from five individuals, with a prevalence of four extensor carpi radialis intermedius muscles (4.9%) and three extensor carpi radialis accessorius muscles (3.6%).

Anomalies

Description

Smith et al. (2015) describe extensor carpi radialis accessorius as superficial to extensor carpi radialis.

Prevalence

Smith et al. (2015) note that this muscle was present in 5 out of 26 individuals with trisomy 18 (19.2%).

Clinical Implications

Extensor carpi radialis accessorius may contribute to lateral epicondylitis (tennis elbow) or nerve entrapment (West et al. 2017).

EXTENSOR CARPI ULNARIS (FIGURE 3.15)

See also: Ulnaris digiti quinti

Synonyms

This muscle is also referred to as ulnaris externus or cubito sus-metacarpien (Todd 1839).

Typical Presentation

Description

Extensor carpi ulnaris originates from the lateral epicondyle of the humerus and the posterior margin of the ulna (Standring 2016). It inserts via a tendon onto the base of the fifth metacarpal (Standring 2016).

Innervation

Extensor carpi ulnaris is innervated by the posterior interosseous nerve (Standring 2016).

Comparative Anatomy

Extensor carpi ulnaris has a similar typical presentation in the apes, extending from the lateral epicondyle and the ulna to the fifth metacarpal (Gratiolet and Alix 1866; Champneys 1872; Kohlbrügge 1890–1892; Beddard 1893; Primrose 1899, 1900; Sonntag 1923, 1924; Sullivan and Osgood 1927; Straus 1941; Raven 1950; Miller 1952; Swindler and Wood 1973; Gibbs 1999; Michilsens et al. 2009; Diogo et al. 2010, 2012, 2013a,b, 2017). The ulnar origin may be absent in orangutans (Kallner 1956; Diogo et al. 2013b). The humeral origin may be absent in bonobos (Diogo et al. 2017).

Variations

Description

The insertion tendon of extensor carpi ulnaris can also attach to the bases of metacarpal three or four, or the proximal phalanx of the fifth digit (Bergman et al. 1988; Akita and Nimura 2016b). A second tendon of extensor carpi ulnaris can replace the tendon of extensor digiti minimi (Macalister 1875; Bergman et al. 1988; Akita and Nimura 2016b). A slip may connect extensor carpi ulnaris to triceps brachii (Macalister 1875). Abductor digiti

minimi may originate from the tendon of extensor carpi ulnaris (Macalister 1875). Extensor carpi ulnaris may be doubled (Bergman et al. 1988; Akita and Nimura 2016b). The tendon of extensor carpi ulnaris may split distally close to insertion (Erickson et al. 2019). Extensor carpi ulnaris is associated with an accessory slip, ulnaris digiti quinti (see the entry for this muscle).

Prevalence

In a study of 17 extensor carpi ulnaris tendons, Erickson et al. (2019) found that 11 specimens demonstrated at least one split in the distal tendon (64.7%), with seven specimens having one split, one specimen having two splits, and three specimens having three splits.

Anomalies

Description

In a fetus with trisomy 18 and cyclopia, the proximal end of extensor carpi ulnaris was fused with extensor digiti minimi and extensor digitorum on the left side (Smith et al. 2015). Bersu et al. (1976) describe a male infant with Hanhart syndrome. On the right side of this specimen, the wrist and hand were deficient. Extensor carpi ulnaris had a normal insertion onto the base of the fifth metacarpal.

Prevalence

In their literature review, Smith et al. (2015) found that extensor carpi ulnaris had a variable insertion (onto the medial aspect of the fifth metacarpal distal to its base) in 1 out of 24 individuals with trisomy 13 (4.2%).

Clinical Implications

Erickson et al. (2019) note that distal splitting of the extensor carpi ulnaris tendon may mimic tears or tendinopathy in MRI and ultrasound imaging of the wrist.

ULNARIS DIGITI QUINTI (FIGURE 3.15)

See also: Extensor carpi ulnaris

Synonyms

This muscle is also referred to as ulnaris digiti minimi (Bergman et al. 1988) or ulnaris quinti (Macalister 1875).

Typical Presentation

This muscle is only present as a variation or anomaly.

Comparative Anatomy

Macalister (1871) observed the presence of an ulnaris digiti quinti tendon in a chimpanzee that inserted on the proximal phalanx of digit five (Diogo et al. 2013a).

Variations

Description

Ulnaris digiti quinti originates from the dorsal surface of the ulna and inserts onto the base of the proximal phalanx of the fifth digit (Bergman et al. 1988; Akita and Nimura 2016b). It can be represented by a bundle from the belly of extensor carpi ulnaris, or more often by a slip from the tendon of extensor carpi ulnaris, which can insert onto the metacarpal, proximal phalanx, or extensor tendon of the fifth digit (Barfred and Adamsen 1986; Bergman et al. 1988). In many cases, a slip can extend from the extensor carpi ulnaris tendon and insert into the fascia covering the metacarpal, the capsule of the metacarpophalangeal joint, or the proximal phalanx of the fifth digit (Macalister 1875; Barfred and Adamsen 1986; Bergman et al. 1988). This slip can also be joined or replaced by a bundle originating from the pisiform (Bergman et al. 1988). Barfred and Adamsen (1986) observe the presence of this muscle, described as a duplication of the extensor carpi ulnaris tendon, in three patients. Pınar et al. (2012) describe in three arms the presence of tendinous accessory slips that originate from the head of extensor carpi ulnaris and insert onto the extensor apparatus of the fifth digit.

Innervation

N/A

Prevalence

Macalister (1875) notes that Wood found "ulnaris quinti" in 12% of subjects. Pınar et al. (2012) found three accessory slips that likely correspond to ulnaris digiti quinti in 3 out of 54 arms (5.6%).

Anomalies

Description

Aziz (1980) observed the bilateral presence of ulnaris digiti quinti in a neonate with trisomy 13. On the right side, it arose as a tendinous slip from extensor carpi ulnaris and inserted onto the proximal phalanx of the fifth digit. On the left side, it consisted of two slips.

Prevalence

In their literature review, Smith et al. (2015) noted that ulnaris digiti quinti was only present in 1 out of 20 individuals with trisomy 13 (5%).

Clinical Implications

The presence of ulnaris digiti quinti may lead to the impairment of the wrist joint and fifth digit (Barfred and Adamsen 1986; Pınar et al. 2012).

EXTENSOR DIGITORUM (FIGURE 3.17)

Synonyms

This muscle is also referred to as extensor digitorum communis (Knott 1883a).

Typical Presentation

Description

Extensor digitorum originates from the lateral epicondyle of the humerus and the neighboring intermuscular septum (Standring 2016). It typically inserts via four tendons onto the extensor expansions, and thus to the middle and distal phalanges, of digits two through five (Standring 2016). Intertendinous connections between the terminal tendons are referred to as juncturae tendinae (Standring 2016; Akita and Nimura 2016b).

Innervation

Extensor digitorum is innervated by the posterior interosseous nerve (Standring 2016).

Comparative Anatomy

Extensor digitorum has a similar typical presentation in the apes with similar variations in tendon absence, duplication, and insertions (Owen 1868; Macalister 1873; Chapman 1878; Kohlbrügge 1890–1892; Hepburn 1892; Sommer

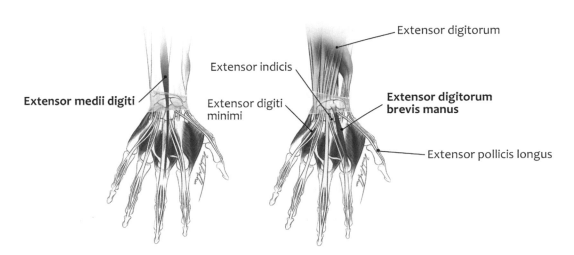

FIGURE 3.17 Extensor muscles on the dorsal (posterior) aspect of the hand and wrist. Extensor medii digiti is illustrated on the left side, and the other finger extensors are illustrated on the right side.

1907; Sonntag 1923, 1924; Straus 1941; Raven 1950; Miller 1952; Preuschoft 1965; Kaneff 1979; Gibbs 1999; Diogo et al. 2010, 2012, 2013a,b, 2017). Additional origins from the radius and/or ulna have been observed in all apes except bonobos (Deniker 1885; MacDowell 1910; Sonntag 1924; Straus 1941; Michilsens et al. 2009; Diogo et al. 2010, 2012, 2013a,b).

Variations

Description

The extensor digitorum tendon to any digit may be doubled, tripled, or quadrupled (Wood 1868; Macalister 1875; Knott 1883a; Mori 1964; Mestdagh et al. 1985; Godwin and Ellis 1992; von Schroeder and Botte 1995; el-Badawi et al. 1995; Hirai et al. 2001; Zilber and Oberlin 2004; Akita and Nimura 2016b; Standring 2016; Bharambe et al. 2017). Occasionally, the tendon to digit five is missing, or there may also be a tendon that acts on the first digit (Macalister 1875; Knott 1883a; Sato 1969; Kaneff 1979; Bergman et al. 1988; Lewis 1989; Zilber and Oberlin 2004; Standring 2016). The muscle belly itself can be split into up to four bellies, one for each target digit (Macalister 1875; Mori 1964; Bergman et al. 1988; Akita and Nimura 2016b). Extensor digitorum may be connected to extensor indicis, extensor digiti minimi, or extensor pollicis longus (Macalister 1875; Bergman et al. 1988; Akita and Nimura 2016b; Standring 2016).

Prevalence

Mori (1964) found that the extensor muscle belly of extensor digitorum had three separations in 90% of cases and four separations in 10% of cases. Doubling of the tendons was reported as follows: tendon to digit three in 2.5% of cases, tendon to digit four in 5% of cases, tendon to digit five in 12.5% of cases, tendons to digits two and four in 2.5% of cases, tendons to digits four and five in 2.5% of cases, tendons to digits three, four, and five in 15% of cases, and tendons to digits three and four in 2.5% of cases (Mori 1964). The juncturae tendinae were absent between the tendons to digits two and three in 10% of cases, the tendons to digits three and four in 10% of cases, and the tendons to digits four and five in 2.5% of cases (Mori 1964). The tendon to digit five was absent in 4% of cases.

Sato (1969) found the tendon to digit five missing in 69 out of 366 limbs (18.85%) from Kyushu-Japanese males and missing in 38 out of 242 limbs (15.7%) from females. A tendon to digit one was present in 99 out of 354 limbs (27.97%) from males and present in 63 out of 232 limbs from females (27.16%). Kaneff (1979) found that extensor digitorum sent tendons to digits two, three, and four in all 200 upper limbs examined by this author (100%), while the tendon to digit five was present in about 94% of cases.

In a study of 50 hands (26 left, 24 right), Zilber and Oberlin (2004) found that extensor digitorum sent a single tendon to the second digit in 100% of cases. The tendon to the third digit was single in 67% of right hands and 62% of left hands, doubled in 29% of right hands and 19% of left

hands, tripled in 15% of left hands, and quadrupled in 4% of both right and left hands. The tendon to the fourth digit was single in 17% of right hands and 19% of left hands, doubled in 41% of right hands and 62% of left hands, tripled in 25% of right hands and 19% of left hands, and quadrupled in 17% of right hands. The tendon to the fifth digit was absent in 71% of right hands and 50% of left hands, single in 21% of right hands and 42% of left hands, doubled in 4% of right hands and 8% of left hands, and tripled in 4% of right hands (Zilber and Oberlin 2004).

Zilber and Oberlin (2004) also provide a comprehensive literature review of extensor tendon variation, summarizing results from a study of 150 hands by Mestdagh et al. (1985), a study of 50 hands by Godwin and Ellis (1992), a study of 43 hands by von Schroeder and Botte (1995), a study of 181 hands by el-Badawi et al. (1995), and a study of 548 hands by Hirai et al. (2001). Among these studies, the prevalence ranges are as follows. The extensor digitorum communis tendon for digit two was single in 92%–100% of hands and doubled in 2%–8% of hands. The extensor digitorum communis tendon for digit three was single in 51%–92% of hands, doubled in 4%–39% of hands, tripled in 4%–19% of hands, and quadrupled in 5% of hands. The extensor digitorum communis tendon for digit four was single in 12%–96% of hands, doubled in 2%–63% of hands, tripled in 1%–16% of hands, and quadrupled in 4%–9% of hands. The extensor digitorum communis tendon for digit five was absent in 1%–54% of hands, single in 2%–30% of hands, doubled in 10%–25% of hands, tripled in 1%–2% of hands, and a common tendon for the fourth and fifth digit was present in 41%–96% of hands.

In a study of 41 hands, Tanaka et al. (2007) found that the extensor digitorum tendon to digit five was absent in ten specimens (24.4%) and present as a single slip in 25 specimens (61%). The tendon going to the fifth digit was an independent tendon in 17 specimens (41.5%) and present as a shared slip with the fourth digit in 14 specimens (34.1%).

From dissections of 100 upper limbs, Suwannakhan et al. (2016) found that the extensor digitorum tendon to digit two was a single, invariable tendon in all cases (100%). The tendon to digit three was doubled at its origin in four hands (4%) and single at its origin in 96 hands (96%). In 42 (42%) hands, the tendon to digit three split into two tendons distally, while the tendon split into three in six hands (6%) and into four tendons in two hands (2%) However, in 99 hands (99%), the tendon to digit three inserted as a single tendon while in one hand (1%) it inserted as a double tendon (Suwannakhan et al. 2016). The tendon to digit four originated as a single tendon in 94 hands (94%), a double tendon in five hands (5%), and a triple tendon in one hand (1%). The tendon to digit four inserted as a single tendon in 64 hands (64%), a double tendon in 30 hands (30%), a triple tendon in five hands (5%), and a quadruple tendon in one hand (1%). The tendon to digit five was absent in 50 hands (50%). In 49 hands (49%), the tendon to digit five originated as a single tendon and in one hand (1%) it originated as a double tendon (Suwannakhan et al. 2016).

In a study of 110 upper limbs, Bharambe et al. (2017) found that the tendon to digit five was absent in 28% of cases. In 2% of cases, both the tendons to the third and fourth digit were tripled. Duplication of the tendon to digit two was seen in 1% of cases, the tendon to digit three in 1% of cases, the tendon to digit four in 12% of cases, and the tendon to digit five in 2% of cases. Triplication of the tendon to the third digit was seen in 1% of cases and of the tendon to the fourth digit in 5% of cases.

Anomalies

Description

On the right upper limb of a fetus with craniorachischisis, Alghamdi et al. (2017) noted that a muscle that seemed to correspond to extensor digitorum originated from the lateral epicondyle and had three tendons, one that inserted on the ulnar styloid process, one that inserted onto digit three, and one that inserted onto digit five. On the left side, the muscle had a more typical presentation, but the fourth tendon attached to both digits four and five and the first tendon was joined with that of extensor indicis (Alghamdi et al. 2017).

In a trisomy 18 cyclopic fetus dissected by Smith et al. (2015) extensor digitorum did not send a tendon to digit five in both upper limbs. On the left side, the proximal end of extensor digitorum was fused with extensor digiti minimi and extensor carpi ulnaris (Smith et al. 2015).

In a female fetus with triploidy, Moen et al. (1984) found that the extensor digitorum tendons were doubled bilaterally. Doubling of the extensor digitorum tendon to the fourth finger and the fifth finger tendon arising from the fourth has been observed in infants with Neu-Laxova syndrome (Shved et al. 1985).

Mieden (1982) describes two male fetuses with cyclopia and alobar holoprosencephaly. On the right side of one specimen, the tendon of extensor digitorum to the fourth digit on the right side was doubled. Bersu et al. (1976) describe a male infant with Hanhart syndrome. On the right side of this specimen, the wrist and hand were deficient. Extensor digitorum had a normal attachment to the distal phalanx of the fifth digit, but the tendons to the other digits were fused and attached to connective tissue distal to the carpus.

Prevalence

Extensor digitorum was variable (e.g., extra slips/tendons, medio-lateral displacement of the extensor hood) in 1 out of 24 individuals with trisomy 13 (4.2%) and in 9 out of 26 individuals with trisomy 18 (34.6%). Extensor digitorum sent a tendon to the fifth digit in all individuals with trisomy 13, 18, and 21 (Smith et al. 2015). In a study of six upper limbs from three infants with Neu-Laxova syndrome, Shved et al. (1985) found that the tendon of extensor digitorum to the fourth finger was doubled in two upper limbs (33%) and the tendon to the fifth finger arose from the tendon to the fourth finger in three upper limbs (50%).

Clinical Implications

Understanding variation in extensor digitorum tendons is important for planning and performing tendon transfer surgery (Zilber and Oberlin 2004).

Extensor digiti minimi (Figure 3.17)

Synonyms

This muscle is also referred to as extensor digiti minimi proprius, extensor digiti minimi manus (Bergman et al. 1988), or extensor digiti quinti proprius (Aziz 1979).

Typical Presentation

Description

Extensor digiti minimi originates from the common extensor tendon and neighboring intermuscular septa (Standring 2016). It inserts via a bifurcated tendon that often joins with the extensor digitorum tendon to insert onto the dorsal digital expansion of digit five (Standring 2016).

Innervation

Extensor digiti minimi is innervated by the posterior interosseous nerve (Standring 2016).

Comparative Anatomy

Extensor digiti minimi is similarly variable in the apes, with frequent connections to digit four (Barnard 1875; Chapman 1878, 1879, 1880, 1900; Kohlbrügge 1890–1892; Hepburn 1892; Beddard 1893; Dwight 1895; Primrose 1899, 1900; Sonntag 1923, 1924; Sullivan and Osgood 1927; Straus 1941; Raven 1950; Miller 1952; Kallner 1956; Preuschoft 1965; Kaneff 1980a; Lewis 1989; Gibbs 1999; Michilsens et al. 2009; Oishi et al. 2009; Diogo et al. 2010, 2012, 2013a,b, 2017). Additional origins from the ulna have been observed in gibbons, orangutans, and common chimpanzees (Deniker 1885; Kohlbrügge 1890–1892; MacDowell 1910; Straus 1941; Michilsens et al. 2009; Gibbs 1999; Diogo et al. 2012, 2013a,b).

Variations

Description

The entire muscle may be absent (Macalister 1875; Knott 1883a; Kaneff 1980a; Bergman et al. 1988; Akita and Nimura 2016b; Standring 2016). When absent, it may be replaced by a slip of extensor digitorum or extensor carpi ulnaris (Macalister 1875; Bergman et al. 1988). The muscle belly or tendon may be doubled (Macalister 1875; Knott 1883a; Mori 1964; Bergman et al. 1988; Perkins and Hast 1993; Zilber and Oberlin 2004; Akita and Nimura 2016b). The tendon may also be tripled (Macalister 1875; Mori 1964; Perkins and Hast 1993; Zilber and Oberlin 2004). Extensor digiti minimi often sends a slip to digit four (Macalister 1875; Knott 1883a; Le Double 1897; Mori 1964; Kaneff 1980a; Bergman et al. 1988; Standring 2016). Le Double (1897) noted a case in which this muscle had four tendons and sent two to digit five, one to digit four, and one to digit three. When the muscle is divided into two, extensor digiti minimi accessorius (Krause) may be used to refer to the radial slip that inserts onto the dorsal carpal ligament (Knott 1883a; Mori 1964; Akita and Nimura 2016b).

This muscle may be fused with extensor digitorum or its tendon (Macalister 1875; Bergman et al. 1988; Akita and Nimura 2016b; Standring 2016). There may be a slip to extensor digiti minimi from the lateral epicondyle of the humerus or an additional origin from the posterior aspect of the ulna (Bergman et al. 1988; Akita and Nimura 2016b). Another slip from the ulna may be present, which attaches to the base of the fifth metacarpal (Bergman et al. 1988; Akita and Nimura 2016b). Sato (1969) notes that this muscle can attach elsewhere without passing into the aponeurosis of the fifth digit.

Prevalence

Macalister (1875) notes that Wood found that extensor digiti minimi sent a tendon to both digits four and five in 13 out of 106 cases (12.3%). Macalister (1875) observed a tendon to both digits four and five in 1 out of 14 Irish individuals (7.1%). Le Double (1897) noted that extensor digiti minimi sent a tendon to digit four in 12 out of 144 cases (8.3%).

Mori (1964) found that the tendon of extensor digiti minimi was single in 6% of cases, doubled in 82% of cases, and tripled in 12% of cases. Extensor digiti minimi accessorius (see description above) was present in 4% of cases (Mori 1964). Mori (1964) also noted a slip to the fourth digit (extensor digiti minimi et quarti) in 2% of cases. The attachment variation described by Sato (1969) was present in 2 out of 344 limbs (0.87%) from Kyushu-Japanese males and present in 2 out of 236 limbs (0.85%) from females. An accessory head of extensor digiti minimi was present in 19 out of 312 limbs (6.09%) from males and present in 13 out of 220 limbs (5.91%) from females.

Kaneff (1980a) examined 300 upper limbs and found that extensor digiti minimi was absent in 1% of cases, sent a tendon to digit five only in about 94% of cases, and sent tendons to both digits four and five in about 5% of cases. Based on dissections of 80 hands from 40 individuals, Perkins and Hast (1993) found that the tendon of extensor digiti minimi split into two or three slips in 77 hands (96%). In a study of 50 hands (26 left, 24 right), Zilber and Oberlin (2004) found that the insertion tendon of extensor digiti minimi was single in 25% of right hands and 31% of left hands, doubled in 71% of right hands and 69% of left hands, and tripled in 4% of right hands. Extensor digiti minimi set a tendon to digit four in one hand (2%) of cases (Zilber and Oberlin 2004).

Zilber and Oberlin (2004) also provide a comprehensive literature review of extensor tendon variation, summarizing results from a study of 150 hands by Mestdagh et al. (1985), a study of 50 hands by Godwin and Ellis (1992), a study of 43 hands by von Schroeder and Botte (1995), a study of 181 hands by el-Badawi et al. (1995), and a study of 548 hands by Hirai et al. (2001). Among these studies, the prevalence ranges are as follows. The extensor digiti minimi tendon was single in 2%–35% of hands, doubled in 63%–87% of hands, tripled in 2%–8% of hands, and quadrupled in 7%–10% of hands.

In a study of 41 hands, Tanaka et al. (2007) found that extensor digiti minimi had a single tendon in one specimen (2.4%), double tendon in 29 specimens (70.7%), and a triple tendon in nine specimens (21.9%). From dissections of 100 upper limbs, Suwannakhan et al. (2016) found that the extensor digiti minimi was absent in one hand (1%). The tendons split at insertion into two tendons in 75 hands (75%), remained single in 16 hands (16%), and inserted as a triple tendon in four hands (4%). In four hands (4%), the tendon originated as single, split into two, then rejoined to insert as one tendon (Suwannakhan et al. 2016). In a study of 110 upper limbs, Bharambe et al. (2017) found that in 16% of cases the tendon to digit five split into two and in 3% of cases three tendons were present, two going to digit five and one going to digit four.

Anomalies

Description

In a fetus with craniorachischisis, Alghamdi et al. (2017) observed that the left extensor digiti minimi attached to both digits four and five. Similarly, in a trisomy 18 cyclopic fetus, Smith et al. (2015) found that the left extensor digiti minimi attached to both digits four and five. "Extensor digiti quinti proprius" was absent bilaterally in a neonate with trisomy 18 (Aziz 1979). It was also absent bilaterally in a neonate with trisomy 13 (Aziz 1980). Doubling of the extensor digiti minimi tendon and an origin of this muscle from extensor digitorum has been observed in infants with Neu-Laxova syndrome (Shved et al. 1985). Bersu et al. (1976) describe a male infant with Hanhart syndrome. On the right side of this infant, the wrist and hand were deficient. Extensor digiti minimi was absent.

Prevalence

In their literature review, Smith et al. (2015) found that extensor digiti minimi was variable (e.g., gives off extra tendons, tendon splits into thirds, medio-lateral displacement of tendons, tendons doubled) in 2 out of 24 individuals with trisomy 13 (8.3%), 12 out of 26 individuals with trisomy 18 (46.2%), and one out of seven individuals with trisomy 21 (14.3%). These authors also found that extensor digiti minimi was absent in 1 out of 24 individuals with trisomy 13 (4.2%) and in 2 out of 26 individuals with trisomy 18 (7.7%). In a study of six upper limbs from three infants with Neu-Laxova syndrome, Shved et al. (1985) found that the tendon of extensor digiti minimi was doubled in three upper limbs (50%), and this muscle took an origin from extensor digitorum in all six upper limbs (100%).

Clinical Implications

Understanding variation in extensor digiti minimi tendons is important for planning and performing tendon transfer surgery (Zilber and Oberlin 2004; Tanaka et al. 2007).

EXTENSOR INDICIS (FIGURES 3.16 AND 3.17)

See also: Extensor medii digiti, Extensor digitorum brevis manus

Synonyms

This muscle is also referred to as extensor indicis proprius (Bergman et al. 1988) or the indicator (Todd 1839).

Typical Presentation

Description

Extensor indicis originates from the posterior aspect of the ulna and the neighboring interosseous membrane (Standring 2016). It inserts via a tendon onto the extensor expansion of digit two (Standring 2016).

Innervation

Extensor indicis is innervated by the posterior interosseous nerve (Standring 2016).

Comparative Anatomy

Extensor indicis has a similar typical presentation in the apes, and accessory insertions onto digits three, four, and/or five are common (Bischoff 1870; Macalister 1871; Chapman 1880, 1900; Deniker 1885; Kohlbrügge 1890–1892; Hepburn 1892; Beddard 1893; Primrose 1899, 1900; MacDowell 1910; Sullivan and Osgood 1927; Straus 1941; Raven 1950; Kallner 1956; Jouffroy 1971; Kaneff 1980a,b; Gibbs 1999; Michilsens et al. 2009; Oishi et al. 2009; Diogo et al. 2010, 2012, 2013a,b, 2017). Origins from the radius and/or humerus have been observed in all apes except bonobos (Gratiolet and Alix 1866; Barnard 1875; Deniker 1885; Sonntag 1923; Diogo et al. 2010, 2012, 2013a,b).

Variations

Description

Extensor indicis may instead originate from the radius, carpal bones, or the interosseous membrane (Wood 1868; Macalister 1875; Bergman et al. 1988; Akita and Nimura 2016b). Occasionally this muscle may be doubled or have two distinct heads, and its tendon may also be duplicated (Wood 1865, 1866, 1867b, 1868; Macalister 1875; Cauldwell et al. 1943; Mori 1964; Bergman et al. 1988; Perkins and Hast 1993; Tountas and Bergman 1993; Standring 2016). Its tendon may also be tripled (el-Badawi et al. 1995; von Schroeder and Botte 1995). It may receive a slip from extensor digitorum or join with extensor medii digiti (Wood 1868; Macalister 1875). Extensor indicis may be absent (Macalister 1875; Mestdagh et al. 1985; Bergman et al. 1988; Tountas and Bergman 1993; el-Badawi et al. 1995; Zilber and Oberlin 2004; Akita and Nimura 2016b; Fernandes et al. 2016; Bharambe et al. 2017).

Suwannakhan et al. (2020) report the presence of what they term an extensor digitorum profundus complex with two bellies originating from the distal ulna in a cadaver. The first belly resembled extensor indicis, and the second belly gave off one tendon slip that inserts onto the second

and third digits, and another tendon slip that inserts onto the fourth and fifth digits (Suwannakhan et al 2020). Kaneff (1980a) suggested that during human development, extensor indicis can extend from digits two through four, and usually reduces to the region of digit two only in later ontogenetic stages.

Accessory muscles and tendons associated with extensor indicis have been designated as distinct muscles. Extensor pollicis-et-indicis has attachments to digits one and two (Macalister 1875; Cauldwell et al. 1943). Extensor digiti quarti sends a slip to digit four (Cauldwell et al. 1943). Extensor indicis is also associated with extensor digitorum brevis manus (extensor indicis brevis) and extensor medii digiti (see the entries for these muscles).

Prevalence

Extensor indicis goes to digit two in 87%–95% of humans according to Straus (1941). Wood (1865, 1866, 1867b, 1868) found that out of 276 upper limbs, 6.5% had duplicated tendons to digit two, 6.9% had an abbreviated extensor indicis, 1.8% had attachments to both digits 1 and 2 (extensor-pollicis-et-indicis), 7.2% had attachments to digit three (extensor digiti medii), and 0% of cases exhibited a complete absence of this muscle. Cauldwell et al. (1943) found that within 263 upper limbs, 2.7% had duplicated tendons to digit two, 1.1% had an abbreviated extensor indicis, 0.7% had an extensor pollicis-et-indicis, 6.5% had an extensor digiti medii, 0.38% had an attachment to digit four (extensor digiti quarti), and 0% of cases exhibited a complete absence of extensor indicis. Kaneff (1980b) found that out of 300 upper limbs, extensor indicis was missing in 1% of cases, and an attachment to digit three was exhibited in 12.97% of cases.

Mori (1964) observed that the distal end of the muscular portion of extensor indicis was distal to the radiocarpal joint in 48% of cases, was on the radiocarpal joint in 8% of cases, and did not reach the radiocarpal joint in 44% of cases. Mori (1964) also observed that the insertion tendon was doubled in 12% of cases and that the distal half the muscle was doubled, and each portion had its own tendon in 8% of cases.

In a study of 50 hands (26 left, 24 right), Zilber and Oberlin (2004) found that extensor indicis was absent in two hands (4%), the insertion tendon was single in 79% of right hands and 77% of left hands, and the tendon was doubled in 17% of right hands and 19% of left hands. These authors also provide a comprehensive literature review of extensor tendon variation, summarizing results from a study of 150 hands by Mestdagh et al. (1985), a study of 50 hands by Godwin and Ellis (1992), a study of 43 hands by von Schroeder and Botte (1995), a study of 181 hands by el-Badawi et al. (1995), and a study of 548 hands by Hirai et al. (2001). Among these studies, the prevalence ranges are as follows. The tendon of extensor indicis was single in 77%–93% of hands, doubled in 5%–16% of hands, and tripled in 4%–7% of hands. Extensor indicis was absent in 1% of hands.

Based on dissections of 80 hands from 40 individuals, Perkins and Hast (1993) found that the tendon of extensor indicis split into two slips in 30 hands (37.5%). From a study of 34 upper limbs from 17 cadavers, extensor indicis was absent in two upper limbs (5.9%) from the same cadaver, and extensor indicis brevis was present on the right side (Fernandes et al. 2016). From dissections of 100 upper limbs, Suwannakhan et al. (2016) found that extensor pollicis et indicis was present in six hands (6%) from four cadavers (7.7%), and in four cases (4%), extensor indicis was absent and replaced by either extensor pollicis et indicis or extensor indicis et medii communis. In a study of 110 upper limbs, Bharambe et al. (2017) found extensor indicis proprius was duplicated in 1% of cases and absent in 2% of cases.

Based on a study of 176 upper limbs, Georgiev et al. (2018b) found that extensor indicis exhibited the typical presentation in 147 cases (83.5%) In the 29 other limbs (16%), variations included the replacement of extensor indicis with extensor indicis brevis, the coexistence of those two muscles, and the presence of accessory tendons.

Anomalies

Description

Mieden (1982) describes two male fetuses with cyclopia and alobar holoprosencephaly. On the left side of one specimen, the tendon of extensor indicis was doubled. On the right side of a male infant with Hanhart syndrome, the wrist and hand were deficient and extensor indicis was absent (Bersu et al. 1976). In a study of specimens with triploidy, extensor indicis had an extra tendon to the extensor retinaculum bilaterally in a male fetus and was absent bilaterally in a female fetus (Moen et al. 1984).

In a male neonate with Meckel syndrome, Pettersen (1984) observed that extensor indicis blended into fascia on the dorsum of the right hand where it partly attached to a small fleshy mass, from which a tendon arose that attached normally onto digit two. On the left side, extensor indicis was represented by a diminutive slip on the dorsum of the wrist and had no insertion tendon. In a trisomy 18 cyclopic fetus, the extensor indicis tendon was doubled and went to both digits two and three (Smith et al. 2015). In a fetus with craniorachischisis dissected by Alghamdi et al. (2017), the left extensor indicis joined the tendon of extensor digitorum to attach onto digit two. On the right side, extensor indicis only sent a tendon to digit four, not digit two.

Prevalence

In their literature review, Smith et al. (2015) found that extensor indicis was variable (e.g., variable origin, diminutive muscle, doubled muscle or tendons) in 7 out of 24 individuals with trisomy 13 (29.2%), 12 out of 26 individuals with trisomy 18 (46.2%), and 2 out of 7 individuals with trisomy 21 (28.6%). The extensor indicis tendon was doubled and went to both digits two and three in one neonate out of 24 with trisomy 13 (4.2%), 12 out of 26 individuals with

trisomy 18 (46.2%), and 2 out of 7 individuals with trisomy 21 (28.6%). Extensor pollicis-et-indicis was present in one out of seven individuals with trisomy 21 (14.3%). Extensor indicis was absent in 4 out of 24 individuals with trisomy 13 (16.7%).

Clinical Implications

Understanding variations in the extensor indicis tendons is important for planning and performing tendon transfer surgery (Zilber and Oberlin 2004; Fernandes et al. 2016; Matsumae et al. 2018).

Extensor medii digiti (Figure 3.17)

See also: Extensor indicis

Synonyms

This muscle is also referred to as extensor digiti medii (Bergman et al. 1988) or extensor medii proprius (Bharambe et al. 2017).

Typical Presentation

This muscle is only present as a variation or anomaly.

Comparative Anatomy

Extensor medii digiti is usually not present as a distinct muscle in the apes (Diogo et al. 2010, 2012, 2013a,b, 2017).

Variations

Description

Extensor medii digiti is considered a variation of extensor indicis (Macalister 1875). It originates from the ulna distal to the origin of extensor indicis and sends a tendon to digit three, or sometimes to both digits two and three (Macalister 1875; Bergman et al. 1988; Carlos et al. 2011; Akita and Nimura 2016b). It may originate from the radius or the carpus (Macalister 1875). It can insert onto the metacarpophalangeal joint (Lee et al. 2019b) or base of the proximal phalanx (Campos et al. 2011; Carlos et al. 2011) of digit three. Extensor medii digiti can sometimes be fused with extensor indicis (Macalister 1875; Bergman et al. 1988). Extensor indicis et medii communis is a similar muscle that arises from the ulna and inserts onto digits two and three (von Schroeder and Botte 1995; Yammine 2015a; Akita and Nimura 2016b).

Vaida et al. (2021) report a case in which both extensor medii proprius and extensor indicis et medii communis were present in the same forearm. The tendon of the former coursed through the second extensor compartment between the tendons of extensor carpi radialis longus and brevis. The latter had three tendons, two to digit two and one to digit three. A third muscle was present with a common origin from extensor carpi radialis brevis and an insertion into the tendon of extensor indicis et medii communis.

Innervation

Extensor medii digiti is innervated by the posterior interosseous nerve (Carlos et al. 2011).

Prevalence

Le Double (1897) stated that extensor medii digiti occurs in 10% of humans. Wood (1865, 1866, 1867b, 1868) found that within 276 upper limbs, 7.2% of extensor indicis muscles had attachments to digit three. Macalister (1875) states that Wood found extensor medii digiti in 11 out of 102 subjects (10.8%). Cauldwell et al. (1943) found that within 263 upper limbs, 6.5% had an extensor medii digiti. Based on dissections of 80 hands from 40 individuals, Perkins and Hast (1993) found that extensor digiti medii originated with extensor indicis from the ulna and sent a tendon to the dorsal expansion of digit three in 17 hands (21%). Carlos et al. (2011) observed the presence of this muscle in 7 out of 94 limbs (7.4%), from 6 out of 47 cadavers (12.8%). Extensor indicis et medii communis has a prevalence of 1.6% (Yammine 2015a). From dissections of 100 upper limbs from 52 cadavers, Suwannakhan et al. (2016) found that extensor indicis et medii communis was present in six hands (6%) from four cadavers (7.7%) and "extensor medii proprius" was present in eight hands (8%) from five cadavers (9.6%). In a study of 110 upper limbs, Bharambe et al. (2017) found extensor medii proprius in 4% of cases.

Anomalies

Description

Windle (1893) reported the presence of extensor medii digiti in one fetus with anencephaly. This muscle was present bilaterally in a neonate with trisomy 18 (Aziz 1979). Dunlap et al. (1986) also found extensor medii digiti in individuals with trisomy 18. In two cases, it sent an additional tendon to digit two. In another case, the entire extensor medii digiti muscle was doubled. In another case, an "extensor medii digiti et quarti" tendon was present. It branched from the extensor medii digiti tendon over the metacarpal of digit three and inserted on the metacarpophalangeal joint of digit four (Dunlap et al. 1986).

Prevalence

In a sample of 20 limbs from ten individuals with trisomy 18, Dunlap et al. (1986) found that extensor medii digiti was present in ten limbs (50%). Smith et al. (2015) note in their literature review that extensor medii digiti is present in 5 out of 26 individuals with trisomy 18 (19.2%).

Clinical Implications

Campos et al. (2011) argue that understanding the presence and anatomy of supernumerary extensor muscles, including the extensor medii digiti they describe (but do not refer to by name), is important for diagnosing carpal tunnel syndromes.

EXTENSOR DIGITORUM BREVIS MANUS (FIGURE 3.17)

See also: Extensor indicis

Synonyms

This muscle is also referred to as extensor brevis digitorum manus (Knott 1883a), extensor anomalus (Sauser 1935), le muscle manieux (Le Double 1897); extensor indicis brevis (Gahhos and Ariyan 1983), extensor indicis brevis manus (Standring 2016), extensor brevis digiti indicis vel medii (Albinus 1758), indicator biceps (Gantzer), and indicator anomalus brevis (Otto) (Macalister 1875).

Typical Presentation

This muscle is only present as a variation or anomaly.

Comparative Anatomy

Extensor digitorum brevis manus is generally absent in the apes (Diogo et al. 2010, 2012, 2013a,b, 2017). The only cases of its presence were reported by Lewis (1989). Lewis (1989) observed this muscle in an orangutan, and it was associated with the tendon of extensor indicis to the third digit (Diogo et al. 2013b). Lewis (1989) also reported the presence of this muscle in a gorilla where it originated from the extensor indicis tendon to digit two and inserted onto digit three (Diogo et al. 2010).

Variations

Description

Extensor digitorum brevis manus is considered a variation of extensor indicis, and it is often joined with this muscle, particularly upon insertion (Ogura et al. 1987; Yammine 2015b). The presence of extensor digitorum brevis manus may signify the failure of a proximal migration of the ulnocarpal parts of the antebrachial muscle mass (Sauser 1935; Ross and Troy 1969). It may also originate from the deep portion of the forearm extensor precursor muscle, which is prone to variations (Yammine 2015b).

Extensor digitorum brevis manus originates from the ulnar portion of the carpus and the ligaments that connect the bones (capitate, hamate, lunate, triquetrum) on this side of the carpus (Knott 1883a; Cauldwell et al. 1943; Bergman et al. 1988; Akita and Nimura 2016b). It may also originate from the distal radius or ulna (Macalister 1875; Knott 1883a; Ogura et al. 1987; Paraskevas et al. 2002; Gonzalez and Netscher 2016). It can be comprised of between one to four bundles and is most commonly represented by a bundle going to digit two, and sometimes a bundle that goes to digit three, four, and/or five (Macalister 1875; Knott 1883a; Ross and Troy 1969; Ogura et al. 1987; Bergman et al. 1988; Paraskevas et al. 2002; Doyle and Botte 2003; Ranade et al. 2008; Akita and Nimura 2016b; Lee et al. 2019b). The tendon of extensor digitorum brevis manus inserts onto the extensor expansion or the metacarpals of the target digit (Knott 1883a; Ogura et al. 1987; Bergman et al. 1988; Rodríguez-Niedenführ et al. 2002; Akita and Nimura 2016b).

Gahhos and Ariyan (1983) report an "extensor indicis brevis" originating from the joint capsule and ligaments of the scaphoid and lunate that attached to the extensor expansion of the second digit. Fernandes et al. (2016) report the presence of extensor indicis brevis on the right side of one cadaver that was associated with bilateral absence of extensor indicis proprius. Suwannakhan et al. (2016) report a case in which extensor digitorum brevis manus was present with extensor medii proprius and the tendon of the latter inserted onto the tendon of the former.

Innervation

Extensor digitorum brevis manus is innervated by the posterior interosseous nerve (Rodríguez-Niedenführ et al. 2002).

Prevalence

Macalister (1875) found extensor digitorum brevis manus in 1 out of 15 subjects (6.7%) and states that Wood found the muscle in 1 out of 36 (2.8%). Smith (1896) reports a high prevalence (70%) for this muscle, as this author claims to have found it in 35 out of 50 hands. Cauldwell et al. (1943) found that within 263 upper limbs, three cases (1.1%) had an abbreviated extensor indicis, and one of these muscles was designated as an extensor digitorum brevis manus as it was completed separated from the ulna.

Gama (1983) found extensor digitorum brevis manus in 38 out of 3404 adults (1.1%). Ogura et al. (1987) observed this muscle in 17 out of 559 hands from 286 cadavers (3%). Bergman et al. (1988) provide a prevalence of 9%. Perkins and Hast (1993) found extensor digiti brevis manus in 1 out of 80 hands (1.25%). Rodríguez-Niedenführ et al. (2002) observed the presence of extensor digitorum brevis manus in 3 out of 128 cadavers (2.3%). Ranade et al. (2008) found this muscle in 3 out of 72 upper limbs (4.2%).

Yammine (2015b) conducted a meta-analysis of 26 studies and found an overall crude cadaveric prevalence of 4% and an overall true cadaveric prevalence of 2.5%. Akita and Nimura (2016b) list a prevalence of 1.6%–3.2%, citing Kosugi et al. (1984) and Yoshida et al. (1984). Gonzalez and Netscher (2016) list a prevalence of 2%–3% and state that its presence is found more often in males. From dissections of 100 upper limbs, Suwannakhan et al. (2016) found that extensor digitorum brevis manus was present in one cadaver (1%). In a study of 110 upper limbs, Bharambe et al. (2017) found extensor digitorum brevis manus in 2% of cases.

Anomalies

Description

Dunlap et al. (1986) state that individuals with trisomy 13 exhibit a diminution of the extensor digitorum profundus complex, which may lead to the presence of extensor digitorum brevis manus.

Prevalence

In a sample of ten limbs from five individuals with trisomy 13, Dunlap et al. (1986) found that extensor digitorum brevis manus was present in three limbs (30%).

Clinical Implications

Extensor digitorum brevis manus can be mistaken for a dorsal wrist ganglion, tendon sheath cyst, infectious mass, bone spur (exostosis), synovitis, hemangioma, rheumatoid tenosynovitis, or a soft tissue tumor (Gahhos and Ariyan 1983; Rodríguez-Niedenführ et al. 2002; Ammendolia 2008; Ranade et al. 2008; Gonzalez and Netscher 2016). Though largely asymptomatic, extensor digitorum brevis manus may present as a tender, painful, and/or swollen mass (Gahhos and Ariyan 1983), particularly if it is present on the dominant hand, potentially due to compression of the hypertrophied muscle in the fourth dorsal compartment (Ross and Troy 1969; Patel et al. 1989).

Extensor pollicis longus (Figures 3.16 and 3.17)

Synonyms

This muscle is also referred to as extensor pollicis major, extensor secondi internodii pollicis, or cubito susphalangettien du pouce (Todd 1839; Macalister 1875; Bergman et al. 2008).

Typical Presentation

Description

Extensor pollicis longus originates from the middle third of the posterior ulna and from the neighboring interosseous membrane (Standring 2016). It inserts via a tendon onto the base of the distal phalanx of the first digit (Standring 2016).

Innervation

Extensor pollicis longus is innervated by the posterior interosseous nerve (Standring 2016).

Comparative Anatomy

Extensor pollicis longus has a similar typical presentation in the apes, with occasional insertions onto the proximal phalanx, metacarpal, or metacarpophalangeal joint of the first digit (Champneys 1872; Deniker 1885; Sutton 1883; Kohlbrügge 1890–1892; Hepburn 1892; Chapman 1900; Sonntag 1924; Straus 1941; Raven 1950; Kallner 1956; Ziegler 1964; Gibbs 1999; Michilsens et al. 2009; Diogo et al. 2010, 2012, 2013a,b, 2017). A slip to digit two has been observed in gorillas and common chimpanzees (Hepburn 1892; Kaneff 1980a; Gibbs 1999; Diogo et al. 2010, 2013a).

Variations

Description

Extensor pollicis longus may be doubled (Macalister 1875; Bergman et al. 1988; Akita and Nimura 2016b). Its tendon may also be split or doubled (Wood 1868; Macalister

1875; Mori 1964; Palatty et al. 2018). Accessory tendons of this muscle may pass through the first, second, fourth, or an additional separate dorsal compartment (as opposed to the typical third dorsal compartment) (Sevivas et al. 2009; Türker et al. 2010; Rubin et al. 2011; Kim et al. 2016). It may be connected via slips to the proximal phalanx of digit one, extensor digitorum, extensor pollicis brevis, or extensor indicis (Wood 1868; Macalister 1875; Knott 1883a; Mori 1964; Bergman et al. 1988; Akita and Nimura 2016b). An accessory extensor (sometimes termed extensor pollicis tertius) between extensor pollicis longus and extensor indicis can be present as a rare variation (Le Double 1897; Bergman et al. 1988; Bluth et al. 2011; Akita and Nimura 2016b). Extensor pollicis longus may be absent (Bergman et al. 1988; Akita and Nimura 2016b).

Prevalence

Mori (1964) reports that in 5% of cases the insertion tendon of extensor pollicis longus was doubled (misprinted as e. p. brevis). The tendon inserted onto the distal phalanx of digit one in 80% of cases, fused with the tendon of extensor pollicis brevis and inserted into the distal phalanx in 20% of cases, and was doubled with one part inserting onto the proximal phalanx and the other onto the distal phalanx in 15% of cases (Mori 1964). Palatty et al. (2018) studied variations in the extrinsic thumb muscles in 30 adult and 20 fetal hands. The tendon of extensor pollicis longus was single in 43 hands (86%) and doubled in seven hands (14%).

Anomalies

Description

On the left side of one male fetus with anencephaly, Windle (1983) observed that extensor pollicis longus was doubled, with the accessory muscle originating with extensor indicis. On the left upper limb of a fetus with craniorachischisis, Alghamdi et al. (2017) found that the tendon of extensor pollicis longus split at the base of the first metacarpal and then rejoined at the metacarpophalangeal joint before inserting onto the base of the distal phalanx of digit one. This morphology was also observed on both sides of the trisomy 18 cyclopic fetus studied by Smith et al. (2015).

Extensor pollicis longus has been observed to share a common muscular belly with extensor indicis in infants with Neu-Laxova syndrome (Shved et al. 1985). On the left arm of a male neonate with Meckel syndrome, Pettersen (1984) observed that extensor pollicis brevis joined and inserted with extensor pollicis longus. In a male infant with Hanhart syndrome, the wrist and hand were deficient on the right side and extensor pollicis longus inserted into the capsule of the radiocarpal joint (Bersu et al. 1976).

Prevalence

In their literature review, Smith et al. (2015) found that extensor pollicis brevis and longus were variant (e.g., fusion of the two muscles, doubling of the tendons, muscles split into more than one part, variable attachments, connections

with the second digit) in 2 out of 24 individuals with trisomy 13 (8.3%), 13 out of 26 individuals with trisomy 18 (50%), and 1 out of 7 individuals with trisomy 21 (14.3%).

In a study of six upper limbs from three infants with Neu-Laxova syndrome, Shved et al. (1985) found that extensor pollicis longus shared a common muscle belly with extensor indicis in five upper limbs (83%).

Clinical Implications

An accessory extensor pollicis longus may cause pain at the wrist (Beatty et al. 2000). Doubling and/or variable insertion of its tendon may limit the ability to extend the first digit (Masada et al. 2003; Sawaizumi et al. 2003; Türker et al. 2010), cause hyperextension of the first digit (Alsharif et al. 2017), or be mistaken for a ruptured tendon (Masada et al. 2003). Variation in the course of the extensor pollicis longus tendon can also cause tenosynovitis that may mimic intersection syndrome or de-Quervain's disease (Rubin et al. 2011).

EXTENSOR POLLICIS BREVIS (FIGURE 3.16)

Synonyms

This muscle is also referred to as extensor primi minor, extensor primi internodii pollicis, extensor minor pollicis manus, or cubito sus-phalangettien du pouce (Todd 1839; Bergman et al. 2008).

Typical Presentation

Description

Extensor pollicis brevis originates from the posterior aspect of the distal radius and from the neighboring interosseous membrane (Standring 2016). It inserts via a tendon onto the base of the proximal phalanx of digit one (Standring 2016).

Innervation

Extensor pollicis brevis is innervated by the posterior interosseous nerve (Standring 2016).

Comparative Anatomy

Among the apes, extensor pollicis brevis is present as a distinct muscle belly only in gibbons, and it is partially blended with abductor pollicis longus (Bischoff 1870; Kohlbrügge 1890–1892; Michilsens et al. 2009; Diogo et al. 2010, 2012, 2013a,b, 2017).

Variations

Description

The tendon of extensor pollicis brevis may have an additional attachment onto the base of the distal phalanx of the first digit, which commonly presents as a slip that join the tendon of extensor pollicis longus (Wood 1868; Macalister 1875; Knott 1883a; Mori 1964; Bergman et al. 1988; Nayak et al. 2009b; Akita and Nimura 2016b; Standring 2016). The tendon can also bifurcate near its insertion, with the second insertion attaching to the base of the first metacarpal

(Macalister 1875; Dawson and Barton 1986; Bergman et al. 1988; Akita and Nimura 2016b). The tendon may also be tripled (Nayak et al. 2009b).

Extensor pollicis brevis may be fused with abductor pollicis longus (Wood 1867a, 1868; Macalister 1875; Knott 1883a; Inoue 1934; Mori 1964; Dawson and Barton 1986; Bergman et al. 1988; Akita and Nimura 2016b; Standring 2016). It may also be completely absent (Wood 1868; Macalister 1875; Knott 1883a; Stein 1951; Mori 1964; Dawson and Barton 1986; Bergman et al. 1988; Akita and Nimura 2016b; Standring 2016).

Prevalence

Wood (1867a) noted that this muscle was absent in 1 out of 36 cases (2.8%) and later noted that it was absent in 3 out of 36 cases (8.3%) (Wood 1868; Macalister 1875). In a study of 84 wrists, Stein (1951) found that extensor pollicis brevis was absent in 7% of wrists, and an accessory tendon of extensor pollicis brevis was present in 4% of wrists. Mori (1964) found that extensor pollicis brevis was absent in 2% of cases. It was fused with abductor pollicis longus in 10% of cases and extensor pollicis longus in 50% of cases. The insertion tendon was split in 10% of cases. The tendon inserted onto the proximal phalanx of digit one in 58.3% of cases, the distal phalanx in 21% of cases, and both phalanges of digit one in 20.8% of cases.

Dawson and Barton (1986) dissected 16 arms from eight cadavers and found that the muscle belly for extensor pollicis brevis was present in 13 arms (81.25%) and absent in three (18.75%). The tendon of extensor pollicis brevis had the typical presentation in ten arms (62.5%), had a branch joining the tendon of abductor pollicis longus in two arms (12.5%), and was attached to the base of the first metacarpal in one arm (6.25%). In the three specimens where the muscle belly was missing, the tendon was absent and replaced by an accessory tendon of abductor pollicis longus in one arm (6.25%) and arose from the fat at the base of the first metacarpal in two arms (12.5%). Regarding insertion, the tendon inserted partially to the base of the proximal phalanx and partially to the extensor hood of digit one in nine arms (56.25%), entirely to the base of the proximal phalanx in four arms (25%), and entirely to the extensor hood in three arms (18.75%) (Dawson and Barton 1986).

In a study of 156 upper limbs, Nayak et al. (2009b) found that extensor pollicis brevis had a single tendon in 133 limbs (85.3%), double tendon in 17 limbs (10.9%), and triple tendon in 6 limbs (3.8%). In 11 limbs (7%), the accessory tendon inserted onto the distal phalanx of digit one. In two limbs (1.3%), extensor pollicis brevis originated from the abductor pollicis longus tendon. In five limbs (3.2%), the extensor pollicis brevis tendon attached to the base of the first metacarpal bone (Nayak et al. 2009b). Palatty et al. (2018) studied variations in the extrinsic thumb muscles in 30 adult and 20 fetal hands. The tendon of extensor pollicis brevis was single in 47 hands (94%) and doubled in three hands (6%) (Palatty et al. 2018).

Anomalies

Description

On the left upper limb of a fetus with craniorachischisis, Alghamdi et al. (2017) noticed that the muscle belly of extensor pollicis brevis was fused with abductor pollicis longus. This muscle narrowed into three tendons which attached to connective tissue on the palmar surface of the first metacarpal to form a u-shaped structure with the tendon of flexor pollicis longus.

In both a female neonate (Aziz 1979) and a female fetus with trisomy 18 (Alghamdi et al. 2018), the proximal ends of extensor pollicis brevis and abductor pollicis longus were fused on both sides of the body. The extensor pollicis brevis tendon was also bifurcated bilaterally in the neonate, with both tendons inserting onto the distal phalanx (Aziz 1979). On the left side of a trisomy 18 cyclopic fetus, Smith et al. (2015) noted that extensor pollicis brevis was diminutive and was also fused with abductor pollicis longus. On the right side of this specimen, the muscle was absent.

In a male fetus with triploidy, extensor pollicis brevis was absent bilaterally (Moen et al. 1984). Absence or "anomalous structure" of extensor pollicis brevis has been observed in infants with Neu-Laxova syndrome (Shved et al. 1985). In a male neonate with Meckel syndrome, extensor pollicis brevis inserted with abductor pollicis longus into the first metacarpal on the right hand (Pettersen 1984). On the left arm, extensor pollicis brevis joined and inserted with extensor pollicis longus. Bersu et al. (1976) describe a male infant with Hanhart syndrome. On the right side of this infant, the wrist and hand were deficient. Extensor pollicis brevis was absent.

Prevalence

In their literature review, Smith et al. (2015) found that extensor pollicis brevis and longus were variant (e.g., fusion of the two muscles, doubling of the tendons, muscles split into more than one part, variable attachments, connections with the second digit) in 2 out of 24 individuals with trisomy 13 (8.3%), 13 out of 26 individuals with trisomy 18 (50%), and 1 out of 7 individuals with trisomy 21 (14.3%). Extensor pollicis brevis was absent in 4 out of 26 individuals with trisomy 18 (15.4%). In a study of six upper limbs from three infants with Neu-Laxova syndrome, Shved et al. (1985) found that extensor pollicis brevis was aplasic in three upper limbs (50%) and had an "anomalous structure" in three upper limbs (50%).

Clinical Implications

Variation of the course of accessory tendons of extensor pollicis brevis and compression of these tendons can contribute to de Quervain's tenosynovitis (Giles 1960; Nayak et al. 2009b).

Abductor pollicis longus (Figure 3.16)

Synonyms

This muscle is also referred to as extensor ossis metacarpi pollicis or cubito-radi sus-metacarpien (Todd 1839; Macalister 1875).

Typical Presentation

Description

Abductor pollicis longus originates from the posterior surface of the ulnar shaft, the neighboring interosseous membrane, and the middle third of the posterior surface of the radius (Standring 2016). It inserts via a tendon that typically splits into two slips, with the first attaching to the base of the first metacarpal and the second to the trapezium (Standring 2016).

Innervation

Abductor pollicis longus is innervated by the posterior interosseous nerve (Standring 2016).

Comparative Anatomy

Abductor pollicis longus has a similar typical presentation in the apes, extending from the radius and ulna to the first metacarpal and trapezium (Macalister 1871; Champneys 1872; Beddard 1893; Chapman 1900; Straus 1941; Miller 1952; Gibbs 1999; Michilsens et al. 2009; Diogo et al. 2010, 2012, 2013a,b, 2017). An insertion into the sesamoid bone adjacent to the trapezium has been observed in all apes except bonobos (Macalister 1873; Kohlbrügge 1890–1892; Hepburn 1892; Dwight 1895; Sonntag 1923, 1924; Primrose 1899, 1900; Straus 1941; Ziegler 1964; Diogo et al. 2010, 2012, 2013a,b). An insertion into the scaphoid has been observed in orangutans and common chimpanzees (Kallner 1956; Ziegler 1964; Diogo et al. 2013a,b). An insertion into the proximal phalanx of the first digit has been observed in gibbons and gorillas (Owen 1868; Chapman 1878; Bischoff 1880; Deniker 1885; Hepburn 1892; Pira 1913; Straus 1941; Raven 1950; Preuschoft 1965; Kaneff 1980a,b; Diogo et al. 2010, 2012).

Variations

Description

The entire muscle and/or the tendon may be divided or doubled (Macalister 1875; Knott 1883a; Stein 1951; Baba 1954; Bergman et al. 1988; Akita and Nimura 2016b; Standring 2016; Jain et al. 2018). There may be three, four, five, or six tendons (Macalister 1875; Knott 1883a; Mori 1964; Perkins and Hast 1993; El-Beshbishy and Abdel-Hamid 2013; Tewari et al. 2015). Slips from the tendon of abductor pollicis longus may pass to the abductor pollicis brevis, opponens pollicis, the flexor retinaculum, thenar fascia, scaphoid, trapezium, or proximal phalanx of digit one (Macalister 1875; Knott 1883a; Mori 1964; Bergman et al. 1988; El-Beshbishy and Abdel-Hamid 2013; Tewari

et al. 2015; Akita and Nimura 2016b; Standring 2016). It is often fused with extensor pollicis brevis (Macalister 1875; Inoue 1934; Mori 1964; Standring 2016). Opponens pollicis may originate from the tendon of abductor pollicis longus (Bergman et al. 1988; Akita and Nimura 2016b). Abductor pollicis longus may be reduced, only having a radial origin (Bergman et al. 1988; Akita and Nimura 2016b). Palatty et al. (2018) found it absent in a fetus.

Paul and Das (2007) describe a case in which the abductor pollicis longus muscle had a normal origin on the ulna and radius, but after its tendon emerged from the extensor retinaculum it continued as a small muscle belly that then had a tendinous insertion onto the proximal phalanx of digit one. Ranade et al. (2017) also describe a similar case in which abductor pollicis longus had a normal origin, but its tendon split proximal to the wrist and one tendon inserted onto the first metacarpal, while the other tendon converted into a small muscle belly that inserted onto the proximal phalanx.

Abductor pollicis longus is associated with one rare supernumerary muscle, abductor pollicis tertius, which is also referred to as extensor atque abductor pollicis accessorius (Bergman et al. 1988). This muscle originates from the posterior surface of the radius along with abductor pollicis longus, fuses with abductor pollicis brevis, and inserts into the first metacarpal (Bergman et al. 1988; Akita and Nimura 2016b).

Prevalence

According to Macalister (1875), Wood found that abductor pollicis longus sent a slip to the origin of abductor pollicis brevis in 7 out of 36 subjects (19.4%). In a study of 84 wrists, Stein (1951) found that an accessory tendon of abductor pollicis longus was present in 68% of wrists. In a study of 134 wrists, Baba (1954) found that 132 wrists (98.5%) had accessory tendons of abductor pollicis longus. Based on dissections of 80 hands from 40 individuals, Perkins and Hast (1993) found that abductor pollicis longus inserted via two or three tendons in 73 hands (91%).

Mori (1964) found that abductor pollicis longus was fused with extensor pollicis brevis in 10% of cases. The insertion tendon was doubled in 35% of cases, tripled in 46% of cases, quadrupled in 14% of cases, and quintupled in 4% of cases (Mori 1964). The tendon inserted onto the first metacarpal only in 2% of cases, onto the first metacarpal and the tendon of abductor pollicis brevis in 24% of cases, and onto the first metacarpal, the tendon of abductor pollicis brevis, and the trapezium in 40% of cases (Mori 1964).

El-Beshbishy and Abdel-Hamid (2013) examined variations in abductor pollicis longus in 50 upper limbs. The tendon was not found to be single in any case (0%). It had two tendons in 20 cases (40%), three tendons in 17 cases (34%), four tendons in nine cases (18%), five tendons in two cases (4%), and six tendons in two cases (4%). The lateral tendons in all cases inserted onto the base of the first metacarpal bone (100%). The insertion of the medial tendons varied from the antero-lateral surface of the first metacarpal (80%), lateral surface of the first metacarpal (20%), the trapezium (80%), abductor pollicis brevis (60%), thenar fascia (40%), the carpometacarpal joint of digit one (30%), and opponens pollicis (20%).

Tewari et al. (2015) examined variations in abductor pollicis longus in 50 upper wrists. The tendon was single in two cases (4%), doubled in 31 cases (62%), tripled in eight cases (16%), quadrupled in eight cases (16%), and six tendons were present in one hand (2%). At least one attachment onto the first metacarpal was seen in all cases (100%), and an accessory insertion was observed onto the trapezium in 46 cases (92%). Of all 126 tendons observed, 68 (53.9%) inserted onto the base of the first metacarpal, 52 (41.3%) inserted onto the trapezium, 4 (3.2%) inserted onto the opponens pollicis, and 2 (1.6%) inserted onto the thenar fascia.

Jain et al. (2018) examined variations in abductor pollicis longus in 40 forearms from 20 cadavers. The tendon of abductor pollicis longus was single in two cases (5%), doubled in 30 cases (75%), and tripled in eight cases (20%). It inserted onto the first metacarpal in all hands (100%) and had a secondary insertion onto the trapezium in 20 hands (50%) (Jain et al. 2018). Palatty et al. (2018) studied variations in the extrinsic thumb muscles in 30 adult and 20 fetal hands. The tendon of abductor pollicis longus was single in 38 hands (76%) and doubled or tripled in 11 hands (22%). The muscle was absent in one of the fetal hands (2%). In one adult male cadaver, the abductor pollicis longus had three slips of origin on the right side and two slips of origin on the left side (Palatty et al. 2018).

Anomalies

Description

On the left upper limb of a fetus with craniorachischisis, Alghamdi et al. (2017) observed that the tendon of abductor pollicis longus pierced the second tendon of brachioradialis and attached to the palmar fascia. It was also fused with extensor pollicis brevis. In both a female neonate (Aziz 1979) and a female fetus with trisomy 18 (Alghamdi et al. 2018), the proximal ends of extensor pollicis brevis and abductor pollicis longus were fused on both sides of the body. The abductor pollicis longus tendon was also doubled bilaterally in the neonate, one attaching to the first metacarpal and the other attaching to the trapezium (Aziz 1979). On the left side of a trisomy 18 cyclopic fetus, Smith et al. (2015) observed that abductor pollicis longus was fused with a diminutive extensor pollicis brevis. The tendon of this muscle was trifurcated, with a usual insertion onto the first metacarpal and sent two tendons to an abnormal thenar mass of muscles.

Abductor pollicis longus sharing a common muscle belly with extensor pollicis brevis has been observed in infants with Neu-Laxova syndrome (Shved et al. 1985). Bersu et al. (1976) describe a male infant with Hanhart syndrome. On the right side of this infant, the wrist and hand were deficient. Abductor pollicis longus inserted into the trapezium.

Prevalence

In their literature review, Smith et al. (2015) found that abductor pollicis longus was variant (e.g., doubling of the muscle, variable attachments) in 4 out of 24 individuals with trisomy 13 (16.7%) and in 9 out of 26 individuals with trisomy 18 (34.6%), but was normal in seven individuals with trisomy 21. Abductor pollicis longus was absent in 1 out of 26 individuals with trisomy 18 (3.8%). In a study of six upper limbs from three infants with Neu-Laxova syndrome, Shved et al. (1985) found that abductor pollicis longus shared a common muscular belly with extensor pollicis brevis in two upper limbs (33%).

Clinical Implications

Variation of the course of accessory tendons of abductor pollicis longus, and compression of these tendons, can contribute to de Quervain's tenosynovitis (Giles 1960).

MUSCLES OF THE HAND

CONTRAHENTES DIGITORUM MANUS (FIGURE 3.18)

Entry adapted by permission from Springer Nature Customer Service Centre GmbH: Springer Current Molecular Biology Reports, Muscles Lost in Our Adult Primate Ancestors Still Imprint in Us: on Muscle Evolution, Development, Variations, and Pathologies. E. Boyle, V. Mahon, R. Diogo, 2020.

Synonyms

This muscle may also be referred to as transversus manus (Hepburn 1892). Contrahens refers to a singular muscle, and contrahentes refer to multiple muscles (Cihak 1972).

Typical Presentation

This muscle is only present as a variation or anomaly.

Comparative Anatomy

Contrahentes digitorum are sometimes present as adductors of the fingers in nonhuman apes (Diogo and Wood 2011, 2012a). These muscles are present in gibbons in about 60% of cases, and in most cases, they extend from the contrahens fascia to the base of the proximal phalanges and extensor expansions on the ulnar side of digit two (contrahens 1), the radial side of digit 4 (contrahens 2), and the radial side of digit five (contrahens 3) (Deniker 1885; Kohlbrügge 1890–1892; Hepburn 1892; Lewis 1989; Diogo et al. 2012). Contrahentes digitorum are absent in gorillas (Deniker 1885; Macalister 1873; Hepburn 1892; Sommer 1907; Pira 1913; Raven 1950; Preuschoft 1965; Diogo et al. 2010) and rarely present in orangutans (Diogo et al. 2013b). Contrahentes to digits four and five are occasionally present in common chimpanzees and bonobos (Hepburn 1892; Miller 1952; Swindler and Wood 1973; Lewis 1989; Diogo et al. 2013a, 2017).

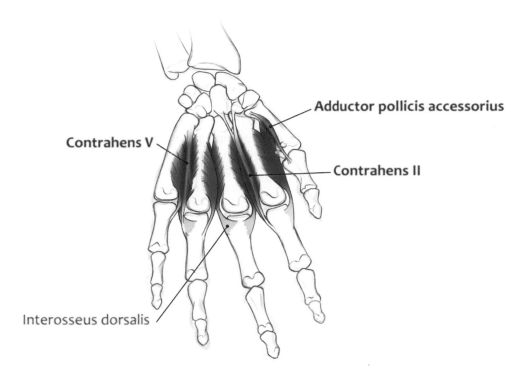

FIGURE 3.18 Interossei and contrahentes muscles of the hand in palmar view.

Variations

Description

Contrahentes of the hand (contrahentes 3, 4, 5) are typically only present in the early stages of human development and then diffuse and/or fuse with the interossei (Cihak 1972; Diogo et al 2019). Adductor pollicis develops from contrahentes 1 and 2 and is present as a differentiated muscle at CR20mm (crown-rump length of 20mm) (Cihak 1972; Diogo et al. 2019). Contrahentes 3, 4, and 5 persist in the embryo until CR36mm (crown-rump length of 36mm), at which point they become undistinguishable (Diogo et al. 2019). Contrahentes are very rare in karyotypically normal humans. Remnants of contrahentes digitorum may present as more proximal and medial attachments of the oblique head of adductor pollicis (Yamamoto et al. 1988; Tubbs et al. 2005b). When present as distinct muscles, contrahentes originate from the carpals, or the bases of the metacarpals, and can have separate distal insertions into the metacarpals and phalanges of digits four and five (Stark et al. 1979; Bergman et al. 1988; Tubbs et al. 2005b). Stark et al. (1979) described the presence of contrahentes in three children, and in each case, the muscle was present unilaterally and was associated with an accessory palmaris brevis.

Innervation

Contrahentes digitorum are innervated by the deep branch of the ulnar nerve (Tubbs et al. 2005b).

Prevalence

N/A

Anomalies

Description

Dunlap et al. (1986) dissected individuals with trisomy 13, 18, and 21 to determine the common forelimb anomalies common to these syndromes. They found that in individuals with trisomy 18, contrahentes muscles extending to digits two, four, and/or five were sometimes present. These muscles originated from the carpal bones, their associated ligaments, and from a median raphe extending from the ventral shaft of the third metacarpal.

Prevalence

In their literature review, Smith et al. (2015) found that out of 26 individuals with trisomy 18, contrahens to digit two was present in four cases (15.4%), contrahens to digit four was present in one case (3.8%), and contrahens to digit five was present in two cases (7.7%).

Clinical Implications

The presence of contrahentes has been associated with problems including cramping of the hand (Stark et al. 1979) or potentially compression of the median nerve (Tubbs et al. 2005b).

PALMARIS BREVIS (FIGURE 3.19)

Synonyms

This muscle is also referred to as palmaris cutaneus, cavo quadrata manus, or Peaucier de la main (Cruveilhier) (Bergman et al. 2008).

Typical Presentation

Description

Palmaris brevis extends from the flexor retinaculum and the medial (ulnar) border of the palmar aponeurosis to the skin on the medial border of the palm (Standring 2016).

Innervation

Palmaris brevis is innervated by the ulnar nerve (Standring 2016).

Comparative Anatomy

Palmaris brevis has a similar typical presentation in the apes, extending from the flexor retinaculum and/or the pisiform to the skin on the medial border of the palm (Raven 1950; Miller 1952; Swindler and Wood 1973; Preuschoft 1965; Gibbs 1999; Diogo et al. 2010, 2012, 2013a,b, 2017). Occasional absence has been observed in all apes (Bischoff 1880; Deniker 1885; Kohlbrügge 1890–1892; Hepburn 1892; Pira 1913; Loth 1931; Kallner 1956; Gibbs 1999; Diogo et al. 2010, 2012, 2013a,b, 2017).

Variations

Description

Palmaris brevis can be variable in its size, length, and orientation (Macalister 1875; Bergman et al. 1988). It may present as several fasciculi or one continuous sheet (Macalister 1875). Palmaris brevis may have a more radial origin via slips from the trapezium or scaphoid (Gonzalez and Netscher 2016). Its insertion may extend to the thenar eminence (Macalister 1875). It may join with flexor digiti minimi brevis or attach to the pisiform (Macalister 1875; Mori 1964; Bergman et al. 1988; Tountas and Bergman 1993; Nayak and Krishnamurthy 2007; Gonzalez and Netscher 2016). It may receive fibers from the flexor carpi ulnaris tendon (Macalister 1875). This muscle may present deeper in the hand without an attachment to the skin (Das and Paul 2006; Gonzalez and Netscher 2016). Palmaris brevis may be absent (Macalister 1875; Bergman et al. 1988; Tountas and Bergman 1993; Gonzalez and Netscher 2016). Palmaris brevis may also be doubled, and the extra muscle can be referred to as palmaris brevis profundus (Bergman et al. 1988; Tountas and Bergman 1993; Gonzalez and Netscher 2016).

Prevalence

Macalister (1875) found palmaris brevis absent in about 1 out of every 45 subjects (2.2%). Mori (1964) did not observe the absence of palmaris brevis in any cases. Mori (1964) did find that palmaris brevis was well-developed in 10% of cases, not well-developed in 32% of cases, and had a slip to the pisiform bone in 16.2% of cases.

Anomalies

Description

In the literature review conducted by Smith et al. (2015), they noted that in one individual with trisomy 13, palmaris brevis ran deep to the ulnar artery and nerve and extended obliquely from the pisiform to the flexor retinaculum. Palmaris brevis was absent bilaterally in two neonates with trisomy 18 and three neonates with trisomy 13 (Aziz 1979, 1980, 1981). It was also absent bilaterally in a fetus with trisomy 18 and cyclopia (Smith et al. 2015). The absence of palmaris brevis has been observed in infants with Neu-Laxova syndrome (Shved et al. 1985).

Prevalence

According to Smith et al. (2015), palmaris brevis was absent in 20 out of 24 individuals with trisomy 13 (83.3%), 15 out of 26 individuals with trisomy 18 (57.7%), and in 1 out of 7 individuals with trisomy 21 (14.3%). This muscle had an abnormal presentation in 1 out of 24 individuals with trisomy 13 (4.2%). In a study of six upper limbs from three infants with Neu-Laxova syndrome, Shved et al. (1985) found that palmaris brevis was absent in all six upper limbs (100%).

Clinical Implications

An accessory palmaris brevis can be mistaken for a soft-tissue tumor of the hand (Bergman et al. 1988; Tountas and Bergman 1993). A hypertrophic palmaris brevis or the presence of an accessory palmaris brevis can compress the ulnar nerve (Tonkin and Lister 1985; Tountas and Bergman 1993; Mackinnon and Dellon 1998; Gonzalez and Netscher 2016).

Lumbricales (Lumbricals) (Figure 3.19)

Synonyms

A singular lumbrical muscle may be referred to as lumbricalis, and multiple lumbrical muscles may be referred to as lumbricales (Bergman et al. 1988; Smith et al. 2015).

Typical Presentation

Description

The lumbricals originate from the tendons of flexor digitorum profundus and attach to the radial sides of the extensor expansions of digits two through five (Standring 2016). The muscles can be either unipennate (single origin) or bipennate (dual origin), and when bipennate, the two heads of the muscle arise from two tendons of flexor digitorum profundus (Standring 2016). The configuration of the lumbricals is variable, but the most common origins are that the first lumbrical arises from the tendon of flexor digitorum profundus to digit two, the second lumbrical from the tendon of flexor digitorum profundus to digit three, the third lumbrical from the tendons of flexor digitorum profundus to digits three and four, and the fourth lumbrical from the tendons of flexor digitorum profundus to digits four and five (Eladoumikdachi et al. 2002b; Standring 2016; Gonzalez and Netscher 2016).

Innervation

The first and second lumbricals are innervated by the median nerve, and the third and fourth lumbricals are innervated by the ulnar nerve (Standring 2016). Occasionally, the first and second lumbricals are supplied by the ulnar nerve, and the third lumbrical may be supplied by the median nerve (Standring 2016).

Comparative Anatomy

Lumbricals have a similar typical presentation in the apes and can have similarly variable origins and insertions (Gibbs 1999; Diogo et al. 2010, 2012, 2013a,b, 2017). The fourth lumbrical (to digit five) in gibbons, gorillas, and bonobos can be reduced or absent (Raven 1950; Gibbs 1999; Diogo et al. 2010, 2012, 2017).

Variations

Description

Variations on the typical origins and insertions are frequent (Bergman et al. 1988; Standring 2016). The first or second lumbrical may be bipennate, and the third or fourth lumbrical may be unipennate (Wood 1866; Macalister 1875; Bergman et al. 1988; Tountas and Bergman 1993; Eladoumikdachi et al. 2002b; Gonzalez and Netscher 2016; Standring 2016). Nation et al. (2019) report a tripinnate first lumbrical in a male cadaver. The first lumbrical may have a second origin from the tendon of flexor pollicis longus (Macalister 1875; Tountas and Bergman 1993; Gonzalez and Netscher 2016; Standring 2016). The third and fourth lumbricals appear to vary more in origin than the first two (Eladoumikdachi et al. 2002b; Gonzalez and Netscher 2016; but see description of studies from Mori 1964, below). The lumbricals may also attach to the proximal phalanges of the target digits (Mori 1964; Bergman et al. 1988; Doyle and Botte 2003; Gonzalez and Netscher 2016).

In some cases, only two or three muscles may be present (Macalister 1875; Knott 1883a; Bergman et al. 1988). In rare cases, all four muscles may be absent, or there could be additional lumbricals due to the presence of accessory slips (Macalister 1875; Bergman et al. 1988; Tountas and Bergman 1993; Gonzalez and Netscher 2016). Sometimes, the lumbricals can bifurcate distally and insert into two digits (Wood 1866, 1868; Bergman et al. 1988; Tountas and Bergman 1993; Doyle and Botte 2003; Gonzalez and Netscher 2016). In the region of the first lumbrical, an accessory slip may join with the tendons of flexor pollicis longus or flexor digitorum superficialis, opponens pollicis, the muscle bellies of flexor digitorum superficialis or flexor digitorum profundus, the first metacarpal, or the palmar carpal ligament (Macalister 1875; Bergman et al. 1988; Tountas and Bergman 1993; Gonzalez and Netscher 2016; Standring 2016). The origins of the lumbrical muscles may be displaced proximally and can arise from the flexor pollicis longus tendon (first lumbrical), from the flexor retinaculum, or an accessory tendon from flexor digitorum superficialis or flexor digitorum profundus (Macalister 1875; Bergman et al. 1988; Tountas and Bergman 1993; Gonzalez and Netscher 2016). The fourth lumbrical may replace the fourth tendon of flexor digitorum superficialis (Macalister 1875; Bergman et al. 1988; Tountas and Bergman 1993; Gonzalez and Netscher 2016).

Silawal et al. (2018) describe an unusual case where the first lumbrical had two muscle bellies connected by a long (16.2 cm) tendon. The first belly was located in the proximal forearm and originated near the medial epicondyle of the humerus with the tendon of flexor digitorum superficialis, and the second belly presented as a typical first lumbrical muscle in the hand (Silawal et al. 2018). The tendon connecting the bellies ran through the carpal tunnel (Silawal et al. 2018).

Prevalence

Macalister (1875) found that the lumbricals were variable in 50 out of 400 subjects (12.5%). In a sample of 34 subjects, Knott (1883a) found that the first lumbrical was absent in two cases (5.9%), and both the first and second lumbrical were absent in one case (2.9%). The third lumbrical bifurcates distally and inserts into two digits in 40% of individuals (Bergman et al. 1988).

Mori (1964) found that the first lumbrical had a typical origin in 100% of cases. The second lumbrical had a typical origin in 78% of cases and was bipennate with origins on digits two and three in 22% of cases (Mori 1964). The third lumbrical had a typical origin in 94% of cases and was unipennate with an origin from digit three only in 6% of cases (Mori 1964). The fourth lumbrical had a typical origin in 98% of cases and was unipennate with an origin from digit four only in 2% of cases. Mori (1964) also found that the tendons of the first two lumbricals were attached along the side of the proximal phalanx to the radial border of the extensor digitorum tendon for digits two and three in 10% of cases. The third lumbrical bifurcated into two slips, with one inserting onto the ulnar surface of extensor digitorum for digit four in 20% of cases (Mori 1964). The tendon for the third lumbrical inserted onto the radial surface of extensor digitorum for digit four in 80% of cases (Mori 1964). The fourth lumbrical bifurcated into two slips that inserted onto the ulnar surface of extensor digitorum for digits four and five in 24% of cases (Mori 1964). The fourth lumbrical inserted onto the ulnar surface of extensor digitorum for digit four in 4% of cases and onto the radial surface of extensor digitorum for digit five in 96% of cases.

Based on dissections of 80 hands from 40 individuals, Perkins and Hast (1993) found that 40 hands (50%) did not have the typical presentation of lumbricals. Twenty-seven (34%) third lumbricals and four (5%) fourth lumbricals bifurcated upon insertion (Perkins and Hast 1993). Four third lumbricals (5%) had a single insertion onto the third digit, and four fourth lumbricals (5%) had a single insertion onto the fourth digit.

Anomalies

Description

Camptodactyly, a congenital flexion deformity typically of the fifth digit, that can be present alone or as part of a suite of malformations (including trisomies), may be caused by variations in lumbrical size, origin, and/or insertions (Eladoumikdachi et al. 2002b; Gonzalez and Netscher 2016; Favril et al. 2019).

In a fetus with craniorachischisis, Alghamdi et al. (2017) observed that, on the right side of the body, flexor digitorum profundus only sent tendons to digits four and five, and thus only two lumbricals were present. On the left side, the lumbricals had a normal presentation. On both sides of a trisomy 18 cyclopic fetus, Smith et al. (2015) observed that the first lumbrical was absent, and the tendon of flexor digitorum profundus to digit five did not contribute to the lumbrical attaching to the fifth digit. In the female fetus with trisomy 18, all four lumbricals were underdeveloped in both hands (Alghamdi et al. 2018). On the right side of a child with trisomy 21, the lumbrical muscles were doubled between the third and fourth digits, and between the fourth and fifth digits (Bersu 1980).

Mieden (1982) describes an infant with median cleft lip, hypotelorism, and alobar holoprosencephaly. The fourth lumbrical muscle was absent on the left side (Mieden 1982). The author does not specify if it was a hand or foot lumbrical. Absence, doubling, and anomalous insertions of one or more of the lumbricals have been observed in infants with Neu-Laxova syndrome (Shved et al. 1985). On the right hand of a male neonate with Meckel syndrome, Pettersen (1984) observed that the fourth lumbrical attached to the ulnar aspect of the fourth digit, and this muscle also had an attachment to the sixth digit. On the left hand, the third lumbrical attached to the ulnar side of the fourth digit.

Prevalence

In their literature review, Smith et al. (2015) found that 5 out of 26 individuals with trisomy 18 had an extra lumbrical between digits one and two (19.2%). They also found that the first lumbrical was variant (e.g., variable origin,

abnormal fusions) in 3 out of 26 individuals with trisomy 18 (11.5%). The fourth lumbrical was variable (variable insertions) in 1 out of 26 individuals with trisomy 18 (3.8%). Overall, the lumbricals were variable (e.g., variable origins and insertions, dual insertions, accessory slips) in 5 out of 24 individuals with trisomy 13 (20.8%), 9 out of 26 individuals with trisomy 13 (34.6%), and 1 out of 7 individuals with trisomy 21 (14.3%) (Smith et al. 2015). These authors also found that the first lumbrical was absent in 3 out of 24 individuals with trisomy 13 (12.5%) and 4 out of 26 individuals with trisomy 18 (15.4%). The second lumbrical was absent in 2 out of 26 individuals with trisomy 18 (7.7%). The third lumbrical was absent in 2 out of 26 individuals with trisomy 18 (7.7%). The fourth lumbrical was absent in 1 out of 24 individuals with trisomy 13 (4.2%) and 2 out of 26 individuals with trisomy 18 (7.7%).

McFarlane et al. (1992) found that the fourth lumbrical muscle had a variant insertion onto digit five in 74 patients (100%) undergoing surgery for camptodactyly. In a study of six upper limbs from three infants with Neu-Laxova syndrome, Shved et al. (1985) found that the first, second, and fourth lumbricals had anomalous insertions in two upper limbs (33%), the fourth lumbrical was absent in two upper limbs (33%), and the fourth lumbrical was doubled in two upper limbs (33%).

Clinical Implications

Variations in the origins and insertions of lumbrical muscles may compress the median nerve and cause carpal tunnel syndrome (Tountas and Bergman 1993; Gonzalez and Netscher 2016).

ADDUCTOR POLLICIS (FIGURE 3.19)

Synonyms

Bergman et al. (1988) refer to this muscle as adductor pollicis brevis.

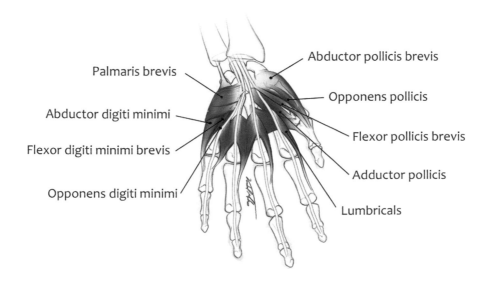

Palmaris brevis

Abductor digiti minimi

Flexor digiti minimi brevis

Opponens digiti minimi

Abductor pollicis brevis

Opponens pollicis

Flexor pollicis brevis

Adductor pollicis

Lumbricals

FIGURE 3.19 Intrinsic muscles of the hand and palmaris brevis in palmar view.

Typical Presentation

Description

The oblique head of adductor pollicis originates from the capitate and the bases of the second and third metacarpals. The transverse head originates from the third metacarpal (Standring 2016). Both heads end in tendons that converge to attach together to the base of the proximal phalanx of the first digit (Standring 2016).

Innervation

Adductor pollicis is innervated by the deep branch of the ulnar nerve (Standring 2016).

Comparative Anatomy

Adductor pollicis has a similar typical presentation in the apes with similar variation in origins and insertions (Gibbs 1999; Diogo et al. 2010, 2012, 2013a,b, 2017). Its insertion may extend to the distal phalanx of the first digit (Owen 1868; Macalister 1873; Raven 1950; Preuschoft 1965; Diogo et al. 2010, 2012, 2013a,b, 2017). There may be an extensive attachment to the first metacarpal in gibbons, and partial attachments to this bone in the other apes (Gratiolet and Alix 1866; Michaelis 1903; Raven 1950; Kallner 1956; Preuschoft 1965; Diogo et al. 2010, 2012, 2013a,b, 2017).

Variations

Description

The sizes and extent of the connection between the oblique head and the transverse head are variable (Mori 1964; Bergman et al. 1988; Doyle and Botte 2003; Gonzalez and Netscher 2016; Standring 2016). The oblique head may have connections to the first metacarpal, fourth metacarpal, trapezium, trapezoid, capitate, and hamate (Chang and Blair 1985). The transverse head may have an origin from the second metacarpal or the fourth metacarpal (Mori 1964; Chang and Blair 1985; Gonzalez and Netscher 2016). Adductor pollicis may be divided into multiple bellies or fascicles (Knott 1883a; Tountas and Bergman 1993; Jan and Rooze 1994; Gonzalez and Netscher 2016). An accessory head may originate near the oblique head from the base of the second metacarpal and insert onto the dorsal aponeurosis of the first digit (Doyle and Botte 2003; Gonzalez and Netscher 2016). Priyadharshini et al. (2019) report a case in which adductor pollicis and opponens pollicis lacked fleshy muscle fibers and were replaced with fibrous tissue.

Prevalence

Mori (1964) found that the transverse head of adductor pollicis originated from the third and fourth metacarpal bones in 76% of cases and from the third metacarpal bone only in 24% of cases. The two heads were completely separated in 82% of cases and partially separated in 16% of cases, and the transverse head was divided into two layers in 2% of cases (Mori 1964). Based on dissections of 20 cadaveric hands, Chang and Blair (1985) found that the oblique head of adductor pollicis had origins from the first metacarpal in 17 specimens (85%), the second metacarpal in all 20 specimens (100%), the third metacarpal in 15 specimens (75%), the fourth metacarpal in 17 specimens (85%), the hamate in one specimen (5%), and from the trapezium, trapezoid, and capitate in all 20 specimens (100%). The transverse head had origins from the third metacarpal in all 20 specimens (100%) with an additional origin from the second metacarpal in one specimen (5%).

Anomalies

Description

On the left side of a fetus with craniorachischisis, Alghamdi et al. (2017) observed that the transverse head of adductor pollicis originated from metacarpals three and four, and the oblique head originated from the bases of metacarpals three and four and from the capitate. Both had a normal insertion. On the left side of a fetus with trisomy 18 and cyclopia, the oblique head of adductor pollicis was separated into distinct bundles (Smith et al. 2015). Lack of separation between the heads of adductor pollicis and the absence of the oblique head have been observed in infants with Neu-Laxova syndrome (Shved et al. 1985).

Prevalence

In 2 out of 24 individuals with trisomy 13, the transverse head of adductor pollicis was hypoplastic and originated from the fourth metacarpal (8.3%). The transverse head of adductor pollicis was absent in 1 out of 24 individuals with trisomy 13 (4.2%) and in 2 out of 26 individuals with trisomy 18 (7.7%). In a study of six upper limbs from three infants with Neu-Laxova syndrome, Shved et al. (1985) found absence of the oblique head in two upper limbs (33%) and lack of separation between the heads in three upper limbs (50%).

Clinical Implications

N/A

INTEROSSEI PALMARIS (PALMAR INTEROSSEI) (FIGURE 3.18)

Synonyms

The first palmar interosseus muscle is also referred to as interosseous volaris primus of Henle or adductor pollicis accessorius (Macalister 1875; Bello-Hellegouarch et al. 2013; Smith et al. 2015).

Typical Presentation

Description

There are four palmar interosseous muscles, though many textbooks and anatomy resources often do not consider the first palmar interosseous muscle to be part of the typical presentation of this muscle group (e.g., Gonzalez and Netscher 2016) (Bello-Hellegouarch et al. 2013). The first originates from the ulnar side of the first metacarpal and inserts onto the ulnar sesamoid bone and proximal phalanx of the first digit and eventually into the dorsal digital expansion

(Standring 2016). The second palmar interosseous muscle originates from the ulnar side of the second metacarpal and inserts into the dorsal digital expansion of the second digit (Standring 2016). The third palmar interosseous muscle originates from the radial side of the fourth metacarpal and inserts into the dorsal digital expansion of the fourth digit with the third lumbrical (Standring 2016). The fourth palmar interosseous muscle originates from the radial side of the fifth metacarpal and inserts into the proximal phalanx of the fifth digit and into the dorsal digital expansion with the fourth lumbrical (Standring 2016).

Innervation

The palmar interossei are innervated by the deep branch of the ulnar nerve (Standring 2016).

Comparative Anatomy

In all apes except common chimpanzees, the palmar interossei have a similar configuration as those in humans (Diogo et al. 2010, 2012, 2013a,b, 2017). "Adductor pollicis accessorius" is occasionally present in gorillas, common chimpanzees, and bonobos extending from the ulnar side of the base of the first metacarpal to the base of the first proximal phalanx (Gratiolet and Alix 1966; Champneys 1872; Diogo et al. 2012, 2013a, 2017).

Variations

Description

One or more of the interosseous muscles may be doubled or absent (Macalister 1875; Kaplan 1965; Bergman et al. 1988; Perkins and Hast 1993; Doyle and Botte 2003; Bello-Hellegouarch et al. 2013; Gonzalez and Netscher 2016; Standring 2016). The palmar interossei may also have one or more bellies (Eladoumikdachi et al. 2002a, b; Bello-Hellegouarch et al. 2013; Gonzalez and Netscher 2016). The first palmar interosseous muscle is often diminutive (Standring 2016) and is sometimes considered to be a deep head of flexor pollicis brevis (Kaplan 1965). It may receive a slip from extensor carpi radialis longus (Macalister 1875).

Eladoumikdachi et al. (2002a) state that the first three palmar interossei are often variable in their origins and insertions. In their literature review on the first palmar interosseous muscle, Bello-Hellegouarch et al. (2013) note that this muscle can originate from the capitate, trapezoid, trapezium, first, metacarpal, second metacarpal, and/or third metacarpal, and have insertions onto the ulnar sesamoid, proximal phalanx of digit one, and/or extensor expansion. The second and third palmar interosseous muscle may receive fibers from the third metacarpal (Eladoumikdachi et al. 2002a; Gonzalez and Netscher 2016).

Prevalence

According to Macalister (1875), Wood found the first palmar interosseous muscle in 3 out of 36 cases (8.3%). Based on dissections of 80 hands from 40 individuals, Perkins and Hast (1993) found that the first palmar interosseous muscle was present in 68 hands (85%) and 36 (90%) individuals.

Bello-Hellegouarch et al. (2013) review literature on the prevalence of the first palmar interosseous muscle and list a range of prevalence from 50% to 100% based on seven studies. Out of the 72 hands dissected by Bello-Hellegouarch et al. (2013), the first palmar interosseous muscle was present in 67 hands (93%). The origin and insertion of the muscle were observed in 66 hands. It originated from the first metacarpal only in 25 hands (37.9%); from the first metacarpal and a common origin with the dorsal interosseous in seven hands (10.6%); from the wrist bones/ligaments only in seven hands (10.6%); from the first metacarpal and the wrist bones/ligaments in seven hands (10.6%); from a thin membrane shared with the dorsal interosseous in four hands (6.1%); from the dorsal interosseous in four hands (6.1%); from the first metacarpal and a common origin with the oblique head of adductor pollicis in four hands (6.1%); from the first metacarpal and the thin membrane shared with the dorsal interosseous in three hands (4.5%); from the first and second metacarpals in two hands (3%); from the first metacarpal, wrist bones/ligaments, and the thin membrane shared with the dorsal interosseous in one hand (1.5%); from the wrist bones/ligaments and the thin membrane shared with the dorsal interosseous in one hand (1.5%); and from the first and second metacarpals and the thin membrane in one hand (1.5%) (Bello-Hellegouarch et al. 2013).

This first palmar interosseous inserted onto the proximal phalanx of the first digit only in 34 hands (51.5%), the proximal phalanx of the first digit and a common insertion with the oblique head of adductor pollicis in 18 hands (27.3%), the first metacarpal and the proximal phalanx of the first digit in five hands (7.6%), the first metacarpal only in three hands (4.5%), the first metacarpal and a common insertion with the oblique head of adductor pollicis in three hands (4.5%), fusion and common insertion with the oblique head of adductor pollicis in two hands (3%), and onto the first metacarpal, proximal phalanx of digit one, and a common insertion with the oblique head of adductor pollicis in one hand (1.5%) (Bello-Hellegouarch et al. 2013). Bello-Hellegouarch et al. (2013) also note that out of 66 hands, the muscle presented as a single muscular bundle in 38 hands (57.6%), two muscular bundles in ten hands (15.2%), more than two muscular bundles in ten hands (15.2%), a single thin tendon with no muscle fibers in five hands (7.6%), and both a muscular and tendinous bundle in three hands (4.5%).

Anomalies

Description

On the right side of a fetus with craniorachischisis, Alghamdi et al. (2017) observed that there were only two palmar interossei, which attached to the radial sides of digits four and five. On both sides of a fetus with trisomy 18 and cyclopia, "adductor pollicis accessorius" was present and arose from the proximal portion of the first metacarpal and inserted onto the base of the first proximal phalanx (Smith et al. 2015). Its insertion was blended with the insertion of adductor pollicis on both sides (Smith et al. 2015).

In individuals with camptodactyly, the fourth palmar interosseous muscle can insert onto the fourth digit (Tountas and Bergman 1993). Anomalous insertion of the first palmar interosseous muscle has been observed in infants with Neu-Laxova syndrome (Shved et al. 1985). In a male neonate with Meckel syndrome, Pettersen (1984) found that on the right hand, the third palmar interosseous muscle attached to the sixth digit.

Prevalence

In their literature review, Smith et al. (2015) found that the fourth palmar interosseous muscle originates from opponens digiti minimi in 1 out of 24 individuals with trisomy 13 (4.2%). They also found that the first palmar and dorsal interossei were absent in 2 out of 26 individuals with trisomy 18 (7.7%). "Adductor pollicis accessorius" was present in 5 out of 24 individuals with trisomy 13 (20.8%), 10 out of 26 individuals with trisomy 18 (38.5%), and two out of seven individuals with trisomy 21 (28.6%). In a study of six upper limbs from three infants with Neu-Laxova syndrome, Shved et al. (1985) found that first palmar interosseous muscle had an anomalous insertion in two upper limbs (33%).

Clinical Implications
N/A

INTEROSSEI DORSALIS (DORSAL INTEROSSEI) (FIGURE 3.18)

Synonyms

The first dorsal interosseous muscle may also be referred to as abductor indicis (Standring 2016).

Typical Presentation

Description

There are four dorsal interosseous muscles (Standring 2016). The first originates from sides of the first and second metacarpals and attaches to the proximal phalanx and the metacarpophalangeal joint capsule of digit two (Standring 2016). The second originates from the sides of metacarpals two and three and attaches onto the radial side of the third digit into the proximal phalanx and dorsal digital expansion (Standring 2016). The third originates from the sides of metacarpals three and four and attaches to the ulnar side of the third digit, into the dorsal digital expansion (Standring 2016). The fourth originates from the sides of metacarpals four and five and attaches to the proximal phalanx and digital expansion of digit four (Standring 2016).

Innervation

The dorsal interossei are innervated by the deep branch of the ulnar nerve (Standring 2016). Innervation may vary, with potential innervation by the radial, musculocutaneous, or median nerves (Kaplan 1965; Bergman et al. 1988; Tountas and Bergman 1993; Doyle and Botte 2003; Gonzalez and Netscher 2016).

Comparative Anatomy

In all apes except common chimpanzees, the flexores breves profundi 3, 5, 6, and 8 are fused with the intermetacarpales 1, 2, 3, and 4, forming the interossei dorsales 1, 2, 3, and 4, respectively (Diogo et al. 2010, 2012, 2013a,b, 2017). As in humans, the dorsal interossei in the apes extend from the sides of adjacent metacarpals to insert onto the proximal phalanges and extensor expansions of digits two, three, and four (Diogo et al. 2010, 2012, 2013a,b, 2017). Accessory interosseus muscles to digit two are common in gibbons (Susman et al. 1982; Diogo et al. 2012).

Variations

Description

One or more of the dorsal interossei may be divided, doubled, reduced, or absent (Wood 1868; Macalister 1875; Kaplan 1965; Bergman et al. 1988; Doyle and Botte 2003; Gonzalez and Netscher 2016). They may have additional heads, with the second and third having up to three heads (Macalister 1875; Bergman et al. 1988; Tountas and Bergman 1993; Eladoumikdachi et al. 2002a; Bharambe et al. 2013; Nayak et al. 2016). The first dorsal interosseous muscle may receive a slip from extensor carpi radialis longus, and the third may receive a slip from extensor carpi radialis brevis (Macalister 1875). Slips may pass to extensor digitorum brevis manus (Macalister 1875). The dorsal interossei may also be associated with accessory muscles (Nayak et al. 2016).

Prevalence

Macalister (1875) notes that a split first dorsal interosseous muscle, with one part attaching to the thumb and the other to the index finger, occurs in about 1 out of 120 subjects (0.8%). In dissections of 25 hands, Bharambe et al. (2013) found an additional head of the second dorsal interosseous muscle in three upper limbs (12%) and additional heads of the second, third, and fourth dorsal interossei in one upper limb (4%). In dissections of 30 hands, Nayak et al. (2016) found supernumerary muscles that originated from the third metacarpal in three hands (10%), and the third dorsal interosseous muscle had three heads in one hand (3%).

Anomalies

Description

On the right side of a fetus with craniorachischisis, Alghamdi et al. (2017) observed that there were only three dorsal interossei.

Prevalence

In their literature review, Smith et al. (2015) found that the first palmar and dorsal interossei were absent in 2 out of 26 individuals with trisomy 18 (7.7%).

Clinical Implications

Bharambe et al. (2013) and Nayak et al. (2016) suggest that supernumerary muscles or additional heads of the dorsal interossei may be largely asymptomatic but could potentially lead to chronic compartment syndrome due to increased intracompartmental pressure.

FLEXOR POLLICIS BREVIS (FIGURE 3.19)

Synonyms

The deep head of this muscle can be referred to as the deep head of Cruveilhier (Dunlap et al. 2017).

Typical Presentation

Description

The superficial head of flexor pollicis brevis originates from the flexor retinaculum and trapezium and inserts via a tendon onto the radial side of the base of the proximal phalanx of the first digit (Standring 2016). The deep head originates from the trapezoid and capitate and joins with the superficial head upon its insertion into the base of the proximal phalanx of the first digit (Standring 2016).

Innervation

The superficial head is typically innervated by the median nerve but may also be innervated by the ulnar nerve, or both nerves (Bergman et al. 1988; Tountas and Bergman 1993; Gonzalez and Netscher 2016; Standring 2016; Caetano et al. 2017). The deep head is primarily innervated by the ulnar nerve but is sometimes innervated by the median nerve or by both nerves (Bergman et al. 1988; Tountas and Bergman 1993; Gonzalez and Netscher 2016; Standring 2016; Caetano et al. 2017; Dunlap et al. 2017).

Comparative Anatomy

Flexor pollicis brevis has a similar typical presentation in the apes, and the deep head (corresponding to flexor brevis profundus 2 of lower mammals) is occasionally absent (Gibbs 1999; Diogo et al. 2010, 2012, 2013a,b, 2017). This muscle may also be partially or fully fused with neighboring muscles, including opponens pollicis or abductor pollicis brevis (Gibbs 1999; Diogo et al. 2010, 2012, 2013a,b, 2017).

Variations

Description

The entire flexor pollicis brevis muscle, or sometimes just the deep head, can be absent or doubled (Macalister 1875; Kaplan 1965; Tountas and Bergman 1993; Bergman et al. 1988; Gonzalez and Netscher 2016; Standring 2016; Caetano et al. 2017). The superficial or deep heads may be divided, or there can be an additional third head (Bergman et al. 1988; Doyle and Botte 2003; Dunlap et al. 2017). Dunlap et al. (2017) note an origin of the superficial head from the trapezoid in one case, and additional insertions onto the shaft of the first metacarpal or with opponens

pollicis. The deep head in many cases showed additional origins from the base of the second, third, and/or fourth metacarpals, or from a fibrous extension of the carpal tunnel wall (Dunlap et al. 2017). This muscle, often the superficial head, can be partially or fully blended with opponens pollicis, abductor pollicis brevis, or adductor pollicis (Macalister 1875; Bergman et al. 1988; Tountas and Bergman 1993; Doyle and Botte 2003; Gonzalez and Netscher 2016; Standring 2016).

Prevalence

Caetano et al. (2017) studied this muscle in 60 hands and found that the superficial head was supplied by the median nerve in 42 hands (70%) and was supplied by both the median and ulnar nerves in 18 hands (30%). The deep head was absent in nine hands (15%) and of the remaining 51 hands, one hand was innervated by the median nerve only (1.96%), 10 were supplied by the ulnar nerve only (19.6%), and 40 had dual innervation (78.4%) (Caetano et al. 2017). Dunlap et al. (2017) studied the innervation of both heads in 11 hands and found that the superficial head was innervated by the median nerve in all (100%) hands while the deep head was innervated by the median nerve only in three hands (27.3%) and both the ulnar and median nerves in eight hands (72.7%).

In dissections of 80 hands, Dunlap et al. (2017) note that all superficial heads (100%) originated from the flexor retinaculum and the trapezium and inserted onto the proximal phalanx of the first digit. Additional insertions were present in 36 hands (45%) and include attachments to the shaft of the first metacarpal in 12 hands (15%), with the opponens pollicis in nine hands (11.3%), or both of these insertions in 15 hands (18.8%). The deep heads of the muscle originated from the trapezoid, capitate, and ligamentum carpi radiatum in all but one hand (1.3%), which lacked an origin from the trapezoid. Additional origins of the deep head include from the base of the second metacarpal in one hand (1.3%), the base of the third metacarpal in 20 hands (25%), the bases of both the third and fourth metacarpals in four hands (5%), or from a fibrous extension of the carpal tunnel wall in 43 hands (53.8%). The deep head had two heads in 37 hands (46.3%).

Anomalies

Description

On the left side of a fetus with craniorachischisis, the deep head had an uncommon insertion onto the distal end of the proximal phalanx of digit one, while the superficial head inserted abnormally onto the proximal end of the distal phalanx of digit one (Alghamdi et al. 2017). In a fetus with trisomy 18 and cyclopia, flexor pollicis brevis was absent on the right side (Smith et al. 2015). On the left side of this specimen, flexor pollicis brevis was fused with abductor pollicis brevis and opponens pollicis. The absence of flexor pollicis brevis has been observed in infants with Neu-Laxova syndrome (Shved et al. 1985).

Prevalence

In their literature review, Smith et al. (2015) found that flexor pollicis brevis was variant (e.g., fused with opponens pollicis, diminutive muscle, variable origin) in 2 out of 24 individuals with trisomy 13 (8.3%) and in 10 out of 26 individuals with trisomy 18 (38.5%). These authors also noted that flexor pollicis brevis was absent in 1 out of 24 individuals with trisomy 13 (4.2%) and in 8 out of 26 individuals with trisomy 18 (30.8%). In a study of six upper limbs from three infants with Neu-Laxova syndrome, Shved et al. (1985) found that flexor pollicis brevis was absent in all six upper limbs (100%).

Clinical Implications

N/A

OPPONENS POLLICIS (FIGURE 3.19)

Synonyms

N/A

Typical Presentation

Description

Opponens pollicis originates from the trapezium and flexor retinaculum and inserts onto the lateral (radial) half of the palmar surface of the first metacarpal (Standring 2016).

Innervation

Opponens pollicis is typically innervated by the median nerve, and sometimes by the ulnar nerve (Standring 2016).

Comparative Anatomy

Opponens pollicis has a similar typical presentation in the apes, often with an additional origin from the radial sesamoid bone and/or the scaphoid (Brooks 1887; Miller 1952; Gibbs 1999; Diogo et al. 2010, 2012, 2013a,b, 2017). It may have an origin from the tendon of abductor pollicis brevis in orangutans (Brooks 1887; Primrose 1899, 1900; Diogo et al. 2013b). Its insertion may extend to the proximal and/or distal phalanx of the first digit in gibbons (Kohlbrügge 1890–1892; Hepburn 1892; Diogo et al. 2012).

Variations

Description

Opponens pollicis may be divided into two parts, doubled, or in some cases, it may be absent entirely (Bergman et al. 1988; Doyle and Botte 2003; Gonzalez and Netscher 2016). It may also be divided into multiple bellies or fascicles (Jan and Rooze 1994). It may be partially or fully fused with flexor pollicis brevis (Bergman et al. 1988; Tountas and Bergman 1993; Doyle and Botte 2003; Gonzalez and Netscher 2016; Standring 2016). It may give origin to a third head of abductor pollicis brevis (Wood 1868; Macalister 1875; Bergman et al. 1988; Tountas and Bergman 1993; Gonzalez and Netscher 2016). Priyadharshini et al. (2019) report a case in which opponens pollicis and adductor

pollicis lacked fleshy muscle fibers and were replaced with fibrous tissue.

Prevalence

N/A

Anomalies

Description

On the left side of a fetus with craniorachischisis, opponens pollicis abnormally originated from the second tendon of brachioradialis at the base of the first metacarpal and inserted onto the proximal end of the distal phalanx of digit one (Alghamdi et al. 2017). In a fetus with trisomy 18 and cyclopia, opponens pollicis was absent on the right side and fused with abductor pollicis brevis and flexor pollicis brevis on the left side (Smith et al. 2015). The absence of opponens pollicis has been observed in infants with Neu-Laxova syndrome (Shved et al. 1985).

Prevalence

In their literature review, Smith et al. (2015) found that opponens pollicis was diminutive in 1 out of 24 individuals with trisomy 13 (4.2%) and in 3 out of 26 individuals with trisomy 18 (11.5%). Opponens pollicis was absent in 1 out of 24 individuals with trisomy 13 (4.2%) and in 6 out of 26 individuals with trisomy 18 (23.1%). In a study of six upper limbs from three infants with Neu-Laxova syndrome, Shved et al. (1985) found that opponens pollicis was absent in all six upper limbs (100%).

Clinical Implications

N/A

FLEXOR DIGITI MINIMI BREVIS (FIGURE 3.19)

Synonyms

This muscle may also be referred to as flexor digiti minimi (Gonzalez and Netscher 2016), abductor digiti quinti brevis (Sullivan and Osgood 1927), or flexor brevis minimi digiti (Macalister 1875).

Typical Presentation

Description

Flexor digiti minimi brevis originates from the hook of the hamate and the flexor retinaculum (Standring 2016). It inserts onto the ulnar side of the base of the proximal phalanx of the fifth digit (Standring 2016).

Innervation

Flexor digiti minimi brevis is innervated by the deep branch of the ulnar nerve (Standring 2016).

Comparative Anatomy

Flexor digiti minimi brevis has a similar typical presentation in the apes, extending from the hamate and/or flexor retinaculum to the proximal phalanx of digit five

(Gratiolet and Alix 1866; Macalister 1873; Deniker 1885; Hepburn 1892; Primrose 1899, 1900; Sonntag 1923, 1924; Raven 1950; Miller 1952; Kallner 1956; Swindler and Wood 1973; Diogo et al. 2010, 2012, 2013a,b, 2017). It may have an origin from the pisiform in gibbons and gorillas (Kohlbrügge 1890–1892; Preuschoft 1965; Diogo et al. 2010, 2012). It was completely fused with abductor digiti minimi in one bonobo (Diogo et al. 2017).

Variations

Description

Flexor digiti minimi brevis may be doubled, reduced, or absent (Macalister 1875; Le Double 1897; Bergman et al. 1988; Doyle and Botte 2003; Wingerter et al. 2003; Murata et al. 2004; Gonzalez and Netscher 2016; Standring 2016, May 2020). It may be fused with or replaced by adjacent muscles, including abductor digiti minimi or opponens digiti minimi (Macalister 1875; Le Double 1897; Bergman et al. 1988; Tountas and Bergman 1993; Gonzalez and Netscher 2016; Standring 2016). It could also be replaced by a tendon that originates from flexor carpi ulnaris (Bergman et al. 1988; Doyle and Botte 2003; Gonzalez and Netscher 2016). Flexor digiti minimi brevis may have an origin from the distal antebrachial fascia (Wingerter et al. 2003). It may also originate from the tendon of flexor carpi radialis (Georgiev and Jelev 2011). Georgiev and Jelev (2007) note a case with a triple origin from the hook of the hamate, the flexor retinaculum, and from the fibers forming Guyon's canal. Flexor digiti minimi brevis may be connected via accessory slips to the shaft or distal end of the fifth metacarpal, the hook of the hamate, the palmaris longus tendon, or flexor carpi radialis (Macalister 1875; Kaplan 1965; Tountas and Bergman 1993; Pribyl and Moneim 1994; Spinner et al. 1996; De Smet 2002; Gonzalez and Netscher 2016; Standring 2016).

Madhavi and Holla (2003) note a case in which the muscle was shifted proximally with an origin from the superficial transverse septum in the distal forearm, extended through Guyon's canal above the ulnar nerve and vessels, fused with abductor digiti minimi, and had a typical insertion onto the proximal phalanx of the fifth digit. Nation et al. (2019) describe a muscle with a similar presentation and term it "flexor digiti minimi longus." Flexor digiti minimi brevis is also associated with tensor capsularis articulationis metacarpophalangei digiti minimi, a supernumerary muscle that originates from the ligaments connecting the hamate and pisiform and inserts onto the metacarpophalangeal joint of digit five (Bergman et al. 1988).

Prevalence

In a study of 35 hands, Murata et al. (2004) found that flexor digiti minimi brevis was absent in eight hands (22.9%), had one belly in 24 hands (68.6%), and had two bellies in three hands (8.6%). In a study of 38 individuals, May (2020) found that this muscle had one belly in 22 cases (58%), two bellies in eight cases (21%), and was absent in eight cases (21%).

Anomalies

Description

On the right side of a fetus with craniorachischisis, Alghamdi et al. (2017) observed that the flexor digiti minimi brevis potentially originated from the trapezoid and inserted onto the proximal phalanx of the fourth digit. Flexor digiti minimi brevis was normal on the left side of this specimen. Flexor digiti minimi brevis has been observed to have an anomalous insertion in infants with Neu-Laxova syndrome (Shved et al. 1985).

Prevalence

In a study of six upper limbs from three infants with Neu-Laxova syndrome, Shved et al. (1985) found that flexor digiti minimi brevis had an anomalous insertion in three upper limbs (50%).

Clinical Implications

Variant origins, insertions, or accessory slips associated with flexor digiti minimi brevis can lead to ulnar nerve compression (Spinner et al. 1996; Madhavi and Holla 2003; Wingerter et al. 2003; Georgiev and Jelev 2007) or potentially ulnar artery thrombosis (Pribyl and Moneim 1994).

OPPONENS DIGITI MINIMI (FIGURE 3.19)

Synonyms

This muscle may also be referred to as opponens digiti quinti (Sullivan and Osgood 1927) or opponens minimi digiti (Macalister 1875).

Typical Presentation

Description

Opponens digiti minimi originates from the hook of the hamate and the flexor retinaculum and inserts along the ulnar border and palmar surface of the fifth metacarpal (Standring 2016). It is frequently divided into two layers by the deep branches of the ulnar artery and ulnar nerve (Doyle and Botte 2003; Standring 2016).

Innervation

Opponens digiti minimi is innervated by the deep branch of the ulnar nerve (Standring 2016).

Comparative Anatomy

Opponens digiti minimi generally has a similar typical presentation in the apes, except the division into a superficial and deep layer may be poorly differentiated in some specimens, and the origin is often blended with flexor digiti minimi brevis (Lewis 1989; Gibbs 1999; Diogo et al. 2010, 2012, 2013a,b, 2017).

Variations

Description

Opponens digiti minimi may be absent (Macalister 1875). Opponens digiti minimi may be partially blended with the adjacent muscles, including the flexor digiti minimi brevis or abductor digiti minimi (Macalister 1875; Tountas and Bergman 1993; Doyle and Botte 2003; Gonzalez and Netscher 2016; Standring 2016). This muscle may be functionally related to ulnaris externis brevis, which originates near the distal end of the ulna and inserts onto the fourth and fifth metacarpals (Bergman et al. 1988).

Prevalence

N/A

Anomalies

Description

Opponens digiti minimi had a generally normal presentation on both upper limbs of a fetus with craniorachischisis dissected by Alghamdi et al. (2017), but the right opponens digiti minimi had a connection to the pisiform cartilage in addition to the hamate. The absence of opponens digiti minimi has been observed in infants with Neu-Laxova syndrome (Shved et al. 1985).

Prevalence

In a study of six upper limbs from three infants with Neu-Laxova syndrome, Shved et al. (1985) found that opponens digiti minimi was absent in three upper limbs (50%).

Clinical Implications

An accessory opponens digiti minimi can be mistaken for a soft-tissue tumor of the hand (Tountas and Bergman 1993; Gonzalez and Netscher 2016).

Abductor pollicis brevis (Figure 3.19)

Synonyms

N/A

Typical Presentation

Description

Abductor pollicis brevis originates primarily from the flexor retinaculum, with additional fibers arising from the scaphoid, trapezium, and abductor pollicis longus tendon (Standring 2016). It inserts via a tendon onto the radial side of the base of the proximal phalanx and dorsal digital expansion of the first digit (Standring 2016).

Innervation

Abductor pollicis brevis is innervated by the recurrent branch of the median nerve (Standring 2016).

Comparative Anatomy

Abductor pollicis brevis has a similar typical presentation in the apes, arising from the flexor retinaculum and sometimes the trapezium, adjacent sesamoid bone, and the scaphoid and inserting onto the proximal phalanx of digit one (Gibbs 1999; Diogo et al. 2010, 2012, 2013a, 2017). The muscle

attachment may extend to the distal end of the first metacarpal or distal phalanx of the first digit in gibbons, gorillas, and common chimpanzees (Kohlbrügge 1890–1892; Hepburn 1892; Dwight 1895; Raven 1950; Preuschoft 1965; Diogo et al. 2010, 2012, 2013a).

Variations

Description

Abductor pollicis brevis can be divided into an outer and inner part (Bergman et al. 1988) or into multiple fascicles (Jan and Rooze 1994). The entire muscle may be absent or doubled (Macalister 1875; Bergman et al. 1988; Tountas and Bergman 1993; Doyle and Botte 2003; Gonzalez and Netscher 2016). It may have a third head that originates from opponens pollicis (Wood 1868; Macalister 1875; Bergman et al. 1988; Tountas and Bergman 1993). Abductor pollicis brevis may receive slips from extensor pollicis brevis, extensor pollicis longus, opponens pollicis, scaphoid, or the styloid process of the radius (Macalister 1875; Bergman et al. 1988; Standring 2016; Gonzalez and Netscher 2016). It can also be connected to abductor pollicis longus, adductor pollicis, extensor carpi radialis longus, flexor pollicis brevis, palmaris longus, or the skin over the thenar eminence (Macalister 1875; Bergman et al. 1988; Gonzalez and Netscher 2016).

Prevalence

N/A

Anomalies

Description

On the left side of a fetus with craniorachischisis, Alghamdi et al. (2017) found that abductor pollicis brevis formed a u-shaped structure with the tendons of extensor pollicis brevis and flexor pollicis longus. Abductor pollicis brevis was absent on the right side of a fetus with trisomy 18 and cyclopia studied by Smith et al. (2015). On the left side of this specimen, abductor pollicis brevis was blended with some tendons of abductor pollicis longus. Furthermore, abductor pollicis brevis, opponens pollicis, and flexor pollicis brevis were all fused (Smith et al. 2015). Absence and anomalous insertion of abductor pollicis brevis has been observed in infants with Neu-Laxova syndrome (Shved et al. 1985).

Prevalence

In their literature review, Smith et al. (2015) found that abductor pollicis brevis was diminutive in 5 out of 26 individuals with trisomy 18 (19.2%). They also found that abductor pollicis brevis was absent in 1 out of 24 individuals with trisomy 13 (4.2%) and in 9 out of 26 individuals with trisomy 18 (34.6%). In a study of six upper limbs from three infants with Neu-Laxova syndrome, Shved et al. (1985) found absence of abductor pollicis brevis in two upper limbs (33%) and anomalous insertion in two upper limbs (33%).

Clinical Implications

An accessory abductor pollicis brevis may be mistaken for a soft-tissue tumor of the hand or lead to compression of the recurrent motor branch of the median nerve (Tountas and Bergman 1993; Gonzalez and Netscher 2016).

Abductor digiti minimi (Figure 3.19)

Synonyms

This muscle may also be referred to as abductor minimi digiti (Macalister 1875).

Typical Presentation

Description

Abductor digiti minimi originates from the pisiform, flexor carpi ulnaris tendon, and the ligament that connects the pisiform and hamate (Standring 2016). It ends in a bifurcated tendon that inserts onto the base of the proximal phalanx and the extensor expansion of digit five (Standring 2016).

Innervation

Abductor digiti minimi is innervated by the deep branch of the ulnar nerve (Standring 2016).

Comparative Anatomy

Abductor digiti minimi has a similar typical presentation in the apes, arising from the pisiform and sometimes the flexor retinaculum and/or hamate and inserting onto the proximal phalanx of digit five (Kohlbrügge 1890–1892; Hepburn 1892; Swindler and Wood 1973; Gibbs 1999; Diogo et al. 2010, 2012, 2013a,b, 2017). The insertion may be blended with flexor digiti minimi brevis (Hepburn 1892; Gibbs 1999; Diogo et al. 2012). Preuschoft (1965) observed an additional origin from the triquetrum in one gorilla. There may be an additional insertion onto the distal end of the fifth metacarpal in gibbons (Deniker 1885; Diogo et al. 2012).

Variations

Description

Abductor digiti minimi may be absent (Macalister 1875; Bergman et al. 1988; Tountas and Bergman 1993; Gonzalez and Netscher 2016). Abductor digiti minimi may be divided into two or three slips (Macalister 1875; Knott 1883a; Bergman et al. 1988; Murata et al. 2004; Standring 2016). It may also be fused with flexor digiti minimi brevis (Macalister 1875; Kaplan 1965; Bergman et al. 1988; Tountas and Bergman 1993; Gonzalez and Netscher 2016; Standring 2016). Additional fibers of abductor digiti minimi may originate from the flexor retinaculum, extensor retinaculum, antebrachial fascia, the palmaris longus tendon, the flexor carpi ulnaris tendon, or the extensor carpi ulnaris tendon (Wood 1866, 1868; Macalister 1875; Knott 1883a; Perkins and Hast 1993; Gonzalez and Netscher

2016; Standring 2016). It may have a connection to the fifth metacarpal via a slip from the pisiform (Standring 2016). Macalister (1875) reports an origin entirely from the pisiform.

Bergman et al. (1988), Tountas and Bergman (1993), and many others have described the presentation of an accessory head of this muscle, termed accessorius ad abductorem digiti minimi manus, otherwise known as an accessory abductor digiti minimi muscle or abductor digiti minimi accessorius. When present, it can originate from a variety of structures including from the flexor retinaculum, the tendon of flexor carpi ulnaris, the tendon of palmaris longus, the tendon of pronator quadratus, the antebrachial fascia, the radius, the ulna, or from the intermuscular fascia beneath flexor carpi ulnaris or flexor carpi radialis (Bergman et al. 1988; Tountas and Bergman 1993; Curry and Kuz 2000; Claassen et al. 2013; Gonzalez and Netscher 2016). This accessory head can insert into the main belly of abductor digiti minimi or flexor digiti minimi brevis (Bergman et al. 1988; Gonzalez and Netscher 2016). It can also have insertions into the fifth metacarpal, the proximal phalanx of the fifth digit, or into the palmar ligament of the metacarpophalangeal joint of the fifth digit (Bergman et al. 1988; Sañudo et al. 1993; Curry and Kuz 2000).

Abductor digiti minimi is associated with three other supernumerary slips. Pisimetacarpeus may extend from the pisiform to the fifth metacarpal (Bergman et al. 1988; Tountas and Bergman 1993; Gonzalez and Netscher 2016). Pisiuncinatus has been termed to describe a muscle extending between the pisiform and hamate (Bergman et al. 1988; Tountas and Bergman 1993; Gonzalez and Netscher 2016). Pisiannularis extends from the pisiform to the flexor retinaculum (Bergman et al. 1988; Tountas and Bergman 1993; Gonzalez and Netscher 2016).

Prevalence

Bergman et al. (1988) state that pisiuncinatus has a prevalence of between 2% and 5%. Based on dissections of 80 hands from 40 individuals, Perkins and Hast (1993) found that abductor digiti minimi had extra slips of origin from various structures (e.g., belly or tendon of palmaris longus, fascia of the forearm, flexor retinaculum) in 8 out of 80 hands (10%). Sañudo et al. (1993) note the presence of accessory bundles of abductor digiti minimi in 2 out of 62 forearms (3.2%). In a study of 35 hands, Murata et al. (2004) found that abductor digiti minimi had one belly in six hands (17.1%), two bellies in 28 hands (80%), and three bellies in one hand (2.9%). May (2020) found accessory muscles associated with abductor digiti minimi in 2 out of 76 hands (2.6%).

Anomalies

Description

Abductor digiti minimi with a high insertion has been observed in infants with Neu-Laxova syndrome (Shved et al. 1985).

Prevalence

According to their literature review, Smith et al. (2015) found that abductor digiti minimi had extra slips and tendons in 1 out of 24 individuals with trisomy 13 (4.2%). In a study of six upper limbs from three infants with Neu-Laxova syndrome, Shved et al. (1985) found that abductor digiti minimi had a high insertion in two upper limbs (33%).

Clinical Implications

An accessory abductor digiti minimi may compress the deep palmar branch of the ulnar nerve (Tountas and Bergman 1993; Bergman et al. 1988; Gonzalez and Netscher 2016) or the median nerve (Soldado-Carrera et al. 2000). Accessory heads or muscle bellies of abductor digiti minimi may also compress the ulnar artery or lead to thrombosis or fibrosis of the ulnar artery (Tountas and Bergman 1993; Soldado-Carrera et al. 2000; Gonzalez and Netscher 2016). These accessory tissues may also be mistaken for soft tissue tumors (Soldado-Carrera et al. 2000).

4 Trunk Muscles

Eve K. Boyle
Howard University College of Medicine

Vondel S. E. Mahon
University of Maryland Medical Center

Rui Diogo
Howard University College of Medicine

Rowan Sherwood
University of Michigan

CONTENTS

DOI: 10.1201/9781003083535-4

MUSCLES OF THE ABDOMINAL REGION

OBLIQUUS EXTERNUS ABDOMINIS (EXTERNAL OBLIQUE) (FIGURE 4.1)

See also: Obliquus abdominis externus profundus

Synonyms

N/A

Typical Presentation

Description

External oblique is typically attached superiorly to ribs 5 through 12 (Standring 2016). The fibers from the lowest ribs attach inferiorly to the iliac crest while the fibers from the middle and upper ribs end in the external oblique aponeurosis, which forms the inguinal ligament and the anterior layer of the rectus sheath (Saga and Takahashi 2016; Standring 2016).

Innervation

External oblique is innervated by the lower five intercostal nerves and the subcostal nerve (Standring 2016).

Comparative Anatomy

External oblique has a similar typical presentation in the apes, extending from the lower ribs to the pelvic region, and may vary in which rib provides the superiormost attachment (Diogo et al. 2010, 2012, 2013a,b, 2017). The external

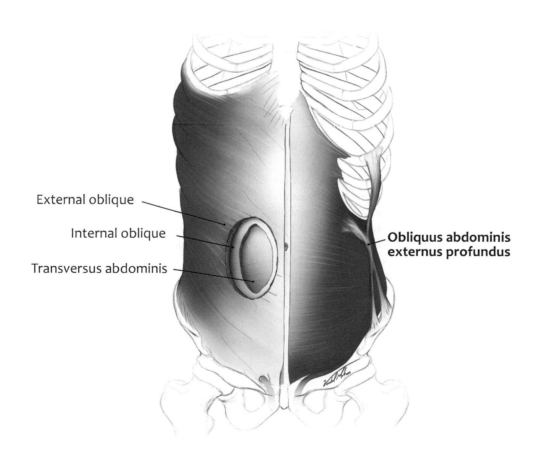

External oblique
Internal oblique
Transversus abdominis

Obliquus abdominis externus profundus

FIGURE 4.1 Lateral abdominal muscles in anterior view.

oblique of bonobos is innervated by the lower intercostal nerves and also by iliohypogastric and ilioinguinal nerves (Miller 1952).

Variations

Description

The external oblique can vary in the number of costal attachments (Macalister 1875; Mori 1964; Rickenbacher et al. 1985; Bergman et al. 1988; Standring 2016; Saga and Takahashi 2016). Some attachments, or even the entire muscle, may be doubled (Knott 1883b; Macalister 1875; Bergman et al. 1988; Standring 2016). The superiormost and inferiormost attachments, or even the entire muscle, can also be absent (Knott 1883b; Macalister 1875; Standring 2016; Dsouza et al. 2017). External oblique can have connections to, or may be continuous with, pectoralis major, serratus anterior, latissimus dorsi, the external intercostals, or serratus posterior inferior (Knott 1883b; Macalister 1875; Bergman et al. 1988; Standring 2016). Additional slips may originate from the lower ribs, the transverse process of the first lumbar vertebra, the lumbar fascia below rib 12, or the fascia over the fifth or sixth intercostal space (Macalister 1875; Rickenbacher et al. 1985; Bergman et al. 1988).

The external oblique is associated with three variable supernumerary muscles. The saphenous muscle refers to a slip of muscle that is attached to the inguinal ligament and loops under the saphenofemoral junction, blending with sartorius and the adductor longus (Tyrie 1894; du Plessis and Loukas 2016; Saga and Takahashi 2016). The interfoveolar muscle refers to muscle fibers within the interfoveolar ligament (Kudo and Otobe 1952; Saga and Takahashi 2016). Obliquus externus abdominis profundus refers to variable bundles that are occasionally associated with the external oblique (see the entry for this muscle).

Prevalence

Based on a sample of 166 Japanese adults (332 sides), Mori (1964) found that the superiormost attachment of the external oblique was from the fourth rib in only 12% of cases on the left side (0% on the right side), the fifth rib in 84.3% of cases on the left side and 81.9% of cases on the right side, the sixth rib in 14.4% of cases on the left side and 18.1% of cases on the right side, and never from the seventh rib (0%). Kudo and Otobe (1952) recorded the presence of the interfoveolar muscle in 46% of their study population.

Anomalies

Description

Poland syndrome can lead to the absence of the external oblique (Cingel et al. 2013). Prune belly syndrome is also associated with the partial reduction or complete absence of this muscle (Adebonojo 1973).

Prevalence

N/A

Clinical Implications

Dsouza et al. (2017) observe that the bilateral absence of the external oblique and its aponeurosis can increase the risk for hernia.

OBLIQUUS ABDOMINIS EXTERNUS PROFUNDUS (FIGURE 4.1)

See also: Obliquus externus abdominis

Synonyms

This muscle is also referred to as obliquus externus secundus s. accessorius (Gruber 1875a), obliquus externus profundus s. minor (Knott 1880), and obliquus externus abdominis minor s. secundus (Knott 1883b) (Saga and Takahashi 2016).

Typical Presentation

This muscle is only present as a variation.

Comparative Anatomy

N/A

Variations

Description

Obliquus abdominis externus profundus refers to distinct muscle bellies that are variably associated with the external oblique. It may present as a deep accessory bundle that originates from the middle/lower ribs or the internal oblique fascia to attach to the anterior superior iliac spine, iliac crest, inguinal ligament, or rectus sheath (Macalister 1875; Knott 1883a,b; Nakayama and Okuda, 1952; Bergman et al. 1988; Saga and Takahashi 2016). This muscle can have two heads (Nakayama and Okuda 1952; Miyauchi et al. 1986). Knott (1883b) records an origin from ribs nine and ten. Nakayama and Okuda (1952) report an origin from the eleventh rib. Miyauchi et al. (1986) record origins from ribs five, six, or seven. It can either be fused with the external oblique or separated from it via a layer of fascia (Macalister 1875; Miyauchi et al. 1986; Bergman et al. 1988).

Miyauchi et al. (1986) note the confusion in the literature of the many variant bundles that have been given the name obliquus abdominis externus profundus, and these authors as well as Kodama (1986) argue for classification of these bundles based on innervation (Saga and Takahashi 2016).

Innervation

Obliquus abdominis externus profundus is supplied by the ramus muscularis externus from the intercostal nerve of the corresponding segment (Miyauchi et al. 1986).

Prevalence

Earlier studies typically report a prevalence for this muscle <10%. Loth (1912, 1931) reports a prevalence of 3.8% in Black individuals and 7% in Europeans. Kudo and Otobe (1952) report a prevalence of 3% in a Chinese population. Nakayama and Okuda (1952) report a prevalence of 1.9%. More recent studies provide higher prevalence rates. Kodama

(1986) reports a prevalence of 36.5%. This muscle was present in 11 out of 50 sides (22%), from 8 out of the 25 Japanese cadavers studied by Miyauchi et al. (1986). Miyauchi et al. (1986) found that the muscle originated via one slip from the fifth rib in two cases, from the sixth rib in six cases, and from the seventh rib in one case. It originated via two slips from the fifth and sixth ribs in two cases. Obliquus abdominis externus profundus was fused with the external oblique in four cases (8%) (Miyauchi et al. 1986).

Anomalies

N/A

Clinical Implications

N/A

OBLIQUUS INTERNUS ABDOMINIS (INTERNAL OBLIQUE) (FIGURES 4.1 AND 4.2)

Synonyms

N/A

Typical Presentation

Description

Internal oblique is deep to external oblique (Standring 2016). It originates from the iliopectineal arch, iliac crest, and the thoracolumbar fascia (Standring 2016). The fibers originating from the iliopectineal arch fuse with the aponeurosis of transversus abdominis and attach to the pubis and pectineal line to form the conjoint tendon (Standring 2016). The fibers that originate from the iliac crest end in the anterior aponeurosis that forms the rectus sheath, and the posterior fibers insert onto the cartilage and inferior borders of ribs 8/9 to rib 12 (Standring 2016).

Innervation

Internal oblique is innervated by the lower five intercostal nerves, the subcostal nerve, the iliohypogastric nerve, and the ilioinguinal nerve (Standring 2016).

Comparative Anatomy

Internal oblique has a similar typical presentation in the apes, extending from the iliac crest, thoracolumbar fascia, and inguinal ligament to join the rectus sheath, lower four ribs, and the pubis via the conjoint tendon (Sonntag 1923; Miller 1952; Gibbs 1999; Diogo et al. 2010, 2012, 2013a,b, 2017).

Variations

Description

Internal oblique can vary in its costal attachments, and the inguinal or anterior superior part of this muscle may be absent (Macalister 1875; Mori 1964; Rickenbacher et al. 1985; Bergman et al. 1988). A fibrous band that is a tendinous connection between internal oblique and the internal intercostal muscles often "interrupts" the muscle, typically opposite the tenth or eleventh rib, but it can also be present opposite the eighth or twelfth rib (Macalister 1875; Knott 1883b; Bergman et al. 1988). The internal oblique muscle fascia may also be connected to the fascia of the external oblique (Tekelioglu et al. 2015).

An additional slip can connect to the eighth costal cartilage or the transverse process of the second lumbar vertebra (Bergman et al. 1988). Internal oblique can be fused with transversus abdominis (Macalister 1875; Knott 1883b; Standring 2016). The portion of the muscle that arises from the iliac crest may be separated into an anterior and posterior part, the latter of which is referred to as accessory internal oblique (Chouke 1935; Bergman et al. 1988). There are variations in how the aponeurosis of internal oblique contributes to the rectus sheath (see prevalence information, below). The rectus sheath can also vary in the degree to which it is aponeurotic, as in some cases the sheath can be more muscular (Monkhouse and Khalique 1986).

Prevalence

Loth (1912) found that the superiormost attachment of the internal oblique was onto rib 11 in 31% of cases, rib 10 in 66.5% of cases, rib 9 in 1% of cases, and rib 8 in 1.5% of cases. In a sample of 200 individuals, Mori (1964) also observed that the most common superior costal attachments were to rib 10 (56% of right sides, 64% of left sides) and rib 11 (34% of right sides, 36% of left sides). According to Monkhouse and Khalique (1986), Chouke (1935) reported an accessory internal oblique with high incidence in a population of 136 cadavers, in which the accessory muscle was only absent four times (97% prevalence).

In a sample of 40 cadavers, Monkhouse and Khalique (1986) found that in 24 cases (60%) the aponeurosis of internal oblique split to enclose rectus abdominis, with the aponeurosis of external oblique remaining anterior and the aponeurosis of transversus abdominis remaining posterior. In 11 cases (27.5%), the aponeurosis of internal oblique passed entirely anterior to rectus abdominis, while the aponeurosis of transversus abdominis remained posterior to rectus abdominis. In five cases (12.5%), the aponeurosis of transversus abdominis split to enclose rectus abdominis, and the anterior layer of this aponeurosis fused with the aponeuroses of both the external and internal obliques. Saga and Takahashi (2016) compare this study with that of McVay and Anson (1940) and note that the latter authors found variations corresponding to the third presentation described by Monkhouse and Khalique (1986) in 43 out of 56 cases (76.8%) and two cases (3.6%) that corresponded to the first presentation described by these authors.

Anomalies

Description

Prune belly syndrome is associated with the partial reduction or complete absence of this muscle (Adebonojo 1973).

Prevalence

N/A

Clinical Implications

Fibrous adhesions between the fascia of the internal oblique and the external oblique and other fibrous bands within this muscle can prevent a successful transverse abdominis plane (TAP) block procedure (Tekelioglu et al. 2015; Lew and Gray 2012).

TRANSVERSUS ABDOMINIS (FIGURE 4.1)

Synonyms

This muscle may also be referred to as transversalis (Macalister 1875) or transversalis abdominis (Knott 1883b).

Typical Presentation

Description

Transversus abdominis is deep to both the internal and external oblique (Standring 2016). It originates from the iliopectineal arch, iliac crest, thoracolumbar fascia, and the lower six costal cartilages (Standring 2016). The muscle ends in an aponeurosis that inserts mostly into the rectus sheath (Standring 2016; Saga and Takahashi 2016). Its lower fibers fuse with the aponeurosis of internal oblique to form the conjoint tendon and insert onto the pubis and pectineal line (Standring 2016).

Innervation

Transversus abdominis is supplied by the lower five intercostal nerves, the subcostal nerve, the iliohypogastric nerve, and the ilioinguinal nerve (Standring 2016).

Comparative Anatomy

Transversus abdominis has a similar typical presentation in the apes, with attachments to the lower costal cartilages, thoracolumbar fascia, and iliac crest and contributions to the conjoint tendon and posterior layer of the rectus sheath (Champneys 1872; Sonntag 1923; Miller 1952; Gibbs 1999; Diogo et al. 2010, 2012, 2013a,b, 2017).

Variations

Description

Transversus abdominis may be absent in rare cases (Macalister 1875; Rickenbacher et al. 1985; Bergman et al. 1988; Saga and Takahashi 2016; Standring 2016). It may also be doubled (Macalister 1875). The attachments of transversus abdominis to the ribs can vary in number, generally ranging from five attachments to seven attachments (Macalister 1875; Knott 1883b; Bergman et al. 1988). Transversus abdominis can be fused with internal oblique (Macalister 1875; Knott 1883b; Standring 2016). A tendinous intersection may be present (Macalister 1875). The spermatic cord may travel through the inferior portion of transversus abdominis (Macalister 1875; Knott 1883b; Saga and Takahashi 2016). There are variations in how the aponeurosis of transversus abdominis contributes to the rectus sheath (see the entry for obliquus internus abdominis for prevalence information).

A supernumerary muscle termed tensor laminae posterioris vaginae musculi rectus or puboperitonealis may be present (Gruber 1873a,b; Macalister 1875; Bergman et al. 1988; Saga and Takahashi 2016). This muscle is comprised of slips that originate inferiorly from the iliopectineal line and transversus fascia and interdigitate with transversus abdominis (Gruber 1873a,b; Macalister 1875; Saga and Takahashi 2016).

Prevalence

Knott (1883b) found that in 29 out of 36 cases (80.6%) transversus abdominis had six costal attachments, in four cases there were seven costal attachments (11.1%), and in three cases there were five costal attachments (8.3%). Anson and McVay (1938) report that transversus abdominis arises from the whole of the inguinal ligament in only 3% of cases.

Anomalies

Description

Macalister (1875) notes that Charvet found the absence of transversus abdominis in ectopia vesicae. Prune belly syndrome is also associated with the partial reduction or complete absence of this muscle (Adebonojo 1973).

Prevalence

N/A

Clinical Implications

N/A

RECTUS ABDOMINIS (FIGURE 4.2)

Synonyms

N/A

Typical Presentation

Description

Rectus abdominis spans the length of the anterior abdominal wall (Standring 2016). It originates by a lateral tendon that is attached to the pubic crest and a medial tendon that is attached closer to the pubic symphysis (Standring 2016). Rectus abdominis typically attaches superiorly to the fifth through seventh costal cartilages and to the xiphoid process (Standring 2016). Rectus abdominis is interrupted by three transverse tendinous intersections that typically intersect the muscle at (1) the level of umbilicus, (2) the level of the end of the xiphoid process, and (3) the area approximately midway between those two (Standring 2016).

Innervation

Rectus abdominis is innervated by the lower six or seven thoracic spinal nerves and sometimes the ilioinguinal nerve (Standring 2016).

Comparative Anatomy

Rectus abdominis has not been described in gibbons (Diogo et al. 2012). In gorillas, it extends from the xiphisternum and

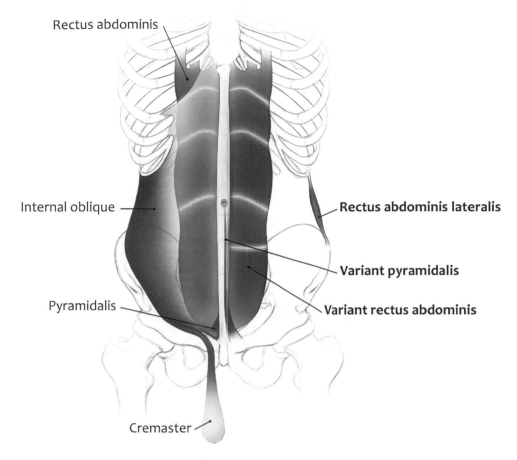

Rectus abdominis

Internal oblique

Pyramidalis

Cremaster

Rectus abdominis lateralis

Variant pyramidalis

Variant rectus abdominis

FIGURE 4.2   Medial abdominal muscles and rectus abdominis lateralis in anterior view.

costal cartilages five through nine to the ventral spine of the pubis and symphyseal ligament (Gibbs 1999; Diogo et al. 2010). In common chimpanzees and bonobos, it extends from the costal cartilages five through seven to the pubic crest and has four tendinous intersections (Champneys 1872; Sonntag 1923; Miller 1952; Gibbs 1999; Diogo et al. 2013a, 2017). Similarly, in orangutans, it extends between the lower costal cartilages and pubic crest and has four tendinous intersections (Diogo et al. 2013b).

Variations

Description

Rectus abdominis may be reduced, absent, or doubled (Macalister 1875; Knott 1883b; Bergman et al. 1988; Saga and Takahashi 2016). The tendinous intersections can vary in number and may only extend halfway across the muscle (Macalister 1875; Knott 1883b; Mori 1964; Sato 1968c; Saga and Takahashi 2016; Standring 2016). One or two incomplete intersections may be found below the level of umbilicus (Figure 4.2) (Macalister 1875; Knott 1883b; Standring 2016). The costal attachments can also vary in number (Macalister 1875; Mori 1964; Bergman et al. 1988; Saga and Takahashi 2016; Standring 2016). The slip to rib five may be absent (Bergman et al. 1988; Standring 2016). The superiormost attachment may extend to ribs two, three, or four, the sternum, or the clavicle (Macalister 1875; Knott

1883b; Bergman et al. 1988; Saga and Takahashi 2016; Standring 2016). Muscular slips may be found between the rectus abdominis and the deep inguinal ring (Bergman et al. 1988; Saga and Takahashi 2016). There are variations in how the aponeuroses of the muscles that surround rectus abdominis contribute to the rectus sheath (see the entry for obliquus internus abdominis for prevalence information).

Prevalence

Knott (1883b) studied the variation in the tendinous inscriptions of rectus abdominis in 60 cases. In two cases (3.3%), the tendinous inscription at the level of the xiphoid was absent unilaterally, and in two other cases, it was absent bilaterally (3.3%). In one case (1.7%), the inscription intermediate between that at the level of the xiphoid and that at the level of umbilicus was absent. In five cases (8.3%), an inscription below the level of umbilicus was present.

In a study of 400 sides from 200 cadavers by Mori (1964), he found that on 313 sides (78.25%), rectus abdominis attached to ribs five, six, and seven, which corresponds to Loth's (1912) "normal type." Three presentations correspond to Loth's (1912) "primitive type" and made up 8.1% of cases, including origin from ribs 4 and 5 on 8 sides (2%), origin from ribs 4, 5, and 6 on 12 sides (3%), and origin from ribs 5 and 6 on 13 sides (3.1%). Two presentations correspond to Loth's (1912) "progressive type" made up 13% of cases and include origin from ribs 6 and 7 in 32 cases

(8%) and origin from ribs 6, 7, and 8 in 20 cases (5%). Mori (1964) also found that tendinous intersections into the muscle varied among two (1% of cases), three (36% of cases), four (61% of cases), and five intersections (2% of cases).

Sato (1968c) reported that in Kyushu-Japanese males, three tendinous intersections were present in 250 out of 416 sides (60%), 4 in 125 sides (30%), 2 in 31 sides (7.45%), and 5 in 10 sides (2.4%). In females, three tendinous intersections were present in 153 out of 268 sides (57.1%), 4 in 83 sides (31%), 2 in 28 sides (10.4%), and 5 in 4 sides (1.5%).

Anomalies

Description

Macalister (1875) notes that Charvet found the absence of rectus abdominis in ectopia vesicae. Prune belly syndrome is associated with the partial reduction or complete absence of this muscle (Adebonojo 1973). Bersu and Ramirez-Castro (1977) and Aziz (1979) note that in individuals with trisomy 18, there may be poor development of the tendinous intersections of rectus abdominis. Diastasis recti can also occur in individuals with trisomy 18 (Aziz 1979; Roberts et al. 2016) and was observed in a female individual with XO/XY mosaicism and partial trisomy 9p (Klasen et al. 1981).

Mieden (1982) describes an infant with median cleft lip, hypotelorism, and alobar holoprosencephaly. On the left side, the intermediate tendinous intersection was 1 cm lower than that of the one on the right side (Mieden 1982). Itoh et al. (1991) describe fetal akinesia/hypokinesia sequence in one male and one female infant, each with a suite of anatomical anomalies. In the male, the rectus abdominis muscles showed focal atrophy.

Prevalence

Roberts et al. (2016) state that diastasis rectus abdominis, among other abdominal wall defects, is present in over 50% of individuals with trisomy 18.

Clinical Implications

N/A

RECTUS ABDOMINIS LATERALIS (FIGURE 4.2)

Synonyms

N/A

Typical Presentation

This muscle is only present as a variation.

Comparative Anatomy

N/A

Variations

Description

Rectus abdominis lateralis (Kelch) is a supernumerary muscle that is situated between the external and internal obliques (Macalister 1875; Saga and Takahashi 2016). It originates from the lower border of rib ten and descends

longitudinally to insert onto the iliac crest (Macalister 1875; Sato 1968c; Saga and Takahashi 2016). Sato (1968c) reported an origin from ribs 10 through 12.

Innervation

N/A

Prevalence

Sato (1968c) found that rectus abdominis lateralis was present in 18 out of 212 sides (8.49%) in Kyushu-Japanese females and in 32 out of 324 sides (9.88%) in males.

Anomalies

N/A

Clinical Implications

N/A

PYRAMIDALIS (FIGURE 4.2)

Synonyms

This muscle is also referred to as pyramidalis abdominis (Knott 1883b).

Typical Presentation

Description

Pyramidalis is a triangular muscle situated anterior to the lower portion of rectus abdominis within the rectus sheath (Standring 2016). It originates from the pubis and in an apex that is attached to the linea alba about halfway between the pubis and umbilicus (Standring 2016).

Innervation

Pyramidalis is typically innervated by the subcostal nerve (Standring 2016). It is occasionally supplied by the iliohypogastric or ilioinguinal nerves (Bergman et al. 1988; Standring 2016).

Comparative Anatomy

Pyramidalis has not been described in orangutans (Ashley-Montagu 1939; Gibbs 1999; Diogo et al. 2013b). It is often absent in the other apes, though its presence has been described in some dissection descriptions for gorillas, gibbons, bonobos, and common chimpanzees (Ashley-Montagu 1939; Miller 1952; Diogo et al. 2010, 2012, 2013a, 2017). Ashley-Montagu (1939) reports that it is present in about 36% of gibbons, 33% of gorillas, and about 60% of chimpanzees.

Variations

Description

Pyramidalis varies substantially in size between individuals (Bergman et al. 1988; Standring 2016). The average length is about 6–7 cm, and the average width is about 1.5–2 cm (Anson et al. 1938; Sinha and Kumar 1985; Saga and Takahashi 2016). Pyramidalis may extend to umbilicus (Macalister 1875) or send a tendinous slip to umbilicus (Knott 1883b) (Figure 4.2). This muscle may also be interrupted by a tendinous intersection (Macalister 1875; Knott 1883b). Pyramidalis can be doubled unilaterally or bilaterally (Winslow 1732; Cruveilhier 1837; Hallett 1848; Macalister 1875; Le Double 1897; Chudzinski 1898; Anson et al. 1938; Saga and Takahashi 2016; Standring 2016).

Pyramidalis is often asymmetric and may be absent unilaterally or bilaterally (Macalister 1875; Knott 1883b; Chouke 1935; Anson et al. 1938; Beaton and Anson 1939; Mori 1964; Sato 1968c; Sinha and Kumar 1985; Monkhouse and Khalique 1986; Bergman et al. 1988; Dickson 1999; Didia et al. 2009; Natsis et al. 2016; Saga and Takahashi 2016; Standring 2016; Das et al. 2017). When it is absent, the size of the lower portion of the rectus abdominis (Bergman et al. 1988) or the internal oblique (Macalister 1875) may be increased.

Prevalence

Saga and Takahashi (2016) report that it is absent in 10% of cases. Knott (1883b) found that this muscle was absent bilaterally in 9 out of 60 subjects (15%) and absent unilaterally in five subjects (8.3%). In six subjects (10%), the left muscle was smaller than the right. A tendinous slip extending to umbilicus was present in one subject (1.7%), and a horizontal tendinous inscription was present bilaterally in another (1.7%) (Knott 1883b). Based on a study of 123 cadavers, Chouke (1935) reported that pyramidalis was absent in over 23% of cases. Anson et al. (1938) reported that this muscle was absent in 10.8% of 165 subjects. Beaton and Anson (1939) reported unilateral or bilateral absence in 20.3% of a White population and in 12.5% of a Black population.

Summarizing the work of other Japanese researchers, Mori (1964) notes that pyramidalis is absent in about 5%–6% of Japanese individuals. Mori (1964) also found that the most common presentation (21.7% of cases) of this muscle was the apex of right pyramidalis being higher than the left, and the origin of the left pyramidalis elongated to the surface of the pubis. Other presentations of this muscle include: the apex of the left pyramidalis is higher than the right, and the origin of the right muscle is elongated to the surface of the pubis (19.3%); the apex of the right pyramidalis is higher than the left, and the origin of the right muscle is elongated to the surface of the pubis (15.7%); the apex of the left pyramidalis is higher than the right and its origin is elongated to the pubis (13.3%); the apex of the muscle on both sides is at the same level and the right origin is elongated to the anterior surface of the pubis (9.6%); the apex of the right pyramidalis is higher than the left, and the origin of the muscle on both sides is at the same level (6%); the apex of the left pyramidalis is higher than the right, and the origin of both sides is at the same level (3.6%), the apex of the muscle on both sides is at the same level, and the left origin is elongated to the anterior surface of the pubis (2.4%); and the pyramidalis is divided into two parts (1.1%).

Sato (1968c) reported that pyramidalis is absent in 47 out of 424 sides (11.08%) from Kyushu-Japanese males and absent in 30 out of 274 sides (10.95%) in females. In a study of 31 Indian male cadavers, Sinha and Kumar (1985) found that pyramidalis was absent bilaterally in 5.88% and absent unilaterally in 2.94% of cadavers. Pyramidalis was present on only 4 out of 112 sides (3.6%) of the 56 cadavers examined Monkhouse and Khalique (1986). Dickson (1999) found that pyramidalis was absent in 42 out of 60 northern European female subjects (70%). Didia et al. (2009) observed that this muscle was absent in 2 out of 24 Nigerian male cadavers (8.33%). In a study of 96 Greek cadavers (50 male, 46 female), Natsis et al. (2016) found that pyramidalis was absent in 6.2% of specimens, was more often present bilaterally, and more often present in females (91.3% of specimens) than in males (68% of specimens). In a study of 25 Indian cadavers (17 male, 8 female), Das et al. (2017) found that pyramidalis was absent in 8% of cases, was more often present bilaterally, and was more often present in males (94.11%) than in females (87.5%).

Anomalies

N/A

Clinical Implications

Understanding variation in the presentation of pyramidalis is important during imaging, so as to not mistake it for a mass (Natsis et al. 2016).

CREMASTER (FIGURE 4.2)

Synonyms

N/A

Typical Presentation

Description

Cremaster covers the spermatic cord and extends to the testis (Standring 2016). It originates from the inferomedial border of the internal oblique and transversus abdominis and attaches medially to the pubis (Standring 2016). In females, cremaster is represented by fibers on the round ligament of the uterus (Bergman et al. 1988; Standring 2016).

Innervation

Cremaster is innervated by the genital branch of the genitofemoral nerve (Standring 2016).

Comparative Anatomy

Cremaster has a similar typical presentation in the apes, extending from the internal oblique and transversus abdominis towards the "inguinal ligament" (Miller 1952; Gibbs 1999; Diogo et al. 2010, 2012, 2013a,b, 2017). As Gibbs (1999) notes, apes do not have a true inguinal ligament but a series of tendinous arches over the femoral vessels and nerves in the inguinal region.

Variations

Description

Cremaster is thickest in younger males (Standring 2016). The medial portion of the muscle that attaches to the pubis may be absent (Standring 2016). Cremaster may originate from the transversalis fascia or fuse with transversus abdominis (Macalister 1875; Knott 1883b; Bergman et al. 1988; Saga and Takahashi 2016). It may also have two heads (Macalister 1875; Bergman et al. 1988).

Prevalence
N/A

Anomalies
N/A

Clinical Implications
N/A

QUADRATUS LUMBORUM (FIGURE 4.3)

Synonyms
This muscle may also be referred to as ileolumbalis (Meyer), scalenus lumborum (Meyer), or rectus abdominis posticus (Luschka) (Knott 1883b; Macalister 1875; Bakkum and Miller 2016).

Typical Presentation
Description
Quadratus lumborum is part of the posterior abdominal wall. It attaches inferiorly to the iliac crest and iliolumbar ligament, medially to the transverses processes of the upper four lumbar vertebrae, and superiorly to the twelfth rib and twelfth thoracic vertebra (Standring 2016).

Innervation
Quadratus lumborum is innervated by the twelfth thoracic nerve and upper three/four lumbar spinal nerves (Standring 2016).

Comparative Anatomy
Quadratus lumborum has a similar typical presentation in the apes, extending from the iliac crest to the upper lumbar vertebrae and last rib (Gibbs 1999; Diogo et al. 2010, 2012, 2013a,b, 2017). In bonobos, the muscle may extend to the penultimate rib (Miller 1952; Diogo et al. 2017).

Variations
Description
The bundles that comprise quadratus lumborum may vary in size and number (Macalister 1875; Knott 1883b; Rickenbacher et al. 1985; Standring 2016). The extent of the development of the attachments to the vertebrae and the number of these attachments may vary (Macalister 1875; Knott 1883b; Rickenbacher et al. 1985; Bergman et al. 1988; Bakkum and Miller 2016). The superior attachment of this muscle may extend to rib eleven, and the superomedial attachment may extend to the tenth and/or eleventh thoracic vertebrae (Knott 1883b; Macalister 1875; Rickenbacher et al. 1985; Bergman et al. 1988; Bakkum and Miller 2016; Saga and Takahashi 2016).

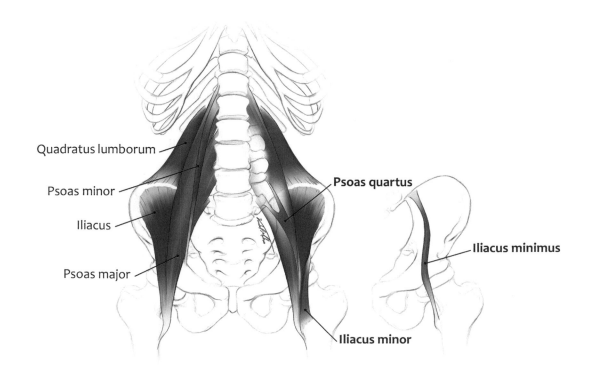

FIGURE 4.3 Posterior abdominal wall muscles in anterior view. Iliacus minimus is illustrated on the right side, and the other muscles are illustrated on the left side.

Prevalence

Knott (1883b) found that the attachment to the body of the twelfth thoracic vertebra was present in 8 out of 30 specimens (26.7%). This author also found that two specimens exhibited a slip to the eleventh thoracic vertebra, one specimen had a slip to the eleventh rib, and three specimens had slips to both the eleventh and twelfth thoracic vertebrae. It is not clear if these six cases are part of the 30 subjects or another unspecified sample size.

Anomalies

Description

Prune belly syndrome may be associated with the partial reduction or complete absence of this muscle (King et al. 1961). Bersu et al. (1976) describe a male infant with Hanhart syndrome. On both sides of this infant, there was an extensive fusion between the lumbar muscular components of the diaphragm, psoas major, and quadratus lumborum.

Prevalence

N/A

Clinical Implications

N/A

ILIACUS (FIGURE 4.3)

See also: Iliacus minor

Synonyms

N/A

Typical Presentation

Description

Iliacus originates from the upper two-thirds of the iliac fossa, the iliac crest, and the lateral aspect of the sacrum (Standring 2016). Iliacus forms the iliopsoas muscle with psoas major as the two insert together via a tendon onto the lesser trochanter of the femur (Standring 2016). Some fibers attach to the femur below the lesser trochanter (Standring 2016).

Innervation

Iliacus is innervated by branches of the femoral nerve (Standring 2016).

Comparative Anatomy

Iliacus has a similar typical presentation in the apes, extending from the iliac fossa to join with psoas major to insert onto the lesser trochanter (Champneys 1872; Hepburn 1892; Beddard 1893; Sigmon 1974; Gibbs 1999; Diogo et al. 2010, 2012, 2013a,b, 2017). Fibers may extend distally onto the femoral shaft in gibbons, orangutans, and bonobos (Hepburn 1892; Beddard 1893; Boyer 1935; Miller 1952; Sigmon 1974; Diogo ct al. 2012, 2013b, 2017).

Variations

Description

Iliacus may present as a completely separate muscle from psoas major (Macalister 1875; Bergman et al. 1988) or be completely fused with it (Aleksandrova et al. 2013; Saga and Takahashi 2016). The origin of iliacus may be fused with fibers from quadratus lumborum (Macalister 1875). The iliopsoas tendon may be partially or completely divided into one, two, or three tendons (Tatu et al. 2002; Polster et al. 2008; Shu and Safran 2011; Crompton et al. 2014; Philippon et al. 2014; Saga and Takahashi 2016). Macalister (1875) found the muscle itself divided in two. One or more accessory slips/muscle bundles may be present medial or lateral to iliacus (Macalister 1875; Bergman et al. 1988; Spratt et al. 1996; Jelev et al. 2005; Vázquez et al. 2007; Astik and Dave 2011; Saga and Takahashi 2016). Aleksandrova et al. (2013) categorize the variations of iliacus into ten types including partial agenesis, complete separation from psoas major, complete fusion with psoas major, the presence of accessory slips/muscle bundles, the presence of iliacus minor, the presence of iliacus minimus, and the division of the muscle into superficial and deep fibers.

Iliacus is associated with several named accessory slips and muscles (see the entry for iliacus minor). Also see the entry for psoas major for information on psoas quartus and psoas tertius. Jelev et al. (2005) describe an accessory iliopsoas muscle that resulted from the connection between an accessory iliacus muscle and an accessory psoas major. Iliacus minimus (Figure 4.3) refers to a slip that pierces the femoral nerve and inserts onto the lesser trochanter or joins the iliopsoas muscle or its tendon (Spratt et al. 1996; Tubbs and Salter 2006a; Aristotle et al. 2013; Aleksandrova et al. 2013; Saga and Takahashi 2016). It may originate from the iliolumbar ligament (Spratt et al. 1996; Tubbs and Salter 2006a) or from the iliac crest (Aristotle et al. 2013). In the case described by Spratt et al. (1996), the muscle divided into two tendons that inserted onto the lesser trochanter and the medial thigh.

Prevalence

Tatu et al. (2002) found that the iliopsoas tendon completely split into two bundles in 2 out of 24 cases (8.3%) and partially split into two bundles in two other cases (8.3%). Crompton et al. (2014) studied the iliopsoas tendon via MRI images in 50 children and found that at least one bifid tendon was present in 13 children (26%), and 5 out of the 37 children that were imaged bilaterally had bilateral bifid tendons (13.5%). Out of the total sample of 87 hips, 18 had two distinct distal iliopsoas tendons (20.7%) (Crompton et al. 2014). Philippon et al. (2014) found that the iliopsoas tendon was single-banded in 15 out of 53 cadaver hemipelves (28.3%), double-banded in 34 hemipelves (64.2%), and triple-banded in four hemipelves (7.5%).

Based on dissections of 68 cadavers, Spratt et al. (1996) found four variant slips (5.9%) which included one case of iliacus minimus, another accessory iliacus slip that extended between the sacrum and the lesser trochanter, and two accessory lateral slips of psoas major. Jelev et al. (2005) found what they define as an accessory iliopsoas in only 1 out of 108 cadavers over the course of 22 years of dissection (0.9%).

Vázquez et al. (2007) found accessory slips or sheets of iliacus and psoas piercing or covering the femoral nerve in 19 out of 242 specimens (7.9%) from 121 cadavers. The femoral nerve was pierced by a muscular slip in 17 specimens (7%), in a sample composed of 12 iliacus slips, four psoas slips, and a slip from both in one specimen. The femoral nerve was covered by a sheet or slip in two specimens (0.8%). Astik and Dave (2011) dissected 64 lumbar plexuses from 32 cadavers and found accessory slips of iliacus in two plexuses (3.1%). The slips originated from the transverse process of the fifth lumbar vertebra and iliolumbar ligament and split the femoral nerve into two branches.

Anomalies

Description

Iliacus can be very small in cases of congenital absence of the femur (Manohar 1939). Itoh et al. (1991) describe fetal akinesia/hypokinesia sequence in one male and one female infant, each with a suite of anatomical anomalies. The iliopsoas muscle in the male contained irregular small fibers while the muscle in the female showed focal atrophy.

Prevalence

N/A

Clinical Implications

A divided iliopsoas tendon may contribute to snapping at the hip joint (Tatu et al. 2002; Shu and Safran 2011; Philippon et al. 2014; Saga and Takahashi 2016). An accessory iliacus tendon can mimic a tear of the iliopsoas tendon on MRI (Nguyen et al. 2013). The presence of accessory muscles or slips, such as iliacus minimus, may put tension on the femoral nerve that can result in pain at the hip or knee joints or the L2-L4 dermatomes (Spratt et al. 1996). Accessory slips of iliacus can compress the femoral nerve (Vázquez et al. 2007). Hypertrophy of iliacus and psoas major can distort the shape of the bladder and may be mistaken for pelvic lipomatosis (Chang 1978).

Iliacus minor (Figure 4.3)

See also: Iliacus

Synonyms

This muscle may also be referred to as iliocapsularis (Harrison) (Macalister 1875; Bergman et al. 1988; Saga and Takahashi 2016), iliotrochantericus (Babst et al. 2011), iliocapsulotrochanteric muscle (Cruveilhier), or iliacus brevis (Putti) (Ward et al. 2000).

Typical Presentation

This muscle may be only present as a variation or anomaly, but see prevalence information below, as well as the discussions of Ward et al. (2000) and Babst et al. (2011).

Comparative Anatomy

Das and Singh (1950) suggest that iliacus minor corresponds to the iliacus externus of lower animals. Citing three German anatomy texts and Gregory and Camp (1818), Babst et al. (2011) state that iliocapsularis can be found in primates, rats, reptiles, and birds.

Variations

Description

A detached portion or third head of iliacus is referred to as iliacus minor (Winslow) (Macalister 1875; Bergman et al. 1988; Saga and Takahashi 2016). Iliacus minor originates from the anterior inferior iliac spine, passes deep to iliopsoas in front of the hip joint capsule, and attaches to the lower portion of the intertrochanteric line on the femur and/ or into the iliofemoral ligament (Macalister 1875; Knott 1883a; Das and Singh 1950; Bergman et al. 1988; Saga and Takahashi 2016). Macalister (1875) notes that the insertion is "always above the main iliacus tendon" but Ward et al. (2000) and Babst et al. (2011) state that the insertion of iliocapsularis is distal to the lesser trochanter.

Das and Singh (1950) suggest that iliacus minor and iliocapsularis are separate muscles, the former inserting completely into the intertrochanteric line and the latter inserting completely into the iliofemoral ligament. These authors observed a case in which the muscle had a partial attachment into both structures (Das and Singh 1950). Smith-Petersen (1949) considers iliacus minor to be the acetabular origin of iliacus (Ward et al. 2000).

Innervation

Das and Singh (1950) note that iliacus minor is innervated by the nerves to iliacus. Therefore, this muscle is likely innervated by branches from the femoral nerve.

Prevalence

Ward et al. (2000) and Babst et al. (2011) suggest that iliocapsularis is uniformly present in all humans but may be atrophied in stable hips and hypertrophied in dysplastic hips. Ward et al. (2000) found iliocapsularis in all 20 cadaveric hips they examined, and Babst et al. (2011) found this muscle in all 85 hips from the 82 patients included in their study.

Anomalies

Description

Mieden (1982) describes an infant with median cleft lip, hypotelorism, and alobar holoprosencephaly. Iliacus minor was present bilaterally, extending between the iliac fossa and the intertrochanteric line. Bersu et al. (1976) describe a male infant with Hanhart syndrome. The femora of this specimen were normally developed but distal secondary ossification centers were absent. The left leg stump had a patella and a small rudiment of the proximal tibia but no fibular rudiment. The right leg stump was less developed and had a patella, smaller tibial rudiment, and no fibular rudiment. On both sides of the body, iliacus minor was present. On the right side, it extended from an origin it shared with rectus femoris to the intertrochanteric line. On the left side, it originated medial and inferior to rectus femoris and inserted onto the lesser trochanter with psoas major.

Prevalence

N/A

Clinical Implications

In cases of hip dysplasia, the presence of iliocapsularis may help to stabilize the femoral head (Ward et al. 2000; Babst et al. 2011). This muscle serves as an important landmark in hip surgery (Ward et al. 2000; Babst et al. 2011). Ward et al. (2000) note that surgeons may fail to distinguish this muscle from rectus femoris and iliacus.

PSOAS MAJOR (FIGURE 4.3)

Synonyms

This muscle can also be referred to as psoas magnus (Knott 1883b; Macalister 1875).

Typical Presentation

Description

Psoas major arises from between the last thoracic and all lumbar vertebrae via five digitations that attach to the vertebral bodies, transverse processes, and intervertebral discs (Standring 2016). Psoas major passes over the pelvic brim and forms the iliopsoas muscle with iliacus as the two insert together via a tendon onto the lesser trochanter of the femur (Standring 2016).

Innervation

Psoas major is primarily innervated by the first two lumbar spinal nerves, with some supply from the third lumbar spinal nerve (Standring 2016).

Comparative Anatomy

Psoas major has a similar typical presentation in the apes, extending from the lumbar vertebrae and intervertebral discs to join with iliacus to insert onto the lesser trochanter (Champneys 1872; Hepburn 1892; Beddard 1893; Boyer 1935; Sigmon 1974; Gibbs 1999; Diogo et al. 2010, 2012, 2013a,b, 2017). The origin may extend to the twelfth thoracic vertebra or first sacral vertebra in all species (Gibbs 1999; Diogo et al. 2010, 2012, 2013a,b, 2017). Fibers may extend distally onto the femoral shaft in gibbons, orangutans, and bonobos (Hepburn 1892; Beddard 1893; Boyer 1935; Miller 1952; Sigmon 1974; Diogo et al. 2012, 2013b, 2017).

Variations

Description

The vertebral attachments of psoas major may vary in number (Standring 2016) and the origin from the fifth lumbar vertebra may be absent (Rickenbacher et al. 1985). Psoas major may be completely separate from iliacus (Macalister 1875; Bergman et al. 1988) or be completely fused with it (Aleksandrova et al. 2013; Saga and Takahashi 2016). It may be divided into longitudinal bundles (Macalister 1875; Bergman et al. 1988; Jelev et al. 2005; Saga and Takahashi 2016). It may receive a slip from the tendon of psoas minor, or some of its fibers may be continuous with the fleshy fibers of the diaphragm or the right crus (Macalister 1875; Rickenbacher et al. 1985). One or more accessory slips/muscle bundles may be present medial or lateral to this muscle (Macalister 1875; Rickenbacher et al. 1985; Bergman et al. 1988; Jelev et al. 2005; Saga and Takahashi 2016). The iliopsoas tendon may be partially or completely divided into one, two, or three tendons (Tatu et al. 2002; Polster et al. 2008; Shu and Safran 2011; Crompton et al. 2014; Philippon et al. 2014; Saga and Takahashi 2016).

Psoas major is associated with several named accessory slips and muscles. Jelev et al. (2005) describe an accessory iliopsoas muscle that resulted from the connection between an accessory iliacus muscle and an accessory psoas major. Psoas quartus (Figure 4.3) has been observed originating from the medial aspect of quadratus lumborum and the transverse process of the fifth lumbar vertebra on the right side of one cadaver, and via two slips from the transverse processes of the fourth and fifth lumbar vertebrae on the left side (Clarkson and Rainy 1889). The muscle on both sides fused with the tendons of psoas major and psoas tertius. Tubbs et al. (2006c) note an origin from quadratus lumborum and the transverse process of the third lumbar vertebra. This muscle joins with iliacus and psoas or the tendon of psoas major at the level of the inguinal ligament (Tubbs et al. 2006c; Wong et al. 2019).

Clarkson and Rainy (1889) also describe the presence of psoas tertius in the same cadaver, which originated from the inner aspect of rib twelve and the transverse processes of the upper four lumbar vertebrae on the right side, passed in front of quadratus lumborum and iliacus, and culminated in tendinous fibers that fused with the psoas major and psoas quartus tendons. On the left side of this cadaver, the muscle originated from the transverse processes of the third and fourth lumbar vertebrae and had the same insertion. Khalid et al. (2017) note a psoas tertius with the same origin as the right side of Clarkson and Rainy's (1889) specimen that pierced the femoral nerve and joined the tendon of iliopsoas.

Prevalence

See iliacus entry for prevalence information regarding splitting of the iliopsoas tendon and the presence of accessory slips associated with iliacus and psoas major. Astik and Dave (2011) dissected 64 lumbar plexuses from 32 cadavers and found that psoas major split the femoral nerve into medial and lateral slips in three plexuses (4.7%).

Knott (1883b) examined psoas major bilaterally in 40 subjects and noted that some fibers took origin from the neck of rib 12 in 3 subjects (7.5%). As this variant occurred bilaterally in two subjects, it was found in 5 out of 80 sides (6.25%). In four cases (10%), fibers of origin came from the right crus of the diaphragm, and in one case (2.5%) from the left crus. The origin from the last lumbar vertebra was absent in five subjects (12.5%). As this variant occurred bilaterally in three subjects, this absence was noted in 8 out of 80 sides (10%). Mori (1964) noted that the superiormost origin of psoas major was from the first lumbar vertebra on 150 sides (98.7%) and from the second lumbar vertebra on two sides (1.3%). This author did not observe an origin from the thoracic vertebrae (Mori 1964).

Anomalies

Description

On the right side of an anencephalic male fetus, Windle (1893) observed that psoas major was divided into two portions (one being deficient) that shared an insertion. In a case of congenital absence of the femur, Manohar (1939) reports that psoas was very small, being well-developed near the vertebral column and inserting via a tendon onto the middle of the iliac crest. Pirani et al. (1991) describe soft tissue anatomy associated with cases of proximal femoral focal deficiency (PFFD). In Aitken type B PFFD, psoas major is smaller than typical. Itoh et al. (1991) describe fetal akinesia/hypokinesia sequence in one male and one female infant, each with a suite of anatomical anomalies. The iliopsoas muscle in the male contained irregular small fibers while the muscle in the female showed focal atrophy.

Bersu et al. (1976) describe a male infant with Hanhart syndrome. On both sides of this infant, there was an extensive fusion between the lumbar muscular components of the diaphragm, psoas major, and quadratus lumborum. The femora of this specimen were normally developed but distal secondary ossification centers were absent. The left leg stump had a patella and a small rudiment of the proximal tibia but no fibular rudiment. The right leg stump was less developed and had a patella, smaller tibial rudiment, and no fibular rudiment. On both sides of the body, a small muscle distinct from quadratus lumborum originated from the lateral aspect of psoas major and inserted onto the dorsal third of the iliac crest.

Prevalence

N/A

Clinical Implications

Hypertrophy of iliacus and psoas major can distort the shape of the bladder and may be mistaken for pelvic lipomatosis (Chang 1978). Accessory slips of psoas major can compress the femoral nerve (Vázquez et al. 2007). A divided iliopsoas tendon may contribute to snapping at the hip joint (Tatu et al. 2002; Shu and Safran 2011; Philippon et al. 2014; Saga and Takahashi 2016).

The presence of psoas quartus may split the femoral nerve and/or contribute to femoral nerve compression (Tubbs et al. 2006c; Wong et al. 2019).

PSOAS MINOR (FIGURE 4.3)

Synonyms

This muscle can also be referred to as psoas parvus (Knott 1883b; Macalister 1875).

Typical Presentation

Description

Psoas minor originates from the bodies of the twelfth thoracic and first lumbar vertebrae, and their shared intervertebral disc, courses along the anterior surface of psoas major, and inserts via a tendon onto the pecten pubis and iliopubic ramus (Standring 2016).

Innervation

Psoas minor is innervated by the first lumbar spinal nerve (Standring 2016).

Comparative Anatomy

Psoas minor has a similar typical presentation in the apes, running from the first lumbar vertebra and often the last thoracic vertebra to the iliopubic eminence (Champneys 1872; Hepburn 1892; Miller 1952; Swindler and Wood 1973; Sigmon 1974; Gibbs 1999; Diogo et al. 2010, 2012, 2013a,b, 2017). An origin from the second lumbar vertebra may be present in gibbons, orangutans, and common chimpanzees and an origin from the eleventh thoracic vertebra may be present in gorillas (Kohlbrügge 1890–1892; Hepburn 1892; Gibbs 1999; Diogo et al. 2010, 2012, 2013a,b). In gibbons and bonobos, the origin may extend to the third lumbar vertebra (Kohlbrügge 1890–1892; Gibbs 1999; Diogo et al. 2012, 2017), and in gibbons alone, this muscle is often fused with psoas major (Sigmon 1974; Diogo et al. 2012).

Variations

Description

Psoas minor may be absent (Macalister 1875; Knott 1883b; Seib 1934; Mori 1964; Sato 1968c; Rickenbacher et al. 1985; Bergman et al. 1988; Hanson et al. 1999; Joshi et al. 2010; Farias et al. 2012; Guerra et al. 2012; Gandhi et al. 2013; Saga and Takahashi 2016; Standring 2016; Dragieva et al. 2018). It may arise from the first lumbar vertebra only or the second lumbar vertebra and the disc above it (Bergman et al. 1988). It can have two heads or be doubled throughout its length (Macalister 1875; Bergman et al. 1988; Gandhi et al. 2013; Saga and Takahashi 2016; Protas et al. 2017). Protas et al. (2017) describe a two-headed psoas minor with a lateral head that originated from the body of the first lumbar vertebra and a medial head that originated from the bodies of the fourth and fifth lumbar vertebrae. The two heads joined at the level of the first sacral vertebra and continued as a single tendon to insert onto the iliopectineal eminence (Protas et al. 2017).

The psoas minor insertion tendon may also bifurcate (Macalister 1875; Bergman et al. 1988). Its insertion may vary, ranging from attachments to the inguinal ligament, iliac fascia, femoral neck, lesser trochanter, pectineal line of the femur, pectineal ligament, junction of the third and fourth lumbar vertebrae, or the junction of the fifth lumbar vertebra and the sacrum (Knott 1883b; Macalister 1875; Bergman et al. 1988; Guerra et al. 2012; Gandhi et al. 2013; Saga and Takahashi 2016). The ratio of tendinous to muscular fibers may vary, and the entire muscle may be replaced by a tendon (Macalister 1875; Guerra et al. 2012; Gandhi et al. 2013; Saga and Takahashi 2016). Accessory psoas major fibers ("psoas accessorius") may originate from the underside of the psoas minor tendon (Joshi et al. 2010; Saga and Takahashi 2016).

Prevalence

Knott (1883b) found this muscle present in 7 out of 40 subjects (17.5%). As this muscle was present bilaterally in five subjects, it was found in 12 out of 80 sides (15%). Seib (1934) found that on 1000 sides from 500 cadavers, psoas minor was present in 386 sides (38.6%). Summarizing other research, Seib (1934) also notes that psoas minor is absent in 57.3% of 5903 sides. Mori (1964) summarized the work of other Japanese researchers and calculated an absence of psoas minor in 513 out of 958 sides (53.5%). Mori himself noted the absence of this muscle in 67 out of 100 sides (67%). Sato (1968c) reported that psoas minor is absent in 163 out of 424 sides (38.4%) from Kyushu-Japanese males and absent in 116 out of 256 sides (45.3%) in females. Hanson et al. (1999) found that psoas minor was absent in 3 out of 23 (13%) White male subjects and absent in 19 out of 21 (91%) Black male subjects. In a study of 30 Brazilian cadaver pelves by Farias et al. (2012), psoas minor was absent in 22 cases (73.33%).

In a study of 30 cadavers, Joshi et al. (2010) found that psoas minor was present in nine subjects (30%). As it was present on eight sides bilaterally and one side unilaterally, psoas minor was present in 17 out of 60 sides (28.3%). In 4 of the 17 cases (23.5%), "psoas accessorius" was present (see description above) (Joshi et al. 2010). In a study of 22 fetuses (11 male, 11 female), Guerra et al. (2012) found that psoas minor was present in 13 out of 22 fetuses overall (59%), being present in eight male fetuses (72.7%) on 15 out of 22 sides (68.2%) and present in five female fetuses (45.5%) on 8 out of 22 sides (36.4%). These authors also noted that the tendon made up 60% of the muscle in females and 54% of the muscle in males (average of 57%) (Guerra et al. 2012). Dragieva et al. (2018) found that psoas minor was present in six out of ten cadavers (60%). As the muscle was present bilaterally in three subjects and unilaterally in three subjects, it was present in 9 out of 20 sides (45%).

Anomalies

Description

In an anencephalic female fetus, Windle (1893) noted the bilateral presence of an accessory muscle lying in front of psoas major that occupied the position of psoas minor and inserted onto the lesser trochanter. Psoas minor was absent bilaterally in a neonate with trisomy 18 (Aziz 1979). Among individuals with trisomy 21, psoas minor was absent on the left side of one child, bilaterally in another child, and bilaterally in a fetus (Bersu 1980).

Prevalence

In the literature review conducted by Smith et al. (2015), the authors state that psoas minor was absent in 9 out of 17 individuals with trisomy 18 (52.9%) and 3 out of 5 individuals with trisomy 21 (60%).

Clinical Implications

Gandhi et al. (2013) note that variations of psoas minor may be mistaken for retroperitoneal lymphadenopathy.

PERINEAL, COCCYGEAL, AND ANAL MUSCULATURE

COCCYGEUS (FIGURE 4.4)

Synonyms

Coccygeus is sometimes considered to be the ischiococcygeal part of levator ani and is thus sometimes referred to as ischiococcygeus (Standring 2016).

Typical Presentation

Description

Coccygeus is a musculotendinous sheet that extends from the coccyx and the fifth sacral segment to the ischial spine (Liu and Salem 2016; Standring 2016).

Innervation

Coccygeus is innervated by branches of the sacral plexus from the third and fourth sacral spinal segments (Standring 2016).

Comparative Anatomy

In orangutans, coccygeus is mostly replaced by the sacrospinous ligament (Diogo et al. 2013b). In gibbons, gorillas, and common chimpanzees, coccygeus is well-developed but primarily tendinous (Elftman 1932; Diogo et al. 2010, 2012, 2013a). In common chimpanzees and bonobos, coccygeus is partially blended with levator ani (Elftman 1932; Miller 1952; Diogo et al. 2013a, 2017).

Variations

Description

Coccygeus may be entirely tendinous instead of muscular (Knott 1883b; Bergman et al. 1998; Liu and Salem 2016; Standring 2016). When tendinous, it is fused with the sacrospinous ligament (Standring 2016). It may only originate from the sacrum (Macalister 1875). Coccygeus is rarely absent (Knott 1883b; Bergman et al. 1988; Standring 2016). It may be doubled or tripled (Macalister 1875; Bergman et al. 1998). Coccygeus is associated with two accessory muscles, curvator coccygeus accessorius or sacrococcygeus

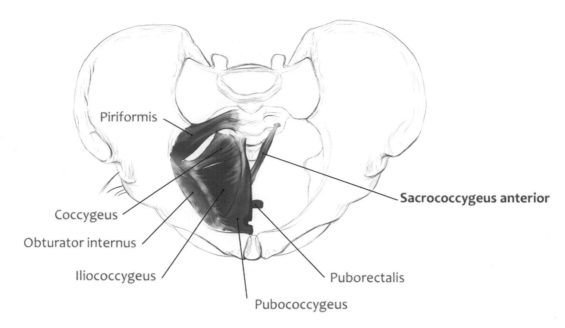

FIGURE 4.4   Pelvic diaphragm muscles in superior view.

anterior (von Luschka 1870; Bergman et al. 1988) (see the entry for this muscle), and a rectococcygeus muscle of Treitz which originates from the anterior surface of the coccyx and partially fuses with the muscle coats of the rectum (Liu and Salem 2016).

Prevalence

Knott (1883b) found that coccygeus was absent in three subjects he examined (no information on total sample size). One individual exhibited bilateral absence of fleshy muscle and replacement of this muscle with tendinous fibers.

Anomalies

N/A

Clinical Implications

As perineal hernias can emerge through defects in the perineal muscles, or in gaps between the muscles, congenital variations in muscular anatomy and any abnormal openings in the muscles or fascia can contribute to the etiology of perineal hernias (Trackler and Koehler 1968).

SACROCOCCYGEUS ANTERIOR (FIGURE 4.4)

See also: Coccygeus, Sacrococcygeus posterior

Synonyms

Sacrococcygeus anterior is also referred to as curvator coccyges (Watson 1880), curvator coccygeus accessorius or sacrococcygeus anterior (von Luschka 1870; Bergman et al. 1988), sacrococcygeus anticus (Knott 1883b), or sacrococcygeus ventralis (Niikura et al. 2010).

Typical Presentation

This muscle is only present as a variation or anomaly.

Comparative Anatomy

Nair et al. (2011) state that sacrococcygeus anterior represents the remnants of tail musculature found in lower animals. Knott (1883b) notes that Krause suggests that this muscle is homologous to flexor caudae. Flexor caudae is present as a vestigial muscle in gorillas and extends from the last sacral vertebra to the middorsal fascia (Raven 1950; Diogo et al. 2010). Remnants of flexor caudae have been reported in orangutans, but there is no trace of flexor caudae in gibbons or chimpanzees (Elftman 1932; Gibbs 1999; Diogo et al. 2012, 2013a,b, 2017).

Variations

Description

Sacrococcygeus anterior is an accessory muscle that originates from the anterior surface of the transverse process of one or two sacral vertebrae and inserts onto the coccyx (von Luschka 1870; Watson 1880; Knott 1883b; Bergman et al. 1988; Nair et al. 2011; Liu and Salem 2016). In the cases described by Watson (1880), the muscles arose in between the third and fourth sacral foramina. Knott (1883b) observed an origin from both the fourth and fifth sacral segments. In the case observed by Nair et al. (2011), the muscle arose from the anterolateral surface of the sacrum at the level of the third sacral vertebra. See the entry for sacrococcygeus posterior for a similar muscle on the posterior aspect of the sacrum.

Niikura et al. (2010) found that this muscle is typically not present in adults. It appears during fetal week 12, and between weeks 18 and 20, it increases in size and fuses with the levator ani. Nair et al. (2011) conclude that the presence of sacrococcygeus anterior in adult humans indicates the failure of the fusion of the dorsal part of levator ani.

Innervation

Sacrococcygeus anterior is innervated by a branch from the sacral plexus (Nair et al. 2011).

Prevalence

Knott (1883b) found fleshy fibers corresponding to "sacrococcygeus anticus" in 2 out of 16 subjects (12.5%).

Anomalies

Description

In a child with trisomy 21, Bersu (1980) found sacrococcygeus anterior extending from the lower sacral vertebrae to the coccyx.

Prevalence

In their literature review, Smith et al. (2015) found that sacrococcygeus anterior was present in one out of five individuals with trisomy 21 (20%).

Clinical Implications

Nair et al. (2011) suggest that fascia can fill the gap between sacrococcygeus anterior and the dorsal part of levator ani, creating an area that may be prone to prolapse of the pelvic organs.

LEVATOR ANI (FIGURE 4.4)

Synonyms

Pubococcygeus may also be referred to as pubovisceralis (Standring 2016; Liu and Salem 2016).

Typical Presentation

Description

Levator ani forms a large part of the pelvic floor and is comprised of small muscles that are not easily differentiated (Standring 2016). The muscles that comprise levator ani vary considerably between individuals, and these muscles are described differently by different researchers (Bergman et al. 1988). Levator ani is typically described as being comprised of iliococcygeus, pubococcygeus, and puborectalis, though some include ischiococcygeus (coccygeus, see the entry above) as part of the levator ani (Standring 2016), or puborectalis as part of pubococcygeus (Standring 2016).

Iliococcygeus attaches to the inner surface of the ischial spine and extends to the obturator fascia (Standring 2016). It also attaches to the sacrum and coccyx and joins with fibers from the opposite side to form a raphe that is continuous with the anococcygeal ligament (Standring 2016). Pubococcygeus is the main part of levator ani (Liu and Salem 2016). It attaches to the posterior surface of the pubis and its fibers run lateral to the urethra and the urethral sphincter along the pelvic floor (Standring 2016). Fibers that attach to the perineal body are referred to as puboperinealis, and some fibers are sometimes referred to as puboanalis as they insert between the external and internal anal sphincters (Liu and Salem 2016; Standring 2016).

In males, fibers inferolateral to the prostate are referred to as puboprostaticus or levator prostate (Standring 2016; Liu and Salem 2016). In females, the fibers attach to the lateral walls of the vagina and are referred to as pubovaginalis (Standring 2016; Liu and Salem 2016). Puborectalis is sometimes considered part of pubococcygeus (Standring 2016). It originates from the pubic bones and forms a muscular sling that wraps around the anorectal junction, and some of these fibers may mix with those of the external anal sphincter (Standring 2016; Liu and Salem 2016).

Innervation

Iliococcygeus, pubococcygeus, and puborectalis are innervated by branches of the sacral plexus from the third and fourth sacral spinal segments (Standring 2016). Pubococcygeus may also be supplied by branches of the pudendal nerve (Standring 2016).

Comparative Anatomy

Most portions of levator ani are missing and replaced with fascia in gibbons, but pubococcygeus has been recorded in some specimens (Elftman 1932; Diogo et al. 2012). The levator ani of gorillas is largely similar to that in humans and iliococcygeus sometimes extends to the sacrum (Gibbs 1999; Diogo et al. 2010). In orangutans, most of the levator ani as it appears in humans is present, but iliococcygeus is usually aponeurotic and puborectalis is homologous with the inferior fibers of pubococcygeus (Elftman 1932; Diogo et al. 2013b). The levator ani in common chimpanzees and bonobos is similar to that of orangutans (Elftman 1932; Diogo et al. 2013a), but Diogo et al. (2017) did not record information for pubococcygeus in bonobos.

Variations

Description

A slip named iliosacralis may arise from the posterior part of iliococcygeus (Standring 2016). Parts of pubococcygeus and puborectalis can be variable in their attachments, while iliococcygeus is typically not (Liu and Salem 2016). Levator ani is rarely absent. One absence was reported by Shepherd (1889), where levator ani was replaced with pelvic fascia. Substantial variation in levator ani among women has been noted, and this variation may be caused by childbirth and aging (Tunn et al. 2003; Hoyte et al. 2004; Delancey et al. 2007).

Prevalence

Tunn et al. (2003) used MRI to study the levator ani in females and found that this muscle did not attach to the pubis in 4 out of 20 subjects (20%). Arakawa et al. (2004) found that the connection between puboanalis and its insertion was via a tight connection with smooth muscle in 37 out of 46 cadavers (80.4%) and via little or no tissue connection in nine cadavers (19.6%). Tansatit et al. (2013) found that puborectalis attached to the superior pubic ramus in six out of ten hemipelves (60%) and to the obturator internus fascia in four hemipelves (40%).

Anomalies

Description

Hoyte et al. (2004) suggest that genetic defects are more likely to occur in iliococcygeus than other parts of levator ani. Anorectal malformations are common congenital anomalies that are often present with many other anomalies (e.g., cardiovascular, gastrointestinal, musculoskeletal, spinal cord, and urogenital) and are associated with several syndromes (e.g., trisomies and other multisystemic conditions) (Alamo et al. 2013). They can prevent the normal appearance and function of levator ani and sphincter ani externus until treated with surgery (Alamo et al. 2013).

Prevalence

Anorectal malformations occur in about 1 out of 5,000 live births and are slightly more common in males (Alamo et al. 2013). In 23 patients with anorectal anomalies studied by Kohda et al. (1985), only ten patients (43.5%) had normal development of the anorectal sphincter muscles (internal anal sphincter, external anal sphincter, and levator ani), while four had intermediate development of these muscles (17.4%) and the remaining nine had poor development of these muscles (39.1%). Among 20 patients with Down syndrome that had anorectal malformations, Torres et al. (1998) found that only one of them (5%) had poorly developed perineal muscles (specific muscles not indicated).

Clinical Implications

Weakness in levator ani and loss of ani volume can contribute to incontinence, constipation, and pelvic organ prolapse (Tunn et al. 2003; Hoyte et al. 2004; Delancey et al. 2007; Alamo et al. 2013). As perineal hernias can emerge through defects in the perineal muscles, or in gaps between the muscles, congenital variation in muscular anatomy and any abnormal openings in the muscles or fascia can contribute to the etiology of perineal hernias (Trackler and Koehler 1968). The classifications of anorectal malformations and the surgical approaches to repair them are often dependent upon their position relative to the levator ani muscle (Nievelstein et al. 1998; Alamo et al. 2013).

Sphincter ani externus (Figure 4.5)

Synonyms

N/A

Typical Presentation

Description

The external anal sphincter is a circular muscle that surrounds the anus (Liu and Salem 2016; Standring 2016). It extends between the perineal body and the anococcygeal raphe (Liu and Salem 2016; Standring 2016). The deep part of the external anal sphincter blends with puborectalis (Liu and Salem 2016; Standring 2016). Fibers from the transverse perineal muscles and bulbospongiosus pass to the external anal sphincter (Peikert et al. 2015; Standring 2005, 2016). The anterior portion of the muscle is shorter in females (Sultan et al. 1994).

Innervation

Sphincter ani externus is innervated by the inferior rectal branch of the pudendal nerve, the perineal nerve, or the anococcygeal nerve (Sato 1980; Liu and Salem 2016; Standring 2016).

Comparative Anatomy

Sphincter ani externus is similar in the apes, and the extension of some fibers to bulbospongiosus has been observed in gibbons, orangutans, and gorillas (Elftman 1932; Diogo et al. 2010, 2012, 2013a,b, 2017).

Variations

Description

Anterior muscle extensions of sphincter ani externus may occur to the corpus cavernosum or to the ischial tuberosity (Sultan et al. 1994; Liu and Salem 2016; Tubbs and Watanabe 2016). Fibers from the superficial surface of the sphincter ani externus can pass to the medial aspect of ischiocavernosus via one or more bundles (Tubbs and Watanabe 2016). Slips may also pass from sphincter ani externus to the

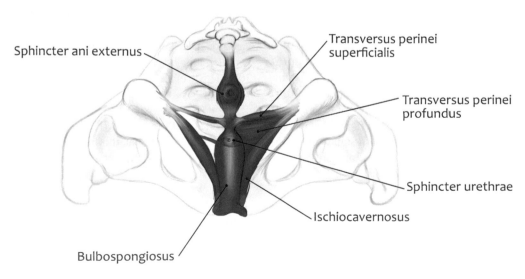

FIGURE 4.5   Perineal muscles in inferior view.

coccyx (Macalister 1875; Liu and Salem 2016). Retractor scroti refers to a bundle that extends from the superficial portion of sphincter ani externus to bulbospongiosus, or to the base of the scrotum (Tubbs and Watanabe 2016).

Prevalence

Sultan et al. (1994) used endosonography to study the external anal sphincter in 93 nulliparous females and 21 males. The authors found that the deep (or proximal) portion of the external sphincter was annular in 72% of females and 76% of males, the superficial anal sphincter was elliptical in 76% of females and 86% of males, and the subcutaneous portion was conical in 56% of females and 57% of males (Sultan et al. 1994). Anterior muscle extensions from this muscle occurred in 13% of females and 14% of males (Sultan et al. 1994).

Peikert et al. (2015) studied the relationship between bulbospongiosus and the external anal sphincter through MRI of 43 male individuals and the study of six male cadavers and classified the relationship into five variants. Variant 1 was present in 2 out of 6 cadavers (~33%) and 14 out of 43 MRI patients (32.6%) and demonstrated a bridge-like muscular connection between the two muscles with connective tissue separating the muscles cranially. Variant 2 was present in 2 out of 6 cadavers (~33%) and 6 out of 43 MRI patients (~14%) and demonstrated direct contact between the two muscles. Variant 3 was present in none of the cadavers (0%) and in 9 out of 43 MRI patients (~21%) and demonstrated ventral fibers of the external anal sphincter reaching the bulbospongiosus muscle median raphe via connective tissue without forming a muscular continuity. Variant 4 was present in 1 out of 6 cadavers (~16.7%) and 7 out of 43 MRI patients (~16.3%) and demonstrated a combination of variants 1 and 2, or 2 and 3. Variant 5 was present in 1 out of 6 cadavers (~16.7%) and 7 out of 43 MRI patients (~16.3%) and demonstrated no muscular or connective tissue connection between the bulbospongiosus and the external anal sphincter (Peikert et al. 2015).

Anomalies

Description

Anorectal malformations are common congenital anomalies that are often present with many other anomalies (e.g., cardiovascular, gastrointestinal, musculoskeletal, spinal cord, and urogenital) and are associated with several syndromes (e.g., trisomies and other multisystemic conditions) (Alamo et al. 2013). They can prevent the normal appearance and function of levator ani and sphincter ani externus until treated with surgery (Alamo et al. 2013).

In a case of a female infant with trisomy 9 studied by Annerén and Sedin (1981), sphincter ani externus was missing and the distance between the anus and vulva was shortened. Bersu et al. (1976) describe a male infant with Hanhart syndrome. In this infant, the external anal sphincter was comprised of two flat and parallel muscular bands that extended between the coccyx to the muscles of the penis with no decussating fibers.

Prevalence

Anorectal malformations occur in about 1 out of 5,000 live births and are slightly more common in males (Alamo et al. 2013). In 23 patients with anorectal anomalies studied by Kohda et al. (1985), only ten patients (43.5%) had normal development of the anorectal sphincter muscles (internal anal sphincter, external anal sphincter, and levator ani), while four had intermediate development of these muscles (17.4%) and the remaining nine had poor development of these muscles (39.1%). Among 20 patients with Down syndrome that had anorectal malformations, Torres et al. (1998) found that only one of them (5%) had poorly developed perineal muscles (specific muscles not indicated). However, the authors state that the sphincter mechanism in all 20 patients was normal (Torres et al. 1998).

Clinical Implications

Variations and anomalies in the development and presentation of this muscle can affect continence (Alamo et al. 2013).

Transversus perinei profundus (Deep transverse perinei) (Figure 4.5)

Synonyms

N/A

Typical Presentation

Description

The deep transverse perinei comprise a sheet of muscle that lies across the urogenital triangle and extends from the ischiopubic ramus (Standring 2005). The muscle sheet attaches to the perineal body posteriorly, and its fibers are deficient anteriorly (Standring 2005). Its fibers join with the fibers of the corresponding muscle on the opposite side (Standring 2005). Some fibers extend to the deep part of the external anal sphincter and the sphincter urethrae (Standring 2005).

Innervation

The deep transverse perinei are innervated by the perineal branch of the pudendal nerve (Standring 2005).

Comparative Anatomy

There are no descriptions of the deep transverse perinei in gibbons, orangutans, or bonobos (Diogo et al. 2012, 2013b, 2017). This muscle is present in gorillas and exhibits a presentation similar to that in humans (Gibbs 1999; Diogo et al. 2010). In common chimpanzees, Elftman (1932) suggested that some fibers of bulbospongiosus that insert into the ischium may be homologous with the deep transverse perinei (Diogo et al. 2013a).

Variations

Description

The deep transverse perineal muscle frequently varies among individuals (Bergman et al. 1988). This muscle may be absent, particularly in females (Knott 1883b; Bergman et al. 1988; Tubbs and Watanabe 2016). An accessory muscle named transversus perinei alter may be present in front of this muscle (Tubbs and Watanabe 2016).

Prevalence

Knott (1883b) found transversus perinei profundus absent in 3 out of 30 bodies (10%).

Anomalies

N/A

Clinical Implications

As perineal hernias can emerge through defects in the perineal muscles, or in gaps between the muscles, congenital variation in muscular anatomy and any abnormal openings in the muscles or fascia can contribute to the etiology of perineal hernias (Trackler and Koehler 1968).

TRANSVERSUS PERINEI SUPERFICIALIS (SUPERFICIAL TRANSVERSE PERINEI) (FIGURE 4.5)

Synonyms

N/A

Typical Presentation

Description

The superficial transverse perinei are muscular slips that course transversely across the superficial perineal space anterior to the anus (Standring 2016). The slips extend between the ischial tuberosity and the perineal body (Standring 2016). The transverse perineal muscles send fibers to bulbospongiosus and the external anal sphincter (Standring 2016).

Innervation

The superficial transverse perinei are innervated by a branch of the pudendal nerve (Standring 2016).

Comparative Anatomy

There are no descriptions of transversus perinei superficialis in gibbons, orangutans, or bonobos (Diogo et al. 2012, 2013b). This muscle is present in some gorillas and exhibits a presentation similar to that in humans (Gibbs 1999; Diogo et al. 2010). Sonntag (1923) states that this muscle is absent in common chimpanzees.

Variations

Description

The superficial transverse perinei may be reduced or absent (Knott 1883b; Bergman et al. 1988; Standring 2016; Tubbs and Watanabe 2016). It can consist of many distinct fasciculi (Bergman et al. 1988; Tubbs and Watanabe 2016). It may connect with puborectalis or the ischiopubic rami (Knott 1883b; Tubbs and Watanabe 2016). It can also be doubled bilaterally (Tubbs and Watanabe 2016).

Prevalence

Knott (1883b) found transversus perinei superficialis present only in 6 out of 30 subjects (20%). Knott (1883b) also notes that transversus perinei medius—"the muscle more generally known as the t. p. superficialis"—was absent in 8 out of 30 subjects (26.7%).

Anomalies

N/A

Clinical Implications

As perineal hernias can emerge through defects in the perineal muscles, or in gaps between the muscles, congenital variation in muscular anatomy and any abnormal openings in the muscles or fascia can contribute to the etiology of perineal hernias (Trackler and Koehler 1968). Perineal hernias are defined based on their position (anterior or posterior) relative to the superficial transverse perineal muscle (Trackler and Koehler 1968), so understanding potential variations in this muscle is important for classifying these hernias.

SPHINCTER URETHRAE (FIGURE 4.5)

Synonyms

N/A

Typical Presentation

Description

The external urethral sphincter varies in presentation between males and females (Jung et al. 2012; Standring 2016). In males, the fibers inferior to the prostate compose the external sphincter of the membranous urethra (Jung et al. 2012). The muscle fibers originate from the junction of the inferior pubic rami and ischium (Jung et al. 2012). In females, the urethral sphincter is found at the distal end of the bladder and is referred to as a urogenital sphincter that has three components (Jung et al. 2012). The urogenital sphincter contains (1) the true sphincter that surrounds the urethra, (2) a compressor urethral muscle that arises from the ischiopubic ramus and passes anterior to the urethra below sphincter urethrae, and (3) the urethrovaginal sphincter, a muscle below compressor urethrae that extends from the ventral and lateral walls of the urethra to the vagina, up to the vestibular bulb (Oelrich 1983; Jung et al. 2012; Standring 2016).

Innervation

Sphincter urethrae is innervated by a branch of the pudendal nerve (Standring 2016).

Comparative Anatomy

There are no descriptions of sphincter urethrae in gibbons, orangutans, or bonobos (Diogo et al. 2012, 2013b, 2017). According to Gibbs (1999), this muscle is a true sphincter in male gorillas with no invasion of the prostate. Roberts and Seibold (1971) state that the fibers of this muscle extend to the vaginal wall in female chimpanzees, as it does in humans.

Variations

Description

Bergman et al. (1988) state that there is frequent variation in the muscles that compose the urethral sphincter, but do not list any specific variations. Variations of sphincter urethrae are not described in Liu and Salem (2016) or Tubbs and Watanabe (2016). Oelrich (1983) states that in females, compressor urethrae may sometimes join the urethrovaginal sphincter near the anterior border of the vagina, instead of joining it ventral to the urethra.

Prevalence

N/A

Anomalies

N/A

Clinical Implications

Variation or weakening of the external sphincter urethrae can lead to urinary incontinence (Jung et al. 2012; Standring 2016).

Ischiopubicus (Not Illustrated)

Synonyms

N/A

Typical Presentation

This muscle is only present as a variation.

Comparative Anatomy

Bardeen (1921) states that ischiopubicus is homologous to the compressor of the dorsal vein of the penis or clitoris found in lower mammals.

Variations

Description

Ischiopubicus originates from the sides of the deep perineal pouch and the inferior rami of the ischium and pubis (Bardeen 1921; Tubbs and Watanabe 2016). It inserts onto the inferior pubic ligament (arcuate ligament of the pubis) (Oelrich 1983; Tubbs and Watanabe 2016). This muscle is frequently absent in humans (Tubbs and Watanabe 2016).

Innervation

N/A

Prevalence

N/A

Anomalies

N/A

Clinical Implications

N/A

Ischiocavernosus (Figure 4.5)

Synonyms

N/A

Typical Presentation

Description

In males, ischiocavernosus covers the crus penis and attaches to the medial surface of the ischial tuberosity and to the ischial ramus (Standring 2016). The muscle is similar in females and is associated with the crus of the clitoris (Standring 2016). Ischiocavernosus is larger in males (Bergman et al. 1988; Tubbs and Watanabe 2016).

Innervation

Ischiocavernosus is innervated by a branch of the pudendal nerve (Standring 2016).

Comparative Anatomy

There are no descriptions of ischiocavernosus in gibbons, orangutans, or bonobos (Diogo et al. 2012, 2013b, 2017). This muscle is present in gorillas and exhibits a presentation similar to that in humans (Diogo et al. 2010). Sonntag (1923) states that the origin of this muscle is from the ascending pubic ramus in common chimpanzees.

Variations

Description

Ischiocavernosus may receive fibers from sphincter ani externus (Tubbs and Watanabe 2016). Ischiocavernosus is associated with two named muscular variations. Compressor venae dorsalis refers to fasciculi that originate from the sheath of the corpus cavernosum urethrae and the median raphe (Houston 1831; Bergman et al. 1988; Tubbs and Watanabe 2016). These fasciculi join with their counterparts on the other side of the body via a tendon that courses over the dorsal vein (Houston 1831; Bergman et al. 1988; Tubbs and Watanabe 2016). Pubocavernosus or levator penis refers to anterior bundles of ischiocavernosus that attach to the dorsal surface of the penis (Bergman et al. 1988; Tubbs and Watanabe 2016).

Prevalence

N/A

Anomalies

N/A

Clinical Implications

N/A

BULBOSPONGIOSUS (FIGURE 4.5)

Synonyms

This muscle is sometimes referred to as bulbocavernosus (Tubbs and Watanabe 2016).

Typical Presentation

Description

In males, bulbospongiosus is comprised of two parts joined by a median fibrous raphe (Standring 2016). The fibers blend with the perineal body and are attached to the superficial transverse perineal muscle and the external anal sphincter (Standring 2016). The middle fibers encircle the bulb of the penis and corpus spongiosum (Standring 2016). The anterior fibers extend over and insert partly into the sides of the corpus cavernosum, and also partially insert into a tendinous expansion over the dorsal vessels of the penis (Standring 2016). In females, bulbospongiosus attaches to the perineal body but the muscle on each side of the body is separate (Standring 2016). It covers the superficial portions of the vestibular bulbs and greater vestibular glands (Standring 2016). It attaches onto the corpus cavernosum clitoridis (Standring 2016).

Innervation

Bulbospongisosus is innervated by a branch of the pudendal nerve (Standring 2016).

Comparative Anatomy

Bulbospongiosus has a similar typical presentation in the apes (Elftman 1932; Diogo et al. 2010, 2012, 2013a,b). There is a connection to the ischium in gibbons, gorillas, and common chimpanzees (Elftman 1932; Diogo et al. 2010, 2012). There is no data on this muscle for bonobos (Diogo et al. 2017).

Variations

Description

The posterior part of bulbospongiosus may be separate from the anterior part, or is absent altogether, particularly in females (Tubbs and Watanabe 2016). Fibers that extend from the ischial tuberosity to bulbospongiosus may be referred to as ischiobulbosi (Tubbs and Watanabe 2016). In males, gluteoperinealis (Krause) refers to a slip that originates from the gluteus maximus fascia or upper fascia lata and inserts beneath the origin of bulbocavernosus in the albuginea of the penile urethra (Knott 1883b; Bergman et al. 1988; Nicholson et al. 2016; Tubbs and Watanabe 2016).

Prevalence

Peikert et al. (2015) studied the relationship between bulbospongiosus and the external anal sphincter through MRI of 43 male individuals and the study of six male cadavers and classified the relationship into five variants. Variant 1 was present in 2 out of 6 cadavers (~33%) and 14 out of 43 MRI patients (32.6%) and demonstrated a bridge-like muscular connection between the two muscles with connective tissue separating the muscles cranially. Variant 2 was present in 2 out of 6 cadavers (~33%) and 6 out of 43 MRI patients (~14%) and demonstrated direct contact between the two muscles. Variant 3 was present in none of the cadavers (0%) and in 9 out of 43 MRI patients (~21%) and demonstrated ventral fibers of the external anal sphincter reaching the bulbospongiosus muscle median raphe via connective tissue without forming a muscular continuity. Variant 4 was present in 1 out of 6 cadavers (~16.7%) and 7 out of 43 MRI patients (~16.3%) and demonstrated a combination of variants 1 and 2, or 2 and 3. Variant 5 was present in 1 out of 6 cadavers (~16.7%) and 7 out of 43 MRI patients (~16.3%) and demonstrated no muscular or connective tissue connection between the bulbospongiosus and the external anal sphincter. In this last case, the origin of the bulbospongiosus muscle was in the dense connective tissue of the body of the perineum (Peikert et al. 2015).

Anomalies

N/A

Clinical Implications

N/A

THORAX, SPINE, AND BACK MUSCLES

DIAPHRAGM (FIGURE 4.6)

Synonyms

N/A

Typical Presentation

Description

The diaphragm is a continuous musculofibrous sheet that has three portions (Standring 2016). The sternal portion originates from the xiphoid process (Standring 2016). The costal portion originates from the lower six costal cartilages and their corresponding ribs on each side of the thorax (Bergman et al. 1988; Standring 2016). The lumbar portion originates from the medial and lateral arcuate ligaments and from the first three lumbar vertebrae via left and right crura (Standring 2016). The muscle fibers converge into a central tendon near the center of the muscle (Standring 2016).

Innervation

The diaphragm is innervated by the phrenic nerves (Standring 2016).

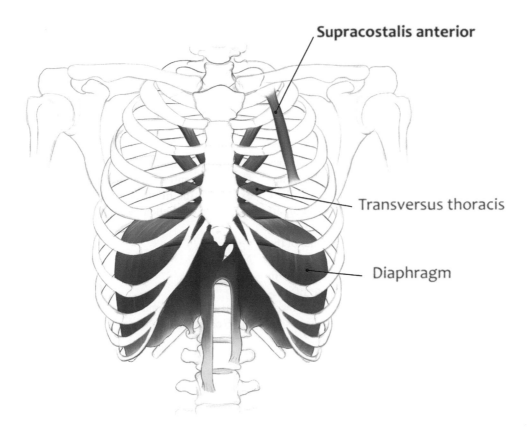

Supracostalis anterior

Transversus thoracis

Diaphragm

FIGURE 4.6 Anterior thoracic wall muscles and diaphragm in anterior view.

Comparative Anatomy

The diaphragm has a similar typical presentation in the apes (Gibbs 1999; Diogo et al. 2010, 2012, 2013a,b, 2017). The costal portion originates from the lower seven ribs in gorillas, common chimpanzees, and bonobos (Sonntag 1923; Miller 1952; Diogo et al. 2010, 2013a, 2017). Accessory slips may be present near the lumbar portion in common chimpanzees (Sonntag 1923). The sternal portion originates from the xiphoid process in bonobos and from the sternum in common chimpanzees (Sonntag 1923; Miller 1952; Diogo et al. 2013a, 2017).

Variations

Description

The diaphragm is variable in size, position, thickness, ratio of tendon to muscle, and in its attachments (Knott 1883b; Snosek and Loukas 2016; Standring 2016). The sternal portion of the muscle varies in attachments and may be absent (Bergman et al. 1988; Standring 2016). The costal portion can potentially extend to the fifth or sixth rib, and the slip to the twelfth rib may not be present (Macalister 1875; Bergman et al. 1988). The crura may be divided into separate bundles (Botros et al. 1990; Snosek and Loukas 2016). Fibers from the diaphragm can occasionally extend to psoas major or quadratus lumborum (Macalister 1875; Bergman et al. 1988). Accessory muscle slips may be found, often near the central tendon (Macalister 1875; Knott 1883b; Rickenbacher et al. 1985;

Bergman ct al. 1988). A slip may connect the right crus to the duodenum, and a fibrous band can extend from the medial borders of the crura to the surface of the esophagus (Bergman et al. 1988).

The diaphragm is associated with a few named accessory muscles. As described by Allen (1950), transpleuralis subclavius presents as two bands of muscle that pass through the oblique fissure of the right lung. The bands originate from the sixth rib and attach onto the central tendon of the diaphragm, just behind the caval opening (Allen 1950; Bergman et al. 1988; Snosek and Loukas 2016). Diaphragmaticoretromediastinalis (Eppinger) extends from the superior end of the medial crus to the posterior mediastinum (Rickenbacher et al. 1985). See the entry for hepatodiaphragmaticus.

Prevalence

In a sample of 50 diaphragms, Botros et al. (1990) found that the right crus divided into a medial, middle, and lateral bundle in 98% of cases. They also found that the left crus only had two bundles, a medial and lateral bundle, in 90% of cases (Botros et al. 1990). Yeh et al. (1990) describe variant anatomy of the diaphragm that was detected with abdominal ultrasonography in 74 patients. Among other abnormalities, 34 patients (45.9%) had a diaphragmatic slip, 10 patients (13.5%) exhibited scalloping of the diaphragm that was associated with slips, and 3 patients (4%) had hypertrophic crura (Yeh et al. 1990).

Anomalies

Description

The diaphragm may be absent as an anomaly (Macalister 1875), particularly in cases of anencephaly (Rickenbacher et al. 1985). Congenital or age-related defects of the diaphragm can lead to thinning or fissure of the musculofibrous sheet (Macalister 1875; Snosek and Loukas 2016). Accessory diaphragms may be present (Hollinshead 1956; Wille et al. 1975; da Silva et al. 2012; Snosek and Loukas 2016). Anomalous presentations of the diaphragm can also involve the presence of slips of muscle fibers to other structures (Smith et al. 2015).

Bersu et al. (1976) describe a male infant with Hanhart syndrome. On both sides of this infant, there was an extensive fusion between the lumbar muscular components of the diaphragm, psoas major, and quadratus lumborum. Itoh et al. (1991) describe fetal akinesia/hypokinesia sequence in one male and one female infant, each with a suite of anatomical anomalies. The diaphragm in both infants showed focal atrophy.

Prevalence

In their literature review, Smith et al. (2015) found several anomalous slips of muscle originating from the diaphragm in 1 out of 20 individuals with trisomy 13 (5%). These slips include a slip from the right crus to psoas major, a slip present on the central tendon, and a slip from the central tendon to the pericardium just below the left inferior pulmonary vein (Smith et al. 2015). In the study and literature review completed by Wille et al. (1975), they found that out of 21 cases, accessory diaphragms were more frequent on the right side (20 cases) than the left side (1 case) and also more common in males (13 cases) than in females (8 cases).

Clinical Implications

Bergman et al. (1988) state that detached or aberrant muscle slips from the diaphragm can compress the renal artery. Accessory slips of the diaphragm may be mistaken for intrahepatic masses (Yeh et al. 1990). Congenital or age-related defects of the diaphragm can lead to herniation of abdominal organs into the thorax (Snosek and Loukas 2016). Age-related changes of the diaphragm are strongly associated with emphysema (Caskey et al. 1989). An accessory diaphragm can lead to pulmonary maldevelopment and some associated symptoms are respiratory distress, recurrent respiratory infection, and/or chronic pulmonary inflammation (Wille et al. 1975).

HEPATODIAPHRAGMATICUS (NOT ILLUSTRATED)

See also: Diaphragm

Synonyms

This muscle may also be referred to as hepaticodiaphragmaticus (Knox) (Macalister 1875).

Typical Presentation

This muscle is only present as a variation or anomaly.

Comparative Anatomy

N/A

Variations

Description

Hepatodiaphragmaticus is a muscular band that originates from the central tendon anterior to the esophagus and extends to the hilum of the liver (Knott 1883b; Macalister 1875; Von der hellen 1903; Bergman et al. 1988).

Innervation

N/A

Prevalence

Knott (1883b) found "hepatico-diaphragmaticus" in 1 out of 36 cases (2.8%).

Anomalies

Description

In a neonate with trisomy 13, Pettersen et al. (1979) found that "hepaticodiaphragmaticus" extended as a band of striated muscle from the undersurface of the diaphragm, into the gastrohepatic ligament and then into the hilum of the liver.

Prevalence

According to the literature review completed by Smith et al. (2015), this muscle was present in 1 out of 20 individuals with trisomy 13 (5%).

Clinical Implications

N/A

TRANSVERSUS THORACIS (FIGURE 4.6)

Synonyms

This muscle is also referred to as sternocostalis or triangularis sternae (Snosek and Loukas 2016; Standring 2016), infra-costalis anterior, or transversus thoracis anterior (Macalister 1875).

Typical Presentation

Description

Transversus thoracis is located on the inner surface of the anterior thoracic wall (Standring 2016). It originates from the sternum, xiphoid process, and the sternal ends of the costal cartilages of ribs four through seven (Standring 2016). The muscle fibers separate into slips that typically attach to the costal cartilages of ribs two through six (Standring 2016).

Innervation

Transversus thoracis is innervated by adjacent intercostal nerves (Standring 2016).

Comparative Anatomy

In gorillas, transversus thoracis has been observed to run between ribs one and eight (Raven 1950; Diogo et al. 2010). In common chimpanzees, it runs between the second and sixth ribs (Diogo et al. 2013a). In bonobos, it runs between the second and seventh ribs (Miller 1952; Diogo et al. 2017). Gibbs (1999) and Diogo et al. (2012, 2013b) have stated that no information is available for gibbons or orangutans. However, Satoh (1971) has stated that the superior most costal attachment is to the second or third rib in the gibbon, and to the third rib in the orangutan.

Variations

Description

The muscle attachments can occasionally extend up to the first rib or down to the seventh rib (Mori 1964; Satoh 1971; Bergman et al. 1988; Jelev et al. 2011; Snosek and Loukas 2016). Attachments can vary between each side of the body within an individual (Macalister 1875; Jelev et al. 2011; Standring 2016). Transversus thoracis may be continuous with transversus abdominis (Macalister 1875). Macalister (1875) notes that this muscle may be absent.

Prevalence

Mori (1964) studied the attachments of transversus thoracis on 310 sides. The superior most costal cartilage/rib of origin was rib 1 on 7 sides (2.2%), rib 2 on 122 sides (39.3%), rib 3 on 155 sides (50%), rib 4 on 23 sides (7.2%), and rib 5 on 3 sides (0.9%). The inferior most costal cartilage/rib of origin was rib 5 on 50 sides (16.1%), rib 6 on 237 sides (76.5%), and rib 7 on 23 sides (7.4%). The most common morphs of this muscle were separation into 4 slips from rib 3 to 6 in 121 cases (39%) and into five slips from rib 2 to 6 in 86 cases (27.7%).

Jelev et al. (2011) studied transversus thoracis on 240 sides from 120 cadavers and found that the most common spread of this muscle was between ribs two and six, and that there was asymmetry between the left and right side in 44.2% of the cadavers. The superior most costal cartilage/rib of origin was rib 1 in 7.5% of left sides and 0.8% of right sides, rib 2 in 53.3% of left sides and 37.5% of right sides, rib 3 in 29.2% of left sides and 46.7% of right sides, rib 4 in 9.2% of left sides and 14.2% of right sides, and rib 5 in 0.8% of left sides and 0.8% of right sides. The inferior most costal cartilage/rib of origin was rib 5 in 0.8% of left sides and 1.7% of right sides, rib 6 in 94.2% of left sides and 89.2% of right sides, and rib 7 in 5% of left sides and 9.2% of right sides.

Anomalies

N/A

Clinical Implications

Jelev et al. (2011) note that understanding the variation in attachments of transversus thoracis is important due to the close anatomical relationship of this muscle to the internal thoracic artery, which is an important vessel for coronary artery bypass grafting (CABG) surgery.

INTERCOSTALES EXTERNI (EXTERNAL INTERCOSTALS) (FIGURE 4.7)

Synonyms

N/A

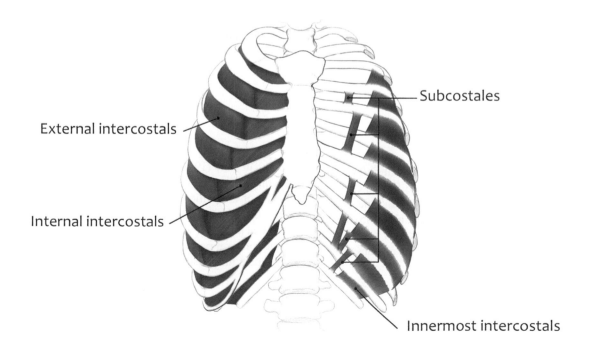

FIGURE 4.7 Intercostal and subcostal muscles in anterior view.

Typical Presentation

Description

Each external intercostal muscle extends from the lower margin of one rib to the superior margin of the rib below it (Standring 2016). Together, the 11 pairs of external intercostals pass from the tubercles of the ribs nearly to the costal cartilages and continue toward the sternum as the external intercostal membrane (Standring 2016).

Innervation

The external intercostal muscles are innervated by the corresponding intercostal nerves (Standring 2016).

Comparative Anatomy

The external intercostals have a similar typical presentation in the apes, attaching between the adjacent margins of each pair of ribs (Diogo et al. 2010, 2012, 2013a,b, 2017). Sonntag (1923) states that in common chimpanzees, the first three and last two external intercostal muscles are fleshy, but the rest are replaced by membranous tissue. In one of the common chimpanzees examined by Diogo et al. (2013a), the external intercostals had a typical presentation.

Variations

Description

One or more external intercostal muscles, particularly the last muscle, may be replaced by a sheet of connective tissue or may be completely absent (Macalister 1875; Rickenbacher et al. 1985). Extra muscle bellies may be present when there are extra ribs (Macalister 1875; Rickenbacher et al. 1985). Fibers from the external intercostal muscles may blend with the internal intercostal muscles, serratus anterior, and/or the external oblique (Macalister 1875; Rickenbacher et al. 1985).

Prevalence
N/A

Anomalies

Description

Itoh et al. (1991) describe fetal akinesia/hypokinesia sequence in one male and one female infant, each with a suite of anatomical anomalies. In the male, the intercostal muscles were slightly atrophic. Paria et al. (2015) describe a case of an infant with congenital absence of the anterior and anterolateral parts of multiple lower ribs and absence of the adjacent intercostal muscles.

Prevalence
N/A

Clinical Implications
N/A

INTERCOSTALES INTERNI (INTERNAL INTERCOSTALS) (FIGURE 4.7)

Synonyms
N/A

Typical Presentation

Description

Each internal intercostal muscle extends from the inner margin of a costal groove and attaches onto the superior margin of the rib below (Standring 2016). Together, the 11 pairs of internal intercostals commence near the sternum and continue to the posterior costal angles as the internal intercostal membrane (Standring 2016).

Innervation

The internal intercostal muscles are innervated by the corresponding intercostal nerves (Standring 2016).

Comparative Anatomy

The internal intercostals have a similar typical presentation in the apes, attaching between the adjacent margins of each pair of ribs (Diogo et al. 2010, 2012, 2013a,b, 2017).

Variations

Description

The internal intercostals may vary in their distance between their dorsal borders and the costal angle (Rickenbacher et al. 1985). These muscles may also show discontinuities as they thin out on the dorsal part of the thorax (Rickenbacher et al. 1985). Macalister (1875) notes that the internal intercostal muscles may join with transversus thoracis ("infracostalis"). Some of the muscles in the eighth through twelfth intercostal spaces may be continuous with the internal oblique (Macalister 1875).

Prevalence
N/A

Anomalies

Description

Itoh et al. (1991) describe fetal akinesia/hypokinesia sequence in one male and one female infant, each with a suite of anatomical anomalies. In the male, the intercostal muscles were slightly atrophic. Paria et al. (2015) describe a case of an infant with congenital absence of the anterior and anterolateral parts of multiple lower ribs and absence of the adjacent intercostal muscles.

Prevalence
N/A

Clinical Implications
N/A

Intercostales intimi (Innermost intercostals) (Figure 4.7)

Synonyms
N/A

Typical Presentation

Description

The innermost intercostal muscles are deep to the internal intercostal muscles and are attached to the internal surfaces of two adjacent ribs (Standring 2016).

Innervation

The innermost intercostal muscles are innervated by the corresponding intercostal nerves (Standring 2016).

Comparative Anatomy

There is no information on the innermost intercostals in the apes (Gibbs 1999), and it is likely that their morphology has been characterized along with the internal intercostals due to the close anatomical association between these muscles.

Variations

Description

The innermost intercostals that occupy the first three intercostal spaces may sometimes extend as far as the vertebral column (Rickenbacher et al. 1985). Standring (2016) notes that the superiormost muscles may be reduced or absent. The innermost intercostals may join with the subcostal muscles posteriorly (Standring 2016).

Prevalence

N/A

Anomalies

Description

Itoh et al. (1991) describe fetal akinesia/hypokinesia sequence in one male and one female infant, each with a suite of anatomical anomalies. In the male, the intercostal muscles were slightly atrophic. Paria et al. (2015) describe a case of an infant with congenital absence of the anterior and anterolateral parts of multiple lower ribs and absence of the adjacent intercostal muscles.

Prevalence

N/A

Clinical Implications
N/A

Subcostales (Subcostal Muscles) (Figure 4.7)

Synonyms

This muscle may also be referred to as infracostales, intracostalis, transversus thoracis posterior, or serratus internus (Macalister 1875).

Typical Presentation

Description

The subcostal muscles are typically only well-developed in the lower part of the posterior thorax (Standring 2016). Each subcostal muscle originates from the inner surface of one rib and crosses one or two intercostal spaces to insert onto the inner surface of the second or third rib below its rib of origin (Rickenbacher et al. 1985; Standring 2016).

Innervation

Subcostales muscles are innervated by the corresponding intercostal nerves (Standring 2016).

Comparative Anatomy

Raven (1950) lists subcostales as absent in the gorilla he dissected. There is no information on this muscle for the other apes (Gibbs 1999; Diogo et al. 2010, 2011, 2013a,b, 2017). Satoh (1974) found three bundles of subcostales in 1 out of 30 macaques (3.3%) and stated that subcostales were absent in the other specimens. Satoh (1974) concludes that subcostales are typically absent in non-human primates.

Variations

Description

The subcostales are often variable in their number and extent of development (Rickenbacher et al. 1985; Standring 2016). Complete absence of subcostales is rare (Rickenbacher et al. 1985). Rickenbacher et al. (1985) state that the bundles of subcostales that are most constant are those between the second and fourth ribs and those between the ninth and twelfth ribs. Satoh (1974) states that the most constant bundles of subcostales are those between the third and fifth ribs, the ninth and eleventh ribs, and the tenth and twelfth ribs.

The lowest subcostal muscle—which attaches onto the internal surface and superior border of the twelfth rib—may also have an attachment onto the body of the twelfth thoracic vertebra (Rickenbacher et al. 1985) or the transverse process of the first lumbar vertebra (Satoh 1974). Satoh (1974) observed that some subcostal muscles radiated over the aponeurosis of transversus abdominis or iliopsoas instead of inserting onto the rib.

Satoh (1974) also categorized bundles of subcostales into six types. In type A, the bundle of subcostales crossed over one rib and ended in the next intercostal space without reaching the next rib. In type B, the muscle crossed two intercostal spaces to insert onto the second rib below its rib of origin. In type C, the muscle spanned 2.5 intercostal spaces. In type D, the muscle spanned three intercostal spaces and inserted onto the third rib below its rib of origin. In type E, the muscle radiated into the aponeurosis of transversus abdominis or iliopsoas. In type F, the muscle inserted onto the transverse process of the last thoracic vertebra or the first lumbar vertebra.

Prevalence

In a sample of 23 Japanese male cadavers, Satoh (1974) found subcostales present on both sides of the body in all cases (100%) The number of subcostales muscles per person ranged from 1 to 14, with an average of five. Satoh's (1974) type A was found in 9 out of 276 cases (3.3%), type B in 216 cases (78.3%), type C in five cases (1.8%), type D in 25 cases (9%), type E in ten cases (3.6%), and type F in 11 cases (4%).

Anomalies
N/A

Clinical Implications
N/A

SUPRACOSTALIS ANTERIOR (FIGURE 4.6)

Synonyms
This muscle may be referred to as supracostalis anterior anomalous (Bochdalek 1867), supra-costalis superficialis (Knott 1883a), or obliques externus thoracis (Keith 1894).

Typical Presentation
This muscle is only present as a variation or anomaly.

Comparative Anatomy
N/A

Variations

Description

Supracostalis anterior may be present unilaterally or bilaterally (Macalister 1875; Nelson et al. 1992; Bergman et al. 1988). When present, supracostalis anterior is situated deep to the pectoral musculature, typically originating from one rib and extending across two or more anterior intercostal spaces to insert onto another rib (Wood 1865; Macalister 1875; Knott 1883a; Eisler 1912; Nelson et al. 1992; Bakkum and Miller 2016; Snosek and Loukas 2016). One or more bundles may be present (Bergman et al. 1988). It may attach onto ribs one through four, the deep fascia of the neck, or the scalene muscles (Macalister 1875; Mori 1964, Bergman et al. 1988; Nelson et al. 1992; Bakkum and Miller 2016; Snosek and Loukas 2016). Some argue that it is derived from remnants of external abdominal oblique (Keith 1894; Bergman et al. 1988; Bakkum and Miller 2016) while others suggest that it arises from the intercostal muscles (Tachibana and Miyauchi 1989; Nelson et al. 1992; Snosek and Loukas 2016).

Innervation

This muscle has been observed to be innervated by the external muscular branch of the first intercostal nerve (Tachibana and Miyauchi 1989), as well as a collateral branch of the second intercostal nerve (Nelson et al. 1992).

Prevalence

Mori (1964) observed that supracostalis anterior was present in 126 cases out of 2,400 sides from 1,200 cadavers (~5.3%). Mori (1964) also noted that the superior most origin of this muscle was at the first rib on 105 sides (~4.4%) and at the second rib on 21 sides (~0.9%). This muscle inserted onto the third rib on 58 sides (~2.4%) and on the fourth rib on 68 sides (~2.8%). Tachibana and Miyauchi (1989) report a similar prevalence, noting the presence of this muscle in 14 out of 316 sides (4.4%). Miyauchi (1982b) found supracostalis anterior in 3 out of 50 sides (6%) from 25 cadavers. Nelson et al. (1992) found this muscle only once out of 317 cadavers (0.3%).

Anomalies

Description

In individuals with trisomy 13 and trisomy 21, supracostalis anterior extends from the first rib to the second, third, or fourth rib (Pettersen 1979; Pettersen et al. 1979; Bersu 1980; Smith et al. 2015).

Prevalence

In their literature review, Smith et al. (2015) found that supracostalis anterior was present in 2 out of 20 individuals with trisomy 13 (10%) and 1 out of 5 individuals with trisomy 21 (20%).

Clinical Implications
N/A

SUPRACOSTALIS POSTERIOR (FIGURE 4.8)

Synonyms
This muscle is also referred to as supracostalis dorsalis (Mori 1964).

Typical Presentation
This muscle is only present as a variation.

Comparative Anatomy
N/A

Variations

Description

Supracostalis posterior may be present unilaterally or bilaterally (Mori 1964). Like its counterpart on the anterior aspect of the thorax, supracostalis posterior originates from one rib and extends across two or more intercostal spaces to insert onto another rib (Eisler 1912; Mori 1964; Rickenbacher et al. 1985; Bakkum and Miller 2016). One or more bundles may be present (Mori 1964). Eisler (1912) notes that bundles of supracostalis posterior are situated medial to the origin of serratus anterior. Mori (1964) provides a review of the three types of supracostalis posterior that Eisler classified. Type I originates from one rib and crosses one or two ribs to insert into another rib, and its fibers are oriented in the same direction as the external intercostal muscles. Type II originates from a rib via one to three fleshy bundles, and its fibers travel

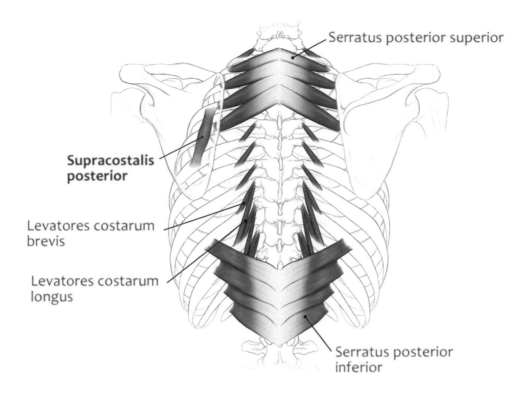

Serratus posterior superior

Supracostalis posterior

Levatores costarum brevis

Levatores costarum longus

Serratus posterior inferior

FIGURE 4.8 Posterior thoracic wall muscles in posterior view.

superomedially to insert onto another rib. Fibers of type II muscles are oriented in the same direction as serratus posterior superior. Type III originate from the eighth, ninth, and tenth ribs and travel superiorly to insert into either the fascia of the ribs or into the fascia of the erector spinae.

Innervation

Bundles of supracostalis posterior are likely innervated by the intercostal nerves.

Prevalence

Mori (1964) observed 65 cases of supracostalis dorsalis and found that type I was present on 19 sides (3.6%), type II was present on 17 sides (3.3%), and type III was present on 29 sides (5.9%). Using these numbers to calculate the total sample size, it is likely that Mori (1964) observed supracostalis posterior in 65 out of around 520–530 sides (about 12% or 12.5%) (Bakkum and Miller 2016).

Anomalies

Description

While supracostalis anterior has been observed in individuals with trisomy 13 and trisomy 21 (Pettersen 1979; Pettersen et al. 1979; Bersu 1980; Smith et al. 2015), supracostalis posterior has not been observed in individuals with trisomy, birth defects, or other congenital disorders, to our knowledge.

Prevalence

N/A

Clinical Implications

N/A

Serratus posterior superior (Figure 4.8)

Synonyms

This muscle is also referred to as serratus posticus superior (Macalister 1875).

Typical Presentation

Description

Serratus posterior superior originates from the nuchal ligament and the spines of the last cervical and upper two or three thoracic vertebrae (Standring 2016). It inserts via four digitations onto the superior margins of the second through fifth ribs (Standring 2016).

Innervation

Serratus posterior superior is innervated by the second through fifth intercostal nerves (Standring 2016).

Comparative Anatomy

Serratus posterior superior originates from the fourth cervical vertebra through the first thoracic vertebra and inserts on the second, third, and fourth ribs in gibbons (Diogo et al. 2012). This muscle is absent or replaced by tendinous threads in orangutans (Gibbs 1999; Diogo et al. 2013b). In gorillas, the muscle extends from all seven cervical vertebrae to ribs two through six (Diogo et al. 2010). In common chimpanzees, the muscle extends from the seventh cervical and first thoracic vertebrae to ribs two through five, and occasionally to rib one, which is the closest to the typical human condition (Sonntag 1923; Diogo et al. 2013a). In bonobos, the origin is variable and can extend superiorly as far as the third cervical vertebra, and its insertion is onto ribs two through four or two through five (Miller 1952; Diogo et al. 2017).

Variations

Description

Serratus posterior superior may be absent (Macalister 1875; Standring 2016), and if so, the muscle is replaced by fibrous tissue (Bergman et al. 1988; Bakkum and Miller 2016). The number of digitations may vary, ranging from three to six (Macalister 1875; Bergman et al. 1988; Bakkum and Miller 2016; Standring 2016), or even only two digitations (Mori 1964). Mori (1964) notes that the origin may extend superiorly up to the fourth, fifth, or sixth cervical vertebra. Satoh (1969) observed an origin as high as the third cervical vertebra. Macalister (1875) states that rhomboatloideus may originate from serratus posterior superior.

Prevalence

Mori (1964) studied the origin and insertion of serratus posterior superior in Japanese cadavers. The most common origin was from between the fifth cervical vertebra and the first thoracic vertebra on 41 out of 99 sides (41%). Other scopes of origin include from the fourth cervical vertebra to the first thoracic vertebra on 33 sides (33%), the fifth cervical vertebra to the seventh cervical vertebra on 12 sides (12%), the fourth cervical vertebra to the seventh cervical vertebra on 4 sides (4%), the fifth cervical vertebra to the second thoracic vertebra on 4 sides (4%), the sixth cervical vertebra to the first thoracic vertebra on 3 sides (3%), and the fourth cervical vertebra to the second thoracic vertebra on 2 sides (2%). Therefore, the upper limit of the origin of this muscle is the fourth cervical vertebra on 42 sides (42%), the fifth cervical vertebra on 57 sides (57%), and the sixth cervical vertebra on 3 sides (3%), while the lower limit of the origin is the seventh cervical vertebra on 16 sides (16%), the first thoracic vertebra on 77 sides (77%), and the second thoracic vertebra on 6 sides (6%).

Serratus posterior superior inserted most frequently onto ribs 2 through 5 on 148 out of 325 sides (46%). The other insertions included from the second through fourth ribs on 84 sides (26%), the third through fifth ribs on 72 sides (23%), the second through sixth ribs on 17 sides (5%), and the third and fourth ribs only on four sides (1%) (Mori 1964).

Satoh (1969) described serratus posterior superior on 20 sides of 10 Japanese cadavers. The upper limit of the origin of this muscle was the third cervical vertebra on two sides (10%), the fourth cervical vertebra on seven sides (35%), the fifth cervical vertebra on nine sides (45%), and the sixth cervical vertebra on two sides (10%). The lower limit of the origin was the first thoracic vertebra on 17 sides (85%) and the second thoracic vertebra on three sides (15%).

It inserted most frequently onto ribs two through five on nine sides (45%). Other insertions included the second through fourth ribs on five sides (25%), the second through sixth ribs on four sides (20%), and second through seventh ribs on one side (5%), and the third through sixth ribs on one side (5%). Therefore, the upper limit of the insertion was the second rib on 19 sides (95%) and the third rib on one side (5%). The lower limit of the insertion was rib five in nine cases (45%), rib four in five cases (25%), rib six in five cases (25%), and rib seven in one case (5%) (Satoh 1969).

Loukas et al. (2008c) studied serratus posterior superior on 100 sides of 50 cadavers. They found that the origin of the muscle was from the seventh cervical through second or third thoracic vertebrae in 65% of specimens, from the sixth cervical through the second thoracic vertebrae in 30% of specimens, and from the fifth cervical through the second or third thoracic vertebrae in 5% of specimens. It inserted onto the second through fifth ribs in 90% of specimens and into the second through sixth ribs in 10% of cases.

Anomalies

Description

Serratus posterior superior may be absent as an anomaly (Colacino and Pettersen 1978; Smith et al. 2015). In a fetus with spina bifida with encephaloceles, the serratus posterior muscles were unidentifiable (Wheeler 1918).

Prevalence

In their literature review, Smith et al. (2015) found that serratus posterior superior was absent in 1 out of 24 cases of trisomy 13 (4.2%)—a case described by Colacino and Pettersen (1978).

Clinical Implications

N/A

SERRATUS POSTERIOR INFERIOR (FIGURE 4.8)

Synonyms

This muscle is also referred to as serratus posticus inferior (Macalister 1875).

Typical Presentation

Description

Serratus posterior inferior originates from the spines of the last two thoracic and upper two or three lumbar vertebrae (Standring 2016). It inserts via four digitations onto the inferior margins of ribs 9 through 12 (Standring 2016).

Innervation

Serratus posterior inferior is supplied by the ninth through twelfth thoracic spinal nerves (Standring 2016).

Comparative Anatomy

Serratus posterior inferior originates from the tenth thoracic vertebra through the second lumbar vertebra and inserts onto ribs 10 through 14 in gibbons (Diogo et al. 2012). It extends from the thoracolumbar fascia to the last four or five ribs in orangutans and common chimpanzees (Sonntag 1923; Diogo et al. 2013ab). In bonobos, it originates from the thoracolumbar fascia, with vertebral attachments as superior as the eighth thoracic vertebra and as inferior as the third lumbar vertebra and attaches to the last four or five ribs (Miller 1952; Diogo et al. 2017). This muscle is absent in gorillas (Raven 1950; Diogo et al. 2010).

Variations

Description

Serratus posterior inferior may be absent (Macalister 1875; Rickenbacher et al. 1985; Standring 2016), and if so, the muscle is replaced by fibrous tissue (Bergman et al. 1988; Bakkum and Miller 2016). The number of digitations may vary (Macalister 1875; Bergman et al. 1988; Standring 2016), ranging from two to five digitations (Macalister 1875; Mori 1964; Rickenbacher et al. 1985; Bakkum and Miller 2016). When it is reduced to only two digitations, often the first and the fourth digitation are absent (Bergman et al. 1988). Mori (1964) notes that the origin may extend up to the tenth thoracic vertebra and the insertion may have an attachment to the eighth rib. Satoh (1970) notes that the origin may extend up to the ninth thoracic vertebra.

The insertion of serratus posterior inferior may extend beneath the external oblique (Rickenbacher et al. 1985). Serratus posterior inferior may have connections to the external intercostal muscles or external oblique (Rickenbacher et al. 1985) or may be fused with latissimus dorsi (Macalister 1875). Accessory muscle bundles may be present at the inferior border of the digitations, forming arches that extend to the next lower digitation (Rickenbacher et al. 1985).

Prevalence

Mori (1964) found that the most common upper limit of the origin of serratus posterior inferior to be the eleventh thoracic vertebra on 60 out of 100 sides (60%). The other upper limits of the origin included the tenth vertebra on 31 sides (31%), the twelfth thoracic vertebra on seven sides (7%), the first lumbar vertebra on one side (1%), and the second lumbar vertebra on one side (1%). The most frequent upper limit of the insertion was to rib 9 on 180 out of 201 sides (90%). The other upper limits of the insertion included rib 10 on 13 sides (6.5%), rib 8 on 5 sides (2.5%), and rib 11 on 3 sides (1.5%). The lower limit of the insertion was to rib 12 on 145 out of 206 sides (70%) and to rib 11 on 61 sides (30%). Thus, serratus posterior inferior inserts most often onto ribs 9 through 12 (Mori 1964).

Satoh (1970) described serratus posterior inferior on 20 sides of 10 Japanese cadavers. The upper limit of the origin of this muscle was the ninth thoracic vertebra on 2 sides (10%), the tenth thoracic vertebra on 4 sides (20%), the eleventh thoracic vertebra on 13 sides (65%), and the twelfth thoracic vertebra on 1 side (5%). It inserted most frequently onto ribs 9 through 12, which was observed on 9 sides (45%). Other insertions include ribs 9 through 11 on 7 sides (35%), ribs 9 and 10 on 2 sides (10%), ribs 10 and 11 on 1 side (5%), and ribs 10 through 12 on 1 side (5%). Therefore, the upper limit of the insertion was to rib 9 in 18 cases (90%) and to rib 10 in 2 cases (10%), while the lower limit of the insertion was to rib 10 on 2 sides (10%), rib 11 on 8 sides (40%), and rib 12 in 10 cases (50%) (Satoh 1970).

Loukas et al. (2008c) studied serratus posterior inferior on 100 sides of 50 cadavers. They found that the origin of the muscle was from the eleventh thoracic through second lumbar vertebrae in 85% of specimens, from the tenth thoracic through second lumbar vertebrae in 10% of specimens, and from the tenth thoracic through third lumbar vertebrae in 5% of specimens. The origins were always blended with the thoracolumbar fascia. It inserted onto the last three ribs in 60% of cases and the last four ribs in 40% of cases.

Anomalies

Description

Serratus posterior inferior was absent bilaterally in both a neonate with trisomy 18 (Aziz 1979) and a neonate with trisomy 13 (Aziz 1980). In a fetus with spina bifida with encephaloceles, the serratus posterior muscles were unidentifiable (Wheeler 1918).

Prevalence

In their literature review, Smith et al. (2015) found that serratus posterior inferior was absent in 4 out of 24 cases of trisomy 13 (16.7%) and 1 out of 26 individuals with trisomy 18 (3.8%).

Clinical Implications

N/A

LEVATORES COSTARUM BREVES AND LONGI (FIGURE 4.8)

Synonyms

N/A

Typical Presentation

Description

The 12 bundles of levatores costarum originate from the transverse processes of the last cervical vertebra and first through eleventh thoracic vertebrae (Standring 2016). Each bundle inserts onto the rib that is immediately below its vertebra of origin (Standring 2016). These bundles insert between the tubercles and the costal angles and are referred to as levatores costarum breves (Standring 2016). The upper eight bundles have only one fascicle. The lowest four bundles have two fasciculi, one corresponding to levatores costarum brevis and the other corresponding to levatores costarum longus, which inserts onto the second rib below its vertebra of origin (Standring 2016).

Innervation

Levatores costarum are innervated by the thoracic spinal nerves (Standring 2016).

Comparative Anatomy

There is no information for levatores costarum in orangutans or common chimpanzees (Gibbs 1999; Diogo et al. 2013a,b) and little information for the other ape species. The muscle seems to have a similar typical presentation to humans in gibbons, gorillas, and bonobos, though the last bundle is attached to the twelfth thoracic vertebra in gorillas and bonobos (Miller 1952; Gibbs 1999; Diogo et al. 2010, 2012, 2017).

Variations

Description

Some bundles of levatores costarum brevis and/or longus may be absent, doubled, or otherwise variable in number (Satoh and Shu 1968; Rickenbacher et al. 1985; Bakkum and Miller 2016). Bundles of levatores costarum breves and longi may unite and present as a sheet (Macalister 1875). Levatores costarum longi may be found in the middle or upper thoracic spine (Satoh and Shu 1968; Rickenbacher et al. 1985). Levatores costarum bundles can send fibers to, or fuse with, the external intercostal muscles, scalenus posterior, or iliocostal muscles (Macalister 1875; Rickenbacher et al. 1985). In some cases, all bundles of levatores costarum may be absent (Rickenbacher et al. 1985).

Satoh and Shu (1968) studied the levatores costarum muscles in a Japanese population and note instances where a muscle originated via tendinous fibers from the lateral side of levator costae brevis and passed over the rib above to insert into the belly of levator costae brevis in the next intercostal space. These authors suggest that it is an inverted and incomplete form of levator costae longus. Satoh and Shu (1968) also categorized bundles of levatores costarum longi into four types. They defined type A as an incomplete form of the muscle which terminated on the external intercostal in the next intercostal space after crossing only over one rib. Type B is the typical presentation of this muscle, which crosses over one rib to insert onto the next rib and thus spans two intercostal spaces. Type C bundles crossed two intercostal spaces and terminated on the external intercostal muscle in the next intercostal space. Type D bundles extended over three intercostal spaces (Satoh and Shu 1968).

Macdonald Brown (1880) describes the bilateral presence of a muscle termed levator costae primae. Levator costae primae originates from the superior border of the scapula and partially from the suprascapular ligament and inserts onto the first rib, immediately external to its cartilage (Macdonald Brown 1880; Snosek and Loukas 2016).

Prevalence

The variable muscle described by Satoh and Shu (1968) that extended from levator costae brevis to the belly of levator costae brevis in the next intercostal space was found in 2 out of 87 cases (2.3%). In two other cases (2.3%), two muscles classified as type B were completely

tendinous. The most common type of levatores costarum longi identified by these authors was type B, found in 51 cases (58.6%).

Anomalies

N/A

Clinical Implications

N/A

INTERSPINALES (FIGURE 4.9)

Synonyms

N/A

Typical Presentation

Description

Interspinales are paired muscular bundles that extend between the tips of adjacent spinous processes throughout the vertebral column (Standring 2016). They are most well-developed in the cervical spine and comprise six pairs of muscles (Standring 2016). In the thoracic spine, the muscles are distinct between the first and second thoracic vertebrae and between the eleventh and twelfth thoracic vertebrae. In the lumbar spine, there are four pairs of muscles (Standring 2016).

Innervation

The interspinales muscles are innervated by the medial branch of the dorsal ramus of the spinal nerve of the corresponding segment (Rickenbacher et al. 1985).

Comparative Anatomy

There is no information about interspinales for gibbons, orangutans, or bonobos (Diogo et al. 2012, 2013b, 2017). Sonntag (1923) states that interspinales in common chimpanzees is similar to those of humans. In gorillas, the muscles have a similar typical presentation to humans and the superiormost attachment of interspinales is to the third cervical vertebra and the inferiormost attachment is to the second thoracic vertebra (Raven 1950; Gibbs 1999; Diogo et al. 2010).

Variations

Description

The interspinales muscles may be doubled or absent (Miyauchi 1976; Bakkum and Miller 2016). In the cervical region, the interspinales muscles may extend across more than two vertebrae (Standring 2016). The muscles in this part of the spine sometimes blend with neighboring muscles (Rickenbacher et al. 1985). The interspinales in the thoracic spine vary substantially in number (Miyauchi 1976; Rickenbacher et al. 1985). In this region, bundles between the second and third thoracic vertebrae are occasionally present (Standring 2016). In the lumbar spine, the interspinales muscles may be present between the last thoracic and

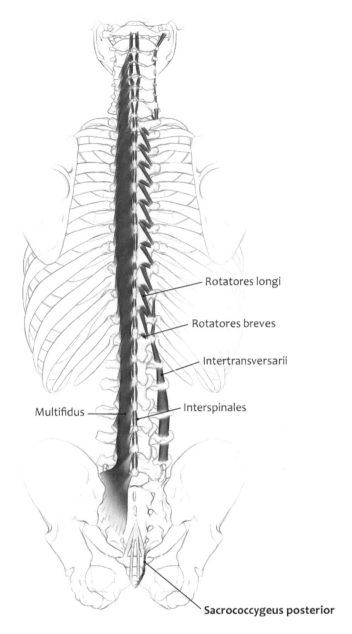

FIGURE 4.9   Interspinal, intertransverse, and caudal spinotransverse muscles in posterior view.

first lumbar vertebrae (Standring 2016). Interspinales muscles may be present in the sacral region (Miyauchi 1976; Standring 2016).

Prevalence

Based on a study of 60 sides from 30 cadavers, Miyauchi (1976) found that all interspinales in the cervical region were present in all cases except for the last (the muscle between the seventh cervical and first thoracic vertebrae), which was absent on three sides (5%). In the upper thoracic region, the interspinales between the first and second thoracic vertebrae were present on only 26 sides (43.3%) and the interspinales between the second and third thoracic vertebrae were present on three sides (5%). These muscles were always absent in the mid-thoracic region. In

the lower thoracic region, the interspinales were always present and the upper limit of these muscles was the tenth thoracic vertebra on 22 sides (36.7%), the eleventh thoracic vertebra on 35 sides (58.3%) and the twelfth thoracic vertebra on three sides (5%). The interspinales in the lumbar region were also present in all cases except for the muscle between the fourth and fifth lumbar vertebrae, which was absent on four sides (6.7%), and the muscle between the last lumbar and first sacral vertebrae, which was absent on 20 sides (33.3%). A muscle was present between the first and second sacral vertebrae on eight sides (13.3%) (Miyauchi 1976).

Anomalies

N/A

Clinical Implications

N/A

SACROCOCCYGEUS POSTERIOR (FIGURE 4.9)

See also: Interspinales; Sacrococcygeus anterior

Synonyms

This muscle may also be referred to as sacrococcygeus posticus, levator coccygis (Morgagni), extensor coccygis (Macalister 1875; Knott 1883b), or sacrococcygeus dorsalis (Rickenbacher et al. 1985).

Typical Presentation

This muscle may be only present as a variation, but Macalister (1875, p. 66) states that it is "a tolerably constant muscle."

Comparative Anatomy

This muscle may be homologous with the extensor (levator) caudae lateralis of other mammals (Knott 1883b; Rickenbacher et al. 1985).

Variations

Description

A variant of interspinales is sacrococcygeus posterior, a musculotendinous bundle that connects the sacrum to the coccyx and has an attachment to the dorsal sacrococcygeal ligaments (Rickenbacher et al. 1985). Sacrococcygeus posterior is covered by strands of the sacrotuberal ligament and by a portion of the gluteus maximus fascia (Rickenbacher et al. 1985). Knott (1883b) observed an origin from the posterior surface of the third and fourth sacral bones in most cases and from the posterior inferior iliac spine in one case. See the entry for sacrococcygeus anterior for a similar muscle on the anterior aspect of the sacrum.

Innervation

N/A

Prevalence

Knott (1883b) found fleshy fibers corresponding to "sacrococcygeus posticus" in 4 out of 30 subjects (13.3%).

Anomalies

While the presence of sacrococcygeus anterior has been recorded in one individual with trisomy 21 (Bersu 1980), the presence of sacrococcygeus posterior has not been recorded in individuals with trisomy, birth defects, or other congenital disorders, to our knowledge.

Clinical Implications

N/A

INTERTRANSVERSARII (FIGURE 4.9)

Synonyms

These muscles may also be referred to as intertransversalis (Macalister 1875).

Typical Presentation

Description

Intertransversarii connect the transverse processes of adjacent vertebrae (Standring 2016). The intertransversarii are most distinct in the cervical spine and are composed of seven pairs of anterior and posterior sets of muscles (Standring 2016). In the thoracic spine, the intertransversarii are single muscles that connect adjacent transverse processes between the last three thoracic vertebrae and the first lumbar vertebra (Standring 2016). In the lumbar spine, the intertransversarii are composed of medial and lateral sets of muscles (Standring 2016).

Innervation

The intertransversarii are innervated by either the ventral or dorsal rami of the spinal nerve of the corresponding segment (Standring 2016).

Comparative Anatomy

There is no information on intertransversarii in gibbons (Gibbs 1999; Diogo et al. 2012), and the intertransversarii in the other ape species are simply described as being similar to those of humans (Sonntag 1923; Raven 1950; Gibbs 1999; Diogo et al. 2010, 2013ab, 2017).

Variations

Description

Any of the intertransverse muscles may be doubled or absent (Macalister 1875; Bakkum and Miller 2016). The anterior set of intertransversarii muscles between the first and second cervical vertebrae are frequently absent (Standring 2016). Accessory intertransverse muscles have been described with attachments from the fourth through sixth to the first three cervical vertebrae (transversalis cervicis anticus of Retzius) and between the third and fifth cervical vertebrae (Sandifort's muscle or musculus singularis) (Macalister 1875; Knott 1883a; Bakkum and Miller 2016). The anterior cervical intertransverse muscles may fuse with the scalene muscles (Rickenbacher et al. 1985).

In rare cases, the intertransverse muscles do not connect to the transverse processes, and instead fuse with the erector spinae (Rickenbacher et al. 1985). Adjacent intertransverse muscles may partially or completely fuse into strands that bridge across one or more segments, a variation that occurs more often in the thoracolumbar region than in the cervical spine (Rickenbacher et al. 1985). The intertransversarii laterales in the lumbar region may fuse with quadratus lumborum (Rickenbacher et al. 1985).

Prevalence

N/A

Anomalies

N/A

Clinical Implications

N/A

ROTATORES LONGUS AND BREVIS (FIGURE 4.9)

Synonyms

These muscles may be referred to as rotatores spinae (Macalister 1875).

Typical Presentation

Description

The rotatores muscles comprise part of the transversospinalis muscular group and are most well-developed in the thoracic spine (rotatores thoracis) (Standring 2016). Rotatores thoracis is comprised of 11 pairs of muscles, each with a longus and brevis portion (Standring 2016). Rotatores breves connect the lamina of a vertebra to the transverse process of the adjacent vertebra below (Standring 2016). Rotatores longi connect the spinous process of a vertebra to the transverse process of the vertebra two segments below (Standring 2016).

Innervation

Rotatores are innervated by medial branches of the dorsal rami of the spinal nerves of the corresponding segment (Standring 2016).

Comparative Anatomy

There is no information on rotatores in gibbons (Gibbs 1999; Diogo et al. 2012). These muscles in the other apes have a similar typical presentation to those of humans, but it is possible that rotatores longi is present only in gorillas and absent in common chimpanzees, bonobos, and orangutans (Sonntag 1923; Raven 1950; Gibbs 1999; Diogo et al. 2010, 2013a,b, 2017).

Variations

Description

One or more of the rotatores muscles may be absent from the upper thoracic vertebrae or the lower thoracic vertebrae (Macalister et al. 1875; Rickenbacher et al. 1985; Standring 2016). The number of rotatores breves in particular may range from 9 to 12 in this region (Rickenbacher et al. 1985). The rotatores longi may be more poorly developed than the rotatores breves (Rickenbacher et al. 1985). The rotatores may be divided into fasciculi (Macalister 1875). Accessory bundles or accessory attachments across two adjacent vertebrae may occur in the thoracic region (Rickenbacher et al. 1985; Cornwall et al. 2011; Bakkum and Miller 2016).

The presence of rotatores muscles in the cervical and lumbar regions are often variable (Rickenbacher et al. 1985), and they may be replaced by deep bundles of multifidus (Standring 2016). They may be completely absent (Rickenbacher et al. 1985; Cornwall et al. 2011). Sometimes, the complete series of rotatores cervicis can be present (Rickenbacher et al. 1985). When present, the rotatores lumborum are represented by strands somewhere between the last thoracic vertebra and the first or second sacral vertebrae and are difficult to separate from interspinales (Rickenbacher et al. 1985).

Prevalence

N/A

Anomalies

N/A

Clinical Implications

N/A

MULTIFIDUS (FIGURE 4.9)

Synonyms

This muscle may also be referred to as multifidus spinae (Macalister 1875).

Typical Presentation

Description

Multifidus is one of the muscles that comprises the transversospinalis muscular group. It is comprised of bundles that lie in the grooves between the spinous processes and transverse processes along the entire vertebral column (Standring 2016). Each bundle extends between the lateral aspect of a vertebral spinous process and the transverse parts of the vertebrae two, four, and five segments below (Standring 2016). Multifidus thus has attachments to the articular processes of the last four cervical vertebrae, to the transverse processes of the thoracic vertebrae, to the mamillary processes of the lumbar vertebrae, to the dorsal surface of the sacrum as far as the fourth sacral foramen, and to the dorsal aspect of the iliac crest (Standring 2016; Rickenbacher et al. 1985).

Innervation

Multifidus is innervated by medial branches of the dorsal rami of the corresponding spinal nerves (Standring 2016).

Comparative Anatomy

There is no descriptive information on multifidus for gibbons (Gibbs 1999; Diogo et al. 2012) or orangutans, though Diogo et al. (2013b) did observe the presence of this muscle in an orangutan. The muscles in gorillas, common chimpanzees, and bonobos have a similar typical presentation to that in humans, but an attachment may extend to the atlas in bonobos (Raven 1950; Miller 1952; Gibbs 1999; Diogo et al. 2010, 2013a, 2017).

Variations

Description

Multifidus is often variable in its configuration and the muscle may be asymmetrical between the sides of an individual (Rickenbacher et al. 1985). One or more digitations may be absent (Macalister 1875). The digitation that originates from the seventh cervical vertebra may be absent (Macalister 1875; Rickenbacher et al. 1985). The digitation that extends between the axis and the fourth cervical vertebra may be attached across the entire breadth of the arch of the axis (Macalister 1875; Rickenbacher et al. 1985). In the cervical region, accessory bundles may be present that attach to the articular and transverse processes and to the capsules of the vertebral joints (Rickenbacher et al. 1985). Willard (1997) reports that multifidus in the lumbar region attaches to the thoracolumbar fascia via a raphe.

Prevalence

N/A

Anomalies

Description

Stevenson et al. (2014) describe cadaver with a severe case of congenital scoliosis. Multifidus was atrophied on the left side and could not be identified above the level of the tenth thoracic spinous process. Multifidus on the right side had a more typical presentation but many digitations were replaced by tendinous slips (Stevenson et al. 2014).

Prevalence

N/A

Clinical Implications

N/A

SEMISPINALIS (FIGURE 4.10)

Synonyms

Semispinalis capitis may also be referred to as complexus major (Krause) (Macalister 1875), complexus (Cowper), and grand complexus (Cruveilhier) (Bakkum and Miller 2016). Semispinalis cervicis may also be referred to as semispinalis colli, and semispinalis thoracis as semispinalis dorsi (Macalister 1875). The medial portion of semispinalis capitis in the cervical region may be referred to as biventer cervicis because its superficial bundles appear distinct from the rest of the muscle and because it has an incomplete tendinous intersection, giving it the appearance of two distinct bellies (Bergman et al. 1988; Standring 2016).

Typical Presentation

Description

The semispinalis muscles are part of the transversospinalis muscular group and are divided into three portions (Standring 2016). Semispinalis capitis originates from the occipital bone between the superior and inferior nuchal lines (Standring 2016). It inserts via tendons onto the articular processes of cervical vertebrae four through seven and the transverse processes of the first six or seven thoracic vertebrae (Standring 2016). Semispinalis cervicis is covered by semispinalis capitis (Standring 2016). It originates from the spinous processes of the second to fifth cervical vertebrae (Standring 2016). Its bundles insert onto the transverse processes of the upper five or six thoracic vertebrae (Standring 2016). Semispinalis thoracis originates via tendons from the spinous processes of the last two cervical and the first four thoracic vertebrae and inserts via tendons

onto the transverse processes of the sixth through tenth thoracic vertebrae (Standring 2016).

Innervation

Semispinalis capitis is innervated by the greater occipital nerve and the third cervical nerve (Standring 2016). Semispinalis cervicis and semispinalis thoracis are innervated by medial branches of the dorsal rami of the corresponding spinal nerves (Standring 2016).

Comparative Anatomy

In common chimpanzees, semispinalis cervicis and thoracis are difficult to separate and semispinalis capitis is often fused with parts of longissimus and spinalis (Sonntag 1923; Diogo et al. 2013a). There is no information for semispinalis thoracis in bonobos (Miller 1952; Diogo et al. 2017), but the other portions of semispinalis resemble those of humans. Sonntag (1924) has noted the presence of the "biventer cervicis" bundle in an orangutan.

Variations

Description

The slips of semispinalis capitis to the vertebrae may vary in number (Macalister 1875; Bergman et al. 1988; Bakkum and Miller 2016). A slip may extend from the third cervical vertebra or from the eighth thoracic vertebra (Rickenbacher et al. 1985). Semispinalis capitis may be partially divided into two bellies with separate tendons of origin that insert together onto the occiput (Çelik et al. 1997). Semispinalis capitis may receive slips from longissimus or spinalis thoracis (Macalister 1875; Rickenbacher et al. 1985; Bergman et al. 1988; Bakkum and Miller 2016). Semispinalis capitis is often blended with spinalis capitis (Bakkum and Miller 2016).

A second lamella under the medial part of semispinalis capitis extending from one or more of the thoracic vertebrae to the occipital bone may be present (Bergman et al. 1988; Bakkum and Miller 2016). There may be accessory bundles that connect to the nuchal ligament or run between semispinalis capitis and rectus capitis posterior major (Macalister 1875; Rickenbacher et al. 1985). An accessory muscle that runs parallel to semispinalis capitis may be present extending between the transverse process of the axis to the occipital bone (Macalister 1875; Rickenbacher et al. 1985).

Semispinalis cervicis and semispinalis thoracis can vary in the number of origins and insertions (Macalister 1875; Rickenbacher et al. 1985). The attachments of semispinalis cervicis may include the seventh cervical or the seventh or eighth thoracic vertebrae (Rickenbacher et al. 1985). Semispinalis thoracis may also vary in the number of vertebrae that its fibers bridge across (Bakkum and Miller 2016). It may be difficult to distinguish the bundles of semispinalis cervicis from those of semispinalis thoracis (Macalister 1875; Rickenbacher et al. 1985).

Semispinalis lumborum may be present as a variation (Rickenbacher et al. 1985). Typically, remnants of semispinalis in the lumbar spine are represented by the mammillo-accessory ligaments (Standring 2016). However, when semispinalis lumborum is present it is covered by fascia that is attached to the mamillary processes of the last four lumbar vertebrae and the first sacral vertebra and is fused to the aponeurosis of longissimus (Rickenbacher et al. 1985). This muscle also has tendinous origins from the mamillary processes of the last thoracic and first lumbar vertebrae and attachments to the spinous processes of the last six thoracic vertebrae and the first lumbar vertebra (Rickenbacher et al. 1985). It may be difficult to separate from multifidus (Rickenbacher et al. 1985).

Prevalence

N/A

Anomalies

Description

On the right side of one male neonate with trisomy 13, Pettersen et al. (1979) found that semispinalis cervicis was connected via an accessory slip to obliquus capitis inferior.

Prevalence

According to the literature review of Smith et al. (2015), the anomalous slip observed by Pettersen et al. (1979) was present in only 1 out of 20 individuals with trisomy 13 (5%).

Clinical Implications

N/A

Splenius capitis and Splenius cervicis (Figure 4.10)

Synonyms

Splenius capitis is also referred to as Riemenmuskeln (Bakkum and Miller 2016). Splenius cervicis is also referred to as Bauschmuskeln or splenius colli (Macalister 1875; Bakkum and Miller 2016).

Typical Presentation

Description

Splenius capitis extends from the mastoid process and the occipital bone to the spinous processes of the last cervical and upper three or four thoracic vertebrae (Standring 2016). Splenius cervicis lies close to the inferior border of splenius capitis, originating from the transverse processes of the first two cervical vertebrae and the posterior tubercle of the third cervical vertebra (Standring 2016). It inserts onto the spinous processes of the third through sixth thoracic vertebrae (Standring 2016).

Innervation

Splenius capitis is innervated by the second and third cervical spinal nerves (Standing 2016). Splenius cervicis is innervated by the lower cervical spinal nerves (Standing 2016).

Comparative Anatomy

Splenius capitis and splenius cervicis have a similar typical presentation in the apes, with similar variations including

variable vertebral attachments in some species and an occasional slip to levator scapulae in common chimpanzees (Sonntag 1923; Diogo et al. 2010, 2012, 2013a,b, 2017).

Variations

Description

The splenius muscles may be absent (Rickenbacher et al. 1985; Bergman et al. 1988). Other variations include proximal displacement of the origin of the splenius muscles by one or two vertebrae, or asymmetric origins (Rickenbacher et al. 1985; Bergman et al. 1988; Bakkum and Miller 2016). Splenius capitis may be divided into a superior and inferior portion (Macalister 1875; Bergman et al. 1988; Bakkum and Miller 2016). Splenius capitis may be blended with splenius cervicis (Macalister 1875; Rickenbacher et al. 1985; Kamibayashi and Richmond 1998; Bakkum and Miller 2016). Slips can connect the splenius muscles to longissimus capitis, iliocostalis, levator scapulae, serratus anterior, or serratus posterior superior (Wood 1870; Macalister 1875; Rickenbacher et al. 1985; Bergman et al. 1988; Bakkum and Miller 2016).

Prevalence

N/A

Anomalies

Description

In a trisomy 18 cyclopic fetus, Smith et al. (2015) found that splenius capitis was closely associated with/fused with trapezius at the midline origin on both sides (Smith et al. 2015).

Prevalence

The close connection between splenius capitis and the trapezius observed by Smith et al. (2015) was not present in any of the trisomy 13, trisomy 18, and trisomy 21 cases included in their literature review.

Clinical Implications

N/A

Rhomboatloideus (Figure 4.10)

See also: Splenius capitis and splenius cervicis

Synonyms

This muscle is also referred to as rhomboaxoideus (Wood 1867a), splenius accessorius (Krause), splenius colli accessorius, splenius capitis accessorius, muscularis singularis splenius accessories (Walther), or adjutor splenii (Macalister 1975; Knott 1883a; Bergman et al. 1988; Bakkum and Miller 2016).

Typical Presentation

This muscle is only present as a variation or anomaly.

Comparative Anatomy

N/A

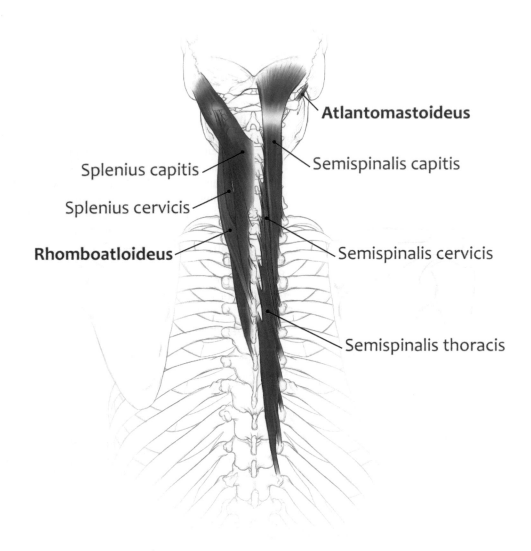

FIGURE 4.10   Splenius, semispinalis, and nearby variations in posterior view.

Variations

Description

Rhomboatloideus describes a slip that originates from the spines of the lower cervical and upper thoracic vertebrae (anywhere from C6 to T3), close to the attachment of rhomboid minor, and passes superficially along the border of splenius to insert on the transverse process of the atlas (Macalister 1866, 1875; Knott 1883a; Bergman et al. 1988; Bakkum and Miller 2016). It can also originate from the fascia of serratus posterior superior or rhomboideus minor (Macalister 1975; Bergman et al. 1988, Beger et al. 2018a). It may have attachments to the mastoid process or occipital bone (Bergman et al. 1988). Rhomboatloideus may have slips that blend with rhomboideus major and serratus posterior superior (Wood 1867a,b; Bakkum and Miller 2016).

Innervation
N/A

Prevalence

Macalister (1875) notes that Wood found rhomboatloideus in 3 out of 36 subjects (8.3%). Knott (1883a) found this muscle in 6 out of 75 subjects (8%).

Anomalies

Description

Beger et al. (2019) observed rhomboatloideus bilaterally in a 26-week old male fetus with CHARGE syndrome. Rhomboatloideus extended from the transverse process of the atlas to the spinous processes of the second, third, and fourth thoracic vertebrae (Beger et al. 2019).

Prevalence
N/A

Clinical Implications

Rhomboatloideus may be incorrectly diagnosed as a tumor or can contribute to myofascial trigger points (Beger et al. 2018a).

Atlantomastoideus (Figure 4.10)

Synonyms

This muscle is also referred to as atlanticomastoideus (Gruber) or rectus lateralis accessorius (Winslow) (Bergman et al. 1988).

Typical Presentation

This muscle is only present as a variation.

Comparative Anatomy

Among the apes, atlantomastoideus has only been reported as a variation in gorillas and common chimpanzees (Gratiolet and Alix 1866; Sommer 1907; Diogo et al. 2010, 2012, 2013a,b, 2017).

Variations

Description

Atlantomastoideus originates from the transverse process of the atlas, courses between the rectus capitis lateralis and obliquus capitis superior, and attaches to the mastoid process (Gruber 1867c; Knott 1883a; Mori 1964; Rickenbacher et al. 1985; Bergman et al. 1988; Bakkum and Miller 2016). Its insertion may occur at the posterior margin of the mastoid process or the lateral or medial margin of the mastoid notch (Rickenbacher et al. 1985). Accessory slips may be present that connect atlantomastoideus to splenius capitis, longissimus capitis, or the axis (Mori 1964). Based on their shared innervation, Mori (1964) suggests that atlantomastoideus derives from the same anlage as longissimus capitis and obliquus capitis superior.

Innervation

Atlantomastoideus is innervated by the dorsal ramus of the first cervical spinal nerve (Mori 1964).

Prevalence

Gruber lists the prevalence of atlantomastoideus as 20%, but Rickenbacher et al. (1985) suggest that this is likely too high. Knott (1883a) found this muscle in 4 out of 33 subjects (12.1%). Mori (1964) found atlantomastoideus bilaterally in 5 out of 54 cadavers (9.3%), on the right side in 5 cadavers (9.3%), and on the left side in 4 cadavers (7.4%). Therefore, out of 108 sides, atlantomastoideus was present in 19 sides (17.6%).

Anomalies

N/A

Clinical Implications

N/A

Spinalis (Figure 4.11)

Synonyms

Miyauchi (1976) refers to spinalis cervicis as interspinalis cervicalis longus. Spinalis thoracis may be referred to as spinalis dorsi and spinalis cervicis may be referred to as spinalis colli (Macalister 1875).

Typical Presentation

Description

Spinalis is partitioned into spinalis thoracis, spinalis cervicis, and spinalis capitis, which are all continuous with each other (Standring 2016). Spinalis thoracis is the best-developed and most constant of the three portions (Standring 2016). Bundles of spinalis thoracis extend between the spinous processes of the lower two thoracic and upper two lumbar vertebrae and the spinous processes of the upper thoracic vertebrae (Standring 2016).

When present, spinalis cervicis extends from the spinous processes of the second through fourth cervical vertebrae to the ligamentum nuchae and spine of the last cervical vertebra (Standring 2016). When present, spinalis capitis is represented by fibers of semispinalis capitis that attach to the spinous processes of the last cervical and first thoracic vertebrae (Standring 2016).

Innervation

The erector spinae group is innervated by the lateral branches of the dorsal rami of the corresponding cervical, thoracic, and lumbar spinal nerves (Standring 2016).

Comparative Anatomy

Spinalis has a similar typical presentation in the apes, often with fusion to semispinalis in gorillas (Gibbs 1999; Diogo et al. 2010, 2012, 2013a,b, 2017).

Variations

Description

Spinalis is rarely completely absent but is also rarely symmetrical on the left and right sides (Rickenbacher et al. 1985). Spinalis thoracis can vary in its number of digitations and attachments (Macalister 1875; Rickenbacher et al. 1985; Bakkum and Miller 2016; Standring 2016). Spinalis thoracis is typically blended with longissimus thoracis and may be considered a part of this muscle (Standring 2016). Spinalis cervicis can send attachments to the spines of the first two thoracic vertebrae (Standring 2016) and may be fused with semispinalis cervicis (Greiner et al. 2004; Bakkum and Miller 2016). Spinalis capitis is often fused with semispinalis capitis and can also be fused with rectus capitis posterior minor (Rickenbacher et al. 1985; Martin 1994; Greiner et al. 2004; Bakkum and Miller 2016). Eister (1912) considers the presence of spinalis capitis to be a variant and not part of the typical presentation of spinalis (Rickenbacher et al. 1985). Spinalis lumborum, which extends between the spinous processes of the lower two lumbar vertebrae and some of the lower thoracic vertebrae, may also be present as a rare variation (Rickenbacher et al. 1985).

Labranche et al. (2017) describe what they believe to be a distinct and unilateral bundle of spinalis capitis. Acknowledging that this muscle has a presentation that

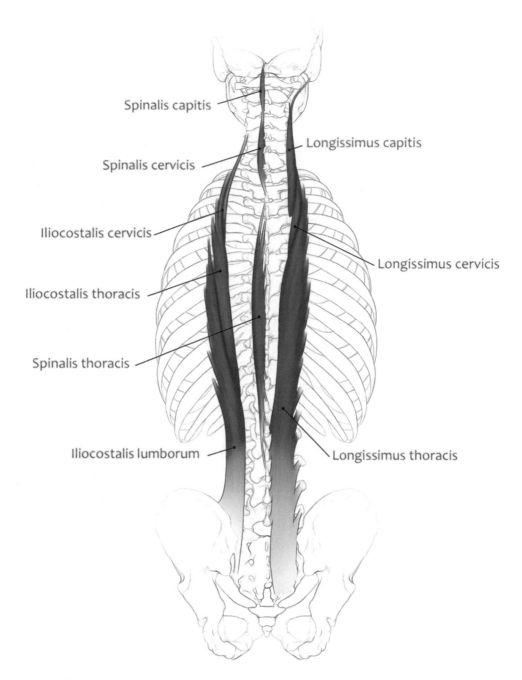

FIGURE 4.11 Erector spinae muscles in posterior view.

does not match previous descriptions, they state a bundle of spinalis capitis arose deep to semispinalis capitis and was on the same fascial plane as spinalis cervicis. The muscle originated from the ligamentum nuchae at the level of the third and fourth cervical vertebrae and attached to the occiput just superficial to the rectus capitis posterior minor at the inferior nuchal line.

Prevalence

In a study of 60 sides from 30 Japanese cadavers, Miyauchi (1976) reports that spinalis cervicis was present in 49 sides (81.7%) and absent on 11 sides (18.3%). Miyauchi (1976) also found that the upper limit of spinalis cervicis was the second cervical vertebra on 36 sides (73.5%), the third cervical vertebra on 8 sides (16.3%), and the fourth cervical

vertebra on 5 sides (10.2%). The lower limit of this muscle was the fourth cervical vertebra on 2 sides (4.1%), the fifth cervical vertebra on 12 sides (24.5%), the sixth cervical vertebra on 18 sides (36.7%), the seventh cervical vertebra on 11 sides (22.4%), and the first thoracic vertebra on 6 sides (12.2%) (Miyauchi 1976).

Based on dissections of 142 cadavers (284 sides), Greiner et al. (2004) found that spinalis cervicis was absent on 102 sides (35.9%), blended with semispinalis cervicis on 51 sides (18%), and distinct from semispinalis cervicis on 131 sides (46.1%). Based on dissections of the 279 sides that would have allowed for the observation of spinalis capitis, Greiner et al. (2004) found that spinalis capitis was absent on 196 sides (70.3%), blended with semispinalis capitis on 80 sides (28.7%), and distinct from semispinalis capitis on 3 sides (1%).

Anomalies

Description

Stevenson et al. (2014) describe a cadaver with a severe case of congenital scoliosis. The erector spinae muscles were severely atrophied on the left side and many parts were replaced by tendinous insertions. Erector spinae on the right side was comprised of typical fleshy muscle fibers but the tendons of iliocostalis inserted in a radial manner due to the abnormal thoracolumbar curvature (Stevenson et al. 2014).

Prevalence

N/A

Clinical Implications

Labranche et al. (2017) note that somatic dysfunction of spinalis capitis can contribute to compressive neuropathy of the dorsal rami of the cervical spinal nerves. Asymmetry of spinalis capitis may unilaterally strain the ligamentum nuchae and lead to the development of cervicogenic headaches or occipital headaches (Labranche et al. 2017).

Longissimus (Figure 4.11)

Synonyms

Longissimus thoracis may be referred to as longissimus dorsi (Macalister 1875).

Typical Presentation

Description

Longissimus is partitioned into longissimus thoracis, longissimus cervicis, and longissimus capitis, which are all continuous with each other (Standring 2016). Longissimus capitis originates from the mastoid process and attaches via tendons to the transverse processes of the first four thoracic vertebrae and the lower three or four cervical vertebrae (Standring 2016). Longissimus cervicis originates via tendons from the posterior tubercles of cervical vertebrae two through six and inserts via tendons onto the transverse processes of the first four or five thoracic vertebrae (Standring 2016).

The thoracic portion of longissimus thoracis originates from the transverse processes of the first four thoracic vertebrae and from the transverse processes and corresponding ribs in the next eight thoracic segments (Standring 2016). It inserts onto the spinous processes of the lumbar vertebrae, the sacrum, and the iliac crest (Standring 2016). The lumbar portion of longissimus thoracis originates from the accessory process and transverse process of each lumbar vertebrae, and inserts onto the ilium, either directly or via a tendon termed the lumbar intermuscular aponeurosis (Standring 2016).

Innervation

The erector spinae group is innervated by the lateral branches of the dorsal rami of the corresponding cervical, thoracic, and lumbar spinal nerves (Standring 2016). In the lumbar region, intermediate branches supply longissimus (Standring 2016).

Comparative Anatomy

Longissimus has a similar typical presentation in the apes (Sonntag 1923; Miller 1952; Gibbs 1999; Diogo et al. 2010, 2012, 2013ab, 2017). It may be fused with iliocostalis and semispinalis capitis in orangutans (Diogo et al. 2013b).

Variations

Description

Longissimus thoracis can be variable in the number of its costal attachments and which ribs it is attached to (Macalister 1875; Rickenbacher et al. 1985; Bergman et al. 1988). Longissimus cervicis can extend to the transverse processes of the tenth or eleventh thoracic vertebrae or have a reduced number of bundles (Rickenbacher et al. 1985; Bergman et al. 1988). Longissimus capitis can be diminished, absent, divided into two parts, or can occasionally be attached to the atlas (Macalister 1875; Rickenbacher et al. 1985; Bergman et al. 1988; Bakkum and Miller 2016). The attachment of longissimus capitis may extend to the fifth thoracic vertebra or can be reduced to just the last two cervical vertebrae (Macalister 1875; Rickenbacher et al. 1985). Longissimus capitis may also fuse with the splenius (Macalister 1875; Rickenbacher et al. 1985).

Accessory slips are occasionally present on the underside of the lumbar portion longissimus (Bergman et al. 1988; Bakkum and Miller 2016). These slips can fuse to form a supernumerary muscle termed transversalis dorsi (or transversalis thoracis) that can attach to the first two or three thoracic vertebrae (Bergman et al. 1988; Bakkum and Miller 2016). Accessory slips can also be found near the cervical portion of longissimus and can form a supernumerary muscle termed transversalis cervicis posticus minor (Knott 1883a; Bergman et al. 1988; Bakkum and Miller 2016). Transversalis cervicis posticus minor (tra chelomastoideus minor or trachelomastoideus accessorius) arises from the transverse processes of the second thoracic through fifth cervical vertebrae and inserts into the transverse process of the first cervical vertebra and the mastoid process (Knott 1883a). Slips from longissimus capitis may originate from the transverse process of the first cervical vertebra, or from the longissimus cervicis tendon near this vertebra and insert onto the mastoid process (Bergman et al. 1988).

Prevalence

N/A

Anomalies

Description

Stevenson et al. (2014) describe a cadaver with a severe case of congenital scoliosis. The erector spinae muscles were severely atrophied on the left side, and many parts were replaced by tendinous insertions. Erector spinae on the right side was comprised of typical fleshy muscle fibers but the tendons of iliocostalis inserted in a radial manner due to the abnormal thoracolumbar curvature (Stevenson et al. 2014).

Prevalence

N/A

Clinical Implications

N/A

ILIOCOSTALIS (FIGURE 4.11)

Synonyms

N/A

Typical Presentation

Description

Iliocostalis is partitioned into iliocostalis lumborum, iliocostalis thoracis, and iliocostalis cervicis, which are all continuous with each other (Standring 2016). The lumbar portion of iliocostalis lumborum originate from the transverse processes of the first four lumbar vertebrae and the thoracolumbar fascia and inserts onto the iliac crest (Standring 2016). The thoracic portion of iliocostalis lumborum originates via tendons from the angles of the lower eight or nine ribs, and its bundles converge into an aponeurosis that inserts onto the iliac crest (Standring 2016). Iliocostalis thoracis originates from the transverse process of the last cervical vertebra and from the first six ribs and inserts onto the lower six ribs (Standring 2016). It also has fascicular attachments to the common erector spinae tendon (Gale et al. 2016). Iliocostalis cervicis originates from the posterior tubercles of the transverse processes of cervical vertebrae four through six and attaches to the angles of ribs three through six (Standring 2016).

Innervation

The erector spinae group is innervated by the lateral branches of the dorsal rami of the corresponding cervical, thoracic, and lumbar spinal nerves (Standring 2016).

In the lumbar region, lateral branches supply iliocostalis (Standring 2016).

Comparative Anatomy

Iliocostalis has a similar typical presentation in the apes, with similar variations in costal and vertebral attachments (Diogo et al. 2010, 2012, 2013a,b, 2017).

Variations

Description

Iliocostalis can vary in the number of its vertebral and costal attachments (Macalister 1875; Rickenbacher et al. 1985; Bakkum and Miller 2016). The digitations to the first, eleventh, and twelfth ribs are most commonly absent (Macalister 1875). Accessory slips may be attached to the middle ribs (Macalister 1875). In the lumbar portion of iliocostalis, there may be a slip to the lumbocostal ligament (Rickenbacher et al. 1985).

Prevalence

N/A

Anomalies

Description

Stevenson et al. (2014) describe a cadaver with a severe case of congenital scoliosis. The erector spinae muscles were severely atrophied on the left side, and many parts were replaced by tendinous insertions. Erector spinae on the right side was comprised of typical fleshy muscle fibers, but the tendons of iliocostalis inserted in a radial manner due to the abnormal thoracolumbar curvature (Stevenson et al. 2014).

Prevalence

N/A

Clinical Implications

N/A

5 Lower Limb Muscles

Eve K. Boyle
Howard University College of Medicine

Vondel S. E. Mahon
University of Maryland Medical Center

Rui Diogo
Howard University College of Medicine

Malynda Williams
Howard University College of Medicine

CONTENTS

DOI: 10.1201/9781003083535-5

GLUTEAL AND THIGH MUSCLES

GLUTEUS MAXIMUS (FIGURE 5.1)

Entry adapted by permission from Springer Nature Customer Service Centre GmbH: Springer Current Molecular Biology Reports, Muscles Lost in Our Adult Primate Ancestors Still Imprint in US: on Muscle Evolution, Development, Variations, and Pathologies. E. Boyle, V. Mahon, R. Diogo, 2020.

See also: Tenuissimus

Synonyms

N/A

Typical Presentation

Description

Gluteus maximus originates from the ilium, sacrum, coccyx, aponeurosis of erector spinae, sacrotuberous ligament, and the gluteal aponeurosis (Standring 2016). It inserts into the iliotibial tract and onto the gluteal tuberosity of the femur (Standring 2016).

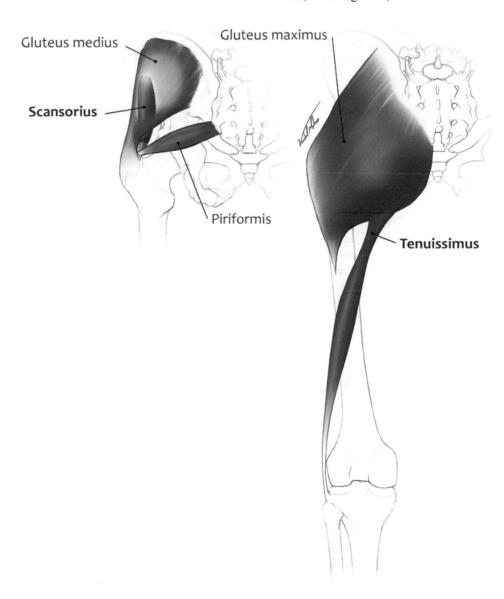

FIGURE 5.1 Gluteal muscles in posterior view. The more superficial muscles of the gluteal region are illustrated on the right side and the deeper muscles are illustrated on the left side.

Innervation

Gluteus maximus is innervated by the inferior gluteal nerve (Standring 2016).

Comparative Anatomy

Gluteus maximus has similar origins and attachments in the apes, but compared with humans, gluteus maximus in the apes is reduced in size and thickness and is more developed in its distal portions (Hepburn 1892; Sonntag 1924; Stern 1972; Sigmon 1974; Diogo et al. 2010, 2012, 2013a,b, 2017; Ferrero 2011; Ferrero et al. 2012).

In the apes, it originates from the posterior iliac crest, including the posterior superior iliac spine, the thoracolumbar fascia, sacrum, coccyx, sacrotuberal ligament, gluteus medius fascia, and ischial tuberosity, and inserts onto the femur in the region of the gluteal tuberosity, into the aponeurosis of vastus lateralis, into the iliotibial tract (when present), and sometimes onto the hypertrochanteric fossa (Champneys 1872; Hepburn 1892; Beddard 1893; Sonntag 1924; Raven 1950; Stern 1972; Sigmon 1974; Brown 1983; Gibbs 1999; Diogo et al. 2010, 2012, 2013a,b, 2017; Ferrero 2011; Ferrero et al. 2012; Standring 2016).

The ischial origin of gluteus maximus is recognized as a distinct, well-developed muscle in orangutans and is present but frequently blended with gluteus maximus in the other apes (Ferrero et al. 2012; Diogo et al. 2010, 2012, 2013a,b, 2017). When present, the ischiofemoralis muscle originates from the ischial tuberosity and inserts on the lateral aspect of the proximal femoral shaft and the aponeurosis of vastus lateralis, with some fibers going to the tensor fasciae latae (Ferrero et al. 2012; Diogo et al. 2010, 2012, 2013a,b, 2017).

The insertion of gluteus maximus inserts more distally onto the femur in the apes than in humans, extending two-thirds down the femur in gibbons and orangutans (Stern 1972; Sigmon 1974), four-fifths down the femur in siamangs (Hepburn 1892; Sigmon 1974), and almost to the distal end of the femur in common chimpanzees and bonobos (Hepburn 1892; Dwight 1895; MacDowell 1910; Miller 1952; Sigmon 1974; Diogo et al. 2013a, 2017). Gluteus maximus may also be divided into multiple bellies or bundles in all apes (Hepburn 1892; Sonntag 1924; Gibbs 1999; Diogo et al. 2012, 2013a,b, 2017).

Variations

Description

Gluteus maximus may be split into two laminae (Macalister 1875; Knott 1883b; Le Double 1897; Standring 2016). It may also be doubled (Macalister 1867b; Nicholson et al. 2016). The extent of the origin from the sacrum, coccyx, or gluteal aponeurosis may vary (Macalister 1875; Le Double 1897; Knott 1883b; Stern 1972; Nicholson et al. 2016). Gluteus maximus may have additional origins from the thoracolumbar fascia, multifidus fascia, sacroiliac ligaments, aponeurosis of iliocostalis lumborum, or aponeurosis of latissimus dorsi (Macalister 1875; Knott 1883b; Testut 1884; Stern 1972; Nicholson et al. 2016; Standring 2016). The femoral insertion may extend proximally to

the upper aspect of the greater trochanter or distally down the femur (Macalister 1875; Stern 1972; Nicholson et al. 2016). Medial fibers of gluteus maximus may have a separate insertion onto the lateral margin of the linea aspera (Bergman et al. 1988). Gluteus maximus may be fused with tensor fasciae latae (Bergman et al. 1988; du Plessis and Loukas 2016).

Taylor et al. (2015) describe an accessory muscle in a female cadaver that was surrounded by a fascial sheath. It arose from the deep fibers of the inferior portion of gluteus maximus and converged into a tendon that had a contribution from the iliotibial tract. The tendon inserted onto the proximal aspect of the femur lateral to the intertrochanteric crest just superior to the gluteal tuberosity.

An additional bundle may be present connecting gluteus maximus to the ischial tuberosity (Macalister 1875; Testut 1884; Bergman et al. 1988; Nicholson et al. 2016; Standring 2016). When this bundle is an independent muscle, it is referred to as ischiofemoralis. This muscle is homologous to the ischiofemoralis of orangutans (Brown 1983; Ferrero 2011, Ferrero et al. 2012; Diogo et al. 2013b) and is likely equivalent with, or a variant of, coccygeofemoralis.

When present, coccygeofemoralis extends from the sacrum and coccyx to the femur just at the lower border of gluteus maximus and may represent a caudal head of this muscle (Macalister 1875; Bergman et al. 1988; Nicholson et al. 2016). The adult human coccygeofemoralis (and potentially the adult human ischiofemoralis) derives from the embryonic coccygeofemoralis, which originates from the coccyx and inserts onto the femur near the distal margin of gluteus maximus and is innervated by a branch of the inferior gluteal nerve. This muscle persists as a distinct structure until CR40–45 mm (crown-rump length of 40–45 mm) and then fuses with gluteus maximus (Tichý and Grim 1985). As noted by Morimoto (2018), the presence of both gluteus maximus and coccygeofemoralis is similar to the configuration seen in adult apes, in which gluteus maximus consists of a proximal portion (gluteus maximus proprius) and a distal portion (ischiofemoralis).

However, Tichý and Grim (1985) suggest that there is little evidence that coccygeofemoralis corresponds to any muscle in normal adult humans. They note that Testut (1884) described a coccy-femoralis muscle, and Le Double (1897) described a femoro-coccygeus muscle. Testut (1884) suggests coccy-femoralis is homologous to caudofemoralis in other mammals, and Tichý and Grim (1985) argue that their coccygeofemoralis corresponds to this structure in adults with incomplete fusion of this muscle and gluteus maximus.

Kirici and Ozan (1999) report a bilateral variation of gluteus maximus in which the muscles had a fibrous sacroiliac part that was separated from a muscular coccygeofemoral part and was associated with a doubled piriformis muscle on the right side. On both sides of the body, coccygeofemoralis originated from the base of the coccyx. On the right side, tendons arose from this muscle, one inserting into the linea aspera 5 cm below the greater trochanter, and the other inserting onto the origin of the short head of biceps femoris

11 cm below the grater trochanter. On the left side, the muscle inserted onto the gluteal tuberosity 7.5 cm below the greater trochanter. These authors conclude that this morphology results from the failure of the fusion of gluteus maximus proprius (the sacroiliac part) and the coccygeofemoralis muscle during embryonic development (Kirici and Ozan 1999).

Prevalence

Knott (1883b) found that in 5 out of 40 subjects (12.5%), a thin deep lamina was formed by the gluteus maximus fibers that originated from the sacrosciatic and posterior sacroiliac ligaments and was separated by the superficial portion of the muscle by a layer of connective tissue. An accessory slip from the lumbar aponeurosis was also present in five subjects (total sample size not specified). Taylor et al. (2015) found an accessory muscle extending from the deep inferior fibers of gluteus maximus to the proximal femur in 1 out of 77 hips (1.3%).

Anomalies

Description

Gluteus maximus may be absent as a rare congenital anomaly (Tagliapietra et al. 1989). On the right side of a fetus with craniorachischisis dissected by Alghamdi et al. (2017), gluteus maximus was difficult to separate from gluteus medius. Gluteus maximus may also have extra slips or tendons (Smith et al. 2015). Pirani et al. (1991) describe soft tissue anatomy associated with cases of proximal femoral focal deficiency (PFFD). In Aitken type D PFFD, the gluteal muscles insert onto the proximal femoral ossicle.

Bersu et al. (1976) describe a male infant with Hanhart syndrome. The femora of this infant were normally developed, but distal secondary ossification centers were absent. The left leg stump had a patella and a small rudiment of the proximal tibia but no fibular rudiment. The right leg stump was less developed and had a patella, smaller tibial rudiment, and no fibular rudiment. On the left side, gluteus maximus had a normal origin but did not insert onto the gluteal tuberosity. It had a normal attachment to the fascia lata but also had a tendinous band that inserted onto the middle third of the linea aspera. The right gluteus maximus had a normal origin but inserted via a tendon onto the distal half of the linea aspera. A small accessory muscle originated from the deep surface of the right gluteus maximus near its origin from the sacrum and inserted onto the ischial tuberosity.

Prevalence

In the literature review conducted by Smith et al. (2015), they found that extra slips or tendons of gluteus maximus were present in only 1 out of 20 individuals with trisomy 13 (5%).

Clinical Implications

Variations in the gluteal muscles including division of the muscle into multiple parts should be acknowledged when considering injections into the gluteal musculature (Kirici and Ozan 1999). Arora et al. (2010) note that accessory slips related to gluteus maximus or piriformis may compress the inferior gluteal nerve and lead to weakness in gluteus maximus. The accessory muscle described by Taylor et al. (2015) (see above) may have caused pain and other symptoms similar to those of Greater Trochanteric Pain Syndrome (GTPS).

Gluteus medius (Figure 5.1)

Synonyms

N/A

Typical Presentation

Description

Gluteus medius originates from the ilium between the posterior gluteal line and the anterior gluteal line (Standring 2016). It inserts via a tendon onto the lateral aspect of the greater trochanter (Standring 2016).

Innervation

Gluteus medius is innervated by the superior gluteal nerve (Standring 2016).

Comparative Anatomy

Gluteus medius has a similar typical presentation in the apes, with similar variations including fusion with nearby muscles and tendons (Beddard 1893; Sigmon 1974; Raven 1950; Diogo et al. 2010, 2012, 2013a,b, 2017). It is often fused with piriformis in gibbons and bonobos (Beddard 1893; Diogo et al. 2017). It may be fused with piriformis, vastus lateralis, or the tensor fasciae latae in orangutans (Diogo et al. 2013b). Its tendon may be fused with that of piriformis in common chimpanzees (Champneys 1872; Hepburn 1892; Dwight 1895).

Variations

Description

Gluteus medius may be divided into two lamellae (Henle 1858; Macalister 1875; Bergman et al. 1988) or into multiple muscle layers (Akita et al. 1993). The extent of the origin from the ilium and the specific location of its insertion onto the greater trochanter may vary (Flack et al. 2012; Nicholson et al. 2016). Deep fibers from gluteus medius may have a separate attachment to the upper border of the greater trochanter (Bergman et al. 1988; Standring 2016). Gluteus medius accessorius may originate from the iliac crest and insert onto the tendon of gluteus medius and the greater trochanter (Henle 1858; Jazuta 1931; Bergman et al. 1988; Nicholson et al. 2016).

The posterior border of gluteus medius may blend with piriformis or send slips to its tendon (Henle 1858; Macalister 1875; Bergman et al. 1988; Akita et al. 1994; Flack et al. 2014; Nicholson et al. 2016; Standring 2016). Gluteus medius may also be partially or completely fused with gluteus minimus or its tendon (Macalister 1875; Knott 1883b; Testut 1884; Akita et al. 1993; Duparc et al. 1997; Flack et al. 2014, Nicholson et al. 2016). The insertion tendon of gluteus medius may also join with the tendon of vastus lateralis (Nazarian et al. 1987; Heimkes et al. 1992; Nicholson et al. 2016).

Heimkes et al. (1992) studied the relationships upon insertion between gluteus medius, gluteus minimus, and vastus lateralis and classified these relationships into five types. In type I, gluteus medius, gluteus minimus, and vastus lateralis formed an ideal joint tendinous junction. In type II, vastus lateralis is connected to gluteus medius and gluteus minimus while gluteus medius and gluteus minimus were not connected with each other. In type III, vastus lateralis connects only to gluteus minimus and gluteus medius has an independent insertion onto the greater trochanter. In type IV, vastus lateralis connects only to gluteus medius and gluteus minimus has an independent insertion onto the greater trochanter. In type V, all three muscles insert independently onto the greater trochanter without connections to each other.

Prevalence

Heimkes et al. (1992) studied the relationships upon insertion between gluteus medius, gluteus minimus, and vastus lateralis in 52 hip specimens. See above for the description of the five types of relationships they identified. Type I was found in 18 cases (34.6%), type II in 13 cases (25%), type III in 11 cases (21.1%), type IV in seven cases (13.5%), and type V in three cases (5.8%).

Akita et al. (1993) studied gluteus medius in 13 hemipelves from 7 cadavers. The anteromedial portion of gluteus medius was comprised of one muscle layer in six specimens (46%), two independent muscle layers in four specimens (31%), and three muscle layers in three specimens (23%). In 12 specimens (92.3%), the inferior aspect of the most anteromedial independent muscle layer inserted onto the gluteus minimus aponeurosis. Flack et al. (2014) studied the morphology of gluteus medius in 12 lower limbs. In 100% of specimens, the tendons of gluteus medius and gluteus minimus fused as they approached the greater trochanter. In four cases (33.3%), gluteus medius fused to piriformis posteriorly.

Anomalies

Description

On the right side of a fetus with craniorachischisis, gluteus medius fused with tensor fasciae latae and was difficult to separate from gluteus maximus (Alghamdi et al. 2017). On both sides of this specimen, the origin of the muscle extended posteriorly so it was wider than normal (Alghamdi et al. 2017). In a female fetus with trisomy 18, gluteus medius fused with tensor fasciae latae bilaterally (Alghamdi et al. (2018). In a male neonate with Meckel syndrome, gluteus medius originated from the ilium below its normal origin and did not extend above the upper margin of gluteus maximus (Pettersen 1984).

Bersu et al. (1976) describe a male infant with Hanhart syndrome. The femora of this infant were normally developed but distal secondary ossification centers were absent. The left leg stump had a patella and a small rudiment of the proximal tibia but no fibular rudiment. The right leg stump

was less developed and had a patella, smaller tibial rudiment, and no fibular rudiment. On the left side, gluteus medius was normal. On the right side, gluteus medius had a normal origin but had an additional insertion onto the gluteal tuberosity. A slip also extended from the posteromedial border of this muscle to the superolateral border of piriformis.

Pirani et al. (1991) describe soft tissue anatomy associated with cases of PFFD. In Aitken type B PFFD, gluteus medius and gluteus minimus are shorter than normal and extend between the ilium and the proximal femoral metaphysis. This latter structure indents these muscles from below. In Aitken type D PFFD, the gluteal muscles insert onto the proximal femoral ossicle.

Prevalence

N/A

Clinical Implications

Acknowledging the variable relationships between gluteus medius, gluteus minimus, and vastus lateralis and the potential independent insertions of these muscles onto the greater trochanter is important for successful hip operations, particularly when using the transgluteal approach (Heimkes et al. 1992).

GLUTEUS MINIMUS (NOT ILLUSTRATED)

See also: Scansorius

Synonyms

N/A

Typical Presentation

Description

Gluteus minimus originates from the ilium between the anterior gluteal line and inferior gluteal line and from the border of the greater sciatic notch (Standring 2016). It inserts via a tendon onto the greater trochanter (Standring 2016). Its insertion expands to the hip joint capsule (Standring 2016).

Innervation

Gluteus minimus is innervated by the superior gluteal nerve (Standring 2016).

Comparative Anatomy

Gluteus minimus has a similar typical presentation in the apes, extending from the ilium to the greater trochanter and hip joint capsule (Champneys 1872; Hepburn 1892; Sonntag 1924; Raven 1950; Miller 1952; Sigmon 1974; Gibbs 1999; Diogo et al. 2010, 2012, 2013a,b, 2017).

Variations

Description

Gluteus minimus can be divided into an anterior part and posterior part (Macalister 1875; Bergman et al. 1988; Standring 2016). The specific location of its insertion onto the greater trochanter may vary (Flack et al. 2012; Nicholson et al. 2016). The insertion onto the hip joint capsule may present as one or more detached muscular bundles or fascicles (Macalister 1875; Bergman et al. 1988; Flack et al. 2014).

Gluteus minimus may send slips to gemellus superior, piriformis, tensor fasciae latae, or vastus lateralis (Macalister 1875; Bergman et al. 1988; Nicholson et al. 2016; Standring 2016). Gluteus medius may be partially fused, or more rarely completely fused, with the muscle belly or tendon of gluteus minimus (Macalister 1875; Knott 1883b; Testut 1884; Akita et al. 1993; Duparc et al. 1997; Flack et al. 2014, Nicholson et al. 2016). Gluteus minimus may also be completely or partially fused with piriformis or its tendon (Knott 1883b; Flack et al. 2014). The insertion tendon of gluteus minimus may also join with the proximal tendon of vastus lateralis (Nazarian et al. 1987; Heimkes et al. 1992; Flack et al. 2014). Heimkes et al. (1992) studied the relationships upon insertion between gluteus medius, gluteus minimus, and vastus lateralis and classified these relationships into five types. See gluteus medius entry for more details and prevalence information.

Prevalence

Flack et al. (2014) studied the morphology of gluteus minimus in 12 lower limbs. In 100% of specimens, the tendons of gluteus medius and gluteus minimus fused as they approached the greater trochanter. In four cases (33.3%), the posterior border of gluteus minimus was fused with the tendon of piriformis. Atrophy of gluteus minimus was observed in eight specimens (66.7%), six cases mild and two extensive.

Anomalies

Description

Pirani et al. (1991) describe soft tissue anatomy associated with cases of PFFD. In Aitken type B PFFD, gluteus medius and gluteus minimus are shorter than normal and extend between the ilium and the proximal femoral metaphysis. This latter structure indents these muscles from below. In Aitken type D PFFD, the gluteal muscles insert onto the proximal femoral ossicle.

Prevalence

N/A

Clinical Implications

Acknowledging the variable relationships between gluteus medius, gluteus minimus, and vastus lateralis and the potential independent insertions of these muscles onto the greater trochanter is important for successful hip operations, particularly when using the transgluteal approach (Heimkes et al. 1992).

PIRIFORMIS (FIGURES 4.4 AND 5.1)

Synonyms

N/A

Typical Presentation

Description

Piriformis originates from the anterior aspect of the sacrum via three digitations, the ilium near the posterior inferior iliac spine, and from the capsule of the sacroiliac joint (Standring 2016). It courses through the greater sciatic foramen to insert onto the greater trochanter (Standring 2016).

Innervation

Piriformis is innervated by the first two sacral spinal nerves, and sometimes the fifth lumbar spinal nerve (Standring 2016).

Comparative Anatomy

Piriformis has a similar typical presentation in the apes, extending from the sacrum, and often the ilium, to the greater trochanter (Raven 1950; Miller 1952; Gibbs 1999; Diogo et al. 2010, 2012, 2013a,b, 2017). It may be fused with gluteus medius in gibbons, orangutans, and common chimpanzees (Champneys 1873; Hepburn 1892; Beddard 1893; Dwight 1895; Sonntag 1924; Sigmon 1974).

Variations

Description

Piriformis may have an origin from the upper part of the pelvic aspect of the sacrotuberous ligament (Standring 2016). Its origin from the sacrum may span from one or two segments up to five segments and may include the coccyx (Macalister 1875; Knott 1883b; Le Double 1897; Bergman et al. 1988; Rickenbacher et al. 1985; Nicholson et al. 2016). The digitations of piriformis can range from two to four (Bergman et al. 1988). Piriformis may have an insertion onto the hip joint capsule (Macalister 1875; Bergman et al. 1988). Piriformis may be partially or entirely absent (Macalister 1875; Rickenbacher et al. 1985; Bergman et al. 1988; Gibbs 1999; Ikidag 2019; Caetano and Seeger 2019). Brenner et al. (2019) describe the right lower limb of a female cadaver in which piriformis and inferior gemellus were missing.

Piriformis may be fused with or receive a slip from gluteus medius or its tendon, gluteus minimus or its tendon, superior gemellus, or obturator internus (Henle 1858; Macalister 1875; Knott 1883b; Le Double 1897; Rickenbacher et al. 1985; Bergman et al. 1988; Chiba 1992; Akita et al. 1994; Flack et al. 2014; Nicholson et al. 2016; Standring 2016). It may also join with coccygeus (Macalister 1875). The tendon of insertion may be blended to some degree with the common tendon of obturator internus, gemellus superior, and gemellus inferior (Macalister 1875; Pine et al. 2011; Standring 2016) or with the insertion tendon of gluteus minimus or gluteus medius (Macalister 1875; Flack et al. 2014). The tendon of gemellus superior may insert onto the piriformis tendon instead of the tendon of obturator internus (Macalister 1875; Knott 1883b).

Piriformis may split into two portions, which is often associated with a high division of the sciatic nerve, often with the peroneal (common fibular) component of the nerve passing between the two portions and the tibial nerve passing inferior to the muscle (type B variation according to Beaton and Anson) (Macalister 1875; Rickenbacher et al. 1985; Bergman et al. 1988; Chiba 1992; Natsis et al. 2014; Nicholson et al. 2016). Other relationships between piriformis and the sciatic nerve include the normal passage of an undivided sciatic nerve below piriformis (type A, typical presentation) or above piriformis (type F), the common fibular nerve passing above piriformis and the tibial nerve passing inferior to it (type C), the entire sciatic nerve passing through a split piriformis (type D), and the common fibular nerve passing above a split piriformis and the tibial nerve passing through the muscle (type E) (Beaton and Anson 1937; Nicholson et al. 2016). In a rare case, the sciatic nerve was observed to travel posterior to piriformis (Sayson et al. 1994). Nicholson et al. (2016) provide a comprehensive review of these relationships and information on the relationships between piriformis and other neurovascular structures. Doubling or division of piriformis may also be associated with doubling or division of the gemelli, quadratus femoris, or gluteus maximus (Kirici and Ozan 1999; Nicholson et al. 2016).

Kirici et al. (2000) report a double piriformis in left lower limbs. In the first case, the common fibular nerve passed between the two portions of piriformis. In the second case, the common fibular and posterior femoral cutaneous nerves passed between the two portions. This second case was associated with the passage of the gemelli, obturator internus, pudendal nerve, and vessels behind the midportion of the sacrotuberous ligament.

An accessory muscle may be present superior to piriformis and may have origins from the sacrotuberous ligament, the greater sciatic foramen, or the posterior end of the ilium, and insertions into the greater trochanter, hip joint capsule, or piriformis tendon (Prasad et al. 2005; Tubbs and Salter 2006b; Ravindranath et al. 2008; Natsis et al. 2014; Nicholson et al. 2016). An accessory digastric muscle may also be present, with a superior belly that arises from or near piriformis and then continues down the thigh as a long intermediate tendon, before ending in an inferior belly (Moore 1922; Suda and Takahashi 1957; Akita et al. 1992; Nicholson et al. 2016). Arora et al. (2010) describe a 5 cm long accessory slip that originated from the inferomedial portion of gluteus maximus and merged with piriformis near the greater trochanter. Although its fibers were parallel to those of piriformis, thus appearing as a second piriformis muscle, the authors suggest that it derived primarily from the gluteus maximus muscle due to its innervation from a branch of the inferior gluteal nerve. They term this slip the "gluteopiriformis" muscle (Arora et al. 2010).

Prevalence

From the examination of 36 bodies, Wood (1868) states that in three males and one female (11%), the tendon of piriformis was blended with that of obturator internus and the two inserted together onto the greater trochanter. Knott (1883b) noted that in 2 out of 40 cases (5%), the iliac origin of piriformis near the upper border of the greater sciatic notch was separated by an areolar layer from the sacral part of piriformis. In three cases (7.5%), piriformis was split by the greater sciatic nerve. Pine et al. (2011) found that out of 29 specimens, the tendons of obturator internus and piriformis were at least partially fused in four specimens (13.8%), with three cases (10.3%) demonstrating insertion of the two as a common tendon, while in one case (3.4%) the combined tendon divided to have separate attachments. Flack et al. (2014) studied the morphology of gluteus medius and gluteus minimus in 12 lower limbs. In four cases each (33.3%), gluteus medius fused to piriformis posteriorly and gluteus minimus was fused with the tendon of piriformis.

Piriformis may be split by the peroneal component of the sciatic nerve in 12.2% of the "normal" population (Mortensen and Pettersen 1966; Bersu 1980). Sato (1970) found that piriformis was split into two portions by the sciatic nerve in 88 out of 418 limbs (21%) from Kyushu Japanese males and in 54 out of 268 limbs (20%) from females. Chiba (1992) found that piriformis was split into three muscle bellies by the branching patterns of the sciatic nerve in 5 out of 514 cases (1%). This author also found that when two bundles of piriformis are present, the tendon of the lower one blends with gemellus superior in five cases (1%).

Natsis et al. (2014) studied the morphology of piriformis on 294 sides from 147 Greek cadavers. Type A anatomy was present on 275 sides (93.6%), and variations were present in 19 cases (6.4%). Type B was present on 12 sides (4.1%) and types C, D, and F each on one side (0.3% each). These numbers are included in the comprehensive review by Nicholson et al. (2016, see next paragraph). Four limbs (1.4%) exhibited other variations. In one case (0.3%), piriformis was divided into three muscle bellies, with the common fibular nerve passing between the superficial and intermediate muscle bellies and the deep muscle belly passing through a branch of the tibial nerve. In another case (0.3%), the common fibular nerve passed between the superficial and deep muscle bellies of a double piriformis and the tibial nerve passed below piriformis. Lastly, on both sides of one cadaver (0.7%), the sciatic nerve traveled below piriformis but there was a bilateral supernumerary muscle just superior to piriformis, extending from the posterior margin of the ilium and inserting onto the greater trochanter. These authors also found that out of the 12 sides that exhibited split piriformis muscles, five of them (41.7%) were positioned as a superficial belly and deep belly and seven (58.3%) were positioned as a superior belly and inferior belly.

Nicholson et al. (2016) summarize information about the relationships between piriformis and the sciatic nerve in 6,466 cases from 43 studies. The normal passage of an undivided sciatic nerve below piriformis, type A or the typical presentation, was present in 5,392 cases (83.4%). Type B variation was present in 827 cases (12.8%), type C in 87 cases (1.3%), type D in 34 cases (0.5%), type E in 5 cases (0.08%), and type F in 7 cases (0.1%). Nicholson et al.

(2016) also review the insertion of piriformis and found that when separated into two muscle bellies, each belly has a tendon that blends with the other to have a common insertion in 41 out of 57 cases (71.9%).

Anomalies

Description

Anomalous presentations of piriformis include variable insertions, the presence of accessory slips, complete absence, or splitting of the muscle belly by the peroneal portion of the sciatic nerve (Bersu et al. 1976; Bersu 1980; Pirani et al. 1991; Smith et al. 2015). Bersu et al. (1976) describe a male infant with Hanhart syndrome. The femora of this infant were normally developed but distal secondary ossification centers were absent. The left leg stump had a patella and a small rudiment of the proximal tibia but no fibular rudiment. The right leg stump was less developed and had a patella, smaller tibial rudiment, and no fibular rudiment. On the left side, piriformis had a normal origin and inserted onto the greater trochanter. It sent a tendinous slip to the tendon of obturator externus. On the right side, piriformis had a normal origin and inserted onto the posterior surface of the capsule of the hip joint. It sent a fascial slip to the lateral aspect of the ischial tuberosity.

Pirani et al. (1991) describe soft tissue anatomy associated with cases of proximal femoral focal deficiency (PFFD). In Aitken type A PFFD, the short external rotators of the hip are larger in cross-sectional diameter than normal and insert onto the posteromedial surface of the greater trochanter. In Aitken type B PFFD, the short external rotators are smaller than normal.

Prevalence

In their literature review, Smith et al. (2015) found that piriformis was absent in 1 out of 17 individuals with trisomy 18 (5.9%). In four out of five individuals with trisomy 21 (80%), piriformis was split by the peroneal portion of the sciatic nerve (as described by Bersu 1980). Per limb, this morphology was found in five out of ten limbs (50%) (Bersu 1980).

Clinical Implications

Knott (1883b) noted that in two cases where the sacral digitations of piriformis were reduced to two, these cases were associated with chronic rheumatoid arthritis on the same side. Variation in how the sciatic nerve relates to piriformis may entrap/compress the sciatic nerve (piriformis syndrome) (Beaton and Anson 1938; Sayson et al. 1994; Natsis et al. 2014; Nicholson et al. 2016). Accessory slips or doubling of piriformis can also compress the sciatic, inferior gluteal, or pudendal nerves (Kirici and Ozan 1999; Ravindranath et al. 2008; Arora et al. 2010) or contribute to superior gluteal nerve entrapment syndrome (Rask 1980). The absence of piriformis on the right side of a patient examined by Ikidag (2019) allowed for the migration of the vermiform appendix to the deep gluteal region. Brenner et al. (2019) suggest that since piriformis is an anatomical landmark for ultrasound investigations, hip surgeries, and other procedures in the deep gluteal region, its absence can influence orientation in the deep gluteal region and affect the identification of target structures.

SCANSORIUS (FIGURE 5.1)

Entry adapted by permission from Springer Nature Customer Service Centre GmbH: Springer Current Molecular Biology Reports, Muscles Lost in Our Adult Primate Ancestors Still Imprint in US: on Muscle Evolution, Development, Variations, and Pathologies. E. Boyle, V. Mahon, R. Diogo, 2020.

See also: Gluteus minimus

Synonyms

This muscle is also referred to as gluteus quartus (Haughton), invertor femoris (Owen) (Macalister 1875; Knott 1883a,b; Sutton 1888), anterior gluteus minimus (Le Double 1897; Testut 1884), the fourth gluteus, marginal gluteus or small anterior gluteus (Ochiltree 1912).

Typical Presentation

This muscle is only present as a variation.

Comparative Anatomy

Scansorius is always present in orangutans, frequently present in bonobos, and occasionally present in gorillas, gibbons, and common chimpanzees (Champneys 1872; Hepburn 1892; Beddard 1893; Sonntag 1923; Raven 1950; Miller 1952; Sigmon 1974; Gibbs 1999; Ferrero et al. 2012; Diogo et al. 2010, 2012, 2013a,b, 2017). When present, it extends from the ilium, including the anterior superior iliac spine, and sometimes from the fascia lata, and inserts onto the greater trochanter, occasionally blending with gluteus minimus (Champneys 1872; Hepburn 1892; Beddard 1893; Sonntag 1923; Raven 1950; Miller 1952; Sigmon 1974; Gibbs 1999; Ferrero et al. 2012; Diogo et al. 2010, 2012, 2013a,b, 2017).

Variations

Description

Scansorius (Traill) is typically not present in adult humans (Sutton 1888; Ferrero et al. 2012). When it is present, the muscle is represented by a bundle considered to derive from the anterior portion of gluteus minimus, or originates from between gluteus minimus and gluteus medius (Macalister 1875; Knott 1883b; Sutton 1888; Bergman et al. 1988; Gibbs 1999). It originates from the anterior superior iliac spine, iliac crest, and sometimes the anterior margin of gluteus minimus and/or the fascia lata and inserts onto the greater trochanter (Macalister 1867b, 1875; Knott 1883a,b; Testut 1884; Gruber 1887; Sutton 1888; Ochiltree 1912; Bergman et al. 1988; Gibbs 1999, du Plessis and Loukas 2016; Nicholson et al. 2016; Orthaber et al. 2020).

It can insert independently onto the greater trochanter or insert with the tendon of gluteus minimus (Knott 1883b). Knott (1883b) also notes that scansorius may insert partially onto the side of vastus lateralis. Macalister (1875) notes that when scansorius is present its tendon may either be continuous with vastus lateralis or be overlapped by it with the vastus lateralis tendon forming an arch over the muscle. Ochiltree (1912) states that the insertion of scansorius corresponds to the normal insertion of gluteus medius and can displace the insertion of the latter more dorsally and proximally than is typical. Sutton (1888) argues that the outer portion of the ilio-femoral band is the fibrous representative of scansorius as (1) the iliofemoral ligament corresponds in its attachments to scansorius and (2) monkeys that have a functional scansorius do not have an iliofemoral band. Orthaber et al. (2020) describe a right lower limb that presented with both gluteus medius accessorius and gluteus quartus. Gluteus quartus extended from the anterior portion of gluteus minimus and the fascia lata to the tip of the greater trochanter.

Innervation

Scansorius is innervated by the superior gluteal nerve (Sutton 1888; Orthaber et al. 2020).

Prevalence

Duparc et al. (1997) found a muscle bundle extending from the anterior superior iliac spine to the anterior margin of the greater trochanter in 3 out of 40 cases from a sample of 24 cadavers (7.5%). Beck et al. (2000) noted the presence of scansorius in 2 out of 16 cadaveric hips (12.5%). Woyski et al. (2012) report a higher prevalence for scansorius in humans. Based on examination of 45 cadaveric hips (29 female, 16 male), these authors found fibers corresponding to scansorius in 41% of female specimens and 44% of male specimens. Scansorius was present as a distinct bundle in 50% of males and 31% of females. The overall prevalence of scansorius was 80% (Woyski et al. 2012).

Anomalies

N/A

Clinical Implications

Orthaber et al. (2020) suggest that the presence of scansorius may contribute to instability in the hip joint on the contralateral side.

TENUISSIMUS (FIGURE 5.1)

See also: Piriformis, Gluteus maximus, Biceps femoris

Synonyms

This muscle may also be referred to as gluteo-cruralis (Klaatsch 1900; Waterman 1929).

Typical Presentation

This muscle is only present as a variation or anomaly.

Comparative Anatomy

Among primates, tenuissimus is present in some Central and South American monkeys (e.g., capuchins) but absent in the lemurs, African and Asian monkeys, and apes (Waterman 1929). Green (1931) notes that in most mammals that possess a tenuissimus, the muscle usually originates from the coccyx, but the origin in monkeys, as observed by Klaatsch (1900), is similar to the origin observed in humans, namely the posterior surface of gluteus maximus and its fascia. When present, the insertion in monkeys is onto the shaft of the fibula (Green 1931).

Variations

Description

There are very few descriptions of muscles that researchers believe correspond to tenuissimus in humans. Green (1931) describes one case in the right thigh of a cadaver. Tenuissimus presented as a fusiform muscle that arose via an expanded aponeurosis and subsequent tendon from the fascia covering the deep surface of gluteus maximus. The muscle belly descended the thigh and inserted onto biceps femoris at the junction of the short head and the long head, with a slightly more extensive attachment to the long head. Green (1931) mentions a similar case that was described by Wood (1867b) as a third head of biceps femoris. It arose via a rounded tendon from the fascia on the deep surface of gluteus maximus and inserted onto the long head of biceps femoris near its junction with the short head.

Arakawa et al. (2017) describe a case in which they conclude that tenuissimus, tensor fasciae suralis, and two other supernumerary muscles are present on the posterior right thigh of a cadaver. Tenuissimus passed between the long and short heads of biceps femoris and fused with the tensor fasciae suralis, which fused with the posterior surface of the crural fascia that covered the lateral head of gastrocnemius. It is possible that the cases described here may be variants of femorococcygeus or coccygeofemoralis (see section on variations for gluteus maximus) (Green 1931). It is also possible that the accessory digastricus muscle often associated with piriformis may be a variant of tenuissimus (see section on variations for piriformis) (Arakawa et al. 2017).

Innervation

Tenuissimus is innervated by a branch of the common fibular nerve (Green 1931; Arakawa et al. 2017).

Prevalence

N/A

Anomalies

Description

On the left side of one female neonate with trisomy 18, Ramirez-Castro and Bersu (1978) found the tenuissimus muscle originating from the coccyx and inferior margin of gluteus maximus, descending along the posterior aspect of the thigh, and inserting into the edge of the lateral condyle of the tibia. Aziz (1979) found the muscle on the right side of another female neonate with trisomy 18, which presented deep to gluteus maximus and originated from the sacrum, coccyx, and sacrotuberous ligament and descended the leg to join the iliotibial tract.

Bersu et al. (1976) describe a male infant with Hanhart syndrome. The femora of this infant were normally developed but distal secondary ossification centers were absent. The left leg stump had a patella and a small rudiment of the proximal tibia but no fibular rudiment. The right leg stump was less developed and had a patella, smaller tibial rudiment, and no fibular rudiment. On the left side, tenuissimus originated from the fascia of the deep surface of gluteus maximus, continued as a slender muscle belly, and joined with the long head of the biceps femoris. On the right side, tenuissimus was larger and originated from the fascia near the insertion tendon of gluteus maximus onto the linea

aspera. It inserted onto the tibia just posterior to the insertion of the long head of the biceps femoris.

Prevalence

In their literature review, Smith et al. (2015) found that tenuissimus was only present in the two cases of trisomy 18 mentioned above, having a prevalence of 2 out of 17 (11.8%) individuals with trisomy 18.

Clinical Implications

N/A

Tensor fasciae latae (Figure 5.2)

Synonyms

This muscle may also be referred to as tensor vaginae femoris (Macalister 1875).

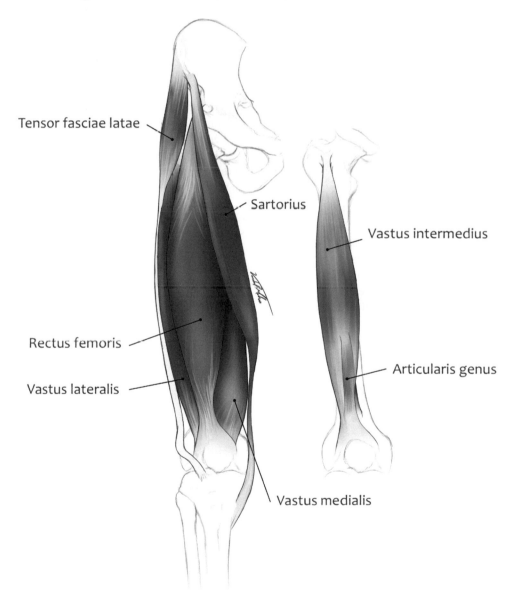

FIGURE 5.2 Anterior thigh muscles in anterior view. The deep anterior thigh muscles are illustrated on the right side and the superficial muscles are illustrated on the left side.

Typical Presentation

Description

Tensor fasciae latae originates from the iliac crest, the anterior superior iliac spine, and from the fascia lata (Standring 2016). It ends in the upper third of the thigh and inserts via the iliotibial tract onto the tibia (Standring 2016).

Innervation

Tensor fasciae latae is innervated by the superior gluteal nerve (Standring 2016).

Comparative Anatomy

Tensor fasciae latae has a similar typical presentation in the apes and has similar variations, including an origin from the gluteal fascia in gibbons and common chimpanzees and occasional fusion with the gluteal muscles in all species (Hepburn 1892; Raven 1950; Sigmon 1974; Gibbs 1999; Diogo et al. 2010, 2012, 2013a,b, 2017). This muscle may be reduced or absent in orangutans and bonobos (Chapman 1880; Sigmon 1974; Diogo et al. 2013b, 2017).

Variations

Description

Tensor fasciae latae may be absent (Bergman et al. 1988; du Plessis and Loukas 2016). The origin of tensor fasciae latae may extend to the fascia superficial to gluteus medius (Standring 2016). Its origin may also be shorter than is typical and not reach the anterior superior iliac spine (Macalister 1875; Knott 1883a). The muscular portion of tensor fasciae latae may extend as far distally as the lateral femoral condyle (Standring 2016). Tensor fasciae latae may be joined with gluteus maximus (Bergman et al. 1988; du Plessis and Loukas 2016). It may be partially or completely divided into bundles (Macalister 1875; Bergman et al. 1988; du Plessis and Loukas 2016). Accessory slips may be present with attachments to the inguinal ligament, abdominal aponeurosis, or iliac crest (Macalister 1875; Bergman et al. 1988; du Plessis and Loukas 2016). Macalister (1875) observed a tendinous band extending from the tensor fasciae latae into the base of the greater trochanter.

Prevalence

N/A

Anomalies

Description

On the right side of a fetus with craniorachischisis dissected by Alghamdi et al. (2017), tensor fasciae latae was fused with gluteus medius. In the female fetus with trisomy 18 dissected by Alghamdi et al. (2018), gluteus medius was fused with tensor fasciae latae bilaterally.

Bersu et al. (1976) describe a male infant with Hanhart syndrome. The femora of this infant were normally developed but distal secondary ossification centers were absent. The left leg stump had a patella and a small rudiment of the proximal tibia but no fibular rudiment. The right leg stump

was less developed and had a patella, smaller tibial rudiment, and no fibular rudiment. On both sides of the body, tensor fasciae latae originated from the fascia at the anterior border of gluteus medius and had normal insertions.

Prevalence

N/A

Clinical Implications

Unilateral hypertrophy of the tensor fasciae latae can simulate a soft tissue tumor (Ilaslan et al. 2003).

SARTORIUS (FIGURE 5.2)

Synonyms

Melling and Zweymüller (1996) refer to a distally divided sartorius muscle as sartorius bicaudatus. A proximally divided sartorius may be referred to as biceps sartorius (Kim and Lee 2019).

Typical Presentation

Description

Sartorius originates from the anterior superior iliac spine (Standring 2016). It inserts onto the medial surface of the proximal tibia via an aponeurosis (Standring 2016). The aponeurosis forms the pes anserinus with the insertions of gracilis and semitendinosus (Standring 2016). It sends a slip to the knee joint capsule and another slip to the deep fascia on the medial side of the leg (Standring 2016).

Innervation

Sartorius is innervated by the femoral nerve (Standring 2016).

Comparative Anatomy

Sartorius has a similar typical presentation in the apes, originating from the lateral ilium near the anterior superior iliac spine and inserting onto the medial aspect of the tibial shaft (Champneys 1872; Hepburn 1892; Beddard 1893; Sonntag 1924; Raven 1950; Sigmon 1974; Gibbs 1999; Diogo et al. 2010, 2012, 2013a,b, 2017). The insertion may be more distal onto the tibia in gibbons (Diogo et al. 2012).

Variations

Description

Sartorius may be absent (Macalister 1875; Bergman et al. 1988; du Plessis and Loukas 2016; Standring 2016). This muscle can vary in its course as it descends in the anterior thigh (Macalister 1875). Sartorius may be partially or fully split into two longitudinal portions, and the additional portion can have a separate insertion onto the tibia, the femur, the fascia lata, the patellar ligament, the semitendinosus tendon, or the tendon of the other sartorius portion (Hallett 1848; Macalister 1875; el-Badawi 1987; Bergman et al. 1988; du Plessis and Loukas 2016; Coban et al. 2019). This bifurcation may be confined to its origin or insertion or comprise over half of the muscle (Hallett 1848; Macalister 1875; Knott 1883b; Kedzia et al. 2011; du Plessis and Loukas 2016; Coban et al. 2019). Macalister (1875) notes that Kelch and Kyrtl observed a central tendinous intersection in sartorius. An extra head of sartorius may originate from the pubis, pectineal line, femoral sheath, below the anterior superior iliac spine, or from the inguinal ligament (Macalister 1875; Bergman et al. 1988; du Plessis and Loukas 2016; Standring 2016).

The insertion of sartorius near the knee may vary (Standring 2016), and insertions range from the fascia lata, fascia of the leg, or knee joint capsule (Macalister 1875; Knott 1883a,b; Bergman et al. 1988; du Plessis and Loukas 2016). Additional insertions may also go to the patella, medial femoral condyle, the knee joint capsule, or medial meniscus (Melling and Zweymüller 1996; Kedzia et al. 2011; du Plessis and Loukas 2016).

Mori (1964) categorized the distal portion of sartorius into five types. In type 1, the boundary of the muscular part and the tendon of insertion is distinct, and the length of the tendon is moderate. In type 2, the boundary of the muscular part and the tendon of insertion is not very clear, but the length of the tendon is moderate. In type 3, the tendon of insertion is short, and the muscle fibers insert directly onto the tibia. In type 4, the distal part of the muscle is divided longitudinally into two portions, and the tendon of the secondary slip is attached to the anterior wall of the adductor canal. In type 5, the muscle fibers typically in the distal portion of sartorius are replaced by a fibrous band, and this band is attached to the vastus medialis fascia.

Kim and Lee (2019) describe a case from a left lower limb in which sartorius split into medial and lateral heads and was associated with an accessory sartorius muscle that originated from the inguinal ligament. The lateral head of sartorius inserted onto the medial aspect of the patella. The medial head merged with the accessory sartorius and the two inserted together onto the medial surface of the tibia, forming the pes anserinus. The medial head also sent a muscular slip to vastus medialis. Sartorius is also associated with the musculus saphenous. It presents as a detached slip that attaches to the inguinal ligament and loops under the saphenofemoral junction, blending with the sartorius laterally and the adductor longus medially (Tyrie 1894; du Plessis and Loukas 2016; Saga and Takahashi 2016).

Prevalence

Mori (1964) classified the distal portions of sartorius into five types (see above for descriptions). Out of 50 thighs, type 1 was found in 31 cases (62%), type 2 in 13 cases (26%), and type 3 in 6 cases (12%). Out of 320 thighs, type 4 was found in 15 cases (4.7%) and type 5 was found in 2 cases (0.6%).

Anomalies

Description

Pirani et al. (1991) describe soft tissue anatomy associated with cases of PFFD. In Aitken type B PFFD, the cross-sectional diameter of sartorius is larger than is typical.

Prevalence

N/A

Clinical Implications

Melling and Zweymüller (1996) note that an attachment of sartorius to the medial meniscus stabilizes and protects this structure in the knee joint and may prevent herniation or injury during sudden extension of the knee.

RECTUS FEMORIS (FIGURE 5.2)

Synonyms

This muscle may also be referred to as quadriceps extensor cruris (Knott 1883b), extensor cruris medialis superficialis, or rectus anterior.

Typical Presentation

Description

Rectus femoris is one component of quadriceps femoris. It has a dual origin, arising from the anterior inferior iliac spine and from the area just above the acetabulum (Standring 2016). Some fibers originate from the capsule of the hip joint (Standring 2016). The muscle ends in a tendon that inserts onto the base of the patella (Standring 2016).

Innervation

Rectus femoris is innervated by the femoral nerve (Standring 2016).

Comparative Anatomy

The typical presentation of rectus femoris in the apes is a muscle with a single head originating from the anterior superior iliac spine that inserts into the patella (Champneys 1872; Hepburn 1892; Beddard 1893; Sonntag 1924; Raven 1950; Sigmon 1974; Gibbs 1999; Diogo et al. 2010, 2012, 2013a,b, 2017). The head from the ilium near the acetabulum is rarely present in orangutans (Gibbs 1999; Diogo et al. 2013b) occasionally present in common chimpanzees and bonobos (Hepburn 1982; Beddard 1893; Miller 1952; Gibbs 1999; Diogo et al. 2013a, 2017), and frequently present in gorillas (Gibbs 1999; Diogo et al. 2010).

Variations

Description

The two origins of rectus femoris may be continuous (Macalister 1875; Knott 1883b; du Plessis and Loukas 2016). A double origin may be present from the anterior inferior iliac spine (Macalister 1875; du Plessis and Loukas 2016). A portion of the insertion tendon may split off from the rest and pass in front of the patella (Macalister 1875). The tendons of the vasti may overlap and form a canal through which the rectus femoris tendon passes (Macalister 1875; Knott 1883b). Vastus lateralis may insert into the tendon of rectus femoris (Macalister 1875). Rectus femoris may be continuous with the vasti (Macalister 1875; Bergman et al. 1988). Stringer et al.

(2012) report two cases in which a shortened rectus femoris narrowed into a tendon at the middle of the thigh before joining the quadriceps tendon. In one of these cases, the tendon also blended with the fascia over vastus medialis and vastus lateralis.

The head of rectus femoris that originates from the acetabulum/capsule of the hip joint may be absent (Macalister 1875; du Plessis and Loukas 2016; Standring 2016). The entire rectus femoris muscle or the whole quadriceps femoris mass may be absent (Bergman et al. 1988; Stringer et al. 2012). A third "femoral" head may be present with a deep attachment to the iliofemoral ligament, a superficial attachment to the tendon of gluteus minimus, and an insertion into the greater trochanter (Tubbs et al. 2006d). Rectus accessorius is an accessory slip that originates from a tendon at the margin of the acetabulum and inserts into the ventral border of vastus lateralis (Bergman et al. 1988). An accessory slip may also be present and extend between the inguinal ligament and vastus medialis (Takeshige et al. 1960).

Prevalence

In a study of 40 specimens, Knott (1883b) reported that three of them (7.5%) exhibited direct continuity of the spinous and acetabular origins. In one case (2.5%), a small, tendinous accessory slip originated from the anterior superior iliac spine. In two cases (5%), the origin from the anterior superior iliac spine was divided into two parts that were separated by a thin layer of connective tissue. In one of these cases (2.5%), and in three other cases which do not appear to be included in the sample of 40 specimens, the insertion tendon of rectus femoris passed through a canal formed by the overlapping of the tendons of the vasti before inserting onto the patella. In a study of 96 sides from 48 cadavers, Tubbs et al. (2006d) found that 80 sides (83%) had a third "femoral" head of rectus femoris. Two sides (2.1%) had third heads that were bilaminar.

Anomalies

Description

In one anencephalic fetus, Windle (1893) found that the straight (spinous) head of rectus femoris was absent on the left side. Pirani et al. (1991) describe soft tissue anatomy associated with cases of proximal femoral focal deficiency (PFFD). In Aitken type B PFFD, rectus femoris is smaller than is typical.

Prevalence

N/A

Clinical Implications

N/A

VASTUS MEDIALIS (FIGURE 5.2)

Synonyms

This muscle may also be referred to as vastus internus (Macalister 1875). Some researchers may refer to the most

inferior fibers that extend between the tendon of adductor magnus and the medial aspect of the patella as vastus medialis obliquus (Standring 2016).

Typical Presentation

Description

Vastus medialis is one component of quadriceps femoris. (Standring 2016). It originates from the femur with attachments to the intertrochanteric line, spiral line, linea aspera, and medial supracondylar line (Standring 2016). It attaches to the medial aspect of the patella and to the quadriceps femoris tendon (Standring 2016).

Innervation

Vastus medialis is innervated by the femoral nerve (Standring 2016).

Comparative Anatomy

Vastus medialis has a similar typical presentation in the apes, extending from the posteromedial femoral shaft near the linea aspera and the iliofemoral ligament to the patella, with a contribution to the knee joint capsule (Champneys 1872; Hepburn 1892; Beddard 1893; Sonntag 1924; Raven 1950; Sigmon 1974; Gibbs 1999; Diogo et al. 2010, 2012, 2013a,b, 2017). The origin is more proximal in gibbons than in the other apes (Sigmon 1974) and can reach the femoral neck in common chimpanzees (Diogo et al. 2013a).

Variations

Description

The vasti may be bilaminar (Macalister 1875; Knott 1883b; Bergman et al. 1988; du Plessis and Loukas 2016). The vasti may be continuous with rectus femoris (Mori 1964; Bergman et al. 1988; du Plessis and Loukas 2016). Vastus medialis is often fused with vastus intermedius (Macalister 1875; Mori 1964). The vasti may merge into one fleshy muscle mass (Bergman et al. 1988). The entire quadriceps femoris muscle may be absent (Bergman et al. 1988). Its lower fibers may have a separate insertion into the medial condyle of the tibia (Macalister 1875). Vastus medialis obliquus (the inferior portion of the muscle) can vary in its extent of its insertion along the medial aspect of the patella (Holt et al. 2008).

Mori (1964) found three types of distal fusion between vastus medialis and rectus femoris. There was either total fusion of the distal portions of both muscles, fusion between the distal part of vastus medialis and the tendon of rectus femoris, or no fusion between the muscles. Mori (1964) also found three types of fusion between vastus medialis and vastus intermedius. There was either total fusion of both muscles, partial fusion, or no fusion.

Prevalence

Mori (1964) reports that out of 50 thighs, there was total fusion of the distal portions of both vastus medialis and rectus femoris in 22% of cases, fusion between the distal part of vastus medialis and the tendon of rectus femoris in 19%, or no fusion between the muscles in 80%. Mori (1964) also found that there was total fusion between vastus medialis and vastus intermedius in 20% of cases, partial fusion in 50%, and no fusion between the muscles in 30%.

Holt et al. (2008) studied the extent of the insertion of vastus medialis obliquus in 65 patients with MRI and in 18 cadavers. The mean insertion was 51% of patellar length (ranging from 13% to 95%) for the MRI cohort, and 52% of patellar length (ranging from 26% to 81%) in the cadaveric study.

Anomalies

Description

In both a male fetus and female fetus with triploidy studied by Moen et al. (1984), the vastus heads of quadriceps femoris were fused bilaterally. Pirani et al. (1991) describe soft tissue anatomy associated with cases of proximal femoral focal deficiency (PFFD). In Aitken type B PFFD, vastus medialis is smaller than is typical.

Prevalence

N/A

Clinical Implications

Variation of the insertion of vastus medialis obliquus into the patella should be acknowledged when choosing a surgical approach for total knee arthroplasty (Holt et al. 2008).

VASTUS LATERALIS (FIGURE 5.2)

Synonyms

This muscle may also be referred to as vastus externus (Macalister 1875). Some may refer to the distal portion of the muscle that inserts into the patella as vastus lateralis obliquus (du Plessis and Loukas 2016).

Typical Presentation

Description

Vastus lateralis is one component of quadriceps femoris (Standring 2016). It originates from the femur with attachments to the intertrochanteric line, greater trochanter, gluteal tuberosity, and linea aspera (Standring 2016). Some fibers originate from the tendon of gluteus maximus and the lateral intermuscular septum (Standring 2016). It inserts onto the lateral aspect of the patella and joins the quadriceps tendon (Standring 2016).

Innervation

Vastus lateralis is innervated by the femoral nerve (Standring 2016).

Comparative Anatomy

Vastus lateralis has a similar typical presentation in the apes, originating from the lateral femur, with attachments to the greater trochanter and lateral lip of the linea aspera,

and inserting into the patella (Hepburn 1892; Beddard 1893; Sonntag 1924; Raven 1950; Sigmon 1974; Gibbs 1999; Diogo et al. 2010, 2012, 2013a,b, 2017).

Variations

Description

The vasti may be bilaminar, which is an accentuation of the normal presentation of the fibers in vastus lateralis (Macalister 1875; Knott 1883b; Bergman et al. 1988). The entire quadriceps femoris muscle may be absent (Bergman et al. 1988). The origin of vastus lateralis may be confined to the gluteal tuberosity (du Plessis and Loukas 2016). Vastus lateralis may also insert into the tendon of rectus femoris (Macalister 1875; Mori 1964). Vastus lateralis may be doubled, presenting as a muscle with two separate heads (Dwight 1887; du Plessis and Loukas 2016).

The vasti may be continuous with rectus femoris (Macalister 1875; Mori 1964; Bergman et al. 1988). Vastus lateralis may be connected to the other vasti, particularly vastus intermedius (Macalister 1875; Mori 1964; Willan et al. 1990; Becker et al. 2009; du Plessis and Loukas 2016). Accessory bellies of vastus lateralis may be present when this muscle is fused with vastus intermedius (du Plessis and Loukas 2016). Vastus lateralis may be connected with articularis genus when this latter muscle consists of two slips (Macalister 1875). The vasti may merge into one fleshy muscle mass (Bergman et al. 1988). Heimkes et al. (1992) studied the relationships upon insertion between gluteus medius, gluteus minimus, and vastus lateralis and classified these relationships into five types. See the gluteus medius entry for more details and prevalence information. Rectus accessorius is an accessory slip that originates from a tendon at the margin of the acetabulum and inserts into the ventral border of vastus lateralis (Bergman et al. 1988).

Mori (1964) found three types of fusion between vastus lateralis and vastus intermedius including total fusion, partial fusion, and no fusion. Mori (1964) also categorized four relationships between the insertions of vastus lateralis and rectus femoris. These relationships include the distal portion of vastus lateralis situated lateral to the distal portion of rectus femoris, the distal portion of vastus lateralis covered by the distal portion of rectus femoris, the distal portion of vastus lateralis fused with the fascia of rectus femoris, and the distal portion of vastus lateralis fused with the tendon of rectus femoris.

Prevalence

Mori (1964) found that in a sample of 50 thighs, vastus lateralis and vastus intermedius were totally fused in 18% of cases, partially fused in 55%, and not fused in 26%. Mori (1964) also found that the distal portion of vastus lateralis was situated lateral to the distal portion of rectus femoris in 52% of cases, the distal portion of vastus lateralis was covered by the distal portion of rectus femoris in 28%, the distal portion of vastus lateralis fused with the fascia of rectus femoris in 12%, and the distal portion of vastus lateralis fused with the tendon of rectus femoris in 8%.

Willan et al. (1990) examined vastus lateralis and vastus intermedius in 75 lower limbs from 40 cadavers. More than three-fourths of the deep surface of vastus lateralis was fused with vastus intermedius in 25 limbs (33.3%), about half of vastus lateralis was fused with vastus intermedius in 32 limbs (42.7%), and less than one-half of vastus lateralis was fused with vastus intermedius in 18 limbs (24%). The anterior edge of vastus lateralis was fleshy in 22 limbs (29.3%), while there was an anterior tendinous lamina wider than 5 mm in 28 limbs (27.3%) and narrower than 5 mm in 24 limbs (32%). There was a separate deep tendinous lamina from either vastus lateralis or vastus intermedius in 22 limbs (29.3%). There was a separate deep fleshy lamina between vastus lateralis and vastus intermedius in 27 limbs (36%), with fusion to the tendinous lamina in 13 limbs (17.3%), fusion to vastus lateralis in 6 limbs (8%), and fusion to vastus intermedius in 8 limbs (10.7%).

Anomalies

Description

Pettersen et al. (1979) found bilateral accessory vastus lateralis muscles in a fetus with trisomy 13. On the left side, the muscle originated from the deep surface of the upper part of the main vastus lateralis muscle and inserted into the patella via fleshy fibers deep to the attachment of rectus femoris. On the right side, the muscle was similar but had originated separately from vastus lateralis. In both a male fetus and female fetus with triploidy studied by Moen et al. (1984), the vastus heads of quadriceps femoris were fused bilaterally.

Prevalence

In their literature review, Smith et al. (2015) found that accessory vastus lateralis muscles have only been recorded in 1 out of 20 individuals with trisomy 13 (5%).

Clinical Implications

Acknowledging the variable relationships between gluteus medius, gluteus minimus, and vastus lateralis and the potential independent insertions of these muscles onto the greater trochanter is important for successful hip operations, particularly when using the transgluteal approach (Heimkes et al. 1992).

Vastus intermedius (Figure 5.2)

Synonyms

This muscle may also be referred to as crureus (Macalister 1875).

Typical Presentation

Description

Vastus intermedius is one component of quadriceps femoris (Standring 2016). It originates from the anterior and lateral surfaces of the proximal femoral shaft (Standring 2016). It inserts onto the lateral edge of patella and lateral condyle of the tibia (Standring 2016).

Innervation

Vastus intermedius is innervated by the femoral nerve (Standring 2016).

Comparative Anatomy

Vastus intermedius has a similar typical presentation in the apes, extending from the ventral surface of the femoral shaft to the patella (Hepburn 1892; Beddard 1893; Sonntag 1924; Raven 1950; Miller 1952; Sigmon 1974; Gibbs 1999; Diogo et al. 2010, 2012, 2013a,b, 2017). The origin may extend to the femoral neck in gorillas (Raven 1950).

Variations

Description

The vasti may be bilaminar (Macalister 1875; Knott 1883b; Bergman et al. 1988). The entire quadriceps femoris muscle may be absent (Bergman et al. 1988). The origin of vastus intermedius may be as high as the intertrochanteric line (Macalister 1875). The vasti may be continuous with rectus femoris (Bergman et al. 1988). Vastus intermedius may be fully or partially fused with vastus lateralis (Macalister 1875; Mori 1964; Willan et al. 1990; Becker et al. 2009; du Plessis and Loukas 2016). Vastus intermedius may also be fused proximally with vastus medialis (Macalister 1875; Standring 2016; du Plessis and Loukas 2016). Vastus intermedius may join with articularis genus, and if the latter muscle is absent, the deep fibers of vastus intermedius can attach in rare cases to the synovial membrane of the knee (Macalister 1875; du Plessis and Loukas 2016). The vasti may merge into one fleshy muscle mass (Bergman et al. 1988).

Prevalence

Mori (1964) found that in a sample of 50 thighs, vastus lateralis and vastus intermedius were totally fused in 18% of cases, partially fused in 55%, and not fused in 26%. Mori (1964) also found that there was total fusion between vastus medialis and vastus intermedius in 20% of cases, partial fusion in 50%, and no fusion between the muscles in 30%.

Willan et al. (1990) examined vastus lateralis and vastus intermedius in 75 lower limbs from 40 cadavers. More than three-fourths of the deep surface of vastus lateralis was fused with vastus intermedius in 25 limbs (33.3%), about half of vastus lateralis was fused with vastus intermedius in 32 limbs (42.7%), and less than one-half of vastus lateralis was fused with vastus intermedius in 18 limbs (24%). There was a separate deep tendinous lamina from either vastus lateralis or vastus intermedius in 22 limbs (29.3%). There was a separate deep fleshy lamina between vastus lateralis and vastus intermedius in 27 limbs (36%), with fusion to the tendinous lamina in 13 limbs (17.3%), fusion to vastus lateralis in six limbs (8%), and fusion to vastus intermedius in eight limbs (10.7%).

Anomalies

Description

In both a male fetus and female fetus with triploidy studied by Moen et al. (1984), the vastus heads of quadriceps femoris were fused bilaterally.

Prevalence

N/A

Clinical Implications

The complex and variable anatomical relationships between articularis genus, vastus intermedius, and subsequently vastus medialis, are important to acknowledge when planning knee surgery (Grob et al. 2017).

ARTICULARIS GENUS (FIGURE 5.2)

Synonyms

This muscle may also be referred to as sub-crураeus (Macalister 1875), subcrurales, tenseur de la synoviale, supragenualis, or suprageniculares (DiDio et al. 1997).

Typical Presentation

Description

Articularis genus is comprised of several bundles that arise deep to vastus intermedius (Standring 2016). The bundles originate from the distal femoral shaft and insert onto the proximal reflection of the synovial membrane (suprapatellar bursa) of the knee joint (Standring 2016).

Innervation

Articularis genus is innervated by the femoral nerve (Standring 2016).

Comparative Anatomy

Hepburn (1892) claims that articularis genus is present in all apes, but this muscle has not been reported or has been found absent in all apes except gorillas (Sonntag 1923; Diogo et al. 2012, 2013a,b, 2017). In gorillas, it extends from the distal part of the femur to the proximolateral aspect of the articular capsule of the knee joint (Raven 1950; Gibbs 1999; Diogo et al. 2010).

Variations

Description

Articularis genus may blend with vastus intermedius (Macalister 1875; du Plessis and Loukas 2016; Standring 2016; Grob et al. 2017). Articularis genus may be reduced, absent, or divided (Macalister 1875; du Plessis and Loukas 2016). It is also variable in shape and size (e.g., DiDio et al. 1967, 1969; Toscano et al. 2004). Its insertion onto the suprapatellar bursa and the knee joint capsule can vary in its specific location (DiDio et al. 1967; Grob et al. 2017). In addition to its typical insertion into the upper portion of the synovial membrane, it can insert onto either side of the knee (Macalister 1875; du Plessis and Loukas 2016).

There is variation in the number of bundles that comprise articularis genus, with some reports finding only one bundle and others finding more than ten bundles (DiDio et al. 1967, 1969; Ahmad 1975; Kimura and Takahashi 1987; Puig et al. 1996; Toscano et al. 2004; Woodley 2016; Woodley et al. 2012; Sakuma et al. 2014; Grob et al. 2017). The bundles may be organized into multiple layers, often recognized as split into superficial and deep layers, and sometimes with a recognized intermediate layer (Kimura and Takahashi 1987; Woodley et al. 2012; Sakuma et al. 2014; Grob et al. 2017). Varying definitions of which fibers constitute articularis genus (Grob et al. 2017) or underestimation of bundles due to using MRI (Puig et al. 1996; Woodley 2016; Woodley et al. 2012) may explain why the number of bundles reported in the literature varies greatly among studies.

Prevalence

Knott (1883b) found that articularis genus was absent in 3 out of 40 limbs (7.5%). DiDio et al. (1967) studied articularis genus in 156 limbs from 78 cadavers. One bundle of articularis genus was found in 70 cases (44.9%), two bundles in 52 cases (33.3%), three bundles in 23 cases (14.7%), four bundles in 9 cases (5.8%), and six bundles in 2 cases (1.3%). The articularis genus muscles were rectangular in 87 cases (55.8%), trapezoidal in 42 cases (26.9%), and had an inverted trapezoidal outline in 27 cases (17.3%). The origin of articularis genus was the lateral and medial aspects of the distal femur in 83 cases (53.5%), the anterior aspect in 26 cases (16.7%), anterior and lateral aspects in six cases (3.8%), medial aspect in four cases (2.6%), anterior and medial aspects in four cases (2.6%), and lateral aspect in two cases (1.3%). Its insertion of its bundles into the suprapatellar bursa varied from the center of its proximal border in 126 out of 401 times (31.4%), medial aspect of its proximal border 117 times (29.2%), lateral aspect 110 times (27.4%), posterior aspect 25 times (6.2%), and the anterior aspect 23 times (5.7%).

DiDio et al. (1969) studied articularis genus in 66 individuals, ranging from fetuses to adults. The shape of the muscle was triangular in 44% of cases, had a lambdoidal outline in 27%, was rectangular in 24%, and had an unclassified shape in 5%. One bundle was found in 66.7% of cases, two partially divided bundles in 27.3% of cases, two bundles in 1.5% of cases, and in 4.5% of cases the number of bundles was not determined. Kimura and Takahashi (1987) studied the number of bundles of articularis genus in 40 thighs from 44 cadavers. One bundle was found in two cases (5%), two bundles in 11 cases (27.5%), three bundles in eight cases (20%), four bundles in seven cases (17.5%), five bundles in five cases (12.5%), six bundles in three cases (7.5%), seven bundles in one case (2.5%), and in three cases (7.5%) the bundles were unable to be properly counted.

Toscano et al. (2004) studied articularis genus in 15 lower limbs. The muscles were trapezoidal in shape in 40% of cases, rectangular in 33%, and in the remaining cases, the muscles were either triangular or irregular. In 57.1% of cases, articularis genus inserted onto the anterior aspect of the proximal edge of the suprapatellar bursa. The most common number of bundles was four bundles (33.3% of cases). Woodley et al. (2012) used MRI and dissection to study articularis genus in 18 lower limbs. Using MRI, these authors found that two bundles were present in one case (5.6%), three bundles in five cases (27.8%), four bundles in nine cases (50%), and five bundles in three cases (16.7%). Using dissection on these same specimens, they found that there were four bundles in one case (5.6%), five bundles in four cases (22.2%), six bundles in one case (5.6%), seven bundles in six cases (33.3%), eight bundles in two cases (11.1%), nine bundles in two cases (11.1%), and ten bundles in two cases (11.1%).

Grob et al. (2017) studied articularis genus in 18 lower limbs from 12 cadavers. They found that bundles of the superficial layer, and in 11 specimens (61.1%) the bundles of the intermediate layer, arose from vastus intermedius and the anterior and anterolateral surfaces of the femurs. The bundles of the deep layer, and in the remaining seven specimens (38.9%), the bundles of the intermediate layer arose from the anterior surface of the femur only. Out of the 18 lower limbs, the articularis genus muscle from one limb had three bundles (5.6%), four limbs had four bundles (22.2%), six limbs had five bundles (33.3%), and seven limbs had articularis genus muscles with six bundles (38.9%).

Anomalies

N/A

Clinical Implications

The complex and variable anatomical relationships between articularis genus, vastus intermedius, and subsequently vastus medialis, are important to acknowledge when planning knee surgery (Grob et al. 2017).

Obturator internus (Figures 4.4 and 5.3)

Synonyms

N/A

Typical Presentation

Description

Obturator internus originates from bony surfaces that surround the obturator foramen including the inferior pubic ramus, the ischial ramus, the pelvic surface of the ilium, and the greater sciatic foramen (Standring 2016). It also originates from the obturator membrane and the obturator fascia (Standring 2016). Its fibers converge into four or five tendinous bands that pass through the lesser sciatic foramen to insert as a single tendon onto the greater trochanter (Standring 2016). The superior gemellus and inferior gemellus fuse with this tendon prior to insertion (Standring 2016).

Innervation

Obturator internus is innervated by the nerve to obturator internus (Standring 2016).

Comparative Anatomy

Obturator internus has a similar typical presentation in the apes, arising from the bones around the internal aspect of the obturator foramen and from the obturator membrane, passing through the lesser sciatic foramen, and inserting with the gemelli onto the trochanteric fossa of the femur (Champneys 1872; Hepburn 1892; Beddard 1893; Raven 1950; Sigmon 1974; Diogo et al. 2010, 2012, 2013a,b, 2017).

Variations

Description

Obturator internus may be divided into two parts (Bergman et al. 1988). Accessory slips may be present (Macalister 1875; Bergman et al. 1988; Nicholson et al. 2016). These slips may originate from the lower margin of the ilio-pectineal line, from the tendon of psoas minor, the ridge above the inner margin of the ischial tuberosity, the inner aspect of the ischium, the third sacral vertebra, the pelvic fascia, or the sacrotuberous ligament (Macalister 1875; Knott 1883b; Nicholson et al. 2016). Some fibers from obturator internus may be continuous with those of gemellus superior or gemellus inferior (Aung et al. 2001; Bergman et al. 1988; Nicholson et al. 2016). The tendon of obturator internus may blend with the tendon of piriformis (Wood 1868; Pine et al. 2011). Obturator internus may be absent (Sato 1970).

Prevalence

From the examination of 36 bodies, Wood (1868) states that in three males and one female (11%), the tendon of piriformis was blended with that of obturator internus—the two

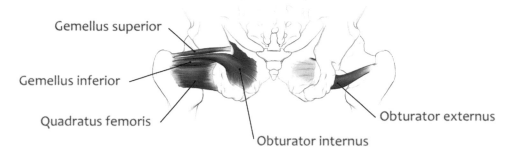

FIGURE 5.3　Lateral rotators of the hip in posterior view.

inserted together onto the greater trochanter. Though total sample size is unclear, Knott (1883b) noted an origin from the sacrotuberous ligament in three cases and a slip from the inner surface of the ischium above the spine in two subjects. Sato (1970) found that obturator internus was absent in 30 out of 410 limbs (7.3%) from Kyushu Japanese males and in 29 out of 250 limbs (11.6%) from females. Aung et al. (2001) found that out of 101 hemipelves from 60 cadavers, two specimens (2%) exhibited a distal extension of obturator internus muscle fibers that continued to join the fibers of inferior gemellus. Pine et al. (2011) found that out of 29 specimens, the tendons of obturator internus and piriformis were at least partially fused in four specimens (13.8%), with three inserting as a common tendon and one dividing to have separate attachments.

Anomalies

Description

Bersu et al. (1976) describe a male infant with Hanhart syndrome. The femora of this infant were normally developed but distal secondary ossification centers were absent. The left leg stump had a patella and a small rudiment of the proximal tibia but no fibular rudiment. The right leg stump was less developed and had a patella, smaller tibial rudiment, and no fibular rudiment. On both sides, obturator internus had normal origins. On the left side, it inserted onto the inferior aspect of the sacrotuberous ligament. On the right side, it inserted into the periosteum of the lesser sciatic notch.

Pirani et al. (1991) describe soft tissue anatomy associated with cases of proximal femoral focal deficiency (PFFD). In Aitken type A PFFD, the short external rotators of the hip are larger in cross-sectional diameter than normal and insert onto the posteromedial surface of the greater trochanter. In Aitken type B PFFD, the short external rotators are smaller than normal. In a female fetus with trisomy 18, obturator internus, superior gemellus, and inferior gemellus were fused laterally on both sides of the body (Alghamdi et al. 2018).

Prevalence

N/A

Clinical Implications

N/A

Obturator externus (Figure 5.3)

Synonyms

N/A

Typical Presentation

Description

Obturator externus originates from the structures that surround the external/anterior surface of the obturator foramen including the pubic ramus, the ischial ramus, and the obturator membrane (Standring 2016). It inserts via a tendon onto the trochanteric fossa of the femur (Standring 2016).

Innervation

Obturator externus is innervated by the posterior branch of the obturator nerve (Standring 2016).

Comparative Anatomy

Obturator externus has a similar typical presentation in the apes, arising from the bones around the external aspect of the obturator foramen and from the obturator membrane and inserting onto the trochanteric fossa of the femur (Champneys 1872; Hepburn 1892; Beddard 1893; Raven 1950; Sigmon 1974; Diogo et al. 2010, 2012, 2013a,b, 2017). It may fuse with obturator internus in gibbons, orangutans, and common chimpanzees (Hepburn 1892; Beddard 1893) and both gemelli in orangutans (Diogo et al. 2013b). It can have an attachment onto the femoral neck in gorillas and common chimpanzees (Hepburn 1892; Gibbs 1999) and from the hip joint capsule in bonobos (Diogo et al. 2017).

Variations

Description

Obturator externus may have a connection with adductor brevis (Bergman et al. 1988; du Plessis and Loukas 2016). Macalister (1875) notes more specifically that adductor brevis may send a slip to the tendon of obturator externus. Macalister (1875) and Knott (1883b) note that the obturator externus tendon may have an attachment or some degree of connection onto the capsule of the hip joint. The muscle may be split into superior and inferior portions by the obturator nerve and vessels (Macalister 1875; Knott 1883b; Bergman et al. 1988; du Plessis and Loukas 2016). The superior portion may arise from the horizontal ramus of the pubis below pectineus and is separated by the rest of the muscle by the obturator nerve and vessels (Macalister 1875; Knott 1883b). Obturator externus may be split into three parts (Bergman et al. 1988; du Plessis and Loukas 2016).

Some authors report accessory muscle slips and/or fasciculi closely associated with obturator externus. Nakamura et al. (1992) and Yatsunami et al. (2004) report accessory muscles occurring between adductor brevis and adductor minimus, originating from the upper part of the inferior pubic ramus and running closely with obturator externus before inserting onto the pectineal line, the lesser trochanter, or the anterior aspect of the aponeurotic insertion of adductor minimus. Nakamura et al. (1992) suggest that these muscles are formed when the superficial fascicle of obturator externus separates from the rest of the muscle during development and forms the supernumerary muscle when it has an insertion other than the trochanteric fossa. In addition to similar accessory muscles, Yatsunami et al. (2004) report accessory fasciculi fused to the posterior surface of adductor minimus, which they suggest are likely homologous to the superficial layer of the main belly of obturator externus.

Upasna et al. (2013) report an accessory muscle in the left leg of a cadaver that also exhibited an adductor longus and pectineus with a combined origin from the pecten pubis, and an adductor brevis that was divided in two and had distal fibers that merged with those of adductor longus. The accessory muscle was located under adductor brevis and lied on top of the obturator externus and the posterior division of the obturator nerve. Its fibers extended between the inferior pubic ramus and merged with the aponeurosis of adductor magnus. A similar muscular slip was also present on the right side but was not described in detail.

Prevalence

Knott (1883b) observed that obturator externus was split into two portions by the obturator nerve and vessels in 4 out of 20 cases (20%). Nakamura et al. (1992) found a supernumerary muscle in 33 out of 100 thighs from 50 cadavers (33%). The muscles had an insertion onto the anterior surface of the insertion aponeurosis of adductor minimus in 17 out of 33 thighs (51.5%), the upper portion of the pectineal line in nine thighs (27.3%), and the posterior aspect of the base of the lesser trochanter in seven thighs (21.2%).

Yatsunami et al. (2004) found that out of 73 thighs from 45 cadavers, the obturator nerve pierced obturator externus in 50 cases (68.5%) and ran over the muscle in 23 cases (31.5%). These authors found accessory muscles occurring between adductor brevis and adductor minimus in 37 thighs (50.7%) and accessory fasciculi fused to the posterior surface of adductor minimus in 18 thighs (24.7%). They suggest that during ontogeny, the superior fasciculus of obturator externus retained its normal morphology in 23 thighs (31.5%), a portion of the superior fasciculus converted into the accessory muscle in 27 thighs (37%), the entire superior fasciculus converted into the accessory muscle in 10 thighs (13.7%), and the entire superior fasciculus disappeared in 13 thighs (17.8%).

Anomalies

Description

Bersu et al. (1976) describe a male infant with Hanhart syndrome. The femora of this infant were normally developed but distal secondary ossification centers were absent. The left leg stump had a patella and a small rudiment of the proximal tibia but no fibular rudiment. The right leg stump was less developed and had a patella, smaller tibial rudiment, and no fibular rudiment. On both sides, obturator externus had normal origins. On the left side, it inserted into a tendon it shared with a slip from piriformis. On the right side, it had a broad aponeurotic insertion onto the lesser trochanter.

Pirani et al. (1991) describe soft tissue anatomy associated with cases of proximal femoral focal deficiency (PFFD). In Aitken type A PFFD, obturator externus is straight. It courses through the concavity of the subtrochanteric varus deformity of the proximal femoral metaphysis and inserts onto the posteromedial surface of the greater trochanter and is muscular nearly up to its insertion. In types B, C, and D, obturator externus is L-shaped. For example, in Aitken type B PFFD, the distal part of obturator externus is oriented 90° cranially and 45° posteriorly and passes between the

dissociated femoral head and proximal femoral metaphysis before inserting onto the posteromedial surface of the proximal end of the shaft of the femur. It is muscular up to its insertion. In Aitken type D PFFD, obturator externus inserts onto the proximal femoral ossicle.

Prevalence

N/A

Clinical Implications

N/A

GEMELLUS SUPERIOR (FIGURE 5.3)

Synonyms

N/A

Typical Presentation

Description

Gemellus superior originates from the ischial spine, blends with the obturator internus tendon, and inserts onto the greater trochanter (Standring 2016).

Innervation

Gemellus superior is innervated by the nerve to obturator internus (Standring 2016).

Comparative Anatomy

Gemellus superior has a similar typical presentation in most apes, arising from the ischium near the ischial spine and having a common insertion onto the trochanteric fossa with the tendon of obturator internus (Diogo et al. 2012, 2013a,b, 2017). Gemellus superior is absent in most gorillas (Gibbs 1999; Diogo et al. 2010).

Variations

Description

Gemellus superior may be reduced or absent (Hallett 1848; Wood 1868; Macalister 1875; Knott 1883a,b; Bergman et al. 1988; Duda et al. 1996; Nicholson et al. 2016; Standring 2016). Absence of both gemelli is rare (Bergman et al. 1988). Gemellus superior can be separated into two parts (Knott 1883b). It may be fused with piriformis or gluteus minimus (Macalister 1875; Bergman et al. 1988; Chiba 1992; Nicholson et al. 2016). Some fibers from obturator internus may be continuous with those of gemellus superior (Aung et al. 2001; Bergman et al. 1988; Nicholson et al. 2016). Macalister (1875) observed it as sometimes inseparable from obturator internus and reports it joining with the lower border of gluteus minimus. Gemellus superior may have an origin from the greater sciatic notch (Aasar 1947; Nicholson et al. 2016). This muscle may have an insertion onto the hip joint capsule (Macalister 1875; Bergman et al. 1988).

Instead of forming a common tendon with obturator internus and inferior gemellus, the tendon of gemellus superior may insert onto the piriformis tendon (Macalister 1875;

Knott 1883b). Furthermore, the gemelli may instead cover the superficial surface of the tendon of obturator internus or extend over this tendon as an aponeurosis (Shinohara 1995; Nicholson et al. 2016). Babinski et al. (2003) describe a case in which a high division of the sciatic nerve caused the common fibular nerve to pass superior to superior gemellus and the tibial nerve to pass inferior to superior gemellus.

Gemellus superior may also be doubled (Macalister 1875; Bergman et al. 1988; Arifoglu et al. 1997; Tanyeli et al. 2006; Nicholson et al. 2016). Ortega et al. (2013) describe a case in which gemellus superior was bilaterally duplicated. The main belly of gemellus superior arose from the ischial spine and inserted onto the greater trochanter with piriformis via a common tendon. The duplicated belly of gemellus superior—along with obturator internus and inferior gemellus—extended from the ischial tuberosity to the quadrate tubercle but was displaced and situated directly on the superior surface of quadratus femoris.

Prevalence

Terry (1942) combines the observations from Wood (1867b and 1868) and finds that out of 70 total subjects, superior gemellus was absent in four bodies (5.7%). It was absent bilaterally in two males and one female, and absent on the right side in one other male and was thus absent in 7 out of 140 sides (5%). Terry (1942) found that superior gemellus was absent in 31 out of 254 total individuals (12.2%) and was absent more often in African Americans (22 out of 150 cases, or 14.7%) than in Whites (9 out of 104, or 8.7%). Sato (1970) found that gemellus superior was absent in 21 out of 390 limbs (5.4%) from Kyushu Japanese males and in 19 out of 260 limbs (7.3%) from females. Shinohara (1995) studied obturator internus and the gemelli on 14 sides from 12 cadavers. This author found that on five sides (36%) the muscle fibers of the superior and inferior gemelli terminated on the obturator internus tendon (the typical presentation). On the nine other sides (64%), the gemelli covered the superficial surface of the obturator internus tendon.

Anomalies

Description

Gemellus superior may be absent in individuals with trisomy 13 or trisomy 18 (Smith et al. 2015). In a female fetus with trisomy 18, obturator internus, gemellus superior, and gemellus inferior were fused laterally on both sides of the body (Alghamdi et al. 2018). Bersu et al. (1976) describe a male infant with Hanhart syndrome. The femora of this infant were normally developed, but distal secondary ossification centers were absent. The left leg stump had a patella and a small rudiment of the proximal tibia but no fibular rudiment. The right leg stump was less developed and had a patella, smaller tibial rudiment, and no fibular rudiment. Gemellus superior was absent bilaterally. Pirani et al. (1991) describe soft tissue anatomy associated with cases of proximal femoral focal deficiency (PFFD). In Aitken type A PFFD, the short external rotators of the hip are larger in cross-sectional diameter than normal and insert onto the posteromedial

surface of the greater trochanter. In Aitken type B PFFD, the short external rotators are smaller than normal.

Prevalence

In their literature review, Smith et al. (2015) found that superior gemellus was absent in 1 out of 24 individuals (4.2%) with trisomy 13 and 3 out of 26 (11.5%) individuals with trisomy 18.

Clinical Implications

If components of the sciatic nerve surround superior gemellus, this morphology could implicate this muscle in piriformis syndrome, coccygodynia, or muscle atrophy (Babinski et al. 2003). Doubling of superior gemellus may compress the sciatic nerve and contribute to piriformis syndrome (Arifoglu et al. 1997). Ortega et al. (2013) note that displacement of a duplicated gemellus superior and nearby muscles can lead to weakness of lateral hip rotation and abduction of the femur.

GEMELLUS INFERIOR (FIGURE 5.3)

Synonyms

N/A

Typical Presentation

Description

Gemellus inferior originates from the ischial tuberosity, blends with the obturator internus tendon, and inserts onto the greater trochanter (Standring 2016).

Innervation

Gemellus inferior is innervated by the nerve to quadratus femoris (Standring 2016).

Comparative Anatomy

Gemellus inferior has a similar typical presentation in the apes, arising from the ischial tuberosity and inserting with obturator internus into the trochanteric fossa, with occasional fusion with nearby muscles (Champneys 1872; Hepburn 1892; Beddard 1893; Raven 1950; Sigmon 1974; Diogo et al. 2010, 2012, 2013a,b, 2017).

Variations

Description

Gemellus inferior may be divided into two or three fasciculi (Knott 1883b). It may also be doubled, and in rare cases, it has been reported absent (Hallett 1848; Knott 1883b; Sato 1970; Bergman et al. 1988; Tanyeli et al. 2006; Nicholson et al. 2016). It is absent less often than is the superior gemellus (Macalister 1875; Bergman et al. 1988; Duda et al. 1996). Absence of both gemelli is rare (Bergman et al. 1988). Wood (1868) found inferior gemellus absent on the right side and superior gemellus absent bilaterally in one female examined by him. Brenner et al. (2019) describe the right lower limb of a female cadaver in which piriformis and inferior gemellus were missing.

Gemellus inferior may be fused with quadratus femoris (Macalister 1875; Knott 1883b; Bergman et al. 1988; Nicholson et al. 2016). Some fibers from obturator internus may be continuous with those of gemellus inferior (Aung et al. 2001; Bergman et al. 1988; Nicholson et al. 2016). Macalister (1875) also observed it as sometimes inseparable from obturator internus. Macalister (1875) reports a case described by Meckel, in which quadratus femoris was absent and gemellus inferior was enlarged. Instead of forming a common tendon with obturator internus, the gemelli may instead cover the surface of the tendon of obturator internus or extend over this tendon as an aponeurosis (Shinohara 1995; Nicholson et al. 2016).

Prevalence

Wood (1868) found inferior gemellus absent in 1 out of 36 individuals (2.8%). Sato (1970) found that gemellus inferior was absent in 14 out of 390 limbs (3.6%) from Kyushu Japanese males and in 12 out of 264 limbs (4.5%) from females. Shinohara (1995) studied obturator internus and the gemelli on 14 sides from 12 cadavers. This author found that on five sides (36%) the muscle fibers of the superior and inferior gemelli terminated on the obturator internus tendon (the typical presentation). On the nine other sides (64%), the gemelli covered the superficial surface of the obturator internus tendon. Aung et al. (2001) found that out of 101 hemipelves from 60 cadavers, two specimens (2%) exhibited a distal extension of obturator internus muscle fibers that continued to join the fibers of inferior gemellus.

Anomalies

Description

Bersu et al. (1976) describe a male infant with Hanhart syndrome. The femora of this infant were normally developed, but distal secondary ossification centers were absent. The left leg stump had a patella and a small rudiment of the proximal tibia but no fibular rudiment. The right leg stump was less developed and had a patella, smaller tibial rudiment, and no fibular rudiment. Gemellus inferior was absent bilaterally. Pirani et al. (1991) describe soft tissue anatomy associated with cases of proximal femoral focal deficiency (PFFD. In Aitken type A PFFD, the short external rotators of the hip are larger in cross-sectional diameter than normal and insert onto the posteromedial surface of the greater trochanter. In Aitken type B PFFD, the short external rotators are smaller than normal. In a female fetus with trisomy 18, obturator internus, gemellus superior, and gemellus inferior were fused laterally on both sides of the body (Alghamdi et al. 2018).

Prevalence

N/A

Clinical Implications

N/A

QUADRATUS FEMORIS (FIGURE 5.3)

Synonyms

N/A

Typical Presentation

Description

Quadratus femoris originates from the ischial tuberosity and inserts onto the quadrate tubercle and onto the femur just below this tubercle (Standring 2016).

Innervation

Quadratus femoris is innervated by the nerve to quadratus femoris (Standring 2016).

Comparative Anatomy

Quadratus femoris has a similar typical presentation in the apes, extending from the ischial tuberosity to the intertrochanteric crest, with occasional extension onto the lesser or greater trochanters (Champneys 1872; Hepburn 1892; Beddard 1893; Sonntag 1924; Raven 1950; Miller 1952; Sigmon 1974; Diogo et al. 2010, 2012, 2013a,b, 2017). There is an attachment to the hip joint capsule in bonobos (Diogo et al. 2017).

Variations

Description

Quadratus femoris may be absent (Macalister 1875; Knott 1880, 1883a,b; Sato 1970; Bergman et al. 1988; Nicholson et al. 2016; Standring 2016). Tubbs and Salter (2006b) describe a case in which an accessory piriformis muscle was present on the same side of a limb where quadratus femoris was absent. Liu et al. (2011) found that in one case, bilateral absence of quadratus femoris was also associated with bilateral absence of semimembranosus. Macalister (1875) reports a case described by Meckel, in which quadratus femoris was absent and gemellus inferior was enlarged. Bergman et al. (1988) note that it can also be replaced by a large obturator internus.

The extent of its insertion onto the femur can vary (Duda et al. 1996; Nicholson et al. 2016). It may also be fused with inferior gemellus or adductor magnus (Macalister 1875; Knott 1883b; Bergman et al. 1988; Nicholson et al. 2016). Quadratus femoris can send a slip to the origin of semimembranosus or have an attachment to the joint capsule of the hip (Macalister 1875; Knott 1883b). Quadratus femoris may be split at its insertion, having a posterior part that inserts normally and an anterior part that inserts onto the intertrochanteric crest (Bergman et al. 1988). Quadratus femoris may be doubled (Tanyeli et al. 2006). Macalister (1875) reports a case observed by Jancke in which quadratus femoris was split into 30 fasciculi.

Prevalence

Sato (1970) found that quadratus femoris was absent in 4 out of 418 limbs (1%) from Kyushu Japanese males and in 13 out of 262 limbs (5%) from females.

Anomalies

Description

Bersu et al. (1976) describe a male infant with Hanhart syndrome. The femora of this infant were normally developed, but distal secondary ossification centers were absent. The left leg stump had a patella and a small rudiment of the proximal tibia but no fibular rudiment. The right leg stump was less developed and had a patella, smaller tibial rudiment, and no fibular rudiment. Quadratus femoris was absent bilaterally. Pirani et al. (1991) describe soft tissue anatomy associated with cases of proximal femoral focal deficiency (PFFD). In Aitken type A PFFD, the short external rotators of the hip are larger in cross-sectional diameter than normal and insert onto the posteromedial surface of the greater trochanter. In Aitken type B PFFD, the short external rotators are smaller than normal. In a fetus with craniorachischisis, quadratus femoris on the right lower limb was smaller than normal and less differentiated (Alghamdi et al. 2017).

Prevalence

N/A

Clinical Implications

Liu et al. (2011) suggest that absence of quadratus femoris may present as muscle weakness of hip lateral rotation. Girolami et al. (2019) describe a case of isolated sciatica in a left leg that was associated with a quadratus femoris muscle with an enlarged belly and narrow origin and insertion.

Gracilis (Figure 5.4)

Synonyms

This muscle may also be referred to as adductor gracilis or rectus femoris internus (Knott 1883b).

Typical Presentation

Description

Gracilis originates from the body of the pubis, the inferior pubic ramus, and the ischial ramus (Standring 2016). It inserts via a tendon onto the medial surface of the proximal tibia just below the medial condyle (Standring 2016). The insertion tendon contributes to the pes anserinus, and some fibers blend with the deep fascia of the lower leg (Standring 2016).

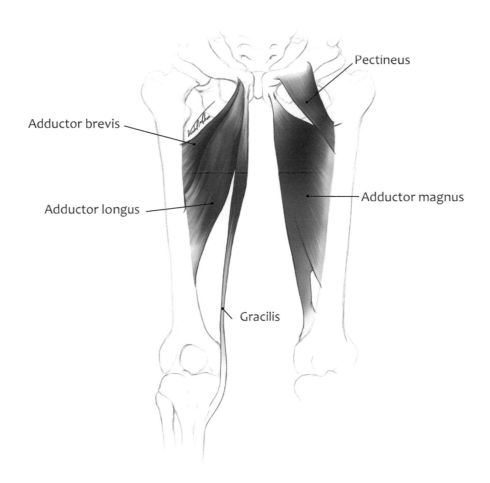

FIGURE 5.4   Medial thigh muscles in anterior view.

Innervation

Gracilis is innervated by the obturator nerve (Standring 2016).

Comparative Anatomy

Gracilis has a similar typical presentation in the apes, extending from the pubis, pubic ramus, and adjoining ischial ramus to the medial aspect of the proximal tibia (Champneys 1872; Hepburn 1892; Beddard 1893; Sonntag 1924; Raven 1950; Miller 1952; Sigmon 1974; Gibbs 1999; Diogo et al. 2010, 2012, 2013a,b, 2017). In bonobos, gracilis has been observed to fuse distally with sartorius, semitendinosus, or adductor brevis (Miller 1952; Diogo et al. 2017).

Variations

Description

Gracilis may be absent (Sainsbury and Wagget 1984). Gracilis may send fibers to the fascia lata or fascia of the leg (Macalister 1875; Knott 1883b; Bergman et al. 1988; du Plessis and Loukas 2016). The extent of its origin may vary (Macalister 1875). It may have a common origin with adductor longus (Tuite et al. 1998). The origin of gracilis may be divided (biceps gracilis), with an upper head that originates from the pubis and a lower head that originates from the ischial ramus (Bergman et al. 1988; du Plessis and Loukas 2016). It may also be split at its insertion (Macalister 1875). Gracilis is frequently associated with a slip that merges with the tendon of the medial head of gastrocnemius (Standring 2016).

Prevalence

Tuite et al. (1998) studied the origin of adductor longus in 37 cadavers. In one case (2.7%), adductor longus had a common origin with gracilis.

Anomalies

N/A

Clinical Implications

If the slip of gracilis that blends with the tendon of the medial head of gastrocnemius is undivided from the main portion of this muscle, there may be complications during surgical harvest of the gracilis tendon (Standring 2016).

ADDUCTOR LONGUS (FIGURE 5.4)

Synonyms

N/A

Typical Presentation

Description

Adductor longus originates via a tendon from the front of the pubis in between the crest and the symphysis (Standring 2016). It has an aponeurotic insertion into the linea aspera on the middle third of the femur and typically blends with vastus medialis, adductor brevis, and adductor magnus (Standring 2016).

Innervation

Adductor longus is innervated by the anterior division of the obturator nerve (Standring 2016).

Comparative Anatomy

Adductor longus has a similar typical presentation in the apes, extending from the pubis to the middle of the medial lip of the linea aspera or posteromedial femoral shaft (Champneys 1872; Hepburn 1892; Beddard 1893; Sonntag 1924; Raven 1950; Miller 1952; Sigmon 1974; Gibbs 1999; Diogo et al. 2010, 2012, 2013a,b, 2017). Adductor longus inserts more proximally in gibbons than in the other apes (Appleton and Ghey 1929). In orangutans, gibbons, common chimpanzees, and bonobos the muscles may be completely or partially fused with the other adductors, vastus medialis, or pectineus (Champneys 1872; Beddard 1893; Sonntag 1924; Miller 1952; Gibbs 1999; Diogo et al. 2017).

Variations

Description

Adductor longus may be doubled (Standring 2016) or bilaminar (Macalister 1875; Knott 1883b). It may be fused with adductor magnus, adductor brevis, or both muscles (Mori 1964; Bergman et al. 1988; du Plessis and Loukas 2016). Adductor longus may insert more distally, as far as the knee (Macalister 1875; Bergman et al. 1988; du Plessis and Loukas 2016). It may receive a slip from pectineus (Macalister 1875). Adductor longus may also send a fasciculus to the inner side of vastus medialis (Macalister 1875; Knott 1883b).

Thomson (1885) reports a case in which adductor longus had a wide origin that extended onto the ilio-pectineal line for 1 inch and blended with the superficial fibers of pectineus. Tuite et al. (1998) found that the origin of adductor longus may have two heads, may be fused with the origin of gracilis, or may be partially muscular. Upasna et al. (2013) describe bilateral variations in the lower limbs of a female cadaver. Adductor longus and pectineus had a combined origin from the pecten pubis, and an adductor brevis was divided in two and had distal fibers that merged with those of adductor longus. These variations were associated with bilateral accessory slips located under adductor brevis.

Prevalence

Knott (1883b) found that adductor longus was bilaminar in 1 out of 40 cases (2.5%). Mori (1964) categorized the fusion of the adductors into eight types. All three adductors fused near their origins in 4% of cases, only adductor longus and adductor brevis fused near their origins in 4% of cases, all three adductors fused near their insertions in 8% of cases, only adductor longus and adductor magnus fused near their insertions in 38% of cases, only adductor brevis and adductor magnus fused near their insertions in 6% of cases, adductor brevis was completely fused with adductor magnus in 8% of cases, adductor magnus fused completely with adductor minimus in 8% of cases, and there was no fusion between any of the adductors in 14% of cases.

Tuite et al. (1998) studied the origin of adductor longus in 37 cadavers. In nine cadavers (24.3%), muscular fibers comprised the lateral origin of adductor longus, ranging in width from 5 to 11 mm. In one case (2.7%), adductor longus had two heads. In one other case (2.7%), adductor longus had a common origin with gracilis.

Anomalies

Description

Aziz (1980) notes that on both sides of one neonate with trisomy 13, a muscular slip arose superficial to the main belly of adductor longus and inserted on the medial surface of the proximal tibia close to the insertion of sartorius. On the right lower limb of a fetus with craniorachischisis dissected by Alghamdi et al. (2017), some fibers of adductor magnus fused with adductor longus. Adductor longus was doubled on the right side in a male fetus with triploidy dissected by Moen et al. (1984). Pirani et al. (1991) describe soft tissue anatomy associated with cases of proximal femoral focal deficiency (PFFD). In Aitken type B PFFD, adductor longus is smaller than normal and oriented more perpendicular to the femur than is typical. In Aitken type D PFFD, adductor longus inserts onto the distal femoral remnant.

Prevalence

An accessory slip associated with adductor longus (Aziz 1980) was only observed in 1 out of 20 individuals with trisomy 13 (5%) included in the literature review of Smith et al. (2015).

Clinical Implications

N/A

ADDUCTOR BREVIS (FIGURE 5.4)

Synonyms

N/A

Typical Presentation

Description

Adductor brevis originates from the body and inferior ramus of the pubis (Standring 2016). It has an aponeurotic insertion into the femur from the lesser trochanter to the linea aspera, and onto the upper aspect of the linea aspera behind pectineus (Standring 2016).

Innervation

Adductor brevis is innervated by the obturator nerve (Standring 2016).

Comparative Anatomy

Adductor brevis has a similar typical presentation in the apes, originating from the pubis and inferior pubic ramus, and sometimes the superior pubic ramus, with an insertion onto the femur below the lesser trochanter and onto the upper third of the medial lip of the linea aspera on the mid-dorsal femoral surface (Champneys 1872; Hepburn 1892; Beddard 1893; Sonntag 1924; Raven 1950; Miller 1952;

Sigmon 1974; Gibbs 1999; Diogo et al. 2010, 2012, 2013a,b, 2017). Adductor brevis may be fused with adductor magnus in all apes (Hepburn 1892; Sigmon 1974; Gibbs 1999; Diogo et al. 2017). In orangutans, it may be divided, with one part arising from the superior pubic ramus and the other from the inferior pubic ramus (Hepburn 1892; Sonntag 1924; Sigmon 1974; Ferrero 2011; Ferrero et al. 2012; Diogo et al. 2013b). It may also be divided into two parts in gorillas (Gibbs 1999; Diogo et al. 2010) and common chimpanzees and bonobos (Champneys 1872; Hepburn 1892; Beddard 1893; Diogo et al. 2017).

Variations

Description

Adductor brevis may be partially or completely divided into two or three parts (Macalister 1875; Knott 1883b; Ochiltree 1912; Bergman et al. 1988; du Plessis and Loukas 2016; Standring 2016). This muscle may be fused with or incorporated into adductor magnus (Macalister 1875; Mori 1964; Bergman et al. 1988; du Plessis and Loukas 2016; Standring 2016). It may also be fused with both adductor longus and adductor magnus or only adductor longus (Mori 1964). Adductor brevis may also have a connection with obturator externus (Bergman et al. 1988; du Plessis and Loukas 2016). Macalister (1875) notes more specifically that adductor brevis may send a slip to the tendon of obturator externus.

Upasna et al. (2013) found bilateral variations in the lower limbs of a female cadaver. Adductor longus and pectineus had a combined origin from the pecten pubis, and an adductor brevis was divided in two and had distal fibers that merged with those of adductor longus. These variations were associated with bilateral accessory slips. The authors describe the accessory muscle on the left side in detail, noting it was located under adductor brevis and overlied obturator externus and the posterior division of the obturator nerve. Its fibers extended between the inferior pubic ramus and merged with the aponeurosis of adductor magnus.

Prevalence

Mori (1964) categorized the fusion of the adductors into eight types. All three adductors fused near their origins in 4% of cases, only adductor longus and adductor brevis fused near their origins in 4% of cases, all three adductors fused near their insertions in 8% of cases, only adductor longus and adductor magnus fused near their insertions in 38% of cases, only adductor brevis and adductor magnus fused near their insertions in 6% of cases, adductor brevis was completely fused with adductor magnus in 8% of cases, adductor magnus fused completely with adductor minimus in 8% of cases, and there was no fusion between any of the adductors in 14% of cases.

Anomalies

Description

Bersu et al. (1976) describe a male infant with Hanhart syndrome. The femora of this infant were normally developed, but distal secondary ossification centers were absent. The left leg stump had a patella and a small rudiment of the proximal tibia but no fibular rudiment. The right leg stump was less developed and had a patella, smaller tibial rudiment, and no fibular rudiment. On the left side, adductor brevis inserted via a tendon it shared with the superior and middle bundles of adductor magnus into the middle third of the linea aspera. On the right side, the origin of this muscle was displaced inferiorly.

Pirani et al. (1991) describe soft tissue anatomy associated with cases of proximal femoral focal deficiency (PFFD). In Aitken type B PFFD, adductor brevis is smaller than normal and oriented more perpendicular to the femur than is typical. In Aitken type D PFFD, adductor brevis inserts onto the distal femoral remnant.

Prevalence

N/A

Clinical Implications

N/A

ADDUCTOR MAGNUS (FIGURE 5.4)

Synonyms

The portion of adductor magnus that extends between the pubic ramus and the gluteal tuberosity may be referred to as adductor minimus, adductor quartus (Macalister 1875; Knott 1883a; Standring 2016; du Plessis and Loukas 2016), pars lateralis, caput superius externum, or premier faisceau du grand adducteur (Tubbs et al. 2011).

Typical Presentation

Description

Adductor magnus originates from the inferior pubic ramus, ischial ramus, and the ischial tuberosity (Standring 2016). The fibers that originate from the pubic ramus insert onto the gluteal tuberosity of the femur (Standring 2016). The fibers that originate from the ischial ramus have an aponeurotic insertion onto the linea aspera and medial supracondylar line (Standring 2016). The fibers that originate from the ischial tuberosity insert via a tendon onto the adductor tubercle on the medial condyle of the femur (Standring 2016).

Innervation

Adductor magnus is innervated by both the obturator nerve and the tibial division of the sciatic nerve (Standring 2016).

Comparative Anatomy

Adductor magnus has a similar typical presentation in the apes, originating from the inferior pubic ramus, ischial ramus, and ischial tuberosity and inserting onto the medial lip of the linea aspera and the adductor tubercle (Champneys 1872; Hepburn 1892; Beddard 1893; Sonntag 1924; Raven 1950; Miller 1952; Sigmon 1974; Gibbs 1999; Diogo et al. 2010, 2012, 2013a,b, 2017). In gibbons, it is often divided into two parts distally (Sigmon 1974; Diogo et al. 2012),

and in orangutans, it may be divided proximally (Ferrero 2011; Ferrero et al. 2012; Diogo et al. 2013b). Adductor minimus is only present as a distinct muscle in about two-thirds of great apes (Hepburn 1892; Sigmon 1974; Gibbs 1999; Diogo et al. 2013, 2013b, 2017). In gibbons, adductor minimus is usually absent or not distinct from the other adductors (Hepburn 1892; Sigmon 1974; Diogo et al. 2012).

Variations

Description

The portion of the muscle referred to as adductor minimus can be variably separated from the rest of the muscle (Macalister 1875; Mori 1964; Tubbs et al. 2011). The portion of adductor magnus that extends between the ischial tuberosity and the medial condyle of the femur is also variably separated from the rest of the muscle (Macalister 1975; Knott 1883b; du Plessis and Loukas 2016; Standring 2016). Adductor magnus may fuse with quadratus femoris, adductor brevis, and/or adductor longus (Macalister 1875; Mori 1964; Bergman et al. 1988; du Plessis and Loukas 2016). There may be accessory slips of adductor magnus that originate from the linea aspera and insert into the adductor magnus tendon and the adductor tubercle (Macalister 1875; Hildebrand 1978; Bergman et al. 1988; Tubbs and Zehren 2006; du Plessis and Loukas 2016).

Prevalence

Knott (1883b) found that the portion of adductor magnus that inserts onto the medial condyle of the femur was completely separate from the rest of the muscle in 1 out of 40 cases (2.5%).

Mori (1964) categorized the fusion of the adductors into eight types. All three adductors fused near their origins in 4% of cases, only adductor longus and adductor brevis fused near their origins in 4% of cases, all three adductors fused near their insertions in 8% of cases, only adductor longus and adductor magnus fused near their insertions in 38% of cases, only adductor brevis and adductor magnus fused near their insertions in 6% of cases, adductor brevis was completely fused with adductor magnus in 8% of cases, adductor magnus fused completely with adductor minimus in 8% of cases, and there was no fusion between any of the adductors in 14% of cases. Adductor magnus was divided into three portions in 70% of cases and divided into two portions in 20% of cases.

Tubbs et al. (2011) studied adductor minimus on 40 sides from 20 adult cadavers and in five fetuses. Adductor minimus was distinct from adductor magnus on 21 sides (52.5%) in the adults. Five out of these 21 sides (24%) had partial fusion to adductor magnus. Adductor minimus was distinct from adductor magnus on all sides of the fetuses (100%).

Anomalies

Description

On the right lower limb of a fetus with craniorachischisis dissected by Alghamdi et al. (2017), some fibers of adductor magnus fused with adductor longus. Bersu et al. (1976) describe a male infant with Hanhart syndrome. The femora of this infant were normally developed but distal secondary ossification centers were absent. The left leg stump had a patella and a small rudiment of the proximal tibia but no fibular rudiment. The right leg stump was less developed and had a patella, smaller tibial rudiment, and no fibular rudiment. On the left side, the inferior bundle of adductor magnus originated from the ischial tuberosity, along with semitendinosus and biceps femoris, and inserted onto the junction of the middle and lower thirds of the linea aspera just above the adductor tubercle. Pirani et al. (1991) describe soft tissue anatomy associated with cases of proximal femoral focal deficiency (PFFD). In Aitken type B PFFD, adductor magnus is oriented more perpendicular to the femur than is typical. In Aitken type D PFFD, adductor magnus inserts onto the distal femoral remnant.

Prevalence

N/A

Clinical Implications

Accessory slips of adductor magnus may compress the proximal popliteal vein and cause an aneurysm (Tubbs and Zehren 2006; du Plessis and Loukas 2016).

PECTINEUS (FIGURE 5.4)

Synonyms

N/A

Typical Presentation

Description

Pectineus originates from the pecten pubis (Standring 2016). It inserts onto the femur between the lesser trochanter and the linea aspera (Standring 2016).

Innervation

Pectineus is typically innervated by the femoral nerve (Standring 2016). It may also be innervated by the accessory obturator nerve, when present, and sometimes from a branch of the obturator nerve (Standring 2016). If divided into two parts or layers, the deep layer (also referred to as dorsal or medial) is innervated by the obturator nerve, and the superficial layer (also referred to as ventral or lateral) is innervated by the femoral nerve (Ochiltree 1912; Bergman et al. 1988; Standring 2016; du Plessis and Loukas 2016).

Comparative Anatomy

Pectineus has a similar typical presentation in the apes, extending from the pubis and/or superior pubic ramus to the femur just below the lesser trochanter (Champneys 1872; Hepburn 1892; Beddard 1893; Sonntag 1924; Raven 1950; Miller 1952; Sigmon 1974; Gibbs 1999; Diogo et al. 2010, 2012, 2013a,b, 2017). It may be fused with adductor longus

in orangutans (Sigmon 1974) or bonobos (Miller 1952). It is divided into two layers/parts in common chimpanzees (Macalister 1871; Gibbs 1999), and also in some gorillas, according to Ochiltree (1912).

Variations

Description

Pectineus may be divided into two layers or parts (Macalister 1875; Knott 1883b; Ochiltree 1912; Bergman et al. 1988; du Plessis and Loukas 2016; Standring 2016). It may receive fibers from adductor longus (Macalister 1875; Bergman et al. 1988). Its origin may be connected with the origin of adductor brevis (Ochiltree 1912). Accessory bundles may connect pectineus with obturator externus, iliacus, the hip joint capsule, or the lesser trochanter (Macalister 1875; Knott 1883b; Bergman et al. 1988; du Plessis and Loukas 2016; Standring 2016). Upasna et al. (2013) describe bilateral variations in the lower limbs of a female cadaver. Adductor longus and pectineus had a combined origin from the pecten pubis, and an adductor brevis was divided in two and had distal fibers that merged with those of adductor longus. These variations were associated with bilateral accessory slips located under adductor brevis.

Prevalence

Knott (1883b) found that pectineus was divided into two parts in 1 out of 40 specimens (2.5%).

Anomalies

Description

Bersu et al. (1976) describe a male infant with Hanhart syndrome. The femora of this infant were normally developed but distal secondary ossification centers were absent. The left leg stump had a patella and a small rudiment of the proximal tibia but no fibular rudiment. The right leg stump was less developed and had a patella, smaller tibial rudiment, and no fibular rudiment. On the right side, the origin of pectineus was shifted medially, and it inserted via a tendon onto the middle third of the linea aspera in close association with adductor brevis and longus. Pirani et al. (1991) describe soft tissue anatomy associated with cases of proximal femoral focal deficiency (PFFD). In Aitken type B PFFD, pectineus is smaller than is typical. In Aitken type D PFFD, pectineus inserts onto the proximal femoral ossicle.

Prevalence

N/A

Clinical Implications

N/A

SEMITENDINOSUS (FIGURE 5.5)

Synonyms

N/A

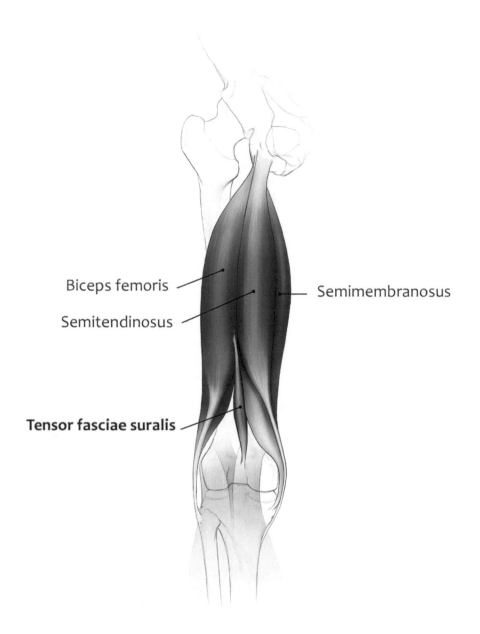

Biceps femoris

Semimembranosus

Semitendinosus

Tensor fasciae suralis

FIGURE 5.5   Posterior thigh muscles in posterior view.

Typical Presentation

Description

Semitendinosus is one of the three hamstring muscles (Standring 2016). It originates via a tendon from the ischial tuberosity (Standring 2016). Its tendon inserts onto the medial aspect of the proximal tibia (Standring 2016). It joins with the tendon of gracilis upon insertion and has an expansion to the deep fascia of the leg and the medial head of gastrocnemius (Standring 2016).

Innervation

Semitendinosus is innervated by the tibial division of the sciatic nerve (Standring 2016).

Comparative Anatomy

Semitendinosus has a similar typical presentation in the apes, originating from the ischial tuberosity with biceps femoris and inserting via a narrow tendon onto the medial tibia (Champneys 1872; Hepburn 1892; Beddard 1893; Sonntag 1924; Raven 1950; Miller 1952; Sigmon 1974; Gibbs 1999; Diogo et al. 2010, 2012, 2013a,b, 2017). A tendinous intersection in the muscle is sometimes present in all apes except gorillas (Macalister 1871; Hepburn 1892; Gibbs 1999). The common origin may include semimembranosus in common chimpanzees, bonobos, and orangutans (Champneys 1872; Hepburn 1892; Beddard 1893; Sonntag 1924; Sigmon 1974; Gibbs 1999; Diogo et al. 2017). The insertion is more distal onto the tibia in common chimpanzees, bonobos, orangutans, and gibbons than in gorillas and humans (Champneys 1872; Hepburn 1892; Gibbs 1999).

Variations

Description

A tendinous inscription is often present near the midpoint of the muscle (du Plessis and Loukas 2016; Standring 2016), and it may be reduced or doubled (Macalister 1875; Knott 1883b). Semitendinosus may be completely separated from biceps femoris (Macalister 1875; Bergman et al. 1988; du Plessis and Loukas 2016). Semitendinosus may receive a slip from the long head of biceps femoris (Bergman et al. 1988; Chakravarthi 2013; du Plessis and Loukas 2016; Standring 2016; Hoban et al. 2019). It may be partially fused with semimembranosus (Bergman et al. 1988; du Plessis and Loukas 2016). It may have an origin from the sacrotuberous ligament (Bergman et al. 1988; du Plessis and Loukas 2016). Accessory slips of semitendinosus may also originate from the sacrotuberous ligament, coccyx, or ischial tuberosity (Bergman et al. 1988; Chakravarthi 2013; Fraser et al. 2013; du Plessis and Loukas 2016).

Gray (1945) reports two cases of semitendinosus variations. In one case, the three hamstring muscles originated from a common tendon that had a superior attachment to the sacrotuberous ligament and fascial sheath of piriformis. The tendon received slips from quadratus femoris, the ischium, and the femur and gave rise to the muscle bellies of the hamstrings at mid-thigh. In the second case, bilateral supernumerary muscles arose from the linea aspera between the short head of biceps femoris and adductor magnus and inserted onto the dorsal aspect of the capsule of the knee joint and into the fascia covering the medial head of gastrocnemius (Gray 1945). Gray (1945) suggests that these bilateral supernumerary muscles should be regarded as femoral heads of semitendinosus.

Paraskevas et al. (2010) report a supernumerary semitendinosus muscle that originated from the lateral lip of the linea aspera between adductor magnus and the short head of biceps femoris and inserted onto the medial tibial condyle. The distal portion of this muscle was covered by the long head of biceps femoris. These authors suggest that an anomaly during the 90° medial rotation of the lower limb bud between weeks 6 and 8 of gestation may have created the supernumerary muscle (Paraskevas et al. 2010).

Prevalence

N/A

Anomalies

Description

Pirani et al. (1991) describe soft tissue anatomy associated with cases of proximal femoral focal deficiency (PFFD). In Aitken type B PFFD, semitendinosus is smaller than normal. In infants with trisomy 18, Ramirez-Castro and Bersu (1978) found two types of accessory bellies associated with semitendinosus. One type originated between semitendinosus and the long head of biceps femoris and inserted onto the semitendinosus tendon. The second type originated from the sacrotuberous ligament and inserted onto the belly of semitendinosus near its origin (Ramirez-Castro and Bersu 1978; Smith et al. 2015).

Prevalence

In their literature review, Smith et al. (2015) found that the accessory belly between semitendinosus and the long head of biceps femoris was present in 3 out of 17 (17.6%) individuals with trisomy 18. An accessory belly between semitendinosus and the sacrotuberous ligament was present in 2 out of 17 (11.8%) individuals with trisomy 18.

Clinical Implications

Attachments of semitendinosus to biceps femoris and gastrocnemius may cause complications when surgically harvesting the semitendinosus tendon (Standring 2016). A supernumerary semitendinosus muscle may compress the sciatic nerve or popliteal artery (Paraskevas et al. 2010). Variation in the origins of the hamstring muscles may predispose individuals to strains and posterior thigh pain (Fraser et al. 2013). An origin of semitendinosus from the ischial tuberosity may predispose individuals to posterior thigh or pelvic floor pain (Fraser et al. 2013). A slip connecting biceps femoris and semitendinosus could compress the sciatic nerve, causing pain, or interfere with popliteal sciatic nerve block (Hoban et al. 2019). Accessory slips or muscles associated with semitendinosus may simulate soft-tissue tumors (Chakravarthi 2013).

SEMIMEMBRANOSUS (FIGURE 5.5)

Synonyms

N/A

Typical Presentation

Description

Semimembranosus is one of the three hamstring muscles (Standring 2016). It originates via a tendon from the ischial tuberosity (Standring 2016). Some fibers blend with biceps femoris and semitendinosus (Standring 2016). Its insertion tendon is divided into five parts (Standring 2016). The main part inserts onto a tubercle on the medial condyle of the tibia (Standring 2016). The other parts of the insertion go to the medial border of the tibia, the posterior side of the medial tibial condyle, the fascia over popliteus, the femoral intercondylar line, and lateral femoral condyle (Standring 2016).

Innervation

Semimembranosus is innervated by the tibial division of the sciatic nerve (Standring 2016).

Comparative Anatomy

Semimembranosus has a similar typical presentation in the apes, extending from the ischial tuberosity to the posterior surface of the medial tibial condyle, with some attachments to the fascia and ligaments of the knee (Champneys 1872; Hepburn 1892; Beddard 1893; Sonntag 1924; Raven 1950; Sigmon 1974; Gibbs 1999; Diogo et al. 2010, 2012, 2013a,b, 2017).

Variations

Description

Semimembranosus is variable in size and may be reduced or absent (Macalister 1875; Bergman et al. 1988; Moncayo et al. 2010; du Plessis and Loukas 2016; Standring 2016). When absent, it may be replaced by a tendon with a small central muscle belly (Macalister 1875). Liu et al. (2011) found that in one case, bilateral absence of semimembranosus was associated with bilateral absence of quadratus femoris. The absence of semimembranosus may also be associated with variations in the length and shape of the other hamstring muscles (Moncayo et al. 2010; Sussmann 2019).

Its proximal attachment may extend to the coccyx (Bergman et al. 1988). Its origin may be primarily from the sacrotuberous ligament in some cases (Macalister 1875). Slips from its insertion may be continuous with the arcuate ligament or end in the popliteal fat (Macalister 1875; Knott 1883b). The distal tendon may course along the tibial collateral ligament and insert more distally than normal (Moncayo et al. 2010). There may be a sixth insertion/tendinous expansion of semimembranosus onto the posterior horn of the lateral meniscus (Kim et al. 1997).

Semimembranosus may send a slip to adductor magnus or the femur (Standring 2016). It may have a slip continuous with quadratus femoris (Macalister 1875). It may be partially fused with semitendinosus (Bergman et al. 1988; du Plessis and Loukas 2016). Gray (1945) reports a case in which the three hamstring muscles originated by a common tendon that had a superior attachment to the sacrotuberous ligament and fascial sheath of piriformis. The tendon received slips from quadratus femoris, the ischium, and the femur. The tendon gave rise to the muscle bellies of the hamstrings at mid-thigh.

Semimembranosus may also be doubled or divided longitudinally (Bergman et al. 1988; du Plessis and Loukas 2016; Standring 2016). The division may be confined to the tendon of origin in some cases (Knott 1883b). When doubled, the accessory belly may present as a fleshy slip with proximal and distal tendons or may arise from the sacrotuberous ligament (Bergman et al. 1988; du Plessis and Loukas 2016). The distal tendon of the accessory belly can have a variable attachment (Bergman et al. 1988; du Plessis and Loukas 2016). Semimembranosus can be comprised of up to four bellies (Bergman et al. 1988; du Plessis and Loukas 2016).

Prevalence

Kim et al. (1997) found a tendinous insertion of semimembranosus onto the posterior horn of the lateral meniscus in 16 out of 37 knees (43.2%).

Anomalies

Description

Bersu et al. (1976) describe a male infant with Hanhart syndrome. The femora of this infant were normally developed but distal secondary ossification centers were absent. The left leg stump had a patella and a small rudiment of the proximal tibia but no fibular rudiment. The right leg stump was less developed and had a patella, smaller tibial rudiment, and no fibular rudiment. Semimembranosus was absent bilaterally. Pettersen et al. (1979) found extra slips of semimembranosus in two neonates with trisomy 13. In one case, the slip was on the right side and originated from the ischial tuberosity anterior to the origin of the normal semimembranosus, and its fibers fused with the main muscle at midthigh. On the left side of the second case, the accessory slip ran along the length of the normal semimembranosus and the two fused upon insertion. On the right side of the second case, the accessory slip was fused anterior to the main muscle. Pirani et al. (1991) describe soft tissue anatomy associated with cases of proximal femoral focal deficiency (PFFD). In Aitken type B PFFD, semimembranosus is smaller than normal.

Prevalence

In their literature review, Smith et al. (2015) found that extra slips of semimembranosus were present in 2 out of 20 individuals (10%) with trisomy 13. An extra slip between the hamstrings was found in 1 out of 17 individuals with trisomy 18 (5.9%).

Clinical Implications

Liu et al. (2011) suggest that the absence of semimembranosus may present as muscle weakness of knee flexion or hypermobility of the posteromedial knee joint. Variation in the origins of the hamstring muscles may predispose individuals to strains and posterior thigh pain (Fraser et al. 2013). Accessory semimembranosus bellies may become entrapped by the semitendinosus tendon and cause pain (Zeren et al. 2009). A tendon attachment to the lateral meniscus may be misdiagnosed as a lateral meniscus tear (Kim et al. 1997).

BICEPS FEMORIS (FIGURE 5.5)

See also: Tenuissimus, Tensor fasciae suralis

Synonyms

This muscle may also be referred to as biceps flexor cruris (Macalister 1875; Knott 1883a,b).

Typical Presentation

Description

Biceps femoris is one of the three hamstring muscles (Standring 2016). The long head originates by a tendon from the ischial tuberosity and from the sacrotuberous ligament (Standring 2016). The short head originates from the linea aspera (Standring 2016). Biceps femoris inserts mainly onto the head of the fibula (Standring 2016). There are additional insertions onto the fibular collateral ligament and lateral tibial condyle (Standring 2016).

Innervation

The long head of biceps femoris is innervated by the tibial division of the sciatic nerve, and the short head is innerved by the common fibular division of the sciatic nerve (Standring 2016).

Comparative Anatomy

Biceps femoris has a similar typical presentation in the apes. The long head originates with semitendinosus from the ischial tuberosity and the short head from the lateral lip of the linea aspera and the intermuscular septum. The long head inserts into the tibial head, lateral tibial condyle, fibular head, iliotibial tract, knee joint capsule, and fascia of the leg while the short head inserts into the fibular head and fascia of the leg (Champneys 1872; Hepburn 1892; Beddard 1893; Sonntag 1924; Raven 1950; Miller 1952; Sigmon 1974; Gibbs 1999; Diogo et al. 2010, 2012, 2013a,b, 2017). The short and long heads are fused in most cases (Hepburn 1892; Sigmon 1974; Gibbs 1999). The origin of the short head extends more distally in great apes than in gibbons or humans (Sigmon 1974). Accessory bellies have been noted in common chimpanzees and bonobos (Diogo et al. 2013a, 2017).

Variations

Description

The short head is sometimes absent (Macalister 1875; Knott 1883a,b; Bergman et al. 1988; du Plessis and Loukas 2016; Standring 2016). The short head may also split into multiple fasciculi (Macalister 1875). The long head and short head can be partially or completely separated (Mori 1964; Bergman et al. 1988; du Plessis and Loukas 2016) and may only unite at their insertion (Macalister 1875; Chakravarthi 2013). The two heads may insert separately (Macalister 1875). Biceps femoris may have a more prominent attachment onto the proximal tibia (Macalister 1875; Knott 1883b; Date et al. 2012; du Plessis and Loukas 2016). It may also not have a fibular insertion and attach entirely onto the proximal tibia (Kristensen et al. 1989; Hernandez et al. 1996).

The long head of biceps femoris may send a slip to semitendinosus (Bergman et al. 1988; Chakravarthi 2013; du Plessis and Loukas 2016; Standring 2016; Hoban et al. 2019). Accessory slips or a third head of biceps femoris originate most commonly from the ischial tuberosity, but may also arise from the coccyx, sacrum, sacrotuberous ligament, gluteus maximus, linea aspera, gluteal tuberosity, fascia lata, adductor magnus, vastus lateralis, gastrocnemius, medial supracondylar line, or the lateral condyle of the femur (Macalister 1875; Knott 1883b; Bergman et al. 1988; du Plessis and Loukas 2016; Standring 2016).

There may be a crural extension of biceps femoris, accessory muscle tensor fasciae suralis, that presents as a slip to the fascia of the leg, the Achilles tendon, and/or gastrocnemius (Knott 1883b; Bergman et al. 1988; du Plessis and

Loukas 2016). See the entry for tensor fasciae suralis for more details. An accessory digastric muscle can also present with a superior belly arising from or near piriformis, continuing down the thigh as a long intermediate tendon, and connecting to an inferior belly that is closely associated with biceps femoris (Moore 1922; Suda and Takahashi 1957; Akita et al. 1992; Nicholson et al. 2016). Tenuissimus, another supernumerary muscle, originates from the fascia on the deep surface of gluteus maximus and often inserts at the junction of the short and long head of biceps femoris (see the entry for this muscle) (Green 1931).

Prevalence

Mori (1964) found that the muscle of the long head of biceps femoris was completely isolated from the muscle of the short head in 30% of cases. The insertion tendon of the long head fused with the muscle of the short head in 70% of cases.

Anomalies

Description

Bersu et al. (1976) describe a male infant with Hanhart syndrome. The femora of this infant were normally developed, but distal secondary ossification centers were absent. The left leg stump had a patella and a small rudiment of the proximal tibia but no fibular rudiment. The right leg stump was less developed and had a patella, smaller tibial rudiment, and no fibular rudiment. On both sides, the long head of biceps femoris inserted onto the lateral surface of the tibia. The short head of the biceps was absent on the right side. On the left side, it inserted into the posterior surface of the knee capsule and the lateral surface of the tibia, independently of the long head. On the right side, an accessory slip originated from the medial portion of the belly of the long head and inserted posterior to the insertion of the main tendon.

In infants with trisomy 18, Ramirez-Castro and Bersu (1978) found two types of accessory bellies associated with semitendinosus. One type originated between semitendinosus and the long head of biceps femoris and inserted onto the semitendinosus tendon (Ramirez-Castro and Bersu 1978; Smith et al. 2015). Pettersen et al. (1979) found an extra belly of the long head (third head) of biceps femoris running lateral to the normal long head in one neonate with trisomy 13. This accessory belly inserted via a tendon onto the short head. Pirani et al. (1991) describe soft tissue anatomy associated with cases of proximal femoral focal deficiency (PFFD). In Aitken type B PFFD, biceps femoris is smaller than normal.

Prevalence

In their literature review, Smith et al. (2015) found that an extra belly of biceps femoris was present in 1 out of 20 individuals (5%) with trisomy 13 (case described by Pettersen et al. 1979). An extra slip between the hamstrings was found in 1 out of 17 individuals with trisomy 18 (5.9%). Smith et al. (2015) also found that the accessory belly between semitendinosus and the long head of biceps femoris was present in 3 out of 17 (17.6%) individuals with trisomy 18.

Clinical Implications

Variation in the origins of the hamstring muscles may predispose individuals to strains and posterior thigh pain (Fraser et al. 2013). An anomalous insertion of the biceps femoris tendon may cause pain and snapping at the knee (Kristensen et al. 1989; Hernandez et al. 1996; Date et al. 2012). A slip connecting biceps femoris and semitendinosus could compress the sciatic nerve, causing pain, or interfere with popliteal sciatic nerve block (Hoban et al. 2019). Accessory bellies of biceps femoris may compress the common fibular nerve and cause foot drop (Kaplan et al. 2008). Accessory slips or muscles associated with biceps femoris may simulate soft-tissue tumors (Chakravarthi 2013).

TENSOR FASCIAE SURALIS (FIGURE 5.5)

See also: Semitendinosus, Biceps femoris, Gastrocnemius

Synonyms

This muscle may also be referred to as ischioaponeuroticus (Bergman et al. 1988). George et al. (2019) propose femeroaponeuroticus for the variant of tensor fasciae suralis described in their study.

Typical Presentation

This muscle is only present as a variation.

Comparative Anatomy

Martinoli et al. (2010) suggest that tensor fasciae suralis may represent a vestigial extension of the hamstrings, as hamstring insertion in some mammals extends more distally to facilitate permanent flexion of the knee.

Variations

Description

When present, tensor fasciae suralis originates from the long head of biceps femoris, occasionally originating from semitendinosus (Kelch 1813; Gruber 1873c, 1879; Knott 1883b; Turner 1884–1885; Barry and Bothroyd 1924; Bergman et al. 1988; Tubbs et al. 2006e; du Plessis and Loukas 2016; Bale and Herrin 2017). It may also originate from a tendon that is continuous with the biceps femoris tendon (Schaeffer 1913). George et al. (2019) report an origin from the lowermost portion of the linea aspera, arising with the fibers of the short head of biceps femoris.

It can also arise via two tendons. Miyauchi et al. (1985) and Somayaji et al. (1998) describe cases in which one tendon arose from semitendinosus and the other from the long head of biceps femoris (Miyauchi et al. 1985). Barry and Bothroyd (1924) also report an origin via two fascial slips, one from the fascia lata at the point of divergence of the biceps femoris and semitendinosus, and the other from the fascia covering the medial and deep surfaces of biceps femoris. Gupta and Bhagwat (2006) report a case in which tensor fasciae suralis originated via two slips, one from semitendinosus and the other from biceps femoris, and gave

rise to a third head of gastrocnemius that inserted into the junction of the two heads of gastrocnemius.

Tensor fasciae suralis ends in a tendon that joins the crural fascia of the lower leg over the gastrocnemius muscle (Knott 1883b; Schaeffer 1913; Barry and Bothroyd 1924; Miyauchi et al. 1985; Bergman et al. 1988; Tubbs et al. 2006e; du Plessis and Loukas 2016; Arakawa et al. 2017; Bale and Herrin 2017; George et al. 2019). Its insertion may also pass distally between the two heads of gastrocnemius and join with the Achilles tendon (Kelch 1813; Gruber 1873c, 1879; Halliburton 1881; Turner 1884–1885; Somayaji et al. 1998).

Tensor fasciae suralis may be digastric (Halliburton 1881; Gruber 1879; Arakawa et al. 2017). Gruber (1879) describes a bilateral case. On the right side, the superior belly originated from the long head of the biceps and ended in a tendon in the popliteal fossa. Across from the intercondylar space, the tendon gave rise to the inferior belly which coursed through the groove between the heads of gastrocnemius and inserted into the Achilles tendon. On the left side, the muscle was similar, but the superior belly received a tendinous bundle from the tendinous inscription of semitendinosus.

Halliburton (1881) describes a similar case in which the superior belly of a supernumerary muscle arose from the long head of biceps femoris. At the top of the popliteal space, it gave rise to a tendon that flattened into an aponeurosis and attached to the fibular head. The inferior belly originated from the tendon where it expanded into the aponeurotic slip and was situated in the groove between the two heads of gastrocnemius. The inferior belly ended in a tendon that inserted into gastrocnemius just below the union of the two heads. Its tendinous fibers ultimately continued into the Achilles tendon.

Arakawa et al. (2017) describe a case in which they conclude that tenuissimus, tensor fasciae suralis, and two other supernumerary muscles are present on the posterior right thigh of a cadaver. Tenuissimus passed between the long and short heads of biceps femoris and fused with the tensor fasciae suralis. Tensor fasciae suralis was digastric with a superior belly that arose from the medial surface of the long head of biceps femoris in the distal third of the muscle. The superior head ended in an aponeurosis, which rotated about 90° and gave rise to the inferior belly that fused with the posterior surface of the crural fascia that covered the lateral head of gastrocnemius.

There may be accessory muscles in the popliteal fossa that could be variants of tensor fasciae suralis or derivatives of nearby muscles (Okamoto et al. 2004; Kim et al. 2009b; Kim et al. 2014). Okamoto et al. (2004) describe a case in which a flat, rectangular muscle extended transversely between the lateral border of the medial head of gastrocnemius and the tendon of biceps femoris, covering the structures in the popliteal fossa. As it was innervated by the common fibular nerve, Okamoto et al. (2004) suggest that it may be derived from the short head of biceps femoris. These authors also note a similar case described by Parsons (1919–1920), who suggested the muscle was the conversion of the popliteal fascia to fleshy fibers.

Kim et al. (2009b) describe a remarkably similar muscle with innervation from the lateral sural cutaneous nerve. Kim et al. (2014) describe another similar case in which the flat transverse muscle was innervated by the tibial nerve. The authors regard it as a third head of gastrocnemius (gastrocnemius tertius) (Kim et al. 2014).

Innervation

Tensor fasciae suralis is typically innervated by a branch from the tibial nerve (Schaeffer 1913; Barry and Bothroyd 1924; Somayaji et al. 1998; Tubbs et al. 2006e; Arakawa et al. 2017). George et al. (2019) found innervation from the common fibular nerve.

Prevalence

Somayaji et al. (1998) found only one case of tensor fasciae suralis out of 300 lower limbs (0.3%) from 150 cadavers compiled from 15 years of dissection. In a study of 236 lower limbs, Bale and Herrin (2019) found three cases of tensor fasciae suralis (1.3%).

Anomalies

N/A

Clinical Implications

Tensor fasciae suralis may appear as a mass or swelling in the popliteal fossa (Montet et al. 2002). As this muscle crosses the popliteal fossa, it may compress the popliteal vein (Somayaji et al. 1998) and/or other neurovascular structures in the fossa. George et al. (2019) describe a laterally displaced variant of tensor fasciae suralis and suggest that its placement may cause compression neuropathy to the common fibular nerve and lateral sural cutaneous nerve.

POSTERIOR MUSCLES OF THE LOWER LEG

GASTROCNEMIUS (FIGURE 5.6)

See also: Tensor fasciae suralis

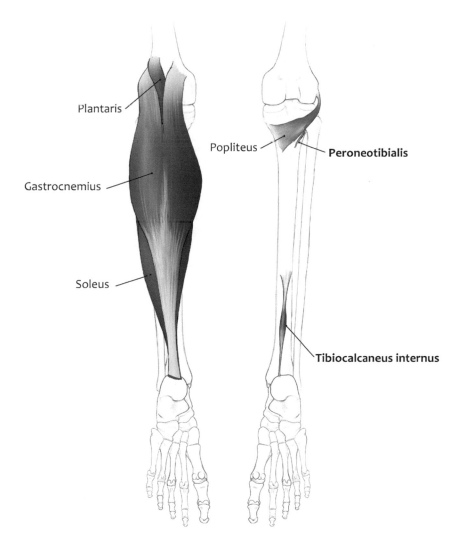

FIGURE 5.6 Superficial muscles of the posterior lower leg in posterior view. The muscles that are typically present are illustrated on the left side. Popliteus and two variations are illustrated on the right side.

Synonyms

N/A

Typical Presentation

Description

The medial head of gastrocnemius originates from the posterior aspect of the medial condyle of the femur and from the popliteal surface (Standring 2016). The lateral head originates from the lateral surface of the lateral femoral condyle (Standring 2016). Fibers from both heads also arise from the knee joint capsule (Standring 2016). Gastrocnemius joins with the tendon of the soleus to form the calcaneal (Achilles) tendon, which inserts onto the calcaneus (Standring 2016).

Innervation

Gastrocnemius is innervated by the tibial nerve (Standring 2016).

Comparative Anatomy

Gastrocnemius in the apes is not as enlarged as it is in humans, but it similarly originates via two heads from the medial and lateral femoral condyles and the knee joint capsule and inserts with soleus into the calcaneus (Hepburn 1892; Beddard 1893; Frey 1913; Sonntag 1924; Raven 1950; Miller 1952; Gibbs 1999; Diogo et al. 2010, 2012, 2013a,b, 2017). Sesamoid bones are present in both heads in gibbons (Hepburn 1892; Frey 1913; Gibbs 1999). The calcaneal tendon is more defined in gibbons and orangutans than in the other apes (Diogo et al. 2012, 2013a,b, 2017).

Variations

Description

The lateral head or the entire muscle may be absent (Bergman et al. 1988; Lambert 2016; Standring 2016). The lateral head may also be reduced and replaced by a fibrous cord (Macalister 1875; Bergman et al. 1988; Lambert 2016). The lateral head may have origins from the lateral collateral ligament or the posterior oblique ligament of the knee (Macalister 1875; Knott 1883b). The medial head may originate higher than usual, from the medial supracondylar line (Stuart 1879). Small accessory slips may be present near the origin of either head (Takase et al. 1997; Liu et al. 2005; Rochier and Sumpio 2009). The length of the gastrocnemius aponeurosis and the extent of its attachments to soleus vary (Blitz and Eliot 2007). The two heads may remain separate until their insertion onto the calcaneus or remain separate from soleus and its tendon (Macalister 1875; Le Double 1897; Bergman et al. 1988; Lambert 2016). A sesamoid bone may be found in either head (Macalister 1875; Mori 1964). The whole muscle may be bilaminar (Macalister 1875; Le Double 1897).

One or both heads may be doubled (Bergman et al. 1988; Ashaolu et al. 2014). Ashaolu et al. (2014) found numerous cases of a "four-headed" gastrocnemius that included the normal medial and lateral heads and smaller intermedio-medial and intermedio-lateral heads. Rodrigues et al. (2016) report a case in which the medial and lateral heads each arose via three bundles from their normal points of origin, giving the appearance of a six-headed muscle. The bundles remained separate until they merged to form the calcaneal tendon.

A third head of gastrocnemius—gastrocnemius tertius—may originate from the popliteal surface of the femur (Macalister 1875; Knott 1883a,b; Iwai et al. 1987; Bergman et al. 1988, 1995; Koplas et al. 2009; Dave et al. 2012; Lambert 2016; Standring 2016). The third head may also originate from the long head or tendon of biceps femoris, the capsule of the knee joint, the crural fascia, the fibula, linea aspera, either supracondylar line, or the lateral epicondyle of the femur (Macalister 1875; Knott 1883b; Le Double 1897; Frey 1919; Mori 1964; Bergman et al. 1988, 1995; Lambert 2016). It may insert into one or both heads of gastrocnemius, or at the junction of these heads (Frey 1919; Mori 1964; Iwai et al. 1987; Bergman et al. 1995; Koplas et al. 2009; Yildirim et al. 2011; Dave et al. 2012; Lambert 2016). Plantaris can present as a third head of gastrocnemius and may blend with the two heads at their junction, merge with only one head, or join the fascia on the deep surface of gastrocnemius (Bergman et al. 1988).

Yildirim et al. (2011) describe a cadaver with bilateral gastrocnemius tertius and a unilateral accessory soleus muscle. On the right side, gastrocnemius tertius originated from the lateral condyle of the femur and inserted onto the medial head of gastrocnemius. On the left, gastrocnemius tertius had two bellies. The deep belly originated from the tendon of plantaris and the superficial belly from just above this tendon. The deep belly inserted onto the inner surface of the medial head of gastrocnemius, and the superficial belly inserted onto the external surface of the lateral head.

Gastrocnemius is associated with accessory muscle tensor fasciae suralis (see the entry for this muscle), which typically extends between the hamstrings and gastrocnemius, the fascia over gastrocnemius, or the Achilles tendon. Given the anatomical similarities between tensor fasciae suralis and gastrocnemius tertius, some authors may designate muscles described as tensor fasciae suralis as the third head of gastrocnemius (Lambert 2016). Gupta and Bhagwat (2006) report a case in which tensor fasciae suralis originated via two slips, one from semitendinosus and the other from biceps femoris, and gave rise to a third head of gastrocnemius that inserted into the junction of the two heads of gastrocnemius.

Okamoto et al. (2004) describe a case in which a flat, rectangular muscle extended transversely between the lateral border of the medial head of gastrocnemius and the tendon of biceps femoris, covering the structures in the popliteal fossa. As it was innervated by the common fibular nerve, Okamoto et al. (2004) suggest that it may be derived from the short head of biceps femoris. These authors also note a similar case described by Parsons (1919–1920), who suggested the muscle was the conversion of the popliteal fascia to fleshy fibers. Kim et al. (2009b) describe a remarkably similar muscle with innervation from the lateral sural cutaneous nerve. Kim et al. (2014) also describe another similar case in which the flat transverse muscle was innervated by the tibial nerve. The authors regard it as a third head of gastrocnemius (Kim et al. 2014).

Prevalence

In a sample of 50 legs, Mori (1964) found a sesamoid bone in the lateral head of gastrocnemius in 14 cases (28%). Mori (1964) also found a third head of gastrocnemius, extending between the capsule of the knee joint and the medial or lateral head in 2.8% of cases. There was muscular fusion between gastrocnemius and soleus in 22 cases (44%) and tendinous fusion between the two muscles in 28 cases (56%). Soleus received a small bundle from the lateral head of gastrocnemius in 2.5% of cases (Mori 1964).

Blitz and Eliot (2007) examined the gastrocnemius aponeurosis in 53 cadaveric specimens. A long aponeurosis was found in 28 specimens (53%), a short aponeurosis was found in five specimens (9%), and direct attachments were found between the deep surface of one of the gastrocnemius heads and soleus in 20 specimens (38%). In an MRI study of 1,039 knees, Koplas et al. (2009) observed a third head of the gastrocnemius arising from the midline of the popliteal surface of the femur in 21 knees (2%). Of these, 20 cases (1.9%) joined the medial aspect of the lateral head and one (0.1%) joined the medial head. Two accessory heads of gastrocnemius were present in one case (0.1%). Ashaolu et al. (2014) studied gastrocnemius in 60 legs from 30 Nigerian cadavers. Typical two-headed gastrocnemius muscles were found in 21 legs (35%). Three-headed gastrocnemius muscles were found in eight legs (13.3%). Four-headed gastrocnemius muscles were found in 31 legs (51.7%).

Anomalies

Description

Bersu et al. (1976) describe a male infant with Hanhart syndrome. The femora of this infant were normally developed, but distal secondary ossification centers were absent. The left leg stump had a patella and a small rudiment of the proximal tibia but no fibular rudiment. The right leg stump was less developed and had a patella, smaller tibial rudiment, and no fibular rudiment. There were no muscle masses suggestive of gastrocnemius at the knee.

In one neonate with trisomy 13, Pettersen et al. (1979) found extra slips of gastrocnemius bilaterally. On the right side, accessory slips originated from the medial and lateral epicondyles of the femur and attached to the normal lateral head of gastrocnemius. On the left side, the extra slip was associated with the lateral head. Mieden (1982) describes two male fetuses with cyclopia and alobar holoprosencephaly. On the left side of one specimen, the medial head of gastrocnemius was split into two heads. In one fetus with trisomy 18 and cyclopia, Smith et al. (2015) found that gastrocnemius and soleus on the right side of the body were fused toward their insertion into the Achilles tendon, while the two muscles on the left side were fused along the majority of their length.

Prevalence

In their literature review, Smith et al. (2015) found that an extra slip of gastrocnemius was present in 1 out of 20 neonates with trisomy 13 (5%).

Clinical Implications

A high origin of the medial head of gastrocnemius was associated with an abnormal course and aneurysm of the popliteal artery in a case described by Stuart (1879). Accessory slips of the medial or lateral head of gastrocnemius may lead to popliteal vascular entrapment syndrome (Takase et al. 1997; Liu et al. 2005; Rochier and Sumpio 2009; Sirasanagandla et al. 2013a). If the third head of gastrocnemius extends across the popliteal fossa, it may compress or entrap the neurovascular structures in this area and impact nerve function and/or cause intermittent claudication, venous stasis, arterial stasis, aneurysms, or thromboembolism (Hamming 1959; Iwai et al. 1987; Bergman et al. 1995; Koplas et al. 2009; Yildirim et al. 2011; Sirasanagandla et al. 2013a; Lambert 2016). Extra heads of gastrocnemius may also cause sural nerve entrapment (Rodrigues et al. 2016). Variation in the length of the gastrocnemius aponeurosis and its attachments to soleus must be considered when planning gastrocnemius recession (Blitz and Eliot 2007).

SOLEUS (FIGURE 5.6)

See also: Peroneotibialis

Synonyms

N/A

Typical Presentation

Description

Soleus originates from the head and the proximal shaft of the fibula (fibular head) and from the soleal line and the medial margin of the tibia (tibial head) (Standring 2016). It also takes origin from a fibrous band connecting the two bones, known as the tendinous arch of the soleus (Standring 2016). Soleus joins with the tendon of gastrocnemius to form the calcaneal (Achilles) tendon, which inserts onto the calcaneus (Standring 2016).

Innervation

Soleus is innervated by the tibial nerve (Standring 2016).

Comparative Anatomy

Soleus inserts into the calcaneus with gastrocnemius in all apes, but the tibial origin of this muscle is typically absent in gibbons, orangutans, and gorillas (Chapman 1878; Hepburn 1892; Beddard 1893; Raven 1950; Lewis 1962; Gibbs 1999; Ferrero 2011; Ferrero et al. 2012; Diogo et al. 2010, 2012, 2013b). The tibial head is sometimes present in common chimpanzees and bonobos (Champneys 1872; Hepburn 1892; Frey 1913; Miller 1952; Lewis 1962; Gibbs 1999; Diogo et al. 2013a, 2017). Accessory soleus muscles have been found in orangutans (Diogo et al. 2013b).

Variations

Description

The tibial head of soleus may be absent (Mori 1964; Bergman et al. 1988). The fibular head may be bilaminar (Macalister 1875; Knott 1883b). The entire soleus or one of the heads may be absent or doubled (Macalister 1875; Le Doublet 1897; Bergman et al. 1988; Lambert 2016). Soleus may remain separate from gastrocnemius and its tendon up to its insertion (Macalister 1875; Knott 1883b; Bergman et al. 1988; Lambert 2016). Soleus is also associated with several named accessory muscles. See the entry for peroneotibialis. Tensor fasciae plantaris or tibiotarsalis is a slip that originates from the soleal line below the attachment of soleus and inserts onto the plantar fascia (Wood 1864; Macalister 1875; Anderson 1880; Knott 1883b; Bergman et al. 1988; Lambert 2016).

Soleus accessorius or accessory soleus is typically found medially and distally in the ankle, often situated between the calcaneal tendon and the flexor tendons or distal tibia (Percy and Telep 1984; Bergman et al. 1988; Sekiya et al. 1994; Brodie et al. 1997; Standring 2016). It may originate from the soleal line, the proximal fibula, or from the deep surface of soleus (Gordon and Matheson 1973; Lorentzon and Wirrell 1987; Bergman et al. 1988; Sekiya et al. 1994; Yu and Resnick 1994; Yildirim et al. 2011; Lambert 2016). It may insert into the calcaneal tendon, upper or medial surfaces of the calcaneus, or tibial collateral ligament of the ankle (Gordon and Matheson 1973; Lorentzon and Wirrell 1987; Bergman et al. 1988; Sekiya et al. 1994; Yu and Resnick 1994; Brodie et al. 1997; Hatzantonis et al. 2011; Yildirim et al. 2011; Lambert 2016; Standring 2016).

Tibiocalcaneus internus (Figure 5.6) originates from medial crest of the tibia and from the soleal line and inserts onto the medial aspect of the calcaneus (Testut 1892; Hecker 1924; Sammarco and Conti 1994; Sookur et al. 2008; Lambert 2016). It also has an origin from the deep fascia of the leg (Sammarco and Conti 1994). While the accessory soleus muscle is superficial to the flexor retinaculum, tibiocalcaneus internus passes deep to the flexor retinaculum and superficial to neurovascular structures in the tarsal tunnel (Hecker 1924; Sookur et al. 2008; Lambert 2016).

Prevalence

In a study of 50 legs, Mori (1964) found that the tibial head of soleus was absent in seven cases (14%). The muscle fibers of soleus extended distal to the talocrural joint in two cases (4%). There was muscular fusion between gastrocnemius and soleus in 22 cases (44%) and tendinous fusion between the two muscles in 28 cases (56%). Soleus received a small bundle from the lateral head of gastrocnemius in 2.5% of cases (Mori 1964).

Luck et al. (2008) found 35 cases of accessory soleus muscles from 4,771 MRI examinations of the ankle (0.73%) over a 10-year duration from a sample of symptomatic adults. Hatzantonis et al. (2011) conducted a literature review and determined that the overall cadaveric prevalence of the accessory soleus muscle was 14 out of 689 cases, or around 2%. The prevalence was 2.4% in males and 2.1% in females. One hundred and fifteen cases of accessory soleus muscles were identified in the clinical literature, 64 of them were male patients (55.6%), 28 were female patients (24%), and 23 were unidentified (20.4%). These authors also found that the most common insertion was onto the medial aspect of the calcaneus via a separate tendon (26.1% of cases). A tendinous insertion into the calcaneal tendon was found in 3.5% of cases, and a fleshy attachment to the medial surface of the calcaneus was found in 4.3% of case. The remaining 66.1% of cases had unidentified attachment types. In their own dissections of 100 legs from 50 cadavers, accessory soleus was found in three legs (3%). In their own imaging study of 100 clinical patients, accessory soleus was found in three cases (3%) (Hatzantonis et al. 2011).

Anomalies

Description

Accessory soleus muscles are sometimes found in individuals with congenital clubfoot (talipes equinovarus) and may cause resistance to correction of this deformity (Sodre et al. 1994; Chotigavanichaya et al. 2000). In a male neonate with Meckel syndrome, Pettersen (1984) observed that soleus was fleshy distal to the usual site of tendon formation at the ankle. In a fetus with trisomy 18 and cyclopia, Smith et al. (2015) found that gastrocnemius and soleus on the right side of the body were fused toward their insertion into the Achilles tendon, while the two muscles on the left side were fused along the majority of their length.

Prevalence

Sodre et al. (1994) noted that accessory soleus muscles were found in 6 out of 72 patients with congenital club foot (8.3%). Porter (1996) reports that an "anomalous calf flexor muscle" (with a description corresponding to that of soleus accessorius) was present in 7 out of 125 feet of children with congenital clubfoot (5.6%).

Clinical Implications

Soleus accessorius becomes hypertrophic with physical activity and therefore often presents in athletes or active individuals as a soft mass in the medial ankle (Percy and Telep 1984; Nelimarkka et al. 1988; Yu and Resnick 1994; Brodie et al. 1997; Lambert 2016). The presence of this muscle may cause pain or swelling during exercise, potentially due to restricted blood supply to the muscle (Gordon and Matheson 1973; Percy and Telep 1984; Nelimarkka et al. 1988; Brodie et al. 1997; Lambert 2016). Symptomatic accessory soleus muscles may simulate retrocalcanear bursitis or peritendinitis of the Achilles tendon (Nelimarkka et al. 1988). Luck et al. (2008) report a high association between the presence of accessory soleus muscles and Achilles tendinopathy. Buschmann et al. (1991) found an association between accessory soleus muscles and pain and tenderness of the tibialis posterior tendon. Accessory soleus may cause compression neuropathy of the posterior tibial nerve and tarsal tunnel syndrome (DosRemedios and Jolly 2000; Kinoshita et al. 2003).

PERONEOTIBIALIS (FIGURE 5.6)

See also: Popliteus, Soleus

Synonyms
N/A

Typical Presentation
This muscle is only present as a variation.

Comparative Anatomy
Peroneotibialis is present in some monkeys (e.g., howler monkeys, macaques). It lies deep to popliteus, originating from the head or neck of the fibula and inserting onto the posterior aspect of the proximal tibial shaft (Howell and Straus 1933; Grand 1968). Grand (1968) describes the muscle as a vestigial rotator of the fibula on the tibia.

Variations
Description

Peroneotibialis originates from the medial aspect of the proximal fibula and inserts into the tendinous arch of the soleus or into the superior end of the soleal line of the tibia (Gruber 1878; Knott 1883a; Bergman et al. 1988; Lambert 2016; Standring 2016). Gruber (1878) refers to this muscle as a tensor of the tendinous arch of the soleus (Bergman et al. 1988; Lambert 2016). Bergman et al. (1988) and Standring (2016) note that it runs deep to popliteus. In the case photographed by Lambert (2016), the muscle has an origin via a tendinous slip from popliteus.

Innervation
N/A

Prevalence

Gruber (1878) found peroneotibialis in 128 out of 860 legs (14.9%), and Knott (1883a) found the muscle in 4 out of 49 subjects (8.2%).

Anomalies
N/A

Clinical Implications
Lambert (2016) notes that since peroneotibialis courses over the neurovascular bundle in the posterior lower leg, it may possibly lead to entrapment of the tibial nerve and the posterior tibial artery.

PLANTARIS (FIGURE 5.6)

Synonyms
Accessory plantaris may be referred to as plantaris minor (Krause), popliteus superior s. minor (Calori) (Knott 1883b), or bicipital plantaris (Hall) (Lambert 2016).

Typical Presentation
Description

Plantaris originates from the lateral supracondylar line of the femur and from the oblique popliteal ligament (Standring 2016). Its tendon courses between gastrocnemius and soleus and inserts onto the calcaneus medial to the insertion of the Achilles tendon (Standring 2016).

Innervation

Plantaris is innervated by the tibial nerve (Standring 2016).

Comparative Anatomy
When present in the apes, plantaris originates runs from the lateral supracondylar line of the femur, lateral epicondyle, lateral tibial condyle, or lateral head of gastrocnemius to the calcaneus (Miller 1952; Vereecke et al. 2005; Ferrero 2011; Ferrero et al. 2012; Diogo et al. 2012, 2013a,b, 2017). Plantaris is typically absent in gibbons, orangutans, and gorillas (Gibbs 1999). It is often present in common chimpanzees and bonobos (Gibbs 1999; Diogo et al. 2013a, 2017).

Variations
Description

Plantaris may be absent (Knott 1883b; Bergman et al. 1988; Daseler and Anson 1943; Mori 1964; Sato 1970; Moss 1988; Saxena and Bareither 2000; Ashaolu et al. 2014; Lambert 2016; Standring 2016; Olewnik et al. 2018b). When absent, it may be replaced by a fibrous band (Bergman et al. 1988). Only the tendon may be absent, the muscle ending in an aponeurosis or fascia between gastrocnemius or soleus (Macalister 1875; Sugavasi et al. 2013). Plantaris may blend with the lateral head of gastrocnemius (Macalister 1875; Freeman et al. 2008; Lambert 2016). It may also send a fibrous expansion to the patella (Freeman et al. 2008; Lambert 2016). The origin may be shifted more distally (Macalister 1875). Plantaris may have an origin from the lateral retinaculum of the knee (Koplas et al. 2009). Plantaris may present as a third head of gastrocnemius and may blend with the two heads at their junction, merge with only one head, or join the fascia on the deep surface of gastrocnemius (Wood 1868; Bergman et al. 1988).

The tendon of plantaris may fuse with the calcaneal tendon upon insertion (Bergman et al. 1988; Nayak et al. 2010; Standring 2016; Olewnik et al. 2018b). It may also join with the flexor retinaculum, tibial collateral ligament of the ankle, or the fascia of the leg (Bergman et al. 1988; Nayak et al. 2010; Standring 2016; Olewnik et al. 2018b). The tendon may have an attachment onto, or send a slip to, the plantar fascia (Macalister 1875; Bergman et al. 1988; Lambert 2016).

An accessory head may be present, making plantaris bicipital (Wood 1868; Macalister 1875; Bergman et al. 1988; Lambert 2016). Plantaris may be doubled, i.e., the accessory head may be entirely separate from the main muscle (Knott 1883b; Standring 2016). Potential origins of the accessory head, or origins of a variable plantaris muscle, include the normal origins of plantaris, the fascia of popliteus, the popliteal surface of the femur, lateral extension of the linea aspera, lateral or medial femoral condyles, the intercondylar fossa, the posterior oblique ligament, the knee joint capsule, the fascia of the leg, the lateral head of gastrocnemius, the soleal line of the tibia, or the proximal fibula (Wood 1868; Macalister 1875; Knott 1883b; Mori 1964; Bergman et al. 1988; Rana et al. 2006; Nayak et al. 2010; Kwinter et al. 2010; Upasna and Kumar 2011; Lambert 2016).

Kotian et al. (2013) report a case where the plantaris muscle originates normally but bifurcates after about 1 cm from its origin. The inferior belly passed posterior to the popliteal neurovasculature and ended in a tendon that joined with the tendon of the superior belly near the origin of soleus. The superior belly ran anterior to the popliteal neurovasculature. The common tendon of the two bellies inserted onto the calcaneus. Kalniev et al. (2014) report an accessory plantaris tendon that originated from soleus and merged with the tendon of the main belly. The two inserted together onto the calcaneal tendon.

Prevalence

Knott (1883b) found plantaris absent in 3 out of 40 subjects (7.5%). Sato (1970) found that plantaris was absent in 43 out of 406 limbs (10.6%) from Kyushu Japanese males and in 36 out of 264 limbs (13.6%) from females. Moss (1988) found that plantaris was absent in 11 out of 150 cadavers (7.3%), and in only four bodies (2.7%) the absence was bilateral. Saxena and Bareither (2000) found that plantaris was absent in 1 out of 40 cadaveric specimens (2.5%). In an MRI study of 1,039 knees, Koplas et al. (2009) found that plantaris originated from the lateral retinaculum in 19 knees (1.8%).

Mori (1964) found that plantaris was absent in 4% of cases. Mori (1964) also found that an accessory head arose from the capsule of the knee joint in 16% of cases and from the upper part of the tibia in 2.5% of cases. Daseler and Anson (1943) found that plantaris was absent in 50 out of 750 lower limbs (6.7%). Insertion of plantaris was examined in 150 cases. In 71 cases (47.3%), plantaris inserted into the medial aspect of the calcaneus medial to the calcaneal tendon. In 48 cases (32%), plantaris inserted into the calcaneus anterior to the calcaneal tendon. In 23 cases (15.3%), the insertion joined blended with the insertion of the calcaneal tendon. In seven cases (4.7%), plantaris inserted into the medial border of the calcaneal tendon. Freeman et al. (2008) studied plantaris in 46 cadaveric knees. Plantaris was absent in six knees (13.04%). In nine knees (19.57%), plantaris interdigitated with the lateral head of gastrocnemius. In five knees (10.87%), there was a strong fibrous extension of plantaris that went to the patella.

Nayak et al. (2010) studied the origin and insertion of plantaris in 52 lower limbs from 26 cadaveric males. Plantaris was completely absent in four limbs (7.69%). Three types of origins were noted: an origin from the lateral supracondylar line, capsule of the knee joint, and lateral head of gastrocnemius in 38 cases (73.08%); from capsule

of the knee joint and lateral head of gastrocnemius in three cases (5.77%); and from the lateral supracondylar line, capsule of the knee joint, lateral head of gastrocnemius, and fibular collateral ligament in seven cases (13.46%).

Three types of insertions were noted: into the flexor retinaculum in 15 cases (28.85%), into the calcaneus in 19 cases (36.54%), and into the calcaneal tendon in 14 cases (26.92%).

Using MRI, Herzog (2011) found accessory plantaris muscles in 63 of 1,000 (6.3%) symptomatic patients. In 62 cases, the normal plantaris and accessory plantaris had merged origins. One accessory plantaris muscle originated with the lateral head of the gastrocnemius muscle. The accessory plantaris muscles had insertions into the iliotibial tract in 5 out of the 63 cases (7.9%), the lateral patellar retinaculum in 15 cases (23.8%), and the iliotibial band in 43 cases (68.3%) (Herzog 2011). Ashaolu et al. (2014) studied gastrocnemius and plantaris in 60 legs from 30 Nigerian cadavers. In the legs with a two-headed gastrocnemius (21 legs), there was 100% simultaneous occurrence of plantaris. In the legs with multi-headed gastrocnemius (39 legs), there was 90% simultaneous occurrence of plantaris. Plantaris was thus present in 56 out of 60 legs (93.3%).

Olewnik et al. (2018b) studied plantaris in 130 cadaveric lower limbs. Plantaris was absent in 14 limbs (10.8%). In 51 out of the 116 cases (44%) in which the muscle was present, plantaris had a wide insertion onto the calcaneus medial to the Achilles tendon. In 26 cases (22.4%), the insertion onto the calcaneus blended with that of the Achilles tendon. In eight cases (6.9%), the insertion was into the calcaneus anterior to the Achilles tendon. In four cases (3.4%), the insertion was into the deep crural fascia. In 21 cases (18.1%), there was a wide insertion onto the posterior and medial aspects of the Achilles tendon. In six cases (5.2%), there was an insertion into the flexor retinaculum.

Anomalies

Description

Plantaris is often reduced or absent as an anomaly (Windle 1893; Bersu et al. 1976; Pettersen et al. 1979; Aziz 1980; Mieden 1982; Urban and Bersu 1897; Smith et al. 2015). Bersu et al. (1976) describe a male infant with Hanhart syndrome. The femora of this infant were normally developed, but distal secondary ossification centers were absent. The left leg stump had a patella and a small rudiment of the proximal tibia but no fibular rudiment. The right leg stump was less developed and had a patella, smaller tibial rudiment, and no fibular rudiment. There were no muscle masses suggestive of plantaris at the knee.

Windle (1893) noted that plantaris was absent in some anencephalic fetuses. Mieden (1982) describes an infant with median cleft lip, hypotelorism, and alobar holoprosencephaly. Plantaris was absent on the right side (Mieden 1982). In one male neonate with trisomy 13, plantaris lacked a tendon on the right side (Pettersen et al. (1979). In one female fetus, plantaris was hypoplastic on the left side (Pettersen et al. 1979). In a female neonate with trisomy 13, plantaris was absent bilaterally (Aziz 1980). In one fetus with mosaic trisomy 18, found that plantaris was absent bilaterally (Urban and Bersu 1987).

Prevalence

Among the limbs of ten anencephalic fetuses, Windle (1893) noted that plantaris was absent unilaterally in two cases (20%). In their literature review, Smith et al. (2015) found that plantaris was absent in 8 out of 20 individuals with trisomy 13 (40%) and in 1 out of 17 individuals with trisomy 18 (5.9%).

Clinical Implications

An extension of plantaris to the patella could have a role in patellofemoral pain syndrome (Freeman et al. 2008). A split plantaris that surrounds the tibial nerve, popliteal vessels, and nerve to soleus may lead to the entrapment of these structures (Kotian et al. 2013). An insertion of the plantaris tendon into the flexor retinaculum may affect the tendinopathy of tibialis posterior and an insertion that blends with the Achilles tendon may increase the risk of Achilles tendinopathy (Olewnik et al. 2018b).

POPLITEUS (FIGURES 5.6 AND 5.7)

See also: Peroneotibialis

Synonyms

An accessory popliteus may be referred to as popliteus biceps (Gruber), proximal popliteus, or popliteus geminus (Fabrice) (Lambert 2016).

Typical Presentation

Description

Popliteus originates via a tendon from the lateral condyle of the femur with supplementary fibers from the arcuate popliteal ligament and the lateral meniscus (Standring 2016). It inserts onto the posterior surface of the tibia just above the soleal line (Standring 2016).

Innervation

Popliteus is innervated by the tibial nerve (Standring 2016).

Comparative Anatomy

Popliteus has a similar typical presentation in the apes, extending from the lateral condyle of the femur to the posterior surface of the tibia (Champneys 1872; Hepburn 1892; Beddard 1893; Sonntag 1924; Raven 1950; Miller 1952; Gibbs 1999; Ferrero 2011; Ferrero et al. 2012; Diogo et al. 2010, 2012, 2013a,b, 2017). An origin from the fibular head and adjacent knee joint capsule is present in orangutans and bonobos (Hepburn 1892; Diogo et al. 2013b, 2017). An origin from the knee joint capsule is also found in gorillas and common chimpanzees (Hepburn 1892; Raven 1950; Gibbs 1999). The muscle in orangutans also has an origin from the oblique popliteal ligament and the lateral meniscus (Ferrero 2011; Ferrero et al. 2012; Diogo et al. 2013b).

Variations

Description

Popliteus may have connections to the posterior capsule of the knee joint, the oblique popliteal ligament, the posterior cruciate ligament, and/or the posterior meniscofemoral ligament (Last 1950; Fetto et al. 1977; Feipel et al. 2003; Lambert 2016). The popliteal tendon near the lateral meniscus may be bifurcated (Burman 1968; Perez Carro et al. 1999; Leal-Blanquet et al. 2009; Lambert 2016). Doral et al. (2006) report a popliteus tendon comprised of three bundles. Popliteus may be absent or doubled (Macalister 1875; Knott 1883b; Le Double 1897; Lambert 2016).

An accessory slip or head of popliteus may originate from the lateral femoral condyle, from the sesamoid bone in the lateral head of gastrocnemius, from the posterior cruciate ligament, or from the posterior knee joint capsule (Macalister 1875; Knott 1883a; Le Double 1897; Bergman et al. 1988; Lambert 2016; Standring 2016). It can insert with popliteus into the tibia and may be situated in front of or behind the vessels in the popliteal fossa (Macalister 1875; Bergman et al. 1988; Lambert 2016). Accessory slips in this region may also extend to the posterior wall of the capsule of the knee joint, the fibular head, or to the tibia near the insertion of the posterior cruciate ligament (Bergman et al. 1988). Using MRI, both Duc et al. (2004) and Hahn et al. (2019) found accessory popliteus muscles with an origin from the lateral head of gastrocnemius and insertion into the posteromedial articular capsule of the knee joint. An accessory slip of popliteus may present as popliteus minor, a muscle situated medial to plantaris that extends from the posterior surface of the lateral condyle of the tibia to the oblique popliteal ligament (Standring 2016). Knott (1883b) describes popliteus minor as an accessory bundle that originates from the lateral tendon of gastrocnemius.

Prevalence

Gruber (1875b) found an accessory popliteus in 11 out of 695 cases (1.6%). In an MRI study of 1,039 knees, Koplas et al. (2009) found an accessory popliteal muscle in three patients (0.3%). In a sample of 42 knees, Feipel et al. (2003) found a fibular attachment of popliteus in 98% of cases, at least one attachment to the lateral meniscus in 95% of cases, and the arcuate ligament in 90% of cases. Additional attachments include the posterior knee joint capsule in 57% of cases, the oblique popliteal ligament in 79% of cases, the posterior cruciate ligament in 5% of cases, and the meniscofemoral ligament in 33% of cases. In a series of 1,569 knee arthroscopies, Leal-Blanquet et al. (2009) found six bifurcated popliteus tendons (0.4%).

Anomalies

Description

Popliteus was absent on the right side of the trisomy 18 cyclopic fetus dissected by Smith et al. (2015). Bersu et al. (1976) describe a male infant with Hanhart syndrome. The femora of this infant were normally developed but distal secondary ossification centers were absent. The left leg stump had a patella and a small rudiment of the proximal tibia but no fibular rudiment. The right leg stump was less developed and had a patella, smaller tibial rudiment, and no fibular rudiment. There were no muscle masses suggestive of popliteus at the knee.

Prevalence

N/A

Clinical Implications

Accessory attachments of popliteus may help to protect the lateral meniscus and the tibiofemoral joint from degenerative disorders and cartilage alterations (Feipel et al. 2003). A popliteus tendon comprised of multiple bundles may be mistaken for tendinosis (Doral et al. 2006).

FLEXOR DIGITORUM LONGUS (FIGURE 5.7)

Synonyms

N/A

Typical Presentation

Description

Flexor digitorum longus originates from the tibia, attaching from just below the soleal line to the distal end of the tibia (Standring 2016). It sends four tendons to digits two through five that pass deep to the tendons of flexor digitorum brevis (Standring 2016). These tendons insert into the bases of the distal phalanges of digits two through five (Standring 2016). These tendons also receive contributions from the quadratus plantae and the tendons of flexor hallucis longus (Standring 2016).

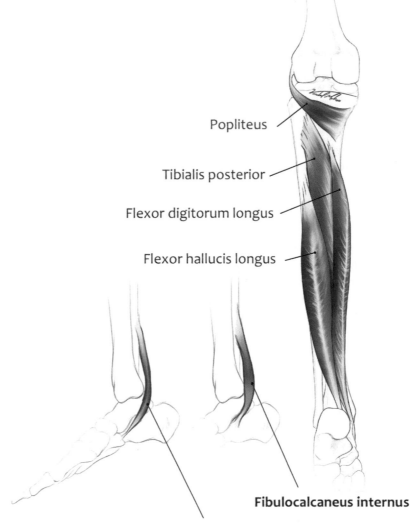

Popliteus

Tibialis posterior

Flexor digitorum longus

Flexor hallucis longus

Fibulocalcaneus internus

Flexor digitorum accessorius longus

FIGURE 5.7   Flexor digitorum accessorius longus (a) and fibulocalcaneus internus (b) in medial view. Deep muscles of the posterior lower leg in posterior view (c).

Innervation

Flexor digitorum longus is innervated by the tibial nerve (Standring 2016).

Comparative Anatomy

Flexor digitorum longus has a similar typical presentation in the apes, extending from the posterior surface of the tibia to the distal phalanges of the lateral digits, with some fusion with nearby muscles and frequent variation in which digits receive tendons (Champneys 1872; Hepburn 1892; Beddard 1893; Sonntag 1924; Raven 1950; Miller 1952; Lewis 1962; Gibbs 1999; Diogo et al. 2010, 2012, 2013a,b, 2017). In gibbons, the tendons to digits two, four, and five are typically present while the tendon to digit three is often absent (Hepburn 1892; Beddard 1893; Lewis 1962; Diogo et al. 2012). In orangutans, digits two, four, and five are typically supplied by the tendons (Gibbs 1999; Diogo et al. 2013b). In gorillas, digits two and five are always supplied by the tendons, and digits three and four are supplied in half of all cases (Gibbs 1999). In common chimpanzees and bonobos, digits two and five are almost always supplied by the tendons while the tendons to digits three and four are typically absent (Champneys 1872; Gibbs 1999; Hepburn 1892; Beddard 1893; Dwight 1895; MacDowell 1910; Miller 1952; Lewis 1962; Diogo et al. 2013a, 2017).

Variations

Description

The lateral portion of flexor digitorum longus or the entire muscle may be absent (Bergman et al. 1988). Accessory slips from the fibula, tibia, tibialis anterior, tibialis posterior, or the crural fascia may join the muscle above the ankle (Macalister 1875; Le Double 1897; Bergman et al. 1988; Lambert 2016). A slip may originate from the fascia over flexor digitorum longus and merge with the tendon of flexor hallucis longus in the foot (Bergman et al. 1988).

The slips that connect the tendon(s) of flexor digitorum longus to the tendon of flexor hallucis longus frequently vary (Macalister 1875; Knott 1883b; Martin 1964; Bergman et al. 1988; Lambert 2016; Standring 2016). The variable blending of the flexor digitorum longus and flexor hallucis longus is referred to as the chiasma plantare or the knot of Henry (e.g., O'Sullivan et al. 2005; LaRue and Anctil 2006; Plaass et al. 2013; Pretterklieber 2017; Beger et al. 2018b; Elvan et al. 2019). This blending often involves quadratus plantae (Pretterklieber 2017). There may also be no connections between the tendons of the long flexors (Knott 1883b; Martin 1964; LaRue and Anctil 2006). See prevalence section below for more information on the anatomical relationships of these tendons.

Some insertion tendons of flexor digitorum longus may be absent or otherwise vary (Macalister 1875; Knott 1883b; Bergman et al. 1988; Lambert 2016). The tendon to digit two may be absent and replaced by a tendon from flexor hallucis longus (Bergman et al. 1988; Lambert 2016). A slip from flexor digitorum longus may replace the tendon to digit

five from flexor digitorum brevis (Bergman et al. 1988). A slip from flexor digitorum longus may pass to join the flexor hallucis longus tendon to digit one (Bergman et al. 1988; Lambert 2016; Lee and Hur 2017). An accessory head of flexor digitorum longus may be present and is referred to as flexor accessorius longus or flexor digitorum accessorius longus (see the entry for this muscle) (Standring 2016).

Prevalence

In a study of 33 feet, Martin (1964) found no connection between the tendons of flexor hallucis longus and flexor digitorum longus in two cases (6.1%) and two other cases (6.1%) where the tendons gave slips to each other. In a study of 16 cadaveric feet, O'Sullivan et al. (2005) identified three patterns of connections between the tendons of flexor digitorum longus and flexor hallucis longus. In 11 feet (68.75%), tendinous fibers passed from the flexor hallucis longus tendon to the flexor digitorum longus tendon. In 2 feet (12.5%), tendinous fibers passed from the flexor digitorum longus tendon to the flexor hallucis longus tendon. In 3 feet (18.75%), tendinous fibers passed from the flexor digitorum longus tendon to the flexor hallucis longus tendon and an additional slip passed from the flexor hallucis longus tendon to the flexor digitorum longus tendon.

In a study of 24 cadaveric legs, LaRue and Anctil (2006) found three patterns of connections between the tendons of flexor digitorum longus and flexor hallucis longus. In 10 feet (41.7%), a tendinous slip passed from the flexor hallucis longus tendon to the flexor digitorum longus tendon. In ten other feet (41.7%), a tendinous slip passed from the flexor hallucis longus tendon to the flexor digitorum longus tendon, and another slip passed from the flexor digitorum longus tendon to the flexor hallucis longus tendon. In 4 feet (16.7%), there was no attachment of the tendons.

Athavale et al. (2012a) studied the connections between the long flexor tendons in sample of 47 lower limbs. In 19 limbs (40.4%), flexor hallucis longus sent a slip to the main tendon of flexor digitorum longus. In 21 limbs (44.7%), the slip from flexor hallucis longus contributed to the digital tendons of flexor digitorum longus, going to the tendon to digit two in two cases (4.3%), the tendons to digits two and three in 14 cases (29.8%), and the tendons to digits two, three, and four in five cases (10.6%). In two cases (4.3%), a slip from flexor digitorum longus went to flexor hallucis longus. In five cases (10.6%), there were no connections between the tendons of these two muscles.

Plaass et al. (2013) studied the connections between the long flexor tendons in sample of 60 feet from 30 cadavers. In 40 feet (67%) there was a proximal slip from flexor hallucis longus to the distal flexor digitorum longus only. Out of these 40 cases, there was a connection to digit two in 18 feet (45%), a connection to digits two and three in 18 feet (45%), and a connection to digits two, three, and four in 4 feet (10%). In 2 feet out of the 60 feet (3%), there was a proximal slip passing from flexor digitorum longus to the distal flexor hallucis longus only. In 18 out of 60 feet (30%), there was a slip from flexor hallucis longus to flexor digitorum longus and additional slips between the proximal flexor digitorum longus and distal flexor hallucis longus. Out of these 18 cases, there was a connection to digit two in three cases (17%) and a connection to digits two and three in 15 cases (83%).

Pretterklieber (2017) studied the chiasma plantare in 100 feet from 50 cadavers and conducted a literature review of previous research. In 61 specimens (61%), the tendon of flexor hallucis longus sent slips to the tendon of flexor digitorum longus. In 39 specimens (39%), the tendons of both muscles exchanged slips with each other. In a review of 14 studies, including the data from Martin (1964), O'Sullivan et al. (2005), LaRue and Anctil (2006), and Plaass et al. (2013), Pretterklieber (2017) found that out of a total of 754 cases, slips from flexor hallucis longus to flexor digitorum longus only were present in 564 cases (74.8%), slips from flexor digitorum longus to flexor hallucis longus only were present in four cases (0.5%), slips exchanged between both tendons were found in 172 cases (22.8%), and no connections between the tendons occurred in 14 cases (1.9%).

Pretterklieber (2017) also examined the contributions of flexor digitorum longus, flexor hallucis longus, and quadratus plantae to the flexor tendons. Flexor digitorum longus contributed to the first tendon in 39 cases (39%), to the second tendon in 98 cases (98%), and to the third, fourth, and fifth tendons in all 100 cases (100%). Elvan et al. (2019) studied the relationships between the tendons of flexor hallucis longus and flexor digitorum longus in 56 feet from 28 fetuses. In 48 feet (85.7%), there was a slip from flexor hallucis longus to the chiasma plantare. In 8 feet (14.3%), there were cross-connections between the tendons of flexor hallucis longus and flexor digitorum longus.

Lee and Hur (2017) found a tendinous slip of flexor digitorum longus going to digit one in 2 out of 66 cadaveric specimens (3%). In a study of 20 feet from 10 cadavers, Beger et al. (2018b) found five patterns of connections between the tendons of flexor hallucis longus and flexor digitorum longus. In 15 feet (75%), there was one slip from flexor hallucis longus to flexor digitorum longus. In two feet (10%), each tendon sent one slip to the other tendon. In one foot (5%), flexor hallucis longus sent two slips to flexor digitorum longus. In one foot (5%), flexor hallucis longus sent two slips to flexor digitorum longus and flexor digitorum longus sent one slip to flexor hallucis longus. In one foot (5%), flexor digitorum longus sent two slips to flexor digitorum longus and flexor hallucis longus sent one slip to flexor digitorum longus.

Anomalies

Description

In a female neonate with trisomy 13, Aziz (1980) found that flexor digitorum longus on the left side had a distally shifted origin. In a male fetus with triploidy studied by Moen et al. (1984), flexor digitorum longus had an extra belly with a tendon attaching to the tendon of flexor hallucis longus on the left side. On the right foot of a male neonate with Meckel syndrome, Pettersen (1984) found that flexor digiti minimi brevis attached to the fifth digit and received a slip from flexor digitorum brevis that did not split to accommodate

the tendon of flexor digitorum longus. Hootnick et al. (1987) describe an individual that had a right limb with congenital tibial aplasia, talocalcaneal synchondrosis, and an adducted foot with five toes. In this limb, flexor digitorum longus originated from the interosseus membrane, became tendinous halfway along its length, and inserted into the common flexor tendon sheet in the foot.

Prevalence

N/A

Clinical Implications

Knowledge of the variation in tendinous connections between flexor digitorum longus and flexor hallucis longus is important for planning tendon transfer to treat tibialis posterior tendon deficiency or dysfunction (O'Sullivan et al. 2005; Plaass et al. 2013).

FLEXOR DIGITORUM ACCESSORIUS LONGUS (FIGURE 5.7)

Synonyms

This muscle may also be referred to as flexor accessorius longus (Standring 2016), accessorius ad accessorium (Turner), accessorius ad flexor accessorium, accessorius ad quadratum plantae, accessorius longus ad flexor digitorum longum, accessorius flexori hallucis longi superior (Reinhart), fibulocalcaneus medialis, flexor accessorius digiti longus, flexor accessorius longus digitorum pedis (Hallett), and peroneocalcaneus internus (Macalister) (Bergman et al. 1988).

Typical Presentation

This muscle is only present as a variation or anomaly.

Comparative Anatomy

The flexor digitorum accessorius longus muscle may represent a remnant of the higher, tibial sided (medial) origin of quadratus plantae (flexor accessorius) present in some lower mammals (Lewis 1962; Jaijesh et al. 2005, 2006). This variant is not found in apes (Jaijesh et al. 2005, 2006).

Variations

Description

Flexor digitorum accessorius longus can originate from any structure or combination of structures in the posterior compartment of the lower leg, with recorded origins including the tibia, fibula, both the tibia and fibula, calcaneus, the deep fascia of the posterior compartment, posterior crural intermuscular septum, flexor retinaculum, flexor digitorum longus, flexor hallucis longus, and/or tibialis posterior (Wood 1868; Hallett 1848; Macalister 1875; Driver and Denison 1914; Nathan et al. 1975; Bergman et al. 1988; Sammarco and Conti 1994; Peterson et al. 1995; Cheung et al. 1999; Gümüşalan and Kalaycioğlu 2000; Sookur et al. 2008; Bowers et al. 2009; Upasna et al. 2011; Standring 2016; Lambert 2016). It can originate via two distinct heads, described as either a long and short head or medial and lateral head (Driver and Denison 1914; Nathan et al. 1975; Pác and Malinovský 1985; Gümüşalan and Kalaycioğlu 2000).

Flexor digitorum accessorius longus passes through the tarsal tunnel to enter the foot (Bergman et al. 1988; Cheung et al. 1999; Sookur et al. 2008; Duran-Stanton and Bui-Mansfield 2010; Lambert 2016). It often has fleshy, muscular fibers as it passes through the tarsal tunnel (Nathan et al. 1975; Cheung et al. 1999; Sookur et al. 2008; Bowers et al. 2009).

It may insert into the main tendon of flexor digitorum longus and/or into quadratus plantae (Hallett 1848; Wood 1864, 1868; Bergman et al. 1988; Sammarco and Conti 1994; Peterson et al. 1995; Cheung et al. 1999; Gümüşalan and Kalaycioğlu 2000; Sookur et al. 2008; Bowers et al. 2009; Georgiev et al. 2009; Upasna et al. 2011; Lambert 2016; Standring 2016). It may also insert into the flexor tendons going to digit two (Georgiev et al. 2009; Upasna et al. 2011), those going to digits two and three (Knott 1883b), or those going to digits three and four (Driver and Denison 1914). Pác and Malinovský (1985) note that the tendon may join the tendons of flexor digitorum longus to digits two, three, and four, and may receive a tendinous slip from flexor hallucis longus. Sookur et al. (2008) state that its tendon splits into four slips and sends a tendon to the distal phalanges of digits two through five.

This accessory muscle may either be separate or attached to flexor digitorum longus (Macalister 1875). Hallett (1848) notes that quadratus plantae may be unusually large when flexor digitorum accessorius longus is present. The presence of flexor digitorum accessorius longus may also be associated with the absence of quadratus plantae (Pác and Malinovský 1985). It may send slips to flexor hallucis longus or tibialis anterior (Standring 2016). Flexor digitorum accessorius longus may present as flexor digiti secundi proprius, which originates from the posterior surface of the tibia (Macalister 1875; Knott 1883b).

Innervation

Flexor digitorum accessorius longus is innervated by the tibial nerve (Driver and Denison 1914; Upasna et al. 2011).

Prevalence

Wood (1868) reports that the muscle was found in 4 out of 68 male subjects (5.9%) and 1 out of 34 female subjects (2.9%). Driver and Denison (1914) found four flexor digitorum accessorius longus muscles from two cadavers in a sample of 50 limbs from 25 cadavers (8%). In a sample of 36 legs from 18 cadavers, Lewis (1962) found the muscle in three legs from two cadavers (8.3%). In a sample of 52 legs from 26 cadavers, Canter and Siesel (1997) found the muscle in two legs (3.8%) from two cadavers. Upasna et al. (2011) found this muscle in 1 out of 60 legs (1.7%). In a sample of 47 lower limbs, Athavale et al. (2012a) found flexor digitorum accessorius longus in two cases (4.3%).

In a sample of 136 lower limbs from 68 cadavers, Peterson et al. (1995) found flexor digitorum accessorius longus in 11 lower limbs (8.1%) from nine cadavers. Five out of the 11 muscles (45.5%) arose from the tibia and deep fascia of the

posterior compartment and six muscles (54.5%) arose from the fibula. The five tendons that had origins from the tibia inserted onto quadratus plantae with two of them having an additional attachment to flexor digitorum longus. Three of the tendons with origins from the fibula inserted onto quadratus plantae, with the remaining three tendons inserting onto flexor digitorum longus.

In a sample of 100 ankle MRI examinations from asymptomatic patients, Cheung et al. (1999) found flexor digitorum accessorius longus in six cases (6%). These authors combined data from these 6 cases and 14 other cases from symptomatic patients to study flexor digitorum accessorius longus in a total sample of 20 cases. Cheung et al. (1999) found that the muscle arose from flexor hallucis longus in 8 out of 20 cases (40%), from the flexor retinaculum in 6 cases (30%), and the other 6 cases (30%) had indeterminate origins.

In a sample of 200 legs from 100 cadavers, Nathan et al. (1975) found flexor digitorum accessorius longus in 14 legs from 12 cadavers (7%). A double origin of the muscle was found in 8 out of the 14 cases (57.1%). Out of a sample of 60 cadavers, Gümüşalan and Kalaycioğlu (2000) found flexor digitorum accessorius longus with two heads bilaterally in only one specimen (1.7%).

In a sample of 44 feet from 37 patients who underwent operations to treat tarsal tunnel syndrome, Sammarco and Conti (1994) found flexor digitorum accessorius longus in 6 feet (13.6%) from five patients. In a sample of 49 feet from 41 patients who underwent operations to treat tarsal tunnel syndrome, Kinoshita et al. (2003) found flexor digitorum accessorius longus in 6 feet (12.2%) from six patients.

Anomalies

Description

Flexor digitorum accessorius longus muscles are sometimes found in individuals born with clubfoot (talipes equinovarus) (Sodre et al. 1994). The muscle was present in the right club foot of an infant with Nager syndrome described by Kubota et al. (2001). It originated from the fascia over flexor hallucis longus and the deep fascia of the lower leg (Kubota et al. 2001).

Urban and Bersu (1987) found extra muscle slips extending between the tibia and quadratus plantae on the right side of a fetus with full trisomy 18 and bilaterally in a fetus with mosaic trisomy 18. Bersu (1980) found a muscle that extended between the fibula and quadratus plantae bilaterally in a child with trisomy 21.

Prevalence

Flexor digitorum accessorius longus muscles were found in 4 out of 72 patients with club foot (5.6%) (Sodre et al. 1994). In their literature review, Smith et al. (2015) found that the extra muscle slips found by Urban and Bersu (1987) were only present in the two fetuses examined by them and were not present in 15 other individuals with trisomy 18, yielding a prevalence of 11.8%. The muscle described by Bersu (1980) was found in one out of five individuals with trisomy 21 (20%).

Clinical Implications

Flexor digitorum accessorius longus can compress the tibial nerve or its branches and cause tarsal tunnel syndrome (Nathan et al. 1975; Sammarco and Stephens 1990; Sammarco and Conti 1994; Canter and Siesel 1997; Kinoshita et al. 2003; Molloy et al. 2015). The presence of this muscle may also cause flexor hallucis syndrome (Eberle et al. 2002).

FIBULOCALCANEUS INTERNUS (FIGURE 5.7)

See also: Flexor digitorum accessorius longus

Synonyms

This muscle may also be referred to as peroneocalcaneus internus (Macalister 1875) or pronator pedis (Knott 1883a). Peroneocalcaneus medialis or fibulocalcaneus medialis may be used as synonyms for this muscle. Although Lambert et al. (2011a) note that the description of fibulocalcaneus medialis by Jackson (1921) best matches descriptions of flexor digitorum accessorius longus, the lateral origins and point of insertion of the fibulocalcaneus medialis muscles described by Pettersen (1979) seem more aligned with descriptions of fibulocalcaneus internus.

Fibulocalcaneus internus is listed as a synonym of flexor digitorum accessorius longus by Bergman et al. (1988). However, some authors note that this synonymy is erroneous as the two muscles are often confused with one another since they both pass deep to the flexor retinaculum (Mellado et al. 1997; Lambert et al. 2011a; Lambert 2016). The two muscles may be distinguished by some key anatomical differences. First, Nathan et al. (1975) suggest that flexor digitorum accessorius longus is the only muscle that retains fleshy fibers within the tarsal tunnel, while only the tendons of other muscles pass through the flexor retinaculum. Second, flexor digitorum accessorius longus has a variable origin from the posterior compartment of the lower leg while fibulocalcaneus internus often originates from the distal fibula (Lambert et al. 2011a; Lambert 2016). Third, while flexor digitorum accessorius longus typically inserts onto quadratus plantae and/or the flexor digitorum longus tendon, fibulocalcaneus internus inserts onto the medial aspect of the calcaneus and is separated from quadratus plantae (Peterson et al. 1995; Mellado et al. 1997; Cheung et al. 1999; Sookur et al. 2008; Lambert et al. 2011a; Lambert 2016). Another way to distinguish the muscles is via their relationships with flexor hallucis longus; flexor digitorum accessorius longus is typically situated medial and posterior to flexor hallucis longus within the tarsal tunnel while fibulocalcaneus internus typically lies lateral to flexor hallucis longus (Lambert 2016; Lambert et al. 2011a). Lastly, flexor digitorum accessorius longus is closely associated with the neurovascular structures in the tarsal tunnel while fibulocalcaneus internus is typically separated from these structures by flexor hallucis longus (Mellado et al. 1997; Sookur et al. 2008; Lambert et al. 2011a; Lambert 2016).

Typical Presentation

This muscle is only present as a variation or anomaly.

Comparative Anatomy

N/A

Variations

Description

Fibulocalcaneus internus typically originates from the distal third of the fibula below the origin of flexor hallucis longus (Macalister 1875; Le Double 1897; Knott 1883a; Mellado et al. 1997; Sookur et al. 2008; Lambert et al 2011a; Lambert 2016). It may also take origin from the posterior intermuscular septum and/or flexor hallucis longus (Perkins 1914; Lambert et al. 2011a). Its origin may interdigitate with flexor hallucis longus (Mellado et al. 1997; Lambert et al. 2011a). The muscle becomes tendinous before entering the tarsal tunnel (Mellado et al. 1997; Howe and Murthy 2012).

The muscle courses lateral to flexor hallucis longus, passes deep to the flexor retinaculum, and inserts via a tendon onto the inferomedial aspect of the calcaneus, typically into a small tubercle below the sustentaculum tali (Macalister 1875; Le Double 1897; Perkins 1914; Mellado et al. 1997; Sookur et al. 2008; Lambert et al 2011a; Howe and Murthy 2012; Lambert 2016). It may insert directly into the sustentaculum tali (Knott 1883a; Best et al. 2005; Seipel et al. 2005; Lambert 2016). Lambert et al. (2011a) observe that the tendon inserts distal to the calcaneal coronoid fossa.

Innervation

Fibulocalcaneus internus is innervated by the branch of the tibial nerve that supplies the distal muscle belly of flexor hallucis longus (Lambert et al. 2011a).

Prevalence

Mellado et al. (1997) found only one case of fibulocalcaneus internus in a sample of MR images from 100 asymptomatic individuals (1%).

Anomalies

Description

Ramirez-Castro and Bersu (1978) report the bilateral presence of "peroneocalcaneus medialis" in three neonates with trisomy 18. These muscles were each innervated by a branch from the tibial nerve. In all three cases, the muscles originated from the posterior aspect of the distal third of the fibula and the corresponding interosseous membrane. The muscles traveled with the tendon of flexor hallucis longus and inserted into the plantar aspect of the calcaneus. In the foot, the peroneocalcaneus medialis muscles sent tendons to nearby structures. In one case, the tendons merged with the medial head of quadratus plantae. In the other two cases, the tendons extended laterally from between the origins of flexor digitorum brevis and quadratus plantae to insert onto the lateral margin of the calcaneus.

Pettersen (1979) reports the presence of "fibulocalcaneus medialis" on both sides of a child with trisomy 13q. On the left side, the muscle originated in the lower third of the posterior lower leg from the fascia of flexor hallucis longus, the fascia of the peroneal muscles, and the lateral intermuscular septum. Its tendon passed under the flexor retinaculum, and it inserted into the deep surface of flexor digitorum brevis near its origin. On the right side, the muscle had a similar insertion but originated from the superficial aspects of fibularis longus and brevis. Pettersen et al. (1979) also found "fibulocalcaneus medialis" bilaterally in a fetus with trisomy 13. The muscle originated from the back of the fibula just above the calcaneus. The muscle ran parallel and posterior to flexor hallucis longus. It inserted via a tendon onto the medial surface of the calcaneus anterior to the tendocalcaneus.

Hootnick et al. (1987) describe an individual that had a right limb with congenital tibial aplasia, talocalcaneal synchondrosis, and an adducted foot with five toes. In this limb, an accessory muscle originated from the distal fibula and interosseous membrane and inserted onto the superior surface of the calcaneus, medial to the insertion of the calcaneal tendon.

Prevalence

In their literature review, Smith et al. (2015) found that peroneocalcaneus medialis was only present in 3 out of 17 individuals with trisomy 18 (17.6%) and 2 out of 20 individuals with trisomy 13 (10%).

Clinical Implications

If fibulocalcaneus internus shifts flexor hallucis longus medially, it may indirectly lead to compression or entrapment of the neurovascular bundle via the displaced flexor hallucis longus (Mellado et al. 1997). The presence of fibulocalcaneus internus has been associated with pain, posterior ankle impingement, and flexor hallucis longus tenosynovitis (Best et al. 2005; Seipet et al. 2005). The presence of this muscle may also contribute to tarsal tunnel syndrome (Duran-Stanton and Bui-Mansfield 2010).

FLEXOR HALLUCIS LONGUS (FIGURE 5.7)

Synonyms

N/A

Typical Presentation

Description

Flexor hallucis longus originates from the fibula, the interosseous membrane, the posterior crural intermuscular septum, and from the tibialis posterior fascia (Standring 2016). Its tendon enters the foot, sends slips to the tendon of flexor digitorum longus, and inserts onto the base of the distal phalanx of digit one (Standring 2016).

Innervation

Flexor hallucis longus is innervated by the tibial nerve (Standring 2016).

Comparative Anatomy

Flexor hallucis longus has a similar typical presentation in most apes, extending from the interosseous membrane, posterior crural intermuscular septum, and/or the fibula to the base of the distal phalanx of digit one (Champneys 1872; Hepburn 1892; Beddard 1893; Sonntag 1924; Raven 1950; Miller 1952; Lewis 1962; Gibbs 1999; Diogo et al. 2010, 2012, 2013a,b, 2017). In orangutans, the tendon inserts onto digits three and four only, with no insertion onto digit one, and there may be an origin from the lateral femoral condyle (Chapman 1880; Hepburn 1892; Beddard 1893; Sonntag 1924; Gibbs 1999; Diogo et al. 2013b).

In gibbons and gorillas, there are often additional insertions onto digits three and four, and sometimes insertions onto digits two and five (Chapman 1878; Hepburn 1892; Beddard 1893; Raven 1950; Lewis 1962; Gibbs 1999; Diogo et al. 2010, 2012). In common chimpanzees and bonobos, there are often additional insertions onto digits three and four, and sometimes an insertion onto digit two (Champneys 1872; Beddard 1893; Miller 1952; Diogo et al. 2013a, 2017).

Variations

Description

Flexor hallucis longus may be doubled, with both tendons ending on the distal phalanx of digit one (Bergman et al. 1988). A slip may originate from the fascia over flexor digitorum longus and merge with the tendon of flexor hallucis longus in the foot (Bergman et al. 1988). The slips that connect the tendon(s) of flexor digitorum longus to the tendon of flexor hallucis longus frequently vary (Macalister 1875; Knott 1883b; Martin 1964; Bergman et al. 1988; Lambert 2016; Standring 2016). The variable blending of the flexor digitorum longus and flexor hallucis longus is referred to as the chiasma plantare or the knot of Henry (e.g., O'Sullivan et al. 2005; LaRue and Anctil 2006; Plaass et al. 2013; Pretterklieber 2017; Beger et al. 2018b; Elvan et al. 2019). This blending often involves quadratus plantae (Pretterklieber 2017). There may also be no connections between the tendons of the long flexors (Knott 1883b; Martin 1964; LaRue and Anctil 2006).

When the tendon of flexor hallucis longus provides slips to the other toes (which occurs in most individuals), it frequently supplies the second and third toes and sometimes extends to the fourth toe (Knott 1883b; Mori 1964; Bergman et al. 1988; Standring 2016). It rarely contributes to the tendon going to digit five (Mori 1964; Bergman et al. 1988; Pretterklieber 2017). Flexor hallucis longus is associated with the supernumerary muscle fibulotarsalis, which extends from the fibula to the plantar aspects of the calcaneus and navicular (Bergman et al. 1988).

Prevalence

Mori (1964) found that flexor hallucis longus sent slips to digits one and two in 8% of cases; to digits one, two, and three in 64% of cases; to digits one through four in 26%

of cases; and to all five digits in 2% of cases. Athavale et al. (2012a) found that slips of flexor hallucis longus gave rise to the first lumbrical muscle in 18 cases (38.3%) and to other lumbrical muscles in nine cases (19.15%). Beger et al. (2018b) classified the contributions of flexor hallucis longus to the flexor tendons of the toes. In 5 feet (25%), flexor hallucis longus sent a slip to the second digit. In 12 feet (60%), flexor hallucis longus sent slips to digits two and three. In 3 feet (15%), flexor hallucis longus sent slips to digits two, three, and four.

Pretterklieber (2017) found that the tendon of flexor hallucis longus sent a slip to digit two in 45 cases (45%), to digits two and three in 46 cases (46%), and to the second through fourth digits in 5 cases (5%). Four cases showed other insertions, including slips to the second and fourth digits, slips to the third and fourth digits, a slip to only digit three, and a slip to only digit four. In a review of nine studies, including the data from Plaass et al. (2013), Pretterklieber (2017) reports that out of 637 total cases, flexor hallucis longus sent a slip to digit two only in 223 cases (35%), digits two and three in 334 cases (52.4%), digits two through four in 75 cases (11.8%), digits two through five in one case (0.16%), and other patterns of insertion in four cases (0.6%). Pretterklieber (2017) also examined the contributions of flexor digitorum longus, flexor hallucis longus, and quadratus plantae to the flexor tendons. Flexor hallucis longus contributed to the first tendon in 100 cases (100%), to the second tendon in 97 cases (97%), to the third tendon in 53 cases (53%), to the fourth tendon in eight cases (8%), and never to the fifth tendon.

Elvan et al. (2019) studied the relationships between the tendons of flexor hallucis longus and flexor digitorum longus in 56 feet from 28 fetuses. In 48 feet (85.7%), there was a slip from flexor hallucis longus to the chiasma plantare. In 8 feet (14.3%), there were cross connections between the tendons of flexor hallucis longus and flexor digitorum longus. See the entry for flexor digitorum longus for more prevalence information regarding the variable the anatomical relationships between the tendons of these muscles.

Anomalies

Description

Mieden (1982) describes two male fetuses with cyclopia and alobar holoprosencephaly. On the right side of one fetus, the tendon of flexor hallucis longus was divided, one tendon having the typical attachment and the other attaching to the tendon of flexor digitorum brevis going to digit two. In a male fetus with triploidy studied by Moen et al. (1984), flexor hallucis longus sent tendons to all phalanges on the left side. In one fetus with full trisomy 18, Urban and Bersu (1987) found that flexor hallucis longus sent a tendon to the navicular. In another fetus with mosaic trisomy 18, flexor hallucis longus sent a tendon to the calcaneus. Slips from this muscle to flexor digitorum longus were present bilaterally in the full trisomy 18 fetus and

on the right side of the mosaic trisomy 18 fetus. Hootnick et al. (1987) describe an individual that had a right limb with congenital tibial aplasia, talocalcaneal synchondrosis, and an adducted foot with five toes. In this limb, flexor hallucis longus was narrow and cord like and inserted onto the calcaneus.

Prevalence

In their literature review, Smith et al. (2015) found that the anomalies described by Urban and Bersu (1987) were only present in the two specimens described by these authors out of a sample of 17 individuals with trisomy 18 (11.8%).

Clinical Implications

Knowledge of the variation in tendinous connections between flexor digitorum longus and flexor hallucis longus is important for planning tendon transfer to treat tibialis posterior tendon deficiency or dysfunction (O'Sullivan et al. 2005; Plaass et al. 2013).

TIBIALIS POSTERIOR (FIGURE 5.7)

Synonyms

This muscle may also be referred to as tibialis posticus (Macalister 1875; Knott 1883b).

Typical Presentation

Description

Tibialis posterior originates via medial and lateral parts (Standring 2016). The medial part originates from the interosseous membrane and from the posterior tibial surface (Standring 2016). The lateral part originates from the posterior fibular surface (Standring 2016). When it reaches the foot, the tendon of tibialis posterior typically divides into two portions (Standring 2016). The superficial portion has insertions onto the navicular, medial cuneiform, and the sustentaculum tali (Standring 2016). The deeper portion has insertions onto the intermediate cuneiform and the bases of metatarsals two through four (Standring 2016). Flexor hallucis brevis partially originates from this portion of the tendon (Standring 2016).

Innervation

Tibialis posterior is innervated by the tibial nerve (Standring 2016).

Comparative Anatomy

Tibialis posterior has a similar typical presentation in the apes, originating from the tibia, fibula, and interosseous membrane and typically inserting into the navicular and metatarsals two through four, with occasional attachments to the cuneiforms and tendon of fibularis longus (Champneys 1872; Hepburn 1892; Beddard 1893; Sonntag 1924; Raven 1950; Miller 1952; Lewis 1964; Gibbs 1999; Vereecke et al. 2005; Diogo et al. 2010, 2012, 2013a,b, 2017).

Variations

Description

Tibialis posterior may be absent (Macalister 1875; Le Double 1897; Lambert 2016). The tendon may be split into three distinct bands (Macalister 1875; Lewis 1964; Bloome et al. 2003; Lambert 2016). The number of slips that arise from the tendon varies (Mori 1964; Bloome et al. 2003; Standring 2016). Its tendon may send slips to the tendon of fibularis longus, tendon of flexor digitorum brevis, flexor hallucis brevis, abductor hallucis, adductor hallucis, the plantar aponeurosis, the spring ligament, capsule of the naviculocuneiform joint, cuboid, lateral cuneiform, or base of the fifth metatarsal (Macalister 1875; Knott 1883b; Lewis 1964; Mori 1964; Gunal et al. 1994; Lohrmann et al. 1997; Bloome et al. 2003; Raheja et al. 2005; Lambert 2016; Standring 2016). The attachment onto the medial cuneiform may be missing (Bergman et al. 1988).

Tibialis posterior is associated with three rare supernumerary muscles. Tensor capsuli tibiotarsalis anterior is considered a variant of tibialis secundus and inserts onto the anterior wall of the ankle joint capsule (Bergman et al. 1988). Macalister (1875) notes that it originates from the lower half of the lateral surface of the tibia below flexor digitorum longus. Tibialis secundus (Bahnsen) or accessory tibialis posterior extends from the posterior surface of the tibia, below tibialis posterior, to the ankle joint capsule or the flexor retinaculum (Bahnsen 1868; Macalister 1875; Knott 1883b; Le Double 1897; Bergman et al. 1988; Lambert 2016; Standring 2016). Accessory tibialis muscles may also have insertions into the tarsals, second metatarsal, and tendons in the foot (Le Double 1897; Lambert 2016). Tibiotarsalis or tensor fasciae plantaris (also described under the entry for soleus) extends from the soleal line of the tibia to insert into the plantar fascia (Wood 1864; Macalister 1875; Anderson 1880; Knott 1883b; Bergman et al. 1988; Lambert 2016).

Prevalence

Mori (1964) found ten different patterns of insertion of the tibialis posterior tendon. In 11% of cases, the tendon inserted onto the navicular, medial cuneiform, and intermediate cuneiform. In 31% of cases, the tendon inserted onto the navicular, intermediate cuneiform, and lateral cuneiform. In 1% of cases, the tendon inserted onto the navicular, medial cuneiform, and first metatarsal. In 2% of cases, the tendon inserted onto the navicular, medial cuneiform, and second metatarsal. In 6% of cases, the tendon inserted onto the navicular, medial cuneiform, and third metatarsal. In 6% of cases, the tendon inserted onto the navicular, medial cuneiform, and fourth metatarsal. In 14% of cases, the tendon inserted onto the navicular, medial cuneiform, and cuboid. In 10% of cases, the tendon inserted onto the navicular, medial cuneiform, and fascia of flexor hallucis brevis. In 10% of cases, the tendon inserted onto the navicular, medial cuneiform, and tendon of fibularis longus. In 5% of cases, the tendon inserted onto the navicular, medial cuneiform, and the plantar aponeurosis.

Bloome et al. (2003) studied the insertions of the tibialis posterior tendon in 11 feet from 10 cadavers. Each tendon had three distinct bands and their insertions included the base of the fifth metatarsal in 7 out of 11 cases (63.6%), the spring ligament in four cases (36.4%), fibularis longus tendon in four cases (36.4%), and flexor hallucis brevis in nine cases (81.2%). Slips to abductor hallucis were found in five cases (45.5%).

Anomalies

Description

Sodre et al. (1994) note that agenesis of tibialis posterior may be found in individuals born with clubfoot (talipes equinovarus). Anomalous insertions of the tibialis posterior tendon are found in cases of congenital metatarsus varus (Browne and Paton 1979). Hootnick et al. (1987) describe an individual that had a right limb with congenital tibial aplasia, talocalcaneal synchondrosis, and an adducted foot with five toes. In this limb, tibialis posterior arose with flexor hallucis longus and inserted by a short tendon onto the common flexor tendon sheet in the foot.

Prevalence

Agenesis of tibialis posterior was found in 1 out of 72 patients born with clubfoot (1.4%) (Sodre et al. 1994). Browne and Paton (1979) operated on 15 feet from ten children to treat congenital metatarsus varus and found anomalous insertions of the tibialis posterior tendon in 14 feet (93.3%).

Clinical Implications

Variations in the insertion of the tibialis posterior tendon may lead to hallux valgus (Bozant et al. 1994; Gunal et al. 1994). Accessory or duplicated tibialis posterior tendons can cause posterior tibial tenosynovitis (Ghormley and Spear 1953).

ANTERIOR AND LATERAL MUSCLES OF THE LOWER LEG

TIBIALIS ANTERIOR (FIGURE 5.8)

Synonyms

This muscle may be referred to as tibialis anticus (Macalister 1875; Knott 1883b).

Typical Presentation

Description

Tibialis anterior originates from the tibia via the lateral condyle and proximal shaft and from the interosseous membrane (Standring 2016). It inserts via a tendon onto the medial cuneiform and base of the hallucal metatarsal (Standring 2016).

Innervation

Tibialis anterior is innervated by the deep fibular nerve (Standring 2016).

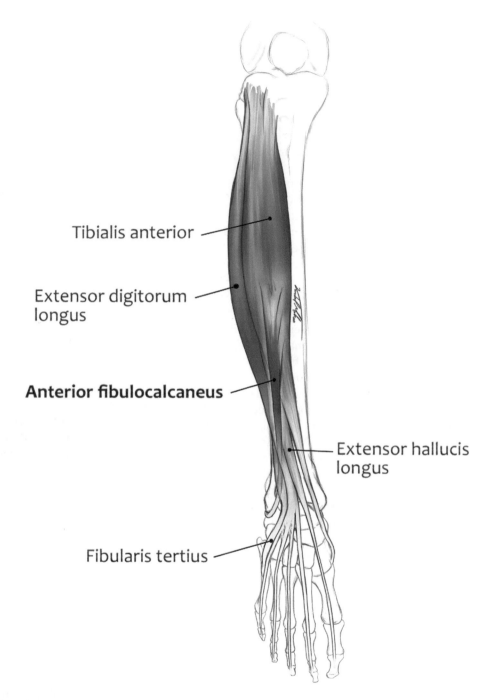

FIGURE 5.8   Anterior muscles of the lower leg in anterior view.

Comparative Anatomy

Tibialis anterior has a similar typical presentation in the apes, extending from the tibia to the medial cuneiform and first metatarsal (Hepburn 1892; Beddard 1893; MacDowell 1910; Sonntag 1924; Raven 1950; Miller 1952; Lewis 1966; Gibbs 1999; Vereecke et al. 2005; Ferrero 2011; Ferrero et al. 2012; Diogo et al. 2010, 2012, 2013a,b, 2017). The muscle is divided into two bellies in gibbons, common chimpanzees, and bonobos (Hepburn 1892; Beddard 1893; MacDowell 1910; Miller 1952; Lewis 1966; Diogo et al. 2017). The insertion onto the first metatarsal in common chimpanzees and bonobos may be considered a separate

muscle, abductor hallucis longus (Gibbs 1999; Diogo et al. 2013a, 2017). There may be an origin from extensor digitorum longus in orangutans (Sonntag 1924; Gibbs 1999; Diogo et al. 2013b).

Variations

Description

Additional fibers of origin may arise from the fibula (Knott 1883b). The origin may also be shifted proximally to the lateral condyle of the femur (Le Double 1897; Lambert 2016). The insertion onto the hallucal metatarsal, or more infrequently the insertion onto the medial cuneiform, may be absent (Hallisy 1930; Arthornthurasook and Gaew-Im 1990; Brenner 2002; Lambert 2016; Olewnik et al. 2019a). Tibialis anterior may have distal attachments to the head of the first metatarsal, base of the proximal phalanx of digit one, talus, navicular, calcaneus, extensor retinaculum, aponeuroses of the foot, or the ankle joint capsule (Macalister 1875; Knott 1883b; Hallisy 1930; Mori 1964; Bergman et al. 1988; Brenner 2002; Lambert 2016; Standring 2016). Ikiz and Üçerler (2005) note an insertion of the tibialis anterior tendon onto the lateral side of the foot, with attachments onto the fifth metatarsal and cuboid.

The entire muscle, or more often just the tendon, may be divided (Macalister 1875; Hallisy 1930; Bergman et al. 1988; Lambert 2016). When the tendon of tibialis anterior is divided into two slips, one slip goes to the medial cuneiform and the other goes to the first metatarsal (Macalister 1875; Mori 1964; Bergman et al. 1988). It may also be divided into three slips (Mori 1964; Olewnik et al. 2019a).

A deep slip of muscle that extends from the distal tibia and interosseous membrane to the neck of the talus may be referred to as tibioastragalus anticus (Gruber) or anterior tibiotalus (Bergman et al. 1988; Berkowitz et al. 2016; Lambert 2016). A separate slip extending from the distal tibia to the annular ligament and/or dorsal fascia of the foot may be referred to as tibiofascialis anticus (Wood) or tibialis anticus accessorius (s. profundus) (Macalister 1875; Knott 1883b; Bergman et al. 1988; Lambert 2016). It may present as a tendinous slip with an origin from tibialis anterior instead of presenting as a separate structure (Macalister 1875; Knott 1883b; Bergman et al. 1988; Jain et al. 2013; Lambert 2016). Although Knott (1883b) lists tensor fasciae dorsalis pedis (Krause) as a synonym of tibiofascialis anticus, Lambert (2016) describes it as a separate slip that has the same insertion onto the inferior extensor retinaculum and dorsal fascia of the foot but with an origin from the distal fibula.

Prevalence

Macalister (1875) notes that Wood found tibiofascialis anticus in 2 out of 36 cases (5.6%). Knott (1883b) found tibiofascialis anticus in 2 out of 40 cases (5%). Out of 30 cases (Knott 1883b), two (6.7%) sent a slip to the extensor retinaculum ("ligamentum cruciatum"), two (6.7%) sent a slip to the head of the first metatarsal, and one (3.3%) sent a slip to the base of the proximal phalanx of digit one. Knott (1883b) notes that Kraus found a slip to the ligamentum cruciatum in 6% of cases.

Hallisy (1930) studied tibialis anterior in 290 feet. In 261 feet (90%), the muscle had the typical insertions onto the first metatarsal and medial cuneiform. In three cases (1%), the tendon split just prior to insertion. In two cases (0.7%), the tendon inserted onto the first metatarsal only. In one case (0.3%), the tendon inserted onto the navicular, medial cuneiform, and first metatarsal. In three cases (1%), the tendon inserted normally and sent a slip to the shaft of the first metatarsal just behind the head. In one case (0.3%), the tendon had a slip with attachments into the head of the first metatarsal

and base of the proximal phalanx of digit one. In seven cases (2.4%), the tendon had an extra slip that inserted onto the medial side of the base of the proximal phalanx of digit one. In two cases (0.7%), a small muscular belly was present that sent a tendon to the base of the proximal phalanx of digit one.

Mori (1964) found that in 78% of cases, an undivided tendon of tibialis anterior coursed over the anterior surface of the tibia to the medial aspect of the foot and inserted into the medial surface of the medial cuneiform and into the base of the first metatarsal. In 20% of cases, the tendon divided into two slips, one inserting onto the medial cuneiform and the other into the first metatarsal. In 2% of cases, the slip was divided into three portions and inserted onto the medial cuneiform, first metatarsal, and navicular.

Arthornthurasook and Gaew-Im (1990) studied the insertion of tibialis anterior in 44 feet from 22 cadavers. In 25 cases (56.8%), the tendon divided into two equal slips, one going to the medial cuneiform and the other to the base of the first metatarsal. In 12 cases (27.3%), the tendon sent a large slip to the medial cuneiform and a small slip to the base of the first metatarsal. In seven cases (15.9%), the tendon inserted onto the medial cuneiform only. Brenner (2002) examined the insertion of tibialis anterior in 156 feet. In two cases (1.3%), there was an insertion only onto the medial cuneiform, and in two other cases (1.3%), there was an insertion only onto the first metatarsal. In one case (0.6%), there was an insertion onto the navicular and medial cuneiform.

Olewnik et al. (2019a) studied the insertion of tibialis anterior in 100 cadaveric lower limbs. In 31 cases (31%), the tendon divided into two equal slips, one going to the medial cuneiform and the other to the base of the first metatarsal (Type I). In 24 cases (24%), the tendon sent a large slip to the medial cuneiform and a small slip to the base of the first metatarsal (Type II). In 11 cases (11%), the tendon sent a small slip to the medial cuneiform and a large slip to the base of the first metatarsal (Type III). In two cases (2%), the tendon trifurcated, sending one slip to the medial cuneiform and two slips to the first metatarsal (Type IV). In 32 cases (32%), the tendon inserted onto the medial cuneiform only (Type V). Olewnik et al. (2019a) also studied the insertion of tibialis anterior in 100 limbs from 50 volunteers using ultrasound. Type I insertion was found in 20 limbs (20%), Type II was found in 35 limbs (35%), Type III was found in 13 limbs (13%), Type IV in no limbs (0%), and Type V in 20 limbs (20%). A sixth type was found in the remaining 12 limbs (12%), which demonstrated two slips of the tendon that both inserted onto the medial cuneiform.

Anomalies

Description

Macalister (1875) notes that in a case of clubfoot, tibialis anterior had a split tendon. One part of the tendon attached to the navicular and medial cuneiform and the other part attached to the talus and calcaneus. Macalister (1875) also notes that in a congenitally deformed limb described by Ringhoffer, tibialis anterior inserted onto the plantar fascia.

Hootnick et al. (1987) describe an individual that had a right limb with congenital tibial aplasia, talocalcaneal synchondrosis, and an adducted foot with five toes. In this limb, tibialis anterior inserted onto a flexor tendon sheet on the plantar aspect of the foot. Tibialis anterior was absent bilaterally in one neonate with trisomy 13 examined by Colacino and Pettersen (1978).

Prevalence

According to their literature review, Smith et al. (2015) found that tibialis anterior was absent in 1 out of 20 individuals (5%) with trisomy 13.

Clinical Implications

Tibioastragalus anticus may be useful for tendon transfer or a graft (Berkowitz et al. 2016).

Extensor hallucis longus (Figure 5.8)

Synonyms

This muscle may also be referred to as extensor proprius hallucis (Macalister 1875; Knott 1883b).

Typical Presentation

Description

Extensor hallucis longus originates from the midportion of the medial fibula and from the interosseous membrane (Standring 2016). The muscle ends in a tendon that inserts onto the base of the distal hallucal phalanx (Standring 2016). The tendon often expands to insert onto the base of the proximal hallucal phalanx (Standring 2016).

Innervation

Extensor hallucis longus is innervated by the deep fibular nerve (Standring 2016).

Comparative Anatomy

Extensor hallucis longus has a similar typical presentation in the apes, extending from the fibula and sometimes the lateral tibial condyle or interosseous membrane to the distal hallucal phalanx (Hepburn 1892; Beddard 1893; Sonntag 1924; Raven 1950; Miller 1952; Lewis 1966; Gibbs 1999; Ferrero 2011; Ferrero et al. 2012; Diogo et al. 2010, 2012, 2013a,b, 2017). There may be an insertion onto the proximal hallucal phalanx in bonobos and gorillas (Raven 1950; Miller 1952; Gibbs 1999; Vereecke et al. 2005; Diogo et al. 2017).

Variations

Description

Extensor hallucis longus may be joined with or send a slip to extensor digitorum longus or its tendon (Macalister 1875; Bergman et al. 1988; Lambert 2016; Standring 2016). It may also be joined with or send a slip to extensor hallucis brevis (Macalister 1875; Knott 1883b; Hallisy 1930; Bergman et al. 1988; Al-Saggaf 2003; Hill and Gerges

2008). The tendon may also have insertions onto the hallucal metatarsal, metatarsophalangeal joint capsule, or both phalanges of digit one (Mori 1964; Hallisy 1930; Bergman et al. 1988; Al-Saggaf 2003; Hill and Gerges 2008; Arora et al. 2011; Lambert 2016). Extensor hallucis longus may send a slip to digit two or join with the common extensor tendons of the toes (Hallisy 1930; Bergman et al. 1988; Lambert 2016; Standring 2016). Extensor hallucis longus may be doubled or tripled, presenting with multiple bellies with separate tendons (Macalister 1875; Hallisy 1930; Bergman et al. 1988; Lambert 2016).

Extensor hallucis longus is also associated with multiple named accessory bellies or tendons. One of these accessory muscles is referred to as extensor ossis metatarsi hallucis or extensor ossis primi metatarsi (Macalister 1875; Lambert 2016). It may present as a slip of extensor hallucis longus or as a distinct accessory muscle (Macalister 1875; Hallisy 1930; Lambert 2016). It may also present as a slip from tibialis anterior or extensor digitorum longus (Macalister 1875; Lambert 2016). This muscle usually inserts onto the distal part of the first metatarsal (Hallisy 1930; Lambert 2016). It may also present only as a tendon originating from the annular ligament with no belly (Macalister 1875).

Another associated muscle is referred to as extensor primi internodii hallucis (Wood) or extensor hallucis longus accessorius (s. minor) (Macalister 1875; Knott 1883b; Lambert 2016). It usually presents as a slip originating from extensor hallucis longus (Macalister 1875; Knott 1883b; Hallisy 1930; Lambert 2016). It can have a separate origin above extensor hallucis longus with an insertion joining extensor hallucis brevis (Macalister 1875). It may originate in the ankle from the tendon of extensor hallucis longus (Macalister 1875; Knott 1883b). It may also arise from extensor digitorum longus or tibialis anterior (Macalister 1875; Knott 1883b; Hallisy 1930; Lambert 2016). Hallisy (1930) notes an origin from the tibia. Extensor primi internodii hallucis typically inserts into the proximal hallucal phalanx (Macalister 1875; Hallisy 1930; Lambert 2016).

Lambert (2016) describes extensor hallucis capsularis as a synonym or variant of extensor primi internodii hallucis. This muscle presents as a slip or accessory tendon of extensor hallucis longus that inserts into the capsule of the first metatarsophalangeal joint (Tate and Pachnik 1976; Lundeen et al. 1983; Bibbo et al. 2004; Boyd et al. 2006; Bayer et al. 2014; Lambert 2016; Natsis et al. 2017). It may also originate from tibialis anterior (Bibbo et al. 2004; Boyd et al. 2006).

Accessory extensor digiti secundus may refer to an accessory slip that is situated between extensor hallucis longus and extensor digitorum longus (Tezer and Cicekcibasi 2012). It may originate from the tendon of extensor hallucis longus (Tezer and Cicekcibasi 2012). The tendon of this muscle joins the tendon of extensor digitorum longus to insert onto the second digit (Tezer and Cicekcibasi 2012). The tendon of extensor digiti secundus may also send a slip to the extensor hallucis longus tendon (Tezer and Cicekcibasi 2012).

Prevalence

Knott (1883b) found a slip extending from extensor hallucis longus to the base of the first metatarsal in 16 out of 40 cases (40%). Mori (1964) found that in 16% of cases, the tendon of extensor hallucis longus inserted onto the distal phalanx of digit one without sending slips to other structures. In 78% of cases, the tendon sent a slip to the proximal phalanx of digit one. In 2% of cases, the tendon divided into two slips that both inserted onto the distal phalanx of digit one. In 4% of cases, the tendon sent a slip to the base of the hallucal metatarsal.

Hallisy (1930) found that in 212 out of 290 feet (73.1%) extensor hallucis longus had a single typical insertion onto the base of the distal hallucal phalanx. In 70 feet (24.1%), the tendon sent a slip to the base of the proximal hallucal phalanx. In two cases (0.7%), the tendon divided into three slips, one going to the base of the distal phalanx of digit one and the other two inserting onto the base of the proximal phalanx. In two cases (0.7%), the tendon sent a slip to the distal part of the dorsal surface of the first metatarsal. In three cases (1%), the tendon sent a slip to the most medial tendon of extensor digitorum brevis (extensor hallucis brevis). In one case (0.3%), the muscle had both the normal tendon and a tendon that split from the normal tendon at the ankle joint to join with the extensor digitorum longus tendon going to digit two.

Hallisy (1930) found slips corresponding to extensor ossis primi metatarsi in 6 out of 290 feet (2.1%). In 3 feet (1%), it presented as a slip from the tendon of tibialis anterior that inserted onto the shaft of the first metatarsal just behind the head. In one case (0.3%), it presented as a separate tendon of tibialis anterior that inserted onto the head of the first metatarsal and base of the proximal hallucal phalanx. In 2 feet (0.7%), it presented as a slip from extensor hallucis longus and inserted onto the distal part of the dorsal surface of the first metatarsal.

Hallisy (1930) found slips corresponding to extensor primi internodii hallucis in 85 out of 290 feet (29.3%). In 72 feet (24.8%), extensor primi internodii hallucis presented as a secondary insertion of the extensor hallucis longus tendon into the base of the proximal phalanx of digit one. In seven cases (2.4%), it presented as a tendon from tibialis anterior that inserted onto the medial aspect of the proximal phalanx. In two cases (0.7%), it presented as a small muscular belly originating from tibialis anterior and inserting onto the medial aspect of the base of the proximal phalanx. In one case (0.3%), it presented as a muscular belly from the lateral aspect of the middle third of the tibia with an insertion onto the medial aspect of the base of the proximal phalanx. In one case (0.3%), it originated as a tendon with a separate muscular belly from extensor hallucis longus in the distal leg and inserted onto the proximal phalanx. In one case (0.3%), it originated as a tendon from extensor hallucis longus in the distal leg and inserted

onto the proximal phalanx. In one case (0.3%), it presented as a common insertion into the base of the proximal phalanx with the extensor ossis metatarsi tendon from tibialis anterior.

Al-Saggaf (2003) studied the insertions of extensor hallucis longus in 60 cadaveric lower limbs. In 39 limbs (65%), the muscle inserted as a single tendon onto the distal hallucal phalanx. In 16 cases (26.7%), the muscle inserted as two tendons. In nine of these 16 cases (15% of all limbs), the accessory tendon inserted onto the base of the proximal hallucal phalanx, distal to the insertion of extensor hallucis brevis. In three cases (5% of all limbs), the accessory tendon inserted with extensor hallucis brevis onto the base of the proximal hallucal phalanx. In two cases (3.3% of all limbs), the accessory tendon inserted onto the base of the proximal hallucal phalanx, medial to the insertion of extensor hallucis brevis. In two cases (3.3% of all limbs), the accessory tendon joined the tendon of extensor hallucis brevis, forming a common tendon that inserted onto the base of the proximal hallucal phalanx. In five cases (8.3%), the muscle had three tendons, with all accessory tendons inserting onto the first metatarsophalangeal joint.

In a sample of 32 cadaveric feet, Bibbo et al. (2004) found extensor hallucis capsularis tendons in 26 feet (81.3%). The tendons originated from extensor hallucis longus in 24 feet (92.3%) and from tibialis anterior in 2 feet (7.7%). In two cases (7.7%), a small muscle belly that was separate from extensor hallucis longus and tibialis anterior gave rise to the tendon. All tendons inserted onto the first metatarsophalangeal joint capsule.

In a sample of 81 cadaveric feet, Boyd et al. (2006) found 73 extensor hallucis capsularis tendons in 71 feet (87.7%). Out of the 73 tendons, 23 arose from the extensor hallucis longus muscle (31.5%), 45 arose from a bifurcation point off of extensor hallucis longus (61.6%), two arose from the tibialis anterior tendon (2.7%), one arose from the extensor hallucis brevis tendon (1.4%), and two tendons had unidentified origins (2.7%). Seventy-two tendons inserted into the metatarsophalangeal joint capsule of digit one (98.6%) and one inserted into the base of the proximal hallucal phalanx (1.4%).

Arora et al. (2011) studied extensor hallucis longus in 60 lower limbs from 30 cadavers. In 54 limbs (90%), the muscle inserted normally but in six limbs (10%) the muscle had doubled tendons. In four limbs (6.7%), the lateral tendon inserted onto the base of the distal hallucal phalanx and the medial tendon inserted onto the base of the proximal hallucal phalanx. In two limbs (3.3%), the lateral tendon inserted onto the base of the distal hallucal phalanx and the medial tendon inserted onto the head of the first metatarsal.

In a sample of 60 patients who underwent operative correction of hallux valgus and interphalangeus, Bayer et al. (2014) found extensor hallucis capsularis tendons in 59 cases (98.3%). In a sample of 98 cadaveric feet, Natsis et al. (2017) found accessory tendons of extensor hallucis longus in 26 feet (26.5%). In all cases, the accessory tendon inserted onto the metatarsophalangeal joint capsule of digit one.

Anomalies

Description

Windle (1893) found an extensor primi internodii hallucis on the left side of one female fetus with anencephaly. In a male fetus with anencephaly, Windle (1893) found that extensor hallucis longus inserted via two tendons. Bersu et al. (1976) describe two infants with Hanhart syndrome. In the infant with an intact right foot, the tendon of extensor hallucis longus fused with the tendon of extensor digitorum longus.

Aziz (1979) described the bilateral presence of extensor primi internodii hallucis in one female neonate with trisomy 18. On the right side, the muscle arose from the anterior surface of the distal tibia (the text says proximal tibia, but the illustration in the paper shows an origin from the distal tibia). The muscle coursed over the ankle joint medial to extensor hallucis longus and then split into three tendons. One tendon inserted onto the medial surface of the proximal hallucal phalanx. The second tendon inserted on the dorsal surface of the proximal hallucal phalanx. The third tendon inserted with the tendon of extensor hallucis longus onto the distal hallucal phalanx. On the left side, the muscle had one tendon that inserted onto the medial surface of the proximal hallucal phalanx.

Hootnick et al. (1987) describe an individual that had a right limb with congenital tibial aplasia, talocalcaneal synchondrosis, and adducted foot with five toes. A tendinous band replaced the tibia. In this limb, extensor hallucis longus originated from the medial side of the tendinous band. Its tendon divided into a main tendon with its usual insertion and two accessory tendons. One accessory tendon inserted onto connective tissue near the talus, and the second accessory tendon traveled with the tibialis anterior tendon to insert onto the common flexor tendon sheet. Extensor hallucis longus also sent a slip to the medial side of the extensor expansion.

Prevalence

In their literature review, Smith et al. (2015) found that extensor primi internodii hallucis was only present in 1 out of 17 individuals with trisomy 18 (5.9%).

Clinical Implications

Accessory tendons of extensor hallucis longus—particularly extensor hallucis capsularis tendons—are often associated with the presence of, but not necessarily the severity of, hallux valgus (Al-Saggaf 2003; Bibbo et al. 2004; Bayer et al. 2014; Natsis et al. 2017). The role of these accessory attachments in the development of hallux valgus is thus unclear.

Extensor digitorum longus (Figure 5.8)

Synonyms

N/A

Typical Presentation

Description

Extensor digitorum longus originates from the lateral tibial condyle, the medial fibular surface, and the interosseous membrane (Standring 2016). The muscle ends in a tendon that divides into four tendinous slips that go to digits two through five (Standring 2016). The tendons to digits two through four receive a contribution from extensor digitorum brevis (Standring 2016). Fibers from the lumbricals and interossei also contribute to form the dorsal digital expansions of each digit (Standring 2016). The dorsal digital expansions divide into three parts, with one slip inserting onto the base of the intermediate phalanx and two slips that unite on the dorsal aspect of the intermediate phalanx to insert onto the base of the distal phalanx (Standring 2016).

Innervation

Extensor digitorum longus is innervated by the deep fibular nerve (Standring 2016).

Comparative Anatomy

Extensor digitorum longus has a similar typical presentation in the apes, extending from the tibia, fibula, and associated fascial and aponeurotic structures to the dorsal aponeuroses of digits two through five (Hepburn 1892; Beddard 1893; MacDowell 1910; Sonntag 1924; Raven 1950; Miller 1952; Lewis 1966; Gibbs 1999; Vereecke et al. 2005; Diogo et al. 2010, 2012, 2013a,b, 2017). In orangutans, the origin may be fused with tibialis anterior and the tendon to digit two may be reduced or absent (Beddard 1893; Gibbs 1999; Ferrero 2011; Ferrero et al. 2012; Diogo et al. 2013b). The tendon to digit two may also be reduced or absent in common chimpanzees (Beddard 1893; Gibbs 1999). Extensor digitorum longus may send extra tendons to digit five in bonobos (Diogo et al. 2017).

Variations

Description

The terminal tendons, especially those going to digits two and five, may be doubled (Macalister 1875; Bergman et al. 1988; Lambert 2016; Standring 2016). The tendons going to digits three, four, or five may be reduced or absent, and in some cases replaced by tendons from other muscles (Macalister 1875; Stevenson 1921; Sakuma et al. 2004; Plochocki and Bodeen 2010; Sirasanagandla et al. 2014; Lambert 2016). The tendons of extensor digitorum longus may send accessory slips to various metatarsals and proximal phalanges, digit one, extensor digitorum brevis, extensor hallucis longus, extensor hallucis brevis, or the interossei (Macalister 1875; Knott 1883b; Bergman et al. 1988; Stevens et al. 1993; Lambert 2016; Standring 2016). The tendon going to digit five may receive contributions from, or join with, the tendon of fibularis tertius (Macalister 1875; Bergman et al. 1988; Stevens et al. 1993; Lambert 2016). Each tendon may have its own muscular belly (Macalister 1875).

Prevalence

In a sample of 30 cases, Knott (1883b) found slips to the medial most tendon of extensor digitorum longus that attached to the proximal phalanx of digit one in two cases (6.7%). Slips to the base of the proximal phalanx of digit two were found in two cases (6.7%). A slip from the tendon to digit five inserted onto the middle of the fifth metatarsal in one case (3.3%) and onto the base of the fifth metatarsal in two cases (6.7%). In one case (3.3%), slips from the tendons to digits three and four inserted onto the bases of the fourth and fifth metatarsals.

Mori (1964) found that in 34% of cases, the distal portion of extensor digitorum longus was divided into two layers, and the tendons to digits two and three arose from the superficial layer while the tendons to digits four and five arose from the deep layer. In 40% of cases, the distal part of the muscle was divided into two layers, and the superficial layer sent tendons to digits one, two, and three while the deep layer sent a tendon to digit five. In 26% of cases, the distal part of the muscle was not divided and sent tendons to digits two through five.

Stevens et al. (1993) studied the relationships between fibularis tertius and extensor digitorum longus in 40 cadaveric lower limbs. The origin of fibularis tertius was continuous with the origin of extensor digitorum longus in 33 limbs (82.5%). In six limbs (15%), the two muscles exchanged fibrous bands. In four limbs (10%), the tendons of the fibularis tertius and extensor digitorum longus were fused. In one limb (2.5%), the tendon of extensor digitorum longus going to digit five originated from the muscle belly of fibularis tertius. In two limbs (5%), extensor digitorum longus sent a slip to the fifth metatarsal. In one limb (2.5%), both muscles gave slips that fused together and then inserted onto the fifth metatarsal.

Anomalies

Description

Macalister (1875) notes that in a deformed limb, Ringhoffer found that extensor digitorum longus sent one tendon to digit two, two tendons to digit four, and one tendon to digit five. Bersu et al. (1976) describe two infants with Hanhart syndrome. In the infant with an intact right foot, the tendon of extensor hallucis longus fused with the tendon of extensor digitorum longus. On the right side of a neonate with trisomy 13, Pettersen et al. (1979) found that extensor digitorum longus sent an extra tendon to the head of the fifth metatarsal.

Mieden (1982) describes an infant with median cleft lip, hypotelorism, and alobar holoprosencephaly. On the left side, the tendons of extensor digitorum brevis and longus were attached to the metatarsophalangeal joints (Mieden 1982). On the left foot of a male neonate with Meckel syndrome, Pettersen (1984) found that the extensor digitorum longus tendon to the second digit was rudimentary and the tendons to digits three and four were absent.

Hootnick et al. (1987) describe an individual that had a right limb with congenital tibial aplasia, talocalcaneal synchondrosis, and an adducted foot with five toes. In this limb, extensor digitorum longus became tendinous just above the ankle joint and entered the dorsal surface of the foot at a right angle as it coursed under the extensor retinaculum. Its tendon split into four slips that entered the extensor expansions of digits two through five. The lateral most slip contributed to the fibularis tertius tendon.

In the fetus with trisomy 18 and cyclopia dissected by Smith et al. (2015), the right extensor digitorum longus exchanged a slip with the tendon of fibularis tertius at the fourth digit and did not send a tendon to digit five. On the right side of a fetus with craniorachischisis dissected by Alghamdi et al. (2017), the tendon of extensor digitorum longus going to digit three sent a slip to the tendon going to digit four. In the female fetus with trisomy 18 dissected by Alghamdi et al. (2018), extensor digitorum longus was proximally fused with fibularis tertius bilaterally.

Prevalence

N/A

Clinical Implications

Understanding variations and potential absences of extensor digitorum longus tendons is important when planning to use these tendons for tendon grafts (Sakuma et al. 2004).

FIBULARIS TERTIUS (FIGURE 5.8)

Synonyms

This muscle may also be referred to as peroneus tertius (Macalister 1875; Standring 2016).

Typical Presentation

Description

Fibularis tertius originates from the distal third of the medial fibula, the interosseous membrane, and the anterior intermuscular septum (Standring 2016). It inserts via a tendon onto the base of the fifth metatarsal (Standring 2016).

Innervation

Fibularis tertius is innervated by the deep fibular nerve (Standring 2016).

Comparative Anatomy

Fibularis tertius is variably present among the apes (Gibbs 1999; Diogo et al. 2010, 2012, 2013a,b, 2017). It seems to be absent in orangutans and present in about half of gibbons, 30% of gorillas, and 5% of common chimpanzees (Gibbs 1999; Diogo et al. 2010, 2012, 2013a,b, 2017). In some bonobos, extensor digitorum longus sends an additional tendon to the fifth metatarsal (Diogo et al. 2017). This extra slip may correspond to fibularis tertius (Diogo et al. 2017).

Variations

Description

Fibularis tertius may be enlarged, reduced, or absent (Hallett 1848; Macalister 1875; Le Double 1897; Bergman et al. 1988; Stevens et al. 1993; Chaney et al. 1996; Joshi et al. 2006; Rourke et al. 2007; Peddity and Velichety 2013; Lambert 2016; Standring 2016; Albay and Candan 2017; Olewnik 2019). Its origin may be shifted more proximally on the fibula (Macalister 1875; Stevens et al. 1993; Joshi et al. 2006; Rourke et al. 2007). Yildiz and Yalcin (2012) report an origin of fibularis tertius from extensor hallucis longus.

The origin of fibularis tertius is often continuous with the origin of extensor digitorum longus (Stevens et al. 1993; Lambert 2016). The tendon of fibularis tertius may be connected or fused with the tendon of extensor digitorum longus going to digit five (Macalister 1875; Bergman et al. 1988; Stevens et al. 1993; Joshi et al. 2006; Lambert 2016). Fibularis tertius may present as a tendinous band that arises from extensor digitorum longus (Macalister 1875; Rourke et al. 2007; Peddity and Velichety 2013; Olewnik 2019). Fibularis tertius may replace the tendon going to digit five when the tendon of extensor digitorum longus to this digit is absent (Macalister 1875; Stevenson 1921; Lambert 2016). Fibularis tertius may send a slip to the digit five tendon of extensor digitorum brevis (Macalister 1875).

Its insertion may expand to the shaft of the fifth metatarsal (Joshi et al. 2006; Lambert 2016; Standring 2016; Olewnik 2019). It may insert onto the extensor aponeurosis or proximal phalanx of digit five (Macalister 1875; Krammer et al. 1979; Joshi et al. 2006; Jana and Roy 2011; Lambert 2016). The tendon of fibularis tertius may be doubled or it may split into two or three parts prior to insertion (Macalister 1875; Stevens et al. 1993; Raheja et al. 2005; Joshi et al. 2006; Rourke et al. 2007; Lambert and Atsas 2010; Jana and Roy 2011; Lambert 2016; Olewnik 2019). It may attach onto or send a slip to the fourth metatarsal or insert entirely onto this bone in some cases (Macalister 1875; Mori 1964; Bergman et al. 1988; Raheja et al. 2005; Joshi et al. 2006; Rourke et al. 2007; Lambert 2016; Standring 2016; Nayak 2017; Olewnik 2019). It may send an accessory tendon to the fascia that covers the fourth interosseus muscle (the fourth interosseous space) (Macalister 1875; Joshi et al. 2006; Lambert 2016; Olewnik 2019). Fibularis tertius may connect with flexor digiti minimi brevis or the tendon of fibularis brevis (Jana and Roy 2011; Olewnik 2019). Sirasanagandla et al. (2014) report a case in which the fibularis tertius tendon divided into three slips, one that inserted on the base of the distal phalanx of digit five, another that inserted onto the base of the fifth metatarsal, and one that inserted into the fascia over the ankle joint capsule.

Fibularis tertius may be doubled (Macalister 1875; Lambert and Atsas 2010; Plochocki and Bodeen 2010; Lambert 2016). Macalister (1875) notes a case in which the posterior muscle of the doubled fibularis tertius sent two tendons to the fifth metatarsal while the anterior muscle sent slips to digit five and to the fourth metatarsal. Plochocki and Bodeen (2010) found a supernumerary fibularis tertius muscle distal to the main muscle. The supernumerary muscle arose from the medial margin and diaphysis of the fibula and the interosseous membrane. It ended in a tendon that passed anterior to the lateral malleolus and deep to the extensor retinaculum and split into two slips that inserted into the calcaneus. It was supplied by the deep fibular nerve.

Prevalence

Macalister (1875) notes that fibularis tertius may be absent in 10% of individuals. Chaney et al. (1996) found that fibularis tertius was absent in 25 out of 282 limbs (8.9%). Albay and Candan (2017) studied the fibular muscles in 200 limbs from 100 fetuses. Fibularis tertius was absent in 40 limbs (20%). Krammer et al. (1979) found that peroneus tertius was present in 157 out of 169 lower limbs, yielding an absence of 7.1% (12 limbs). Mori (1964) found that the tendon of fibularis tertius inserted onto the base of the fifth metatarsal in 68% of cases and onto the base of the fourth metatarsal in 32% of cases.

Stevens et al. (1993) studied fibularis tertius and its relationships with extensor digitorum longus in 40 cadaveric lower limbs. The origin of fibularis tertius was continuous with the origin of extensor digitorum longus in 33 limbs (82.5%). In six limbs (15%), the two muscles exchanged fibrous bands. In four limbs (10%), the tendons of the fibularis tertius and extensor digitorum longus were fused. In one limb (2.5%), the tendon of extensor digitorum longus going to digit five originated from the muscle belly of fibularis tertius. In one limb (2.5%), both muscles gave slips that fused together and then inserted onto the fifth metatarsal. Fibularis tertius was absent in two limbs (5%). In 35 limbs (87.5%), fibularis tertius originated from the lower middle quarter of the fibula. In 37 limbs (92.5%), fibularis tertius had a single tendon, and in one limb (2.5%), it had a double tendon. The insertion of fibularis tertius onto the fifth metatarsal was bifurcated in two limbs (5%) and trifurcated in one limb (2.5%).

Joshi et al. (2006) studied fibularis tertius in 220 lower limbs from 110 cadavers. The muscle was absent in 14 right limbs and nine left limbs, being absent in a total of 23 limbs (10.5%). Out of the 96 right limbs in which the muscle was present, the muscle had a normal origin from the distal third of the fibula in 46 limbs (47.9%), an extensive origin from the lower half of the fibula in 31 limbs (32.3%), and a very extensive origin from the lower three quarters of the fibula in 19 limbs (19.8%). Also out of these 96 right limbs, the muscle inserted onto the base of the fifth metatarsal in 44 limbs (45.8%), onto the base and shaft of the fifth metatarsal in 11 limbs (11.5%), onto the base and shaft of the fifth metatarsal and the fourth interosseous space in 22 limbs (22.9%), and had other insertions in 19 limbs (19.8%). Out of the 101 left limbs in which the muscle was present, the muscle had a normal origin from the distal third of the fibula in 55 limbs (54.5%), an extensive origin from the lower half of the fibula in 29 limbs (28.7%), and a very extensive origin from the lower three quarters of the fibula in 17 limbs (16.8%). Also out of these 101 left limbs, the muscle inserted onto the base of the fifth metatarsal in 55 limbs (54.5%), onto the base and shaft of the fifth metatarsal in 13 limbs (12.8%), onto the base and shaft of the fifth metatarsal and the fourth interosseous space in 14 limbs (13.9%), and had other insertions in 19 limbs (18.8%).

Rourke et al. (2007) examined fibularis tertius in 82 lower limbs from 41 cadavers. The muscle was absent in five limbs (6.1%). In one limb (1.2%), the tendon was doubled and inserted onto the shafts of the fourth and fifth metatarsals. In all other limbs, the tendons had a single insertion onto the shafts of both these bones. Nayak (2017) studied fibularis tertius in 100 cadaveric limbs. Fibularis tertius was present in all limbs (100%). In all limbs (100%), it originated from the distal fourth of the fibula. In 94 limbs (94%), it inserted onto the base of the fifth metatarsal. In four limbs (4%), it inserted onto the fifth metatarsal up to the metatarsophalangeal joint. In two limbs (2%), it inserted near the base of the fourth metatarsal.

Yammine and Erić (2017) conducted a literature review of 35 studies regarding the anatomy of fibularis tertius. Out of 7,601 legs, they found that the muscle was present in 93.2% of cadaveric legs and in 80% of legs examined in clinical studies. Out of the 1,026 legs for which the origin of the muscle was recorded, it originated from the distal half of the fibula in 721 cases (70.3%), the distal third of the fibula in 133 cases (13%), and from extensor digitorum longus in 162 cases (15.8%). Out of the 1,248 limbs for which the insertion was recorded, it inserted on the shaft of the fifth metatarsal in 152 cases (12.2%), the base of the fifth metatarsal in 252 cases (20.2%), both the base and shaft in 292 cases (23.4%), both the fourth and fifth metatarsals in 423 cases (33.9%), the fourth metatarsal in 38 cases (3%), and onto the tendon of extensor digitorum longus in 24 cases (2%). A slip to the head of the fifth metatarsal or to the base of digit five was found in 67 cases (5.3%).

Olewnik (2019) studied fibularis tertius in a sample of 106 cadaveric lower limbs. Fibularis tertius was absent in 15 limbs (14.2%). Out of the 91 limbs in which the muscle was present, it originated from the distal half of the fibula and intermuscular septum in 61 limbs (67%) and the distal third of the fibula and intermuscular septum in 20 limbs (22%). In ten limbs (11%), the muscle belly was missing and the fibularis tertius tendon arose from the extensor digitorum longus tendon. In 41 limbs (45%), the tendon had a single insertion onto the shaft of the fifth metatarsal. In 20 limbs (22%), the tendon had a single insertion onto the base of the fifth metatarsal. In 15 limbs (16.5%), the tendon had a single, broad insertion onto the base and shaft of the fifth metatarsal and the fascia over the fourth interosseous space. In eight limbs (8.8%), the tendon had a split insertion, with one slip going to the base of the fifth metatarsal and an accessory slip going to the shaft of this bone. In five lower limbs (5.5%), the tendon had a split insertion, with one slip inserting onto the base of the fifth metatarsal and

an accessory slip going to the base of the fourth metatarsal. In two limbs (2.2%), the tendon was fused with a slip from the fibularis brevis tendon and the fourth interosseous muscle originated from this fusion.

Several researchers have used clinical assessments to visualize and palpate the fibularis tertius tendon. Witvrouw et al. (2006) used palpation to determine the presence of fibularis tertius in a sample of 200 limbs from 100 individuals. These authors found that fibularis tertius was absent in 37 limbs (18.5%).

Ramirez et al. (2010) used palpation to determine the presence of fibularis tertius in a sample of 336 limbs from 168 individuals from Chile. These authors were able to identify fibularis tertius in 49.11% of limbs. Ashaolu et al. (2013) used palpation to determine the presence of fibularis tertius in a sample of 200 limbs from 100 individuals in Nigeria. These authors were able to identify fibularis tertius in 125 limbs (62.5%). Potu et al. (2016) used palpation to determine the presence of fibularis tertius in a sample of 390 legs from 195 Southeastern Indian individuals. These authors were able to identify the muscle in 203 legs (52.1%). Salem et al. (2018) used palpation to determine the presence of fibularis tertius in a sample of 1,248 Arab patients. The sample included 439 individuals from Bahrain, 208 individuals from Saudi Arabia, 153 individuals from Kuwait, 198 individuals from Tunisia, and 250 individuals from Egypt. The authors were able to identify the presence of fibularis tertius in 42% of the Bahraini individuals, 38.5% of Saudi individuals, 41.2% of Kuwaiti individuals, 67.7% of Tunisian individuals, and 52.8% of Egyptian individuals. Palomo-López et al. (2019) used palpation to determine the presence of fibularis tertius in a sample of 481 individuals in Spain. These authors were able to identify the presence of fibularis tertius in 184 participants (38.3%).

Anomalies

Description

On the left side of a female fetus with anencephaly, Windle (1893) noted that fibularis tertius formed the bulk of the muscle belly of extensor digitorum longus. This author also found that fibularis tertius was enlarged in a male fetus with anencephaly. In a male infant with triploidy studied by Moen et al. (1984), this muscle was absent bilaterally. In a male neonate with Meckel syndrome, Pettersen (1984) observed that peroneus tertius was absent on the right side. On the left side, this muscle was attached to the fifth and sixth metatarsals.

In four neonates with trisomy 13, Colacino and Pettersen (1978) found that fibularis tertius was absent bilaterally in all four cases. Fibularis tertius was absent bilaterally in two neonates with trisomy 18 and three neonates with trisomy 13 (Aziz 1979, 1980, 1981), and in a boy with trisomy 13q described by Pettersen (1979). In the fetus with trisomy 18 and cyclopia dissected by Smith et al. (2015), the right fibularis tertius exchanged a slip with the tendon of extensor digitorum longus at the fourth digit, had a separate fleshy head, and had a distally shifted insertion. In the female fetus with trisomy 18 dissected by Alghamdi et al. (2018), extensor digitorum longus was proximally fused with fibularis tertius bilaterally.

Prevalence

In their literature review, Smith et al. (2015) found that fibularis tertius was absent in 12 out of 20 individuals with trisomy 13 (60%) and absent in 2 out of 17 individuals with trisomy 18 (11.8%).

Clinical Implications

Witvrouw et al. (2006) found that individuals who lack fibularis tertius are not at higher risk for ankle ligament injuries.

ANTERIOR FIBULOCALCANEUS (FIGURE 5.8)

Synonyms
N/A

Typical Presentation
This muscle is only present as a variation.

Comparative Anatomy
N/A

Variations

Description

Anterior fibulocalcaneus is an accessory fibular muscle considered to be in the anterior compartment of the leg (Lambert and Atsas 2010; Lambert et al. 2011b; Upadhyay and Amiras 2015; Lambert 2016). It has been found in association with the doubling of fibularis tertius and its tendon (Lambert and Atsas 2010), as well as the absence of fibularis tertius (Upadhyay and Amiras 2015).

Anterior fibulocalcaneus originates from the fibula, anterior intermuscular septum, and the fascia covering fibularis tertius (Lambert and Atsas 2010; Lambert et al. 2011b; Upadhyay and Amiras 2015; Lambert 2016). Its origin on the fibula varies, with recorded origins ranging from the head to the distal half of the bone (Lambert and Atsas 2010; Lambert et al. 2011b; Lambert 2016). It courses anterior to the lateral malleolus and inserts onto the lateral surface of the calcaneus in the region of the peroneal trochlea (Lambert and Atsas 2010; Lambert et al. 2011b; Upadhyay and Amiras 2015; Lambert 2016). Its tendon may send a slip to the capsule of the talocrural joint (Lambert and Atsas 2010).

Innervation

Anterior fibulocalcaneus is innervated by the deep fibular nerve (Lambert et al. 2011b).

Prevalence

Prevalence is unknown but, to our knowledge, anterior fibulocalcaneus has been only found bilaterally in three individuals (Lambert and Atsas 2010; Lambert et al. 2011b) and unilaterally in one individual (Upadhyay and Amiras 2015).

Anomalies
N/A

Clinical Implications

Clinicians should consider the presence of anterior fibulocalcaneus as a potential cause of ankle pain (Lambert and Atsas 2010; Lambert et al. 2011b; Upadhyay and Amiras 2015).

FIBULARIS LONGUS (FIGURE 5.9)

See also: Fibularis quartus

Synonyms

This muscle may also be referred to as peroneus longus (Macalister 1875; Standring 2016).

Typical Presentation

Description

Fibularis longus originates from the head and lateral surface of the fibula, and from the anterior and posterior intermuscular septa (Standring 2016). It ends in a tendon that inserts by one slip onto the base of the first metatarsal and by another slip onto the medial cuneiform (Standring 2016).

Innervation

Fibularis longus is innervated by the superficial fibular nerve (Standring 2016).

Comparative Anatomy

Fibularis longus has a similar typical presentation in the apes, extending from the proximal fibula to the first metatarsal (Hepburn 1892; Beddard 1893; MacDowell 1910; Sonntag 1924; Raven 1950; Miller 1952; Lewis 1966; Gibbs 1999; Vereecke et al. 2005; Ferrero 2011; Ferrero et al. 2012; Diogo et al. 2010, 2012, 2013a,b, 2017). It may have an additional origin from the lateral condyle of the tibia and have a fibrous connection to the fifth metatarsal in gibbons, common chimpanzees, and bonobos (Miller 1952; Lewis 1966; Gibbs 1999; Diogo et al. 2013a, 2017). In orangutans, it may be fused or otherwise connected with fibularis brevis, extensor digitorum longus, and flexor hallucis longus (Beddard 1893; Sonntag 1924; Gibbs 1999).

Variations

Description

Some fibers from the lateral tibial condyle, and more rarely the lateral femoral condyle, may contribute to the origin of this muscle (Bergman et al. 1988; Standring 2016). Mehta et al. (2011a) report a case in which fibularis longus was divided into superficial and deep portions, with the superficial belly inserting onto the first metatarsal and the deep

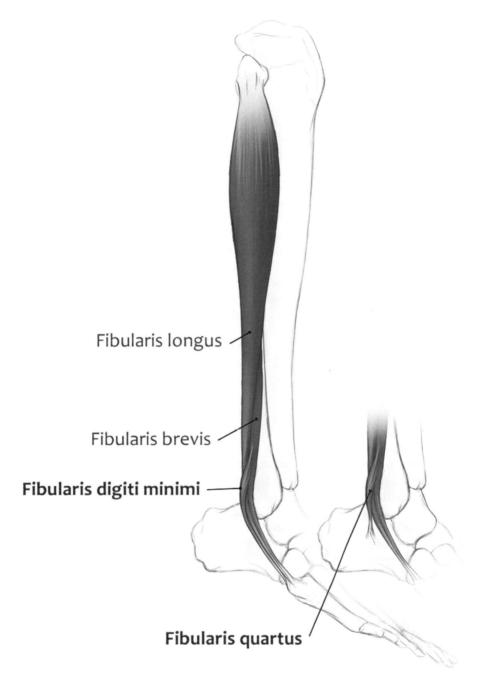

Fibularis longus

Fibularis brevis

Fibularis digiti minimi

Fibularis quartus

FIGURE 5.9 Lateral muscles of the lower leg in lateral view. Fibularis quartus is illustrated on the right side, and the other muscles are illustrated on the left.

belly inserting onto the lateral aspect of the calcaneus. This variation was also associated with a split fibularis brevis.

As many as four slips of insertion may be present (Verma et al. 2011; Verma and Arora 2012). The insertion onto the medial cuneiform may be absent (Mori 1964; Shyamsundar et al. 2012; Chhaparwal et al. 2015; Edama et al. 2020) or doubled (Verma and Arora 2012). Its insertion may have an additional attachment onto the first metatarsal (Macalister 1875; Knott 1883b; Jayakumari et al. 2006; Lambert 2016). Accessory slips may pass to the base of the second, third, fourth, or fifth metatarsals (Macalister 1875;

Knott 1883b; Shyamsundar et al. 2012; Verma and Arora 2012; Lambert 2016; Standring 2016; Edama et al. 2020). Slips may insert onto the navicular or tendon of tibialis posterior (Mori 1964). A slip may pass to the first interosseous space (Jayakumari et al. 2006; Chhaparwal et al. 2015; Edama et al. 2020). It may have an insertion onto the calcaneus (Athavale et al. 2012b; Shyamsundar et al. 2012) or intermediate cuneiform (Lambert 2016). Fibularis longus may connect to the cuboid (Patil et al. 2007; Cromeens and Reeves 2011; Athavale et al. 2012b; Lambert 2016; Edama et al. 2020). It may also send a slip to the lateral malleolus or lateral ligaments of the ankle (Macalister 1875). Via the anterior or posterior frenular ligaments, the tendon of fibularis longus may have connections to flexor digiti minimi brevis, opponens digiti minimi, some interosseous muscles, and the fifth metatarsal (Edama et al. 2020).

In rare cases, fibularis longus may fuse with fibularis brevis (Macalister 1875; Knott 1883b; Jayakumari et al. 2006; Lambert 2016; Standring 2016). A slip may extend to adductor hallucis (Standring 2016) or flexor hallucis brevis (Chhaparwal et al. 2015). Tibialis posterior may send a slip or insert onto the tendon of fibularis longus (Mori 1964; Lohrmann et al. 1997; Bloome et al. 2003; Raheja et al. 2005; Chhaparwal et al. 2015; Lambert 2016; Edama et al. 2020). Flexor digiti minimi brevis, the oblique head of adductor hallucis, and some interosseus muscles may originate from the fibularis longus tendon (Lamont 1908; Ochiltree 1912; Harbeson 1933, 1938; Bergman et al. 1988; Jayakumari et al. 2006; Verma et al. 2011; Chhaparwal et al. 2015; Lambert 2016; Edama et al. 2020).

Prevalence

In a sample of 40 cases, Knott (1883b) found that fibularis longus was fused with fibularis brevis in three cases (7.5%). In two cases (5%), a slip from the tendon went to the base of the fifth metatarsal. In one case (2.5%), a slip passed to the head of the first metatarsal. In one case each (2.5%), a slip passed to the base of the third and fourth metatarsals.

Mori (1964) found that fibularis longus inserted onto the first metatarsal in 64% of cases, the first metatarsal and medial cuneiform in 28% of cases, the first metatarsal and navicular in 2% of cases, and the first metatarsal, medial cuneiform, and tendon of tibialis posterior in 4% of cases. Mori (1964) also found that in 10% of cases, the tendon of tibialis posterior inserted onto the navicular, medial cuneiform, and tendon of fibularis longus.

Bloome et al. (2003) studied the insertions of the tibialis posterior tendon in 11 feet from 10 cadavers. Each tendon had three distinct bands and their insertions included the fibularis longus tendon in four cases (36.4%). Athavale et al. (2012b) studied the peroneal muscles in 92 cadaveric lower limbs. In five cases (5.4%), the fibularis longus tendon split into two slips. The accessory slip inserted into the cuboid in one case, the peroneal trochlea in two cases, and joined with the main tendon of fibularis longus in two cases.

Shyamsundar et al. (2012) studied the insertion of fibularis longus in 26 feet from 14 cadavers. All 26 feet had an insertion onto the first metatarsal, but the insertion onto the medial cuneiform was absent in four specimens (15.4%). Slips passed to the base of the fourth/fifth metatarsals in 12 feet (46.2%), base of the third metatarsal in 2 feet (7.7%), base of the second metatarsal in 8 feet (30.8%), and to the calcaneus in 8 feet (30.8%).

Chhaparwal et al. (2015) studied the insertion of fibularis longus in 38 feet from 19 cadavers. In 15 feet (39.5%), fibularis longus had a normal insertion onto the base of the first metatarsal and the medial cuneiform. In 4 feet (10.5%),

the tendon flared into a triangular expansion and had a normal insertion. In 9 feet (23.7%), the tendon flared into a triangular expansion and had a normal insertion but received a slip from tibialis posterior. In 1 foot (2.6%), the tendon sent a slip to flexor hallucis brevis, and in 3 feet (7.9%), the tendon sent a slip to the first interosseous space. In 4 feet (10.5%), the tendon inserted onto the first metatarsal only. In 2 feet (5.3%), the oblique head of adductor hallucis arose from the tendon.

Edama et al. (2020) studied the insertion of fibularis longus in 104 feet from 52 Japanese cadavers. The fibularis longus tendon received a slip from the tibialis posterior tendon in 32 feet (30.8%). All feet exhibited an insertion into the first metatarsal. Additional insertions were present onto the medial cuneiform in 21 feet (20.2%) and the first dorsal interosseous muscle in 38 feet (36.5%). The anterior frenular ligament was present in 33 feet (31.7%), and it attached to flexor digiti minimi brevis and opponens digiti minimi in 33 feet (31.7%), the second plantar interosseous muscle in 13 feet (12.5%), the third plantar interosseous muscle in 29 feet (27.9%), the fourth dorsal interosseous muscle in 20 feet (19.3%), and the fifth metatarsal in 9 feet (8.7%). The posterior frenular ligament was present in 6 feet (5.8%), and it attached to the fourth metatarsal in 4 feet (3.9%), the fifth metatarsal in 1 foot (1%), and the cuboid in 1 foot (1%).

Anomalies

Description

Macalister (1875) notes that in a case of clubfoot, fibularis longus inserted via three tendons onto the first, third, and fifth metatarsals. Hootnick et al. (1987) describe an individual that had a right limb with congenital tibial aplasia, talocalcaneal synchondrosis, and an adducted foot with five toes. In this limb, fibularis longus became tendinous at midleg. Its tendon inserted onto the distal end of the fibula. Its tendon sent a slip to the connective tissue of the groove posterior to the lateral malleolus.

In a male fetus with triploidy studied by Moen et al. (1984), fibularis longus had an extra slip attaching to the calcaneus on the left side. In a female fetus with trisomy 18, the proximal two thirds of fibularis longus and fibularis brevis were fused bilaterally (Alghamdi et al. 2018). Pettersen et al. (1979) found extra slips of fibularis longus in two male neonates with trisomy 13. On the left side of one specimen, a thin tendon originated from the muscle belly of fibularis longus and crossed the fibularis brevis tendon to insert onto the posterolateral calcaneal surface. On the right side of the second specimen, a supernumerary muscle belly originated from the anterior intermuscular septum just anterior to fibularis longus. This belly became tendinous in the middle of the lower leg and crossed the fibularis brevis tendon to insert onto the anterolateral calcaneal surface. On the left side of this same specimen, two supernumerary muscles originated anterior to fibularis longus. One inserted onto the posterior surface of the lateral malleolus, and the other inserted onto the inferior peroneal retinaculum of the calcaneus.

Prevalence

In their literature review, Smith et al. (2015) found that the extra slips of fibularis longus found by Pettersen et al. (1979) were only present in the two neonates they described, out of a sample of 20 individuals with trisomy 13 (10%).

Clinical Implications

Mehta et al. (2011a) suggest that doubled peroneal muscles and tendons could potentially contribute to ankle instability and lateral ankle pain.

FIBULARIS BREVIS (FIGURE 5.9)

See also: Fibularis quartus

Synonyms

This muscle may also be referred to as peroneus brevis (Macalister 1875; Standring 2016).

Typical Presentation

Description

Fibularis brevis originates from the distal two-thirds of the lateral fibula and from the anterior and posterior intermuscular septa (Standring 2016). Its tendon inserts onto the lateral surface of the base of the fifth metatarsal (Standring 2016).

Innervation

Fibularis brevis is innervated by the superficial fibular nerve (Standring 2016).

Comparative Anatomy

Fibularis brevis has a similar typical presentation in the apes, extending from the distal fibula to the base of the fifth metatarsal (Hepburn 1892; Beddard 1893; MacDowell 1910; Sonntag 1924; Raven 1950; Miller 1952; Lewis 1966; Gibbs 1999; Vereecke et al. 2005; Diogo et al. 2010, 2012, 2013a,b, 2017). It may have an insertion into the tendon of extensor digitorum brevis going to digit five in orangutans and common chimpanzees (Champneys 1872; Hepburn 1892; Beddard 1893; MacDowell 1910; Sonntag 1924; Gibbs 1999; Ferrero 2011; Ferrero et al. 2012). In common chimpanzees, it may have an insertion onto the proximal or intermediate phalanges of digit five (Champneys 1872; MacDowell 1910; Diogo et al. 2013a).

Variations

Description

The tendon of fibularis brevis may insert onto the dorsal surface, shaft, and/or distal aspect of the fifth metatarsal (Knott 1883b; Mori 1964; Bergman et al. 1988; Lambert 2016; Olewnik et al. 2019b; Rosser et al. 2019). The tendon may also insert into the fourth dorsal interosseous muscle (Knott 1883b; Bergman et al. 1988; Lambert 2016). The tendon may also be truncated and insert onto or near the peroneal trochlea without extending into the foot (Athavale et al. 2012b; Lucas

et al. 2013; Cecava and Campbell 2015). It may send a slip to the extensor tendon of digit five (Knott 1883b). It may send a slip to the distal phalanges of digits four or five (Mori 1964). A slip from the fibularis brevis tendon to the metatarsal, dorsal digital expansion, or phalanges of digit five may be designated as fibularis digiti minimi (Cunningham and St. John Brooks 1889–1891; Le Double 1897; Macalister 1867b, 1875; Raheja et al. 2005; Jadhav et al. 2013; Lambert 2016; Chaney et al. 2018; Olewnik et al. 2019b) (see the entry for this muscle).

In rare cases, fibularis brevis may fuse with fibularis longus (Macalister 1875; Knott 1883b; Jayakumari et al. 2006; Lambert 2016; Standring 2016). It may have an attachment with flexor digiti minimi brevis or send a slip to fibularis tertius (Knott 1883b; Bergman et al. 1988; Lambert 2016; Olewnik et al. 2019b). It may contribute to the origin of abductor digiti minimi (Macalister 1875; Lambert 2016) or the fourth dorsal interosseous muscle (Olewnik et al. 2019b). Mehta et al. (2011a) report a case in which fibularis brevis was divided into superficial/lateral and deep/medial portions, with the superficial/lateral belly inserting onto the fifth metatarsal and the deep/medial belly inserting onto the lateral aspect of the calcaneus. This variation was also associated with a split fibularis longus.

Prevalence

Knott (1883b) found that in 6 out of 40 cases (15%), fibularis brevis sent a slip to the extensor tendon of digit five. In a review of 200 MRI examinations, Cecava and Campbell (2015) found two cases (1%) of the fibularis brevis tendon ending on the calcaneus. Mori (1964) found that fibularis brevis inserted onto the base of the fifth metatarsal in 47% of cases, sent a slip to the distal part of the fifth metatarsal in 10% of cases, and sent a slip to the distal phalanx of the fourth digit in 5% of cases. Mori (1964) found that the tendon sent a slip to the distal phalanx of digit five in 20% of cases, with this slip having a separate muscular belly in 8% of cases.

Olewnik et al. (2019b) studied the insertion of fibularis brevis in 102 lower limbs. In 72 cases (70.6%), the tendon had a single insertion onto the base of the fifth metatarsal. In 30 cases (29.4%), the tendon had a bifurcated attachment with the main tendon having a normal insertion onto the fifth metatarsal. In 23 cases (22.5%), the accessory tendon inserted onto the dorsal surface of the base of the fifth metatarsal. In five cases (4.9%), the accessory tendon sent a band to the dorsal surface of the base of the fifth metatarsal and a band to the shaft of the fifth metatarsal. In two cases (2%), the accessory tendon sent a band to the dorsal surface of the base of the fifth metatarsal while another band fused with fibularis tertius and gave origin to the fourth dorsal interosseous muscle.

Anomalies

Description

In a female fetus with trisomy 18, the proximal two-thirds of fibularis longus and fibularis brevis were fused bilaterally (Alghamdi et al. 2018).

N/A

Clinical Implications

Mehta et al. (2011a) suggest that doubled peroneal muscles and tendons could potentially contribute to ankle instability and lateral ankle pain. An insertion of the fibularis brevis tendon onto the calcaneus may be misdiagnosed as a tear of the tendon (Lucas et al. 2013; Cecava and Campbell 2015).

FIBULARIS QUARTUS (FIGURE 5.9)

See also: Fibularis longus, Fibularis brevis

Synonyms

This muscle may also be referred to as peroneus quartus (Macalister 1875; Bergman et al. 1988), peroneocalcaneus externum (Otto) (Donley and Leyes 2001; Sookur et al. 2008; Lambert 2016), or fibulocalcaneus externus (Albay and Candan 2017). Other synonyms include peroneus sextus, peroneus calcaneus externus, or peroneus medius (Le Double 1897; Knott 1883a; Lambert 2016).

Typical Presentation

This muscle is only present as a variation or anomaly.

Comparative Anatomy

Fibularis quartus appears to be a muscle variation unique to humans (Hecker 1923; Athavale et al. 2012b; Lambert 2016). As such, muscles equivalent to fibularis quartus—accessory fibular muscles in the lateral compartment that insert onto the calcaneus—have not been found in the apes (Gibbs 1999; Diogo et al. 2010; 2012, 2013a,b, 2017).

Variations

Description

Fibularis quartus is an accessory muscle found in the lateral compartment of the leg (Chaney et al. 1996; Sookur et al. 2008; Lambert 2016; Standring 2016). It typically originates from the posterior intermuscular septum, from the bellies of fibularis brevis or fibularis longus, and/or from the distal fibula (Wood 1867b; Macalister 1867b, 1875; Knott 1883a; Hecker 1923; Bergman et al. 1988; Sobel et al. 1990; Sammarco and Brainard 1991; Chaney et al. 1996; Chepuri et al. 2001; Donley and Leyes 2001; Zammit and Singh 2003; Sookur et al. 2008; Athavale et al. 2012b; Clarkson et al. 2013; Hur et al. 2015a; Lambert 2016; Standring 2016; Albay and Candan 2017; Mustafa et al. 2017).

The tendon of fibularis quartus courses medial and posterior to the tendons of fibularis brevis and fibularis longus (Macalister 1867b, 1875; Cheung et al. 1997; Sookur et al. 2008). It most often inserts onto the lateral surface of the calcaneus, usually into the retrotrochlear eminence or peroneal trochlea (Macalister 1867b, 1875; Wood 1867b; Knott 1883a; Hecker 1923; Bergman et al. 1988; Sobel et al.

1990; Sammarco and Brainard 1991; Cheung et al. 1997; Chepuri et al. 2001; Zammit and Singh 2003; Sookur et al. 2008; Athavale et al. 2012b; Clarkson et al. 2013; Lambert 2016; Standring 2016; Albay and Candan 2017; Mustafa et al. 2017). This calcaneal insertion (peroneocalcaneus or fibulocalcaneus externum variant) is the most common presentation of fibularis quartus (Hecker 1923; Cheung et al. 1997; Saupe et al. 2007; Lambert 2016). Its insertion onto the calcaneus may be split into two tendons (Knott 1883b). It may have an attachment to flexor hallucis longus (Macalister 1875). Fibularis quartus may be doubled (Hur et al. 2015a).

Fibularis quartus has several other variants that are named for their insertions beyond the calcaneus. Fibularis digiti minimi or fibularis digiti quinti refers to a variant of fibularis quartus that inserts onto the fifth digit (see the entry for this muscle) (Macalister 1875; Bergman et al. 1988; Sookur et al. 2008; Lambert 2016; Olewnik et al. 2019b). Fibularis quartus may insert onto the cuboid, thus having the name peroneocuboideus (fibulocuboideus) (Chudzinski 1875; Macalister 1875; Bergman et al. 1988; Donley and Leyes 2001; Sookur et al. 2008; Clarkson et al. 2013; Lambert 2016; Standring 2016). Tubbs et al. (2008b) use the name peroneotalocalcaneus to describe a muscle that originated from the anterior intermuscular septum and fibularis longus and inserted onto both the calcaneus and talus. Clarkson et al. (2013) use the name peroneocalcaneocuboideus to describe a muscle that originated from fibularis brevis, the distal fibula, and the posterior intermuscular septum and inserted into both the calcaneus and the cuboid.

Fibularis accessorius (peroneoperoneolongus) is regarded as a variant of fibularis quartus that takes origin from either fibularis brevis or fibularis longus and inserts onto the fibularis longus tendon (Macalister 1875; Knott 1883b; Hecker 1923; White et al. 1974; Bergman et al. 1988; Saupe et al. 2007; Sookur et al. 2008; Lambert 2016; Standring 2016). The muscle may also insert into the fibularis brevis tendon (Athavale et al. 2012b; Hur et al. 2015a; Lambert 2016).

Innervation

Fibularis quartus and its variants are innervated by the superficial fibular nerve (Tubbs et al. 2008b; Athavale et al. 2012b).

Prevalence

In a sample of 124 legs from 65 cadavers, Sobel et al. (1990) found fibularis quartus in 27 legs (21.8%). In 17 out of the 27 legs (63%), it originated from the belly of fibularis brevis and inserted into the peroneal trochlea. In 1 out of the 27 legs (3.7%), the muscle originated from fibularis brevis and inserted onto the fibularis longus tendon (fibularis accessorius). In another leg (3.7%), the muscle originated from the fibularis brevis muscle and inserted onto its tendon. In one leg (3.7%), the muscle originated from fibularis longus and inserted into the fibularis longus tendon. In one leg (3.7%), the muscle originated from fibularis longus and inserted into fibularis brevis. In two legs (7.4%), the muscle presented as fibularis digiti minimi (see the entry for this muscle). In two legs (7.4%), fibularis quartus originated from fibularis longus and inserted onto the peroneal trochlea. In three legs (11.1%), the muscle originated from fibularis brevis and inserted onto the lateral retinaculum.

Chaney et al. (1996) found that fibularis quartus was present in 8 out of 269 limbs (3%). In a sample of 92 cadaveric lower limbs, Athavale et al. (2012b) found fibularis quartus in 20 limbs (21.7%). The tendon of fibularis quartus inserted onto the retrotrochlear eminence in 15 out of the 20 cases (75%) and into the peroneal trochlea in three cases (15%). In two cases (10%), it inserted onto the tendon of either fibularis longus or fibularis brevis. In a sample of 277 cadaveric legs, Clarkson et al. (2013) found fibularis quartus in 58 legs (20.9%), with 56 of these muscles presenting as fibulocalcaneus externum, one of 58 these muscles presenting as peroneocuboideus, and another muscle presenting as peroneocalcaneocuboideus. In a sample of Indian cadavers, Prakash et al. (2011) found fibularis quartus in 3 out of 70 specimens (4.3%). In a sample of 20 Saudi Arabian cadaveric lower limbs, Mustafa et al. (2017) found fibularis quartus in four limbs (20%).

In a sample of 80 lower limbs from 40 Korean cadavers, Hur et al. (2015a) found fibularis quartus in 13 specimens (16.3%). In two specimens, fibularis quartus was doubled, thus yielding 15 instances of fibularis quartus within the sample. Fibularis quartus originated from fibularis brevis in 12 cases (15%). The fibularis quartus muscle belly converged into a tendon in eight of these 12 cases, with that tendon inserting into the tendon of fibularis brevis in 3 cases (3.8%), the calcaneus in 2 cases (2.5%), the inferior peroneal retinaculum in 2 cases (2.5%), and the base of the fifth metatarsal in 1 case (1.3%). The fibularis quartus originated from fibularis brevis as a tendon in four of these 12 cases, inserting onto the calcaneus in three of them (3.8%) and into the periosteum of the retromalleolar grove in 1 case (1.3%). The remaining three cases (3.8%) did not arise from fibularis brevis. In one of these cases, it extended from the fibula to the tendon of fibularis brevis. In the second case, it originated from the superior peroneal retinaculum and inserted onto the calcaneus. In the third case, a doubled fibularis quartus was present, with the tendon of one arising from the muscle belly of the other.

Zammit and Singh (2003) searched for the presence of fibularis quartus in 102 legs from 80 cadavers using dissection, and in 80 symptomatic patients using MRI. Fibularis quartus was present in six of the cadaveric legs (5.9%), with two presenting as fibularis digiti quinti and one presenting as peroneocuboideus. Fibularis quartus was also present in six of the MRI images (7.5%). Saupe et al. (2007) used MRI to study the peroneal region in 65 patients with asymptomatic ankles. Fibularis quartus was found in 11 ankles (17%), with ten of these muscles (91%) inserting onto the calcaneus (peroneocalcaneus externum variant) and one muscle (9%) inserting onto the fibularis longus tendon (peroneoperoneolongus variant).

Cheung et al. (1997) studied a sample of 136 ankle MRI studies to determine the prevalence of fibularis quartus. This muscle was found in 14 cases (10.3%), inserting into the calcaneus in 11 of these cases. In a sample of 31 MR images from 27 patients that exhibited longitudinal splits of the fibularis brevis tendon, Rosenberg et al. (1997) found fibularis quartus in two images (6.5%). Using sonography and MRI, Chepuri et al. (2001) found seven instances of fibularis quartus muscles in a sample of 32 patients (21.9%). Nascimento et al. (2012) found 16 instances of fibularis quartus out of a sample of 211 MR examinations (7.6%). Using MRI, Agha et al. (2018) found fibularis quartus in 15 out of 181 patients (8.3%).

Yammine (2015c) conducted a comprehensive review of fibularis quartus. This author found that out of a total of 2,816 feet from 20 cadaveric studies, fibularis quartus has a "true" prevalence of 10.2%. Based on a total of 252 cadavers from five cadaveric studies, fibularis quartus has a "crude" prevalence of 16.6%. Based on a total of 253 operated ankles from six studies, fibularis quartus has a surgical prevalence of 5.5%. Based on a total of 854 legs from 12 studies, fibularis quartus has an MRI prevalence of 10.6%.

Albay and Candan (2017) studied the fibular muscles in 200 limbs from 100 fetuses. In four limbs (2%), "fibularis quartus" muscles were present, with an origin from fibularis brevis and an insertion onto the lateral calcaneal surface. In three limbs (1.5%), they found accessory fibular muscles that originated from the fibula and inserted onto the lateral surface of the calcaneus. These authors deemed these muscles to be examples of "fibulocalcaneus externus."

Anomalies

Description

Pettersen (1979) found peroneus quartus bilaterally in a boy with trisomy 13q. On the left side, it originated in the distal third of the leg with fibularis longus along the posterior intermuscular septum. On the right side, it originated from the distal third of the fibula and along the posteromedial margin of fibularis brevis. On both sides, the tendon inserted onto the peroneal trochlea. Pettersen et al. (1979) found peroneus quartus bilaterally in two male neonates with trisomy 13. These muscles originated from the fibula between fibularis brevis and flexor hallucis longus and inserted onto the calcaneus behind the tendons of fibularis brevis and fibularis longus.

Mieden (1982) describes two male fetuses with cyclopia and alobar holoprosencephaly. On the left side of one specimen, the authors state that peroneus digiti quinti was present, originating from the distal fibula and attaching to the peroneal trochlea. Based on the insertion of this muscle, it should be designated as fibularis quartus instead of the variant that inserts onto digit five.

Prevalence

In their literature review, Smith et al. (2015) found that fibularis quartus was present in 3 out of 20 individuals with trisomy 13 (15%) and in 5 out of 17 individuals with trisomy 18 (29.4%).

Clinical Implications

The presence of fibularis quartus and its variants may lead to lateral ankle pain, weakness, instability, and/or swelling (White et al. 1974; Buschmann et al. 1991; Sammarco and Brainard 1991; Chaney et al. 1996; Trono et al. 1999; Donley and Leyes 2001; Martinelli and Bernobi 2002; Zammit and Singh 2003; Sookur et al. 2008; Lotito et al. 2011; Lambert 2016). Its presence may cause peroneal compartment syndrome (Wenning et al. 2019). Fibularis quartus and its variants may mimic a soft tissue mass during medical imaging (Bergman et al. 1988; Tubbs et al. 2008b). Sookur et al. (2008) note that the fibularis quartus tendon may be mistaken for a longitudinal tear of the fibular tendons. However, fibularis quartus has been found in tandem with longitudinal splitting of the fibularis brevis tendon (Sobel et al. 1990; Rosenberg et al. 1997; Trono et al. 1999; Chepuri et al. 2001; Zammit and Singh 2003). It has also been associated with impingement, subluxation, tendinitis, and tenosynovitis of the fibular tendons (Trono et al. 1999; Chepuri et al. 2001; Lambert 2016; Opdam et al. 2017; Agha et al. 2018).

FIBULARIS DIGITI MINIMI (FIGURE 5.9)

See also: Fibularis quartus

Synonyms

This muscle may also be referred to as peroneus quintus (Knott 1883b), peroneus digiti quinti or peroneus quinti digiti (Macalister 1867b, 1875), or fibularis digiti quanti (Olewnik et al. 2019b).

Typical Presentation

This muscle is present only as a variation or anomaly.

Comparative Anatomy

Muscles and tendinous slips that may correspond to fibularis digiti minimi have been found in gorillas, common chimpanzees, and bonobos (Champneys 1872; Macalister 1873; MacDowell 1910; Raven 1950; Gibbs 1999; Diogo et al. 2010, 2013a, 2017). In gorillas, slips have been found (1) extending between fibularis brevis and the extensor expansion of the fifth digit and (2) inserting onto the proximal and intermediate phalanges of digit five (Macalister 1873; Raven 1950; Gibbs 1999; Diogo et al. 2010). In common chimpanzees, the tendon of fibularis brevis may send a slip to the proximal and/or intermediate phalanges of digit five (Champneys 1872; MacDowell 1910; Diogo et al. 2013a). In one bonobo dissected by Diogo et al. (2017), extensor digitorum longus sent an extra tendon to the fifth digit with attachments onto the metatarsal, proximal phalanx, and extensor expansion of this digit.

Variations

Description

Fibularis digiti minimi is regarded as a variant of fibularis quartus that inserts onto the fifth digit (Bergman et al. 1988; Sobel et al. 1990; Sookur et al. 2008; Lambert 2016).

However, it is possible that the two are entirely separate structures, due to differences in their shape, composition, and prevalence (Yammine 2015c).

Fibularis digiti minimi has multiple presentations. It may present as a tendinous slip that originates from the tendon of fibularis tertius or, more often, the tendon of fibularis brevis (Cunningham and St. John Brooks 1889–1891; Le Double 1897; Macalister 1867b, 1875; Jadhav et al. 2013; Lambert 2016; Chaney et al. 2018; Olewnik et al. 2019b). Alternatively, it may present as an independent muscle belly that originates from fibularis brevis or the distal fibula (Macalister 1875; Mori 1964; Zammit and Singh 2003; Sookur et al. 2008; Lambert 2016). Fibularis digiti minimi may also present as a small, independent muscle belly that arises in the foot from the tendon of fibularis brevis and sends its own tendon to digit five (Cunningham and St. John Brooks 1889–1891; Raheja et al. 2005).

Fibularis digiti minimi has variable insertions onto the fifth digit, including the base and/or head of the fifth metatarsal, the proximal phalanx, or the extensor expansion (Cunningham and St. John Brooks 1889–1891; Le Double 1897; Macalister 1875; Sobel et al. 1990; Zammit and Singh 2003; Raheja et al. 2005; Sookur et al. 2008; Jadhav et al. 2013; Lambert 2016; Chaney et al. 2018; Olewnik et al. 2019b). It may insert via two tendons onto the base and head of the fifth metatarsal (Sobel et al. 1990; Sookur et al. 2008). It may also have an insertion into both the fourth and fifth metatarsals (Jadhav et al. 2013; Demir et al. 2015). It may join with or insert onto the extensor digitorum longus tendon going to digit five (Knott 1883b; Jadhav et al. 2013; Demir et al. 2015; Olewnik et al. 2019b).

Innervation

When it presents as an independent muscle belly, fibularis digiti minimi is likely innervated by the superficial fibular nerve, as are the other variants of fibularis quartus (e.g., Tubbs et al. 2008b; Athavale et al. 2012b).

Prevalence

In a sample of 45 lower limbs, Cunningham and St. John Brooks (1889–1891) found fibularis digiti minimi in well-developed form (a slip from the tendon of fibularis brevis that inserted onto the extensor expansion of digit five) in 21 cases (46.7%) and in rudimentary form (a slip that ended on the dorsal surface of the fifth metatarsal) in five cases (11.1%).

Mori (1964) found "peroneus digiti quinti" extending from the distal fibula to the fifth digit in 2 out of 73 legs (2.7%). Mori (1964) also notes that the fibularis brevis tendon sent a slip to the distal phalanx of digit five in 20% of cases, with this slip having a separate muscular belly in 8% of cases. These could also be presentations of fibularis digiti minimi. Bareither et al. (1984) found fibularis digiti minimi in 178 out of 298 cadaveric feet (59.7%). Sobel et al. (1990) found fibularis digiti minimi extending between fibularis brevis and the fifth metatarsal in 2 out of 124 legs (1.6%). In a sample of 102 legs from 80 cadavers, Zammit and Singh (2003) found fibularis digiti minimi in two legs (2%).

Jadhav et al. (2013) found slips corresponding to fibularis digiti minimi in 51 out of 100 cadaveric lower limbs (51%). They inserted onto the dorsal digital expansion of digit five in 41% of these 51 cases, onto the common extensor tendon in 19% of cases, onto the base of the proximal phalanx of digit five in 16% of cases, onto the head of the fifth metatarsal in 21% of cases, and onto both the shaft of the fourth metatarsal and the head of the fifth metatarsal in 3% of cases.

In a sample of 25 cadaveric lower limbs, Demir et al. (2015) found fibularis digiti minimi in eight limbs (32%). Five of these eight cases (62.5%) had a single tendon and three (37.5%) had a doubled tendon, thus yielding 11 tendons. Out of these 11 tendons, three (27.3%) inserted onto the base of the fifth metatarsal, two (18.1%) inserted onto the "dorsolateral ridge" of the fifth metatarsal, four (36.4%) inserted onto the fifth digit near the proximal phalanx, one (9.1%) inserted onto the extensor digitorum longus tendon going to digit five, and one (9.1%) inserted onto both the fourth metatarsal and the fifth metatarsal.

Yammine (2015c) conducted a comprehensive review of fibularis digiti minimi. This author found that out of a total of 1,112 feet from eight cadaveric studies, fibularis digiti minimi had a "true" prevalence of 34.3%. Based on a total of 194 cadavers from three cadaveric studies, fibularis digiti minimi had a "crude" prevalence of 21.5%.

Chaney et al. (2018) dissected 52 limbs from 26 cadavers to determine the prevalence of fibularis digiti minimi. A fully present fibularis digiti minimi—defined as a tendon that originated from the fibularis brevis tendon and inserted onto the extensor expansion of digit five—was present in 17 limbs (32.7%). A rudimentary fibularis digiti minimi—defined as either a thin tendon or a tendon that did not reach the extensor expansion—was present in 20 limbs (38.5%). Olewnik et al. (2019b) found "fibularis digiti quanti" in 18 out of 102 lower limbs (17.6%). It inserted onto the base of the proximal phalanx of digit five in eight cases (7.8%), onto the extensor expansion of digit five in five cases (4.9%), and fused with the extensor digitorum longus tendon in five cases (4.9%).

Anomalies

Description

Ramirez-Castro and Bersu (1978) found fibularis digiti minimi in five infants with trisomy 18. These muscles originated from the distal fibula and inserted onto the base of the fifth metatarsal and sent tendinous slips to the base of digit five. Aziz (1979) found fibularis digiti minimi bilaterally in one neonate with trisomy 18. It extended from the distal fibula to join the insertion of fibularis brevis onto the fifth metatarsal. Aziz (1979, 1980, 1981) found fibularis digiti minimi in two neonates with trisomy 13 and two neonates with trisomy 18. These muscles originated from the distal fibula and inserted into the fifth metatarsal.

Hootnick et al. (1987) describe an individual that had a right limb with congenital tibial aplasia, talocalcaneal synchondrosis, and an adducted foot with five toes. In this limb, there was an accessory muscle that originated from the fibula deep to fibularis tertius and inserted via a long tendon onto the fifth metatarsal.

Prevalence

Ramirez-Castro and Bersu (1978) found fibularis digiti minimi in five out of eight infants (62.5%) with trisomy 18. In their literature review, Smith et al. (2015) found that fibularis digiti minimi was present in 2 out of 20 individuals with trisomy 13 (10%) and in 3 out of 17 individuals with trisomy 18 (17.6%). It seems like this assessment neglected to include the specimens described by Ramirez-Castro and Bersu (1978).

Clinical Implications

N/A

MUSCLES OF THE FOOT

ABDUCTOR HALLUCIS (FIGURE 5.10)

Synonyms

N/A

Typical Presentation

Description

Abductor hallucis originates from the flexor retinaculum, the plantar aponeurosis, and the medial process of the calcaneal tuber (Standring 2016). Its tendon inserts onto the base of the proximal phalanx of digit one (Standring 2016).

Innervation

Abductor hallucis is innervated by the medial plantar nerve (Standring 2016).

Comparative Anatomy

Abductor hallucis has a similar typical presentation in the apes, originating from the medial and plantar surfaces of the calcaneus and the plantar aponeurosis and inserting onto the base of the proximal hallucal phalanx (Hepburn 1892; Beddard 1893; Sonntag 1924; Raven 1950; Miller 1952; Gibbs 1999; Diogo et al. 2010, 2012, 2013a,b, 2017). It may be blended with flexor hallucis brevis in orangutans and gibbons, and with flexor digitorum brevis in orangutans (Beddard 1893; Sonntag 1924; Gibbs 1999; Diogo et al. 2012, 2013b).

Variations

Description

Abductor hallucis often has an insertion onto the medial sesamoid bone and/or the "medial sesamoidal ligament" (fibers that extend from the medial sesamoid bone to the joint capsule at the head of the first metatarsal) (Brenner 1999; Agawany and Mcguid 2010; Kafka et al. 2016;

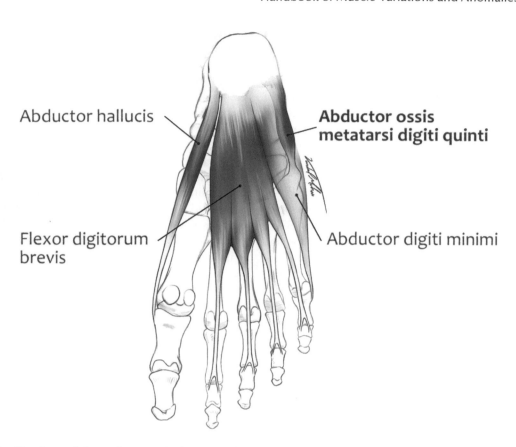

Abductor hallucis

Abductor ossis metatarsi digiti quinti

Flexor digitorum brevis

Abductor digiti minimi

FIGURE 5.10   First layer of plantar foot muscles in plantar (inferior) view.

Standring 2016). Abductor hallucis may send a tendinous slip to the base of the proximal phalanx of digit two (Wood 1868; Macalister 1875; Knott 1883b) or to the proximal phalanges of digits two and three (Bergman et al. 1988; Kafka et al. 2016). It may send a slip to the flexor hallucis longus tendon (Macalister 1875; Knott 1883b). It may also be connected via a slip to the skin on the medial margin of the foot (Macalister 1875; Bergman et al. 1988; Standring 2016). Chittoria et al. (2015) report an unusual case in which abductor hallucis had numerous tendinous slips along three quarters of its internal surface that attached to the medial intermuscular septum arising from the connection of the tibial and central components of the plantar aponeurosis, the medial surface of the hallucal metatarsal, and the intermuscular septum abductor hallucis shares with flexor hallucis brevis.

Edwards et al. (1969) found an accessory belly of abductor hallucis that originated from the interior surface of the navicular. Bhansali and Bhansali (1997) found an accessory muscle that originated from the deep surface of the fascia covering the posterior tibial nerve just above the medial malleolus, passed deep to the nerve, and then coursed through the tarsal tunnel to unite with abductor hallucis.

Prevalence

Wood (1868) found a slip from abductor hallucis going to the base of the proximal phalanx of digit two in 5 out of 40 males (12.5%) and in 1 out of 30 females (3.3%). Knott

(1883b) notes that Krause found a slip from abductor hallucis going to the base of the proximal phalanx of digit two in 9% of cases. Brenner (1999) studied the insertions of abductor hallucis in 109 feet. The muscle inserted onto the proximal phalanx of the hallux in 42 feet (38.5%), into the medial sesamoid ligament and the medial sesamoid bone in 65 feet (59.6%), and into the medial sesamoid bone only in 2 feet (1.8%). Agawany and Meguid (2010) studied the insertions of abductor hallucis in 15 feet. The muscle inserted onto the proximal phalanx of digit one in 7 feet (46.7%), into the base of the proximal phalanx and the sesamoid bone via two slips in 5 feet (33.3%), into the sesamoid bone only in 1 foot (6.7%), and into both the base of the proximal phalanx and the metatarsophalangeal joint capsule of digit one in 2 feet (13.3%).

Anomalies

Description

Mieden (1982) describes two male fetuses with cyclopia and alobar holoprosencephaly. On the left side of one specimen, abductor hallucis was doubled. Hootnick et al. (1987) describe an individual that had a right limb with congenital tibial aplasia, talocalcaneal synchondrosis, and an adducted foot with five toes. In this limb, abductor hallucis was absent. In the female fetus with trisomy 18 dissected by Alghamdi et al. (2018), the distal end of abductor hallucis was fused with the medial head of flexor hallucis brevis bilaterally.

Prevalence

N/A

Clinical Implications

An accessory abductor hallucis can entrap the posterior tibial nerve (Edwards et al. 1969; Bhansali and Bhansali 1997). It is unclear whether variations in the insertion of abductor hallucis contribute to the etiology of hallux valgus (Brenner 1999).

Flexor digitorum brevis (Figure 5.10)

Synonyms

It may also be referred to as flexor brevis digitorum (Macalister 1875).

Typical Presentation

Description

Flexor digitorum brevis originates via a tendon from the medial process of the calcaneal tuber and from the planar aponeurosis (Standring 2016). It ends in four tendons that travel to digits two through five (Standring 2016). These tendons split to accommodate the tendons of flexor digitorum longus and then insert onto both sides of the shaft of the intermediate phalanx of their respective digits (Standring 2016).

Innervation

Flexor digitorum brevis is innervated by the medial plantar nerve (Standring 2016).

Comparative Anatomy

Flexor digitorum brevis has a similar typical presentation in the apes, extending from the calcaneus to various combinations of the intermediate phalanges of the toes (Champneys 1872; Hepburn 1892; Beddard 1893; Dwight 1895; MacDowell 1910; Sonntag 1924; Raven 1950; Miller 1952; Gibbs 1999; Diogo et al. 2010, 2012, 2013a,b, 2017). As in humans, the insertion onto the fifth digit is not constant.

In gibbons, there may be an origin from flexor digitorum longus, and the tendons usually insert onto digits two, three, and four with an occasional insertion onto digit five (Hepburn 1892; Beddard 1893; Diogo et al. 2012). In orangutans, the tendon always inserts onto digits two and three, occasionally onto digit four, and rarely onto digit five (Chapman 1880; Hepburn 1892; Beddard 1893; Primrose 1900; Sonntag 1924; Diogo et al. 2013b). In common chimpanzees and bonobos, the tendons always go to digits two and three and sometimes to digits four and five (Hepburn 1892; Miller 1952; Diogo et al. 2013a, 2017). In gorillas, a superficial head of the muscle inserts onto digits two and three, and a deep head inserts onto digit four and sometimes five (Raven 1950; Diogo et al. 2010). When the tendons to digits four and five are present in the apes besides gorillas, they are often described as deriving from a deep head of flexor digitorum brevis (Hepburn 1892; Primrose 1900; Gibbs 1999; Diogo et al. 2012, 2013a,b).

Variations

Description

The tendons of flexor digitorum brevis may receive accessory slips from other muscles, often flexor digitorum longus or quadratus plantae (Wood 1868; Macalister 1875; Nathan and Gloobe 1974; Bergman et al. 1988; Kafka et al. 2016; Standring 2016). Any of the digital tendons may be absent, but the tendon to digit five is most commonly absent (Wood 1867b, 1868; Macalister 1875; Knott 1883b; Aasar 1947; Mori 1964; Sato 1970; Bergman et al. 1988; Nathan and Gloobe 1974; Chaney et al. 1996; Claassen and Wree 2003; Lobo et al. 2008; Gugapriya 2012; Kafka et al. 2016; Standring 2016).

When a tendon is absent, particularly the tendon going to digit five, it may be replaced by a muscular slip originating from the tendon of flexor digitorum longus, quadratus plantae, tendon of tibialis posterior, the medial process of the calcaneus, the lateral band of the plantar aponeurosis, and/or the lateral intermuscular septum (Wood 1864, 1867b, 1868; Macalister 1875; Knott 1883b; Aasar 1947; Nathan and Gloobe 1974; Bergman et al. 1988; Claassen and Wree 2003; Asomugha et al. 2005; Gugapriya 2012; Kafka et al. 2016; Standring 2016; Ramesh Rao and Rao 2017).

The tendon to digit five may also fail to divide around the tendon of flexor digitorum longus (Macalister 1875). This tendon may also end on the anterior fascia of digit five (Macalister 1875; Bergman et al. 1988). This tendon may be thin or otherwise reduced (Claassen and Wree 2003; Yalçin and Ozan 2005b; Bernhard et al. 2013). The insertion onto digit five may be split into two slips, one going to the proximal phalanx and the other inserting with flexor digitorum longus onto the distal phalanx (Yalçin and Ozan 2005b).

Yalçin and Ozan (2005b) describe a case in which flexor digitorum brevis had a superficial head and a deep head. Both heads contributed to the tendons going to digits three and four, and the deep head formed separate muscle bellies to send tendons to digits two and five. This morphology is similar to that seen in some ape specimens, though different digits are targeted by the superficial and deep heads (see comparative anatomy, above).

Prevalence

Wood (1868) found that the flexor digitorum brevis tendon to digit five was absent in 10 out of 68 males (14.7%) and in 5 out of 34 females (14.7%). Knott (1883b) found that the tendon to digit five was absent in 3 out of 30 cases (10%). Knott (1883b) also notes that Krause found it was absent in 15% of cases. Mori (1964) found that the tendon to digit five was absent in 16% of feet. Sato (1970) found that the flexor digitorum brevis tendon to digit five was absent in 106 out of 380 limbs (27.9%) from Kyushu Japanese males and in 72 out of 252 limbs (28.6%) from females.

Out of a sample of 100 feet, Nathan and Gloobe (1974) found that the flexor digitorum brevis tendon to digit five was absent in 23 cases (23%). The tendons to both the fourth and fifth digits were absent in 3 feet (3%). Flexor digitorum longus sent slips to the flexor digitorum brevis tendon to digit five in 20 cases (20%) and to the brevis tendons to digits four and five in 3 cases (3%). The fifth tendon of flexor digitorum brevis had an origin from flexor digitorum longus in five cases (5%), from the intermuscular septum in one case (1%), and from tibialis posterior in one case (1%).

Chaney et al. (1996) found that the tendon to digit five was absent in 181 out of 284 limbs (63.7%). In a sample of 11 feet from 8 cadavers, Kura et al. (1997) found that the tendon to digit five was absent in 4 feet (36.4%). Out of a sample of 97 feet from 60 cadavers, Bernhard et al. (2013) found that 47 did not have a tendon to the fifth digit (48.4%), 25 feet had small tendons to the fifth digit (25.8%), and the remaining 25 feet (25.8%) demonstrated the typical presentation of flexor digitorum brevis. Yalçin and Ozan (2005b) studied flexor digitorum brevis in 33 feet from 15 cadavers. The muscle had a typical presentation in 15 feet (45.5%). The tendon to digit five was small in 12 feet (36.4%) and absent in 6 feet (18.2%).

In a sample of 60 feet from 30 Nepalese cadavers, Lobo et al. (2008) found that the flexor digitorum brevis tendon for the fifth digit was absent in all 60 feet (100%). Gugapriya (2012) examined flexor digitorum brevis in 30 feet from 15 cadavers from the northern Tamil Nadu region of India. The tendon to digit five was absent in 25 feet (83.3%). In a sample of 270 feet from 135 Sri Lankan cadavers, Ilayperuma (2012) found that the tendon to digit five was absent bilaterally in 194 limbs (71.9%) from 67 cadavers. Ferreira Arquez (2017) studied flexor digitorum brevis in 34 feet from 17 cadavers. In 2 feet (5.9%) the tendon to digit five was absent. In the remaining 32 feet (94.1%), the muscle sent tendons to digits two through five.

Yammine (2015d) conducted a comprehensive review of flexor digitorum brevis. This author found that out of a total of 2,789 feet from 22 studies, the "true" prevalence of the absence of the tendon to digit five was 31.3%. Based on a total of 416 cadavers from six studies, the "crude" prevalence of the absence of the tendon to digit five was 47%. Based on a total of 476 feet from four studies, the "true" prevalence of the tendon to digit five presenting as a thin slip was 47.7%. Based on a total of 223 feet from four studies, the "true" prevalence of variations in origin of the fifth tendon was 12.7%.

Anomalies

Description

On the left foot of a boy with trisomy 13q, Pettersen (1979) found that flexor digitorum brevis only had two tendons of insertion. These tendons inserted onto the middle phalanges of digits three and four. On the right foot of this individual, only the tendon to digit five was absent. Pettersen et al. (1979) found that flexor digitorum brevis lacked a tendon to digit five in two fetuses and two neonates with trisomy 13. In one of these cases, flexor digitorum brevis was a distinctly separate muscle. The tendon to digit five was also absent bilaterally in another neonate with trisomy 13 (Aziz 1980).

Absence of the digit five tendon is also a common feature in individuals with trisomy 18 (Ramirez-Castro and Bersu 1978; Alghamdi et al. 2018) and trisomy 21 (Bersu 1980).

On the right foot of a male neonate with Meckel syndrome, Pettersen (1984) found that flexor digiti minimi brevis attached to digit five and received a slip from flexor digitorum brevis that did not split to accommodate the tendon of flexor digitorum longus. The transverse head of adductor hallucis also a partial origin from the flexor digitorum brevis to the fifth digit. In a fetus with craniorachischisis dissected by Alghamdi et al. (2017), the flexor digitorum brevis tendon to digit five was absent on both sides. Hootnick et al. (1987) describe an individual that had a right limb with congenital tibial aplasia, talocalcaneal synchondrosis, and an adducted foot with five toes. In this limb, flexor digitorum brevis did not send a tendon to the fifth digit.

Prevalence

In their literature review, Smith et al. (2015) found that the flexor digitorum brevis tendon to digit five was absent in 5 out of 20 individuals with trisomy 13 (25%). Based on 16 sides from eight infants with trisomy 18, Ramirez-Castro and Bersu (1978) found that the flexor digitorum brevis tendon to digit five was absent in 11 out of 16 sides (68.75%) and from seven out of eight infants (87.5%). According to Bersu (1980), the tendon to digit five was absent on at least one side in two out of five individuals with trisomy 21 (40%).

Clinical Implications

Understanding variations in the presentation of the flexor digitorum brevis tendons is important for planning tendon transfer surgeries (Ilayperuma 2012).

ABDUCTOR DIGITI MINIMI (FIGURE 5.10)

Synonyms

N/A

Typical Presentation

Description

Abductor digiti minimi originates from the calcaneal tuberosity and the plantar aponeurosis (Standring 2016). Its tendon blends with that of flexor digiti minimi brevis to insert onto the base of the proximal phalanx of digit five (Standring 2016).

Innervation

Abductor digiti minimi is innervated by the lateral plantar nerve (Standring 2016).

Comparative Anatomy

Abductor digiti minimi has a similar typical presentation in the apes, extending from the calcaneus and the plantar aponeurosis to the proximal phalanx of digit five (Champneys 1872; Hepburn 1892; Beddard 1893; Sonntag 1924; Raven 1950; Miller 1952; Gibbs 1999; Vereecke et al. 2005; Diogo et al. 2010, 2012, 2013a,b, 2017). The insertion may be split into two tendons in gibbons and bonobos (Vereecke et al. 2005; Diogo et al. 2012).

Variations

Description

Abductor digiti minimi may be fused with flexor digiti minimi brevis (Macalister 1875; Kopuz et al. 1999). Its insertion onto the proximal phalanx may be separate from the insertion of flexor digiti minimi brevis (Macalister 1875; Knott 1883b). Abductor digiti minimi is associated with several accessory muscles (Bergman et al. 1988; Kafka et al. 2016; Standring 2016). A short and deep accessory head may originate from the tuberosity (styloid process) of the fifth metatarsal and insert onto the base of the proximal phalanx of digit five with abductor digiti minimi (Macalister 1875; Knott 1883b; Bergman et al. 1988; Kopuz et al. 1999; Kafka et al. 2016; Standring 2016). Abductor accessorius digiti minimi arises from the lateral plantar process of the calcaneus and inserts into the lateral aspect of the base of the proximal phalanx of digit five (Bergman et al. 1988; Nayyar et al. 2010; Kafka et al. 2016).

Abductor digiti minimi may send a tendinous slip to the base of the fifth metatarsal (Knott 1883b). In some cases, this slip may present as abductor ossis metatarsi digiti quinti, a supernumerary muscle that extends between the lateral plantar process of the calcaneus and the tuberosity of the fifth metatarsal (see the entry for this muscle) (Wood 1864, 1867b, 1868; Macalister 1875; Knott 1883b; Bergman et al. 1988; Chaney et al. 1996; Kopuz et al. 1999; Kafka et al. 2016; Standring 2016).

Kopuz et al. (1999) report a left foot in which there were multiple accessory muscles present in association with the normal abductor digiti minimi. Abductor ossis metatarsi digiti quinti arose from the lateral process of the calcaneus and inserted onto the tuberosity of the fifth metatarsal. A "distal belly" was present extending between the tuberosity of the fifth metatarsal and the lateral aspect of the base of the proximal phalanx of digit five. Lastly, a medial accessory muscle was present extending between the plantar surface of the calcaneus and the base of the fifth metatarsal.

Boupha and Wree (1995) report a bicipital accessory muscle situated in between the superficial and deep posterior crural muscles that they name "abductor digiti minimi longus." The tibial head originated from the tibia distal to the soleal line. The fibular head originated from the posterior intermuscular septum just proximal to the lateral malleolus. The heads united to end in a tendon that coursed behind the medial malleolus posterior to the tendon of flexor hallucis longus. After entering the plantar aspect of the foot, the tendon passed laterally and inserted with abductor digiti minimi onto the proximal phalanx of the fifth digit. These authors designate this muscle as a novel variation but note that it shares some similarities with other accessory muscles of the calf (e.g., tensor fasciae plantaris (tibiotarsalis), flexor digitorum accessorius longus).

Prevalence

Knott (1883b) found that abductor digiti minimi sent a tendinous slip to the base of the fifth metatarsal in 60% of subjects.

Anomalies

Description

On the left side of a female fetus with trisomy 13, Pettersen et al. (1979) found that abductor digiti minimi had an accessory slip. On the left side of male neonate with trisomy 13, Pettersen et al. (1979) found that abductor digiti minimi attached to the extra digit in that foot instead of onto digit five. On the right foot of a male neonate with Meckel syndrome, Pettersen (1984) observed that abductor digiti minimi went to the sixth digit and sent a small slip to the fifth digit. On the left foot, this muscle (along with flexor digiti minimi brevis) was represented by a mass on the plantar and lateral sides of digit six with vague attachments to this digit and partially to digit five.

Prevalence

In their literature review, Smith et al. (2015) found that abductor digiti minimi had an extra slip in only 1 out of 24 individuals with trisomy 13 (4.2%).

Clinical Implications

An accessory abductor of digit five may present as a soft tissue lump on the lateral border of the foot (Carmont et al. 2002).

ABDUCTOR OSSIS METATARSI DIGITI QUINTI (FIGURE 5.10)

Entry adapted by permission from Springer Nature Customer Service Centre GmbH: Springer Current Molecular Biology Reports, Muscles Lost in Our Adult Primate Ancestors Still Imprint in US: on Muscle Evolution, Development, Variations, and Pathologies. E. Boyle, V. Mahon, R. Diogo, 2020.

See also: Abductor digiti minimi

Synonyms

This muscle is also referred to as abductor ossis metatarsi quinti (Wood 1864), abductor os metatarsi minimi digiti (digiti minimi) (Macalister 1875), or abductor metatarsi quinti (Gruber 1886).

Typical Presentation

This muscle is only present as a variation.

Comparative Anatomy

Ferrero et al. (2012) are the first to report this muscle in gibbons and found an insertion onto the proximal phalanx of the fifth digit. In the other apes, abductor ossis metatarsi digiti quinti is frequently present as a distinct muscle that extends between the calcaneus and the tuberosity of the fifth metatarsal (Champneys 1872; Beddard 1893; Primrose 1899; Raven 1950; Miller 1952; Gibbs 1999; Diogo et al.

2010, 2012, 2013a,b, 2017). Wood (1868) notes that similar muscles have been found monkeys, cats, bears, and other mammals.

Variations

Description

Abductor ossis metatarsi digiti quinti is a variation of abductor digiti minimi that is typically not present in humans (Swindler and Wood 1973). It is a supernumerary muscle that originates from the lateral plantar process of the calcaneus and inserts onto the tuberosity (styloid process) of the fifth metatarsal (Wood 1864, 1867b, 1868; Macalister 1875; Knott 1883b; Bergman et al. 1988; Chaney et al. 1996; Kopuz et al. 1999; Kafka et al. 2016; Standring 2016). It may have an origin from the medial process of the calcaneus (Wood 1867b; Macalister 1875). Its insertion may shift distally to the midsection or the anterior portion of the fifth metatarsal (Wood 1867b; Macalister 1875; Bergman et al. 1988; Kafka et al. 2016). It may be fused with abductor digiti minimi (Macalister 1875; Bergman et al. 1988).

Kopuz et al. (1999) report a left foot in which there were multiple accessory muscles present in association with the normal abductor digiti minimi. Abductor ossis metatarsi digiti quinti arose from the lateral process of the calcaneus and inserted onto the tuberosity of the fifth metatarsal. A "distal belly" was present extending between the tuberosity of the fifth metatarsal and the lateral aspect of the base of the proximal phalanx of digit five. Lastly, a medial accessory muscle was present extending between the plantar surface of the calcaneus and the base of the fifth metatarsal.

Innervation

Abductor ossis metatarsi digiti quinti is innervated by the lateral plantar nerve (Gibbs 1999; Kopuz et al. 1999).

Prevalence

Wood (1867b) found abductor ossis metatarsi digiti quinti in 17 out of 36 subjects (47.2%) and later (Wood 1868) found this muscle in 19 out of 36 subjects (52.8%). Knott (1883b) found this muscle in 3 out of 40 cases (7.5%). Le Double (1897) reports a prevalence of 43% (from examinations of 65 feet) and of 45% (from examinations of 40 feet). Chaney et al. (1996) found this muscle in 125 out of 275 feet (45.5%).

Anomalies

N/A

Clinical Implications

N/A

QUADRATUS PLANTAE (FIGURE 5.11)

Synonyms

This muscle may also be referred to as flexor accessorius pedis (Macalister 1875), flexor accessorius (Standring 2016), flexor digitorum accessorius (Knott 1883b), flexor digitorum accessorius brevis (Verma et al. 2018), moles carnea or

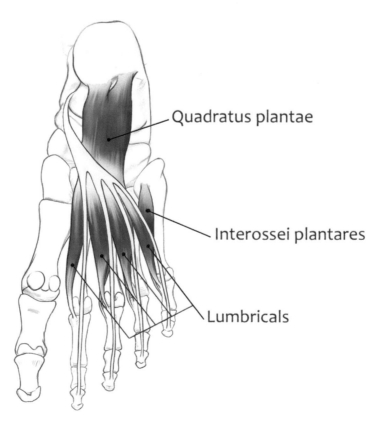

FIGURE 5.11 Second layer of plantar muscles and the plantar interossei in plantar (inferior) view.

massa carnea (Sylvius), caro plantae pedis quadrata, or caro quadrata (Pretterklieber 2018).

Typical Presentation

Description

The medial head of quadratus plantae originates from the medial plantar surface of the calcaneus (Standring 2016). The lateral head originates from the lateral plantar surface of the calcaneus (Standring 2016). Quadratus plantae inserts into the tendon of flexor digitorum longus at the juncture where it splits into four tendons that go to digits two through five (Standring 2016)

Innervation

Quadratus plantae is innervated by the lateral plantar nerve (Standring 2016).

Comparative Anatomy

Quadratus plantae is absent in gibbons but sometimes found in the other apes with an insertion onto the flexor digitorum longus tendon (Gibbs 1999; Diogo et al. 2010, 2012, 2013a,b, 2017). When the muscle is present in orangutans, the lateral head is more common than the medial head (Chapman 1880; Hepburn 1892; Gibbs 1999; Lewis 1962; Diogo et al. 2013b). When present in the gorillas, common chimpanzees, and bonobos, the medial head is absent (Champneys 1872; Hepburn 1892; Gibbs 1999; Diogo et al. 2010, 2013a, 2017).

Variations

Description

Quadratus plantae may be diminutive, missing either the lateral or medial head, or entirely absent (Bergman et al. 1988; Kura et al. 1997; Hur et al. 2011b; Athavale et al. 2012a; Standring 2016; Pretterklieber 2018; Edama et al. 2019). Three heads may be present (Yalçin and Ozan 2005b; Pretterklieber 2018). Its fibers or its insertion may be split into a superficial and deep layer (Bergman et al. 1988; Verma et al. 2018). It may originate more proximally on the calcaneus, from the upper surface of the calcaneal tuber near the insertion of the plantaris tendon or from the Achilles tendon (Macalister 1875; Knott 1883b). It may also originate from the calcaneocuboid ligament (Macalister 1875; Pretterklieber 2018). Pretterklieber (2018) lists several other origins for both the medial and lateral heads (see prevalence information, below).

Its insertion onto the tendon(s) of flexor digitorum longus is variable (Macalister 1875; Lewis 1962; Bergman et al. 1988; Standring 2016; Pretterklieber 2017; Elvan et al. 2019). The tendons of flexor digitorum longus that go digit three (in rare cases), digit four, and digit five (frequently) may be missing contributions from quadratus plantae (Macalister 1875; Lewis 1962; Standring 2016; Pretterklieber 2017, 2018; Edama et al. 2019; Elvan et al. 2019). The quadratus plantae contribution to the flexor tendon going to digit two may also be lacking (Pretterklieber 2017, 2018; Elvan et al. 2019).

Quadratus plantae may insert entirely onto, or connect via an accessory slip to, the tendon of flexor hallucis longus (Macalister 1875; Knott 1883b; Bergman et al. 1988; Tubbs et al. 2004b; Hur et al. 2011b; Athavale et al. 2012a; Gupta and Nasir 2013; Pretterklieber 2017, 2018; Beger et al. 2018b). Hur et al. (2011b) and Beger et al. (2018b) found that the insertion of quadratus plantae into the tendons of both long flexor muscles is common. Quadratus plantae is often involved in the variable blending of the flexor digitorum longus and flexor hallucis longus tendons, which is referred to as the chiasma plantare or the knot of Henry (O'Sullivan et al. 2005; LaRue and Anctil 2006; Plaass et al. 2013; Pretterklieber 2017, 2018; Beger et al. 2018b; Elvan et al. 2019). Quadratus plantae may send an accessory slip to the flexor tendon of digit five or to the flexor digitorum brevis tendon of digit three (Macalister 1875). It may receive a slip from fibularis brevis (Macalister 1875). It may also be associated with a slip that inserts onto the distal phalanx of digit five (Macalister 1875; Claassen and Wree 2003). Its insertion may expand to the lumbricals (Verma et al. 2018).

The accessory muscle flexor digitorum accessorius longus originates from the posterior compartment of the lower leg and usually inserts the main tendon of flexor digitorum longus and/or into quadratus plantae (see the entry for this muscle) (Hallett 1848; Wood 1864, 1868; Bergman et al. 1988; Sammarco and Conti 1994; Peterson et al. 1995; Cheung et al. 1999; Gümüşalan and Kalaycioğlu 2000; Sookur et al. 2008; Bowers et al. 2009; Georgiev et al. 2009; Hur et al. 2011b; Upasna et al. 2011; Standring 2016). This muscle may be described as high origin of quadratus plantae (e.g., Macalister 1875). Hallett (1848) notes that quadratus plantae may be unusually large when flexor digitorum accessorius longus is present. The presence of flexor digitorum accessorius longus may also be associated with the absence of quadratus plantae (Pác and Malinovský 1985).

Prevalence

In a sample of 18 feet, Lewis (1982) found that quadratus plantae contributed to the flexor tendons going to digits two and three in 4 cases (22.2%) and into the flexor tendons going to digits two, three, and four in 14 cases (77.8%). In a sample of 11 feet from eight cadavers, Kura et al. (1997) found that the lateral head of quadratus plantae was absent in 1 foot (9.1%). Hur et al. (2011b) examined quadratus plantae in 50 cadaveric specimens. The muscle was absent on one side of one cadaver (2%). Forty muscles (80%) had two heads of origin, five muscles had a medial head only (10%), and four muscles had a lateral head only (8%). Quadratus plantae inserted onto both the tendon of flexor digitorum longus and tendinous slips of flexor hallucis longus in 48 cases (96%) and into the flexor digitorum longus tendon only in two cases (4%).

Athavale et al. (2012a) studied quadratus plantae in 47 cadaveric limbs. The medial head was absent in five limbs (10.6%). In four limbs (8.5%), the medial head did not unite with the lateral head. Out of the 42 limbs in which it was present, the medial head inserted into the flexor digitorum longus tendon in 35 limbs (83.3%), into the flexor digitorum longus tendon and a slip from flexor hallucis longus in four limbs (9.5%), into a slip from flexor hallucis longus in one limb (2.4%), and into the digital tendons of flexor digitorum longus in two limbs (4.8%). Out of the 47 limbs in which it was present, the lateral head inserted into the flexor digitorum longus tendon in 44 limbs (93.6%) and into the flexor digitorum longus tendon and a slip from flexor hallucis longus in three limbs (6.4%).

Pretterklieber (2017) examined the contributions of flexor digitorum longus, flexor hallucis longus, and quadratus plantae to the long flexor tendons in 100 cases. Quadratus plantae contributed to the first tendon in 14 cases (14%), to the second tendon in 97 cases (97%), to the third tendon in 98 cases (98%), to the fourth tendon in 99 cases (99%), and to the fifth tendon in 51 cases (51%). Pretterklieber (2018) studied quadratus plantae in 100 feet from 50 cadavers. The muscle had one head in 34 cases (34%), two heads in 57 cases (57%), and three heads in 9 cases (9%). In the nine cases where the muscle had three heads, these middle heads originated from the plantar or medial calcaneal surface in five cases (56%), the long plantar ligament in five cases (56%), the medial plantar intermuscular septum in two cases (22%), and the plantar calcaneocuboid ligament in one case (11%).

The medial head was absent in one foot (1%). Out of the 99 cases in which it was present, the medial head had origins from the medial calcaneal surface in all cases (100%), the long plantar ligament in 92 cases (93%) the plantar calcaneocuboid ligament in 79 cases (80%), the plantar calcaneal surface in 62 cases (63%), the medial calcaneal process in 12 cases (12%), the tendon of tibialis posterior in 8 cases (8%), the sheath of the flexor hallucis longus tendon in 8 cases (8%), the medial plantar intermuscular septum in 5 cases (5%), the flexor retinaculum in 2 cases (2%), the lateral plantar intermuscular septum in 2 cases (2%), the connection between quadratus plantae and abductor hallucis in 1 case (1%), and from abductor hallucis in 1 case (1%) (Pretterklieber 2018).

The lateral head was absent in 31 feet (31%). Out of the 69 cases in which it was present, the lateral head had origins from the long plantar ligament in 62 cases (90%), the lateral plantar process in 44 cases (64%), the plantar surface of the calcaneus in 11 cases (16%), the lateral surface of the calcaneus in eight cases (12%), the plantar calcaneocuboid ligament in two cases (3%), the lateral plantar intermuscular septum in two cases (3%), and the medial plantar intermuscular septum in one case (1%) (Pretterklieber 2018).

Pretterklieber (2018) was able to identify the insertions of quadratus plantae onto the long flexor tendons in 44 cases. Quadratus plantae contributed to the first tendon in two cases (5%), the second tendon in 43 cases (98%), the third tendon in 44 cases (100%), the fourth tendon in 42 cases (96%), and the fifth tendon in 19 cases (43%).

Beger et al. (2018b) studied the connections of the master knot of Henry in 20 feet from ten cadavers. In 4 feet (20%), the medial head of quadratus plantae was either mostly tendinous (one case) or half tendinous (three cases). Quadratus plantae attached to the slip of flexor hallucis longus only in

6 feet (30%) and to both this slip and the tendon of flexor digitorum longus in the 14 remaining cases (70%). Edama et al. (2019) studied quadratus plantae in 116 legs from 62 Japanese cadavers. Quadratus plantae was comprised of both the medial and lateral heads in 101 legs (87.1%). In 11 cases (9.5%) the lateral head was absent, and in four cases (3.4%) the medial head was absent.

Out of ten sides from five fetuses, Elvan et al. (2019) found that quadratus plantae contributed to the long flexor tendon going to digit two on one side (10%), to the long flexor tendon going to the third and fourth digits on all ten sides (100%), and to the long flexor tendon going to the fifth digit on four sides (40%).

Anomalies

Description

Pettersen (1979) found that quadratus plantae was rudimentary in both feet of a boy with trisomy 13q. In both feet, the lateral head was absent. In the left foot, the medial head was diminutive and originated from the posteromedial aspect of the calcaneus near the insertion of the calcaneal tendon. The muscle did not have fleshy fibers as it crossed the longitudinal arch of the foot. It had a "weblike" attachment onto the deep surface of flexor digitorum brevis, into the part of the flexor hallucis longus tendon that unites with flexor digitorum longus, and into the deep plantar fascia and ligaments of the foot. In the right foot, the medial head had a similar origin and was also diminutive but sent fleshy fibers across the foot that ended with a tendinous attachment into flexor digitorum longus. Hootnick et al. (1987) describe an individual that had a right limb with congenital tibial aplasia, talocalcaneal synchondrosis, and an adducted foot with five toes. In this limb, quadratus plantae originated from the calcaneus and inserted into the common flexor tendon sheet in the foot.

Prevalence

In their literature review, Smith et al. (2015) found that absence of the lateral head of quadratus plantae was only observed in 1 out of 20 individuals with trisomy 13 (5%).

Clinical Implications

Athavale et al. (2012a) suggest that a bulky medial head of quadratus plantae may cause tarsal tunnel syndrome.

LUMBRICALES (LUMBRICALS) (FIGURE 5.11)

Synonyms

A singular lumbrical muscle may be referred to as lumbricalis, and multiple lumbrical muscles may be referred to as lumbricales or lumbricales pedis (Wood 1868; Macalister 1875).

Typical Presentation

Description

The four lumbrical muscles originate from the digital tendons of flexor digitorum longus at the points where they separate from the common flexor digitorum longus tendon (Standring 2016). The first lumbrical muscle originates from the tendon going to digit two and goes to digit two (Standring 2016). The second lumbrical originates from the tendons going to digits two and three and goes to digit three (Standring 2016). The third lumbrical originates from the tendons going to digits three and four and goes to digit four (Standring 2016). The fourth lumbrical originates from the tendons going to digits four and five and goes to digit five (Standring 2016). Each lumbrical inserts into the dorsal digital expansion on the proximal phalanx of its target digit (Standring 2016).

Innervation

The first lumbrical is innervated by the medial plantar nerve and the others are innervated by the lateral plantar nerve (Standring 2016).

Comparative Anatomy

The lumbrical muscles have similar typical presentations in the apes, with origins from the tendons of flexor digitorum longus and flexor hallucis longus and insertions onto the medial aspects of the dorsal digital expansions of digits two through five (Chapman 1880; Hepburn 1892; Beddard 1893; Dwight 1895; Sonntag 1924; Raven 1950; Miller 1952; Gibbs 1999; Diogo et al. 2010, 2012, 2013a,b, 2017). As in humans, the lumbricals may be missing in some cases (Beddard 1893) or may have double origins from the flexor digitorum longus and flexor hallucis longus tendons (Champneys 1872; Chapman 1880; Hepburn 1892; Beddard 1893; Dwight 1895; Sonntag 1924; Gibbs 1999; Diogo et al. 2012, 2013a,b).

Variations

Description

One or more of the lumbrical muscles may be absent (Wood 1868; Macalister 1875; Knott 1883b; Ochiltree 1912; Bergman et al. 1988; Chaney et al. 1996; Kura et al. 1997; Kafka et al. 2016). Any one of the lumbricals may originate with two bellies (i.e., are doubled) instead of having a unified origin from one or more of the flexor tendons (Wood 1868; Macalister 1875; Bergman et al. 1988; Hur et al. 2015b). The lumbricals may receive contributions from flexor digitorum longus, flexor hallucis longus, and/or quadratus plantae (Macalister 1875; Bergman et al. 1988; Hur et al. 2015b). The lumbricals may also lack origins from the flexor digitorum longus tendons and instead originate from the tendon(s) of flexor digitorum brevis, tibialis posterior (in the case of the first lumbrical), and/or flexor hallucis longus (Wood 1868; Macalister 1875; Bergman et al. 1988; Athavale et al. 2012a; Hur et al. 2015b; Kafka et al. 2016).

The third or fourth lumbricals may be bifurcated at their insertions, particularly when these muscles are doubled, and attach onto the contiguous sides of the corresponding digits (Wood 1868; Macalister 1875; Oukouchi et al. 1992).

The lumbrical muscles may send accessory tendons to the proximal phalanges of their target digit (Oukouchi et al. 1992). Oukouchi et al. (1992) suggest that the insertion onto proximal phalanges and bifurcated insertions onto two adjacent digits may be atavistic presentations of the lumbricals.

Prevalence

In a sample of 102 subjects, Wood (1868) found that the lumbricals only showed variations in seven subjects (6.9%). The second lumbrical was absent bilaterally in one subject. The third lumbrical originated from flexor digitorum brevis in one subject and was doubled bilaterally in another subject. The fourth lumbrical muscle was absent in three subjects (one bilateral case, two unilateral cases) and doubled bilaterally in another subject and had bifurcated insertions that attached onto both digits four and five.

Oukouchi et al. (1992) studied the lumbrical muscles in 25 feet from Japanese cadavers. Accessory slips to the proximal phalanges of the corresponding digit were sent by the first lumbrical in three cases (12%), the second lumbrical in two cases (8%), the third lumbrical in three cases (12%), and the fourth lumbrical in four cases (16%). In one foot (4%), the third and fourth lumbricals were split at their insertions, with the former sending slips to digits three and four and the latter sending slips to digits four and five.

In a sample of 257 cadaveric feet, Chaney et al. (1996) found that all the lumbricals were absent in 8 cases (3.1%). One lumbrical was present in 9 cases (3.5%), two lumbricals were present in 31 cases (12.1%), three lumbricals were present in 70 cases (27.2%), and all four lumbricals were present in 139 cases (54.1%). In a sample of 11 feet from eight cadavers, Kura et al. (1997) found that the third and fourth lumbrical muscles were absent in 1 foot (9.1%).

In a sample of 47 lower limbs, Athavale et al. (2012a) found that slips of flexor hallucis longus gave rise to the first lumbrical muscle in 18 cases (38.3%) and to other lumbrical muscles in 9 cases (19.15%). In a sample of 66 cadaveric specimens, Hur et al. (2015b) found that the first lumbrical had two bellies with origins from the digit two tendon of flexor digitorum longus and a slip of flexor hallucis longus in 55 specimens (83.3%). It originated as a single belly from the digit two tendon of flexor digitorum longus only in one case (1.5%) and as a single belly from the tendinous slip of flexor hallucis longus only in the remaining ten cases (15.2%). The second lumbrical originated from the digit three tendon of flexor digitorum longus and from tendinous slips of flexor hallucis longus going to digits two and three in all specimens (100%). The third lumbrical originated from tendinous slips of flexor hallucis longus going to digits three and four in 46 specimens (69.7%). The fourth lumbrical originated from the tendinous slip of flexor hallucis longus going to digit four in 12 specimens (18.2%). Deep muscle fibers of the fourth lumbrical originated from the tendinous slip of flexor hallucis longus going to digit two in three specimens (4.5%), from the slip going to digit three in 19 specimens (28.8%), and from the slip going to digit four in 10 specimens (15.2%).

Anomalies

Description

Mieden (1982) describes an infant with median cleft lip, hypotelorism, and alobar holoprosencephaly. The fourth lumbrical muscle was absent on the left side (Mieden 1982). The author does not specify if it was a hand or foot lumbrical. On the left side of a child with trisomy 21, there were double lumbrical muscles between digits four and five (Bersu 1980). In the right foot of the fetus with craniorachischisis dissected by Alghamdi et al. (2018), the first lumbrical muscle was absent. Hootnick et al. (1987) describe an individual that had a right limb with congenital tibial aplasia, talocalcaneal synchondrosis, and an adducted foot with five toes. In this limb, the four lumbricals partially arose from the common flexor tendon sheet found in the foot.

Prevalence

Bersu (1980) found double lumbrical muscles in one out of five individuals with trisomy 21 (20%).

Clinical Implications

Chaney et al. (1996) note that the absence of a lumbrical can result in claw toe or a sagittal plane deformity of a digit that can lead to calluses.

FLEXOR HALLUCIS BREVIS (FIGURE 5.12)

Synonyms

This muscle may also be referred to as flexor brevis hallucis (Macalister 1875).

Typical Presentation

Description

Flexor hallucis brevis arises from a bifurcated tendon, with the lateral part originating from the cuboid and the lateral cuneiform and the medial part originating from the tibialis posterior tendon and the medial intermuscular septum (Standring 2016). The muscle splits into medial and lateral portions that each have a tendinous attachment onto their respective side of the base of the proximal hallucal phalanx (Standring 2016). Upon insertion, the medial portion joins with the abductor hallucis tendon and the lateral portion joins with the adductor hallucis tendon (Standring 2016).

Innervation

Flexor hallucis brevis is innervated by the medial plantar nerve (Standring 2016).

Comparative Anatomy

Flexor hallucis brevis has a similar typical presentation in the apes. It has two heads that extend from the medial and/or lateral cuneiform, the first metatarsal, and sometimes the tibialis posterior tendon to the proximal hallucal phalanx, often fusing with abductor hallucis, adductor hallucis, or opponens hallucis and exhibiting additional insertions into the first metatarsal (Champneys 1872; Brooks 1887; Hepburn 1892; Beddard 1893; Dwight 1895; Sonntag 1924; Raven 1950; Miller 1952; Lewis 1964; Gibbs 1999; Vereecke et al. 2005; Diogo et al. 2010, 2012, 2013a,b, 2017). It may have an origin from the calcaneus, first tarsometatarsal

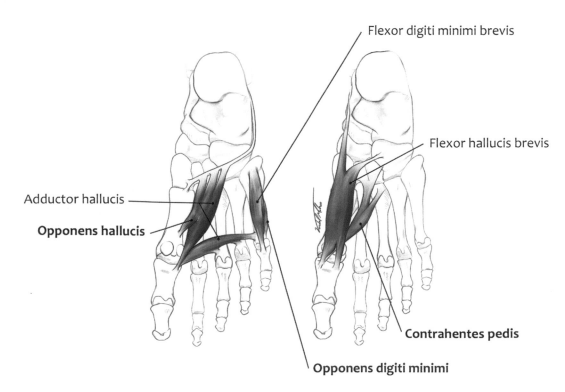

FIGURE 5.12   Third layer of plantar foot muscles in plantar (inferior) view. Contrahentes pedis and flexor hallucis brevis are illustrated on the right side, and the other muscles are illustrated on the left side.

joint, or the navicular in gorillas (Gibbs 1999; Diogo et al. 2010). It may have an origin from the cuboid in common chimpanzees (Beddard 1893).

Variations

Description

The lateral head of flexor hallucis brevis may be fused with adductor hallucis, and the medial head may be fused with abductor hallucis (Macalister 1875; Le Double 1897; Bergman et al. 1988; Kafka et al. 2016). It may receive accessory slips from the calcaneus, medial cuneiform, long plantar ligament, the tendon of flexor digitorum longus, or the tendon of tibialis posterior (Wood 1867b, 1868; Macalister 1875; Le Double 1897; Bergman et al. 1988; Kafka et al. 2016; Standring 2016). It may send a slip to the proximal phalanx of digit two (Wood 1867b; Macalister 1875; Le Double 1897; Bergman et al. 1988; Kafka et al. 2016; Standring 2016).

Prevalence
N/A

Anomalies

Description

Pettersen et al. (1979) found that flexor hallucis brevis had anomalous presentations in one neonate and one fetus with trisomy 13. In the neonate, the left flexor hallucis brevis had an accessory head of origin from the medial cuneiform. The other "normal" heads of this muscle originated from the base of the first metatarsal. In the fetus, the muscle on both sides of the body originated from the first metatarsal distal to its base.

On the right side of the fetus with craniorachischisis dissected by Alghamdi et al. (2017), flexor hallucis brevis was absent. On the left side of the specimen, flexor hallucis brevis extended from the lateral cuneiform and base of the first metatarsal to the base of the proximal hallucal phalanx and sent fibers to the tendon of abductor hallucis. In the female fetus with trisomy 18 dissected by Alghamdi et al. (2018), the distal end of abductor hallucis was fused with the medial head of flexor hallucis brevis bilaterally.

Prevalence

In their literature review, Smith et al. (2015) found that accessory slips of flexor hallucis brevis were only present in 1 of 20 individuals with trisomy 13 (5%).

Clinical Implications
N/A

ADDUCTOR HALLUCIS (FIGURE 5.12)

Synonyms

The transverse head of adductor hallucis was considered a separate muscle in earlier texts and may be referred to as transversalis pedis Casserii (Macalister 1875), transversalis

pedis, transversus pedis, transversus plantae, abducteur transverse, or adductor transversus hallucis (Knott 1883b).

Typical Presentation

Description

The transverse head of adductor hallucis originates from the plantar metatarsophalangeal ligaments of digits three, four, and five and from the deep transverse metatarsal ligaments between these digits (Standring 2016). The oblique head originates from the bases of metatarsals two, three, and four and from the sheath of the fibularis longus tendon (Standring 2016). The medial portion of the oblique head joins with flexor hallucis brevis and inserts onto the lateral sesamoid bone of the hallux (Standring 2016). The lateral portion of the oblique head merges with the transverse head and inserts onto the lateral sesamoid bone and onto the base of the proximal hallucal phalanx (Standring 2016).

Innervation

Adductor hallucis is innervated by the lateral plantar nerve (Standring 2016).

Comparative Anatomy

Adductor hallucis has a similar typical presentation in the apes. In most cases, this muscle has (1) an oblique head that originates from the bases of the second, third, and sometimes fourth metatarsals; (2) a transverse head that originates from the distal plantar surfaces of metatarsals two through four and their corresponding metatarsophalangeal joints and ligaments; and (3) insertions onto the first metatarsal, the base of the proximal hallucal phalanx, and sometimes the lateral hallucal sesamoid bone (Champneys 1872; Brooks 1887; Hepburn 1892; Beddard 1893; Dwight 1895; Sonntag 1924; Raven 1950; Miller 1952; Lewis 1964; Gibbs 1999; Vereecke et al. 2005; Diogo et al. 2010, 2012, 2013a,b, 2017).

The two heads are always fused in gibbons (Brooks 1887) and variably united in common chimpanzees (Gibbs 1999). The oblique head in gorillas and bonobos does not have an origin from the base of the fourth metatarsal (Miller 19552; Vereecke et al. 2005; Diogo et al. 2010, 2017). Attachments to the fourth metatarsal are absent entirely in orangutans (Beddard 1893; Brooks 1887; Gibbs 1999) and in some bonobos (Diogo et al. 2017). The oblique head in orangutans may have an origin from the sheath of the fibularis longus tendon (Beddard 1893; Brooks 1887; Sonntag 1924).

Variations

Description

The central component of the transverse head may be inseparable from the medial and lateral components (Kura et al. 1997). The origin of the transverse head from the fifth digit may be absent (Macalister 1875; Le Double 1897; Bergman et al. 1988; Arakawa et al. 2003; Standring 2016). Macalister (1875) and Knott (1883b) note that the attachments to the third and fourth digits may also be absent. More often, the entire transverse head of adductor hallucis may be absent (Macalister 1875; Knott 1883b; Cralley and Schuberth 1979; Kura et al. 1997; Kafka et al. 2016; Standring 2016).

The oblique head of adductor hallucis may originate entirely from the sheath of the fibularis longus tendon (Macalister 1875). The oblique head of adductor hallucis may send a slip to the base of the proximal phalanx of digit two (Wood 1867b; Macalister 1875; Knott 1883b; Arakawa et al. 2003; Kafka et al. 2016; Standring 2016) or more rarely digit three (Ochiltree 1912; Bergman et al. 1988). The oblique head may receive a slip from the tendon of tibialis posterior (Gunal et al. 1994).

Chouke (1927) uses "adductor hallucis accessorius" to refer to a trigastric supernumerary muscle that has some similarities with the accessory long flexors of the calf. Adductor hallucis accessorius originated as a fleshy belly (first belly) from the medial margin of the tibia below the origin of flexor digitorum longus, about three inches above the medial malleolus. It also had an origin from the deep fascia of the leg. The muscle coursed superficial to the tibial nerve and became tendinous at the level of the medial malleolus. The tendon passed under the flexor retinaculum medial to the synovial sheath of the flexor hallucis longus tendon and posterior to the tibial nerve. The tendon then received a fleshy bundle (second belly) from the posterior portion of the medial surface of the calcaneus that originated from under the origin of abductor hallucis. In the sole of the foot, adductor hallucis accessorius became tendinous again and passed to the plantar surface of the medial cuneiform. At this point, it became fleshy again (third belly) and joined with the oblique head of adductor hallucis just before its insertion.

Arakawa et al. (2003) identified the common origin sites of the oblique head as the sheath of the fibularis longus tendon, the long plantar ligament, the bases of metatarsals two through four and the plantar metatarsal ligaments between them, and the lateral cuneiform. These authors then classified the oblique head into four types. Type A was described as the narrow type and had a confined range of origin. This type was divided into three subtypes. In subtype 1, all the common origins were present. In subtype 2, the origin from the long plantar ligament was missing. In subtype 3, the origin from the lateral cuneiform was missing. Type B was described as the lateral type and exhibited all the common origin sites as well as an origin via an aponeurotic slip from the base of the fifth metatarsal. Type C was described as the wide type and had broad origins. In addition to the common origin sites, type C oblique heads originated laterally from a slip from the base of the fifth metatarsal and had possible medial origins from the tibialis posterior tendon, medial intermuscular septum, plantar tarsometatarsal ligament between the medial cuneiform and the base of the second metatarsal, or the fibularis longus tendon inserting into the first dorsal interosseous muscle. Type D was described as the medial type and exhibited all the common origin sites and had potential medial origins from the medial sites found in Type C.

Arakawa et al. (2003) also identified the common origin sites of the transverse head as the capsules of the third, fourth, and fifth metatarsophalangeal joints and the deep transverse metatarsal ligaments between them. These authors classified the transverse head into three types. Type A was described as the narrow type and had a confined range of origin, only originating from the third, fourth, and fifth metatarsophalangeal joints and the deep transverse metatarsal ligaments between them. Type B was described as the lateral type and originated from the common origin sites only. Type C was described as the wide type and originated from the common origin sites, the aponeurosis between the third plantar and the fourth dorsal interosseous muscles, and the deep band of the fibular portion of the plantar aponeurosis.

Prevalence

Knott (1883b) found that the attachment of "transversus pedis" to the heads of the third and fourth metatarsals was absent in 5 out of 34 cases (14.7%). In a sample of 91 cadaveric feet, Cralley and Schuberth (1979) found that the transverse head of adductor hallucis was absent in 6% of cases. In a sample of 11 feet from eight cadavers, Kura et al. (1997) found that the transverse head of adductor hallucis was absent in 1 foot (9.1%). In 10 feet (90.9%), the central component of the transverse head of adductor hallucis could not be separated from the medial or lateral components.

Arakawa et al. (2003) studied adductor hallucis in 45 feet from 34 cadavers. These authors classified the oblique head into four types (see above for descriptions). Type A was found in 21 cases (46.7%), type B was found in 15 cases (33.3%), type C was found in four cases (8.8%), and type D was found in five cases (11.1%). These authors could only identify the origins and insertions of the transverse head in 34 specimens and classified this head into three types (see above for descriptions). Type A was found in 14 cases (41.2%), type B was found in 10 cases (29.4%), and type C was found in 10 cases (29.4%).

Anomalies

Description

In a study of individuals with trisomy 13, Pettersen et al. (1979) noted that the transverse head of adductor hallucis was absent on the left side of one neonate and bilaterally in one fetus. The muscle was hypoplastic bilaterally in a second neonate and on the right side of a second fetus. On the left side of this second fetus, it originated from the deep surface of the flexor digitorum longus tendon to digit five but had a typical insertion.

On the right foot of a male neonate with Meckel syndrome, Pettersen (1984) observed that the transverse head of adductor hallucis had a partial origin from the flexor digitorum brevis to the fifth digit. On the left foot, the transverse head was joined at its origin to flexor digiti minimi brevis and to the interosseous muscles of digit four. Hootnick et al. (1987) describe an individual that had a right limb with congenital tibial aplasia, talocalcaneal synchondrosis, and an adducted foot with five toes. In this limb, the transverse head of adductor hallucis was absent.

The transverse head of adductor hallucis was absent in the right foot of the fetus with trisomy 18 and cyclopia described by Smith et al. (2015). On the right side of the fetus with craniorachischisis dissected by Alghamdi et al. (2017), the transverse head of adductor hallucis was absent. The oblique head originated from the medial cuneiform and had a typical insertion onto the proximal phalanx of digit one. On the left foot, the oblique head originated from the bases of the third and fourth metatarsals and the transverse head originated from the distal ends of these metatarsals. The heads inserted together onto the base of the proximal phalanx of digit one.

Prevalence

In their literature review, Smith et al. (2015) found that absence of the transverse head of adductor hallucis was noted in 2 out of 20 individuals (10%) with trisomy 13.

Clinical Implications

Expansion of the tibialis posterior tendon into the oblique head of adductor hallucis is associated with hallux valgus (Gunal et al. 1994).

CONTRAHENTES PEDIS (FIGURE 5.12)

Entry adapted by permission from Springer Nature Customer Service Centre GmbH: Springer Current Molecular Biology Reports, Muscles Lost in Our Adult Primate Ancestors Still Imprint in US: on Muscle Evolution, Development, Variations, and Pathologies. E. Boyle, V. Mahon, R. Diogo, 2020.

See also: Adductor hallucis

Synonyms

Contrahens refers to a singular muscle, and contrahentes refer to multiple muscles (Cihak 1972).

Typical Presentation

This muscle is only present as a variation.

Comparative Anatomy

Descriptions of contrahentes of the feet are often neglected in descriptions of ape anatomy. In gibbons, Hirasaki and Kumakura (2010) note the presence of a contrahens muscle originating from the sheath of the fibularis longus tendon and the third metatarsal and inserting onto the tibial side of the proximal phalanx of digit five. In bonobos, the contrahens muscle extending from the contrahens raphe to digit five is often present and well-developed while that to digit four is often thin, reduced, or absent (Hepburn 1892; Miller 1952; Lewis 1989; Diogo et al. 2017). Contrahentes with variable attachments to digits two, four, and five are common in lemuriform primates and some monkeys (Gebo 1985; Hirasaki and Kumakura 2010).

Variations

Description

Contrahentes of the foot (contrahentes 3, 4, 5) are typically only present in the early stages of human development and then disappear completely later in ontogeny (Cihak 1972; Diogo et al 2019). Adductor hallucis derives from contrahentes 1 and 2 (Cihak 1972; Arakawa et al. 2003).

The oblique head develops from the tibial part of the contrahentes layer at CR18 mm (crown-rump length of 18 mm), and the transverse head develops from the fibular part of the contrahentes layer at CR30 mm (crown-rump length of 30 mm) (Cihak 1972; Diogo et al 2019). Contrahentes 3, 4, and 5 persist in the embryo until CR25–35 mm (crown-rump length of 25 to 35 mm) and then become completely lost (Cihak 1972, Diogo et al. 2019).

Contrahentes are very rare in karyotypically normal humans. Hirsch and Vekkos (1984) found contrahentes muscles in 2 feet. In both cases, the contrahentes muscles occupied the approximate position of the oblique head of adductor hallucis but were larger and had more extensive attachments. The transverse head of adductor hallucis was absent in both feet. In one case, the muscle inserted onto the metatarsophalangeal joint capsules of digits one and two. In the second case, the muscle inserted onto the metatarsophalangeal joint capsules of digits two through five.

Innervation

Contrahentes pedis are innervated by the lateral plantar nerve (Miller 1952; Hirch and Vekkos 1984).

Prevalence

N/A

Anomalies

N/A

Clinical Implications

N/A

OPPONENS HALLUCIS (FIGURE 5.12)

Entry adapted by permission from Springer Nature Customer Service Centre GmbH: Springer Current Molecular Biology Reports, Muscles Lost in Our Adult Primate Ancestors Still Imprint in US: on Muscle Evolution, Development, Variations, and Pathologies. E. Boyle, V. Mahon, R. Diogo, 2020.

See also: Adductor hallucis, Flexor hallucis brevis

Synonyms

N/A

Typical Presentation

This muscle is only present as a variation.

Comparative Anatomy

Among the apes, opponens hallucis has been described in detail only in orangutans (Chapman 1880; Brooks 1887; Primrose 1899; Boyer 1935; Diogo et al. 2013b) and seems to be present in some common chimpanzees and bonobos (Chapman 1879; Champneys 1872; Diogo et al. 2013a, 2017). Though it has been described in one gibbon, the presence of this muscle in gibbons has not been confirmed by other dissections (Diogo et al. 2012). When present in orangutans, common chimpanzees, and bonobos, the muscle originates from the medial cuneiform and inserts onto the first metatarsal (Brooks 1887; Primrose 1899; Diogo et al. 2013a,b, 2017). In orangutans, Brooks (1887) notes an origin from a cartilaginous nodule in the tibialis posterior tendon, and Boyer (1935) notes an insertion into the base of the proximal hallucal phalanx. It is also often fused with flexor hallucis brevis in orangutans (Brooks 1887; Primrose 1889; Boyer 1935).

Variations

Description

Opponens hallucis has typically been described as an accessory slip of adductor hallucis that inserts onto the first metatarsal (Macalister 1875; Knott 1883b; Playfair McMurrich 1906; Standring 2016). Kafka et al. (2016) state that opponens hallucis describes a slip originating from either the oblique or transverse head of adductor hallucis that inserts onto the proximal hallucal phalanx. Bergman et al. (1988) state that opponens hallucis is an accessory slip of flexor hallucis brevis that inserts onto the first metatarsal.

Innervation

In orangutans, opponens hallucis is innervated by the medial plantar nerve (Brooks 1887).

Prevalence

No prevalence information is available, but Macalister (1875, p. 129) describes it as a "frequent constituent element in the human foot."

Anomalies
N/A

Clinical Implications
N/A

FLEXOR DIGITI MINIMI BREVIS (FIGURE 5.12)

Synonyms

It may also be referred to as flexor brevis minimi digiti (Macalister 1875) or flexor brevis quinti digiti (Playfair McMurrich 1906).

Typical Presentation

Description

Flexor digiti minimi brevis originates from the base of the fifth metatarsal and from the sheath of fibularis longus (Standring 2016). Its tendon blends with that of abductor digiti minimi to insert onto the base of the proximal phalanx of digit five (Standring 2016).

Innervation

Flexor digiti minimi brevis is innervated by the lateral plantar nerve (Standring 2016).

Comparative Anatomy

Flexor digiti minimi brevis has a similar typical presentation in the apes, originating from the base of the fifth metatarsal and/or the plantar tarsometatarsal ligament extending to the tuberosity of this metatarsal and inserting onto the proximal phalanx of digit five (Champneys 1872; Sonntag 1924; Boyer 1935; Raven 1950; Miller 1952; Gibbs 1999; Vereecke et al. 2005; Ferrero 2011; Ferrero et al. 2012; Diogo et al. 2010, 2012, 2013a,b, 2017). There may be an origin from the fourth metatarsal in gorillas (Raven 1950; Gibbs 1999) and from the sheath of fibularis longus in orangutans (Sonntag 1924; Gibbs 1999). It may be absent in some common chimpanzees (Champneys 1872; Diogo et al. 2013a).

Variations

Description

Flexor digiti minimi brevis may be fused with abductor digiti minimi (Macalister 1875; Kopuz et al. 1999). It may also be fused with the tendon of abductor ossis metatarsi digiti quinti (Macalister 1875). It may originate entirely from the sheath of fibularis longus (Macalister 1875). Jana and Roy (2011) note an unusual case in which flexor digiti minimi brevis arose from the lateral plantar process of the calcaneus with abductor digiti minimi and then passed onto the lateral side of the fifth metatarsal. The tendon of flexor digiti minimi brevis received the lateral slip of the fibularis tertius insertion at the base of the fifth metatarsal (Jana and Roy 2011). The insertion of flexor digiti minimi brevis onto the proximal phalanx may be separate from the insertion of abductor digiti minimi (Macalister 1875; Knott 1883b). A deep fascicle of flexor digiti minimi brevis that inserts onto the fifth metatarsal may be referred to as opponens digiti minimi (see the entry for this muscle) (Wood 1864, Macalister 1875; Playfair McMurrich 1906; Bergman et al. 1988; Kafka et al. 2016; Standring 2016).

Prevalence
N/A

Anomalies

Description

On the right foot of a male neonate with Meckel syndrome, Pettersen (1984) found that flexor digiti minimi brevis attached to the fifth digit and received a slip from flexor digitorum brevis that did not split to accommodate the tendon of flexor digitorum longus. On the left foot, this muscle was fused with the origin of adductor hallucis and was represented by a mass (along with abductor digiti minimi) on the plantar and lateral sides of digit six with vague attachments to this digit and partially to digit five. Hootnick et al. (1987) describe an individual that had a right limb with congenital tibial aplasia, talocalcaneal synchondrosis, and an adducted foot with five toes. In this limb, flexor digiti minimi brevis originated from the calcaneus abnormally deep in the foot and passed deep to quadratus plantae.

Prevalence

N/A

Clinical Implications

N/A

Opponens digiti minimi (Figure 5.12)

Entry adapted by permission from Springer Nature Customer Service Centre GmbH: Springer Current Molecular Biology Reports, Muscles Lost in Our Adult Primate Ancestors Still Imprint in US: on Muscle Evolution, Development, Variations, and Pathologies. E. Boyle, V. Mahon, R. Diogo, 2020.

Synonyms

This muscle is also referred to as opponens quinti digiti (Playfair McMurrich [1906) or opponens minimi digiti (Macalister 1875).

Typical Presentation

This muscle is only present as a variation.

Comparative Anatomy

While typically absent in adult humans, opponens digiti minimi is present in adult apes (Gibbs 1999; Diogo et al. 2010, 2012, 2013a,b, 2017). In most cases, opponens digiti minimi has variable connections to flexor digiti minimi brevis, originates from the base of the fifth metatarsal, and inserts onto to the lateral border of the fifth metatarsal and/or the proximal phalanx of digit five (Primrose 1899; Raven 1950; Miller 1952; Gibbs 1999; Diogo et al. 2010, 2012, 2013a,b, 2017). In orangutans and bonobos, this muscle has an origin from the sheath of the fibularis longus tendon (Miller 1952; Gibbs 1999; Ferrero 2011; Ferrero et al. 2012; Diogo et al. 2013b, 2017).

Variations

Description

Opponens digiti minimi is typically only present in the early stages of human development, and then disappears later during gestation. Bardeen (1906) states that the blastema of opponens digiti minimi and flexor digiti minimi brevis appears at CR12mm, and then the muscles differentiate at CR18mm. Cihak (1972) suggests that this muscle appears at CR20mm (crown-rump length of 20mm) and differentiates from flexor digiti minimi brevis at CR40mm.

Diogo et al. (2019) found that opponens digiti minimi is well-differentiated from flexor digiti minimi brevis at CR 36mm and persists until at least CR51mm, or gestational week 11.

When present in adults, this muscle is a distinct, deep fascicle of flexor digiti minimi brevis that originates from the base of the fifth metatarsal and inserts along the lateral aspect of the shaft of the fifth metatarsal (Wood 1864, Macalister 1875; Playfair McMurrich 1906; Bregman et al. 1988; Kafka et al. 2016; Standring 2016). Another presentation in an adult male cadaver was noted by Rana and Das (2006), where this muscle had the same origin but inserted onto the distal phalanx of the fifth digit. It may be present bilaterally (Wood 1868; Rana and Das 2006). Opponens digiti minimi may receive a slip from the fibularis longus tendon (Edama et al. 2020).

Innervation

Opponens digiti minimi is innervated by the lateral plantar nerve (Gibbs 1999; Rana and Das 2006).

Prevalence

Wood (1868) found opponens digiti minimi in 6 out of 36 subjects (16.7%).

Anomalies

N/A

Clinical Implications

N/A

Interossei plantares (Plantar Interossei) (Figure 5.11)

Synonyms

N/A

Typical Presentation

Description

The plantar interossei are comprised of three muscles that are situated beneath the three lateral metatarsals (Standring 2016). Each muscle originates from the base and medial side of one metatarsal and inserts onto the dorsal digital expansion and base of the proximal phalanx of its corresponding digit (Standring 2016). The first plantar interosseous muscle thus originates and inserts onto digit three, the second plantar interosseous muscle originates and inserts onto digit four, and the third plantar interosseous muscle originates and inserts onto digit five (Standring 2016).

Innervation

The plantar interossei are innervated by the lateral plantar nerve (Standring 2016).

Comparative Anatomy

While the functional axis of the foot is digit two in humans, in the apes, the digit around which the interosseous muscles are arranged is typically digit three (Dwight 1895; Boyer 1935; Sonntag 1924; Raven 1950; Miller 1952; Gibbs 1999; Diogo et al. 2010, 2012, 2013a,b, 2017; Hirasaki and Oishi 2018). In most apes, the plantar interossei are attached along the lateral side of digit two and the medial sides of digits four and five (Dwight 1895; Boyer 1935; Sonntag 1924; Raven 1950; Miller 1952; Gibbs 1999; Diogo et al. 2010, 2012, 2013a,b, 2017; Hirasaki and Oishi 2018). Accessory attachments to metatarsals one and three have been observed in gorillas and orangutans (Raven 1950; Gibbs 1999; Ferrero 2011; Ferrero et al. 2012; Diogo et al. 2010, 2013b). Two accessory plantar interossei attached to the medial and lateral sides of the third metatarsal were observed by Dwight (1895) in common chimpanzees. Hirasaki and Oishi (2018) found that the interossei exhibited the human presentation and were thus arranged around digit two in two out of ten chimpanzees (20%), one out of three gorillas (33.3%), and in one bonobo.

Variations

Description

The second and third plantar interosseous muscles may receive a slip from the tendon of fibularis longus (Edama et al. 2020). The interossei may have accessory origins from the plantar ligaments and/or the fascia of adjacent muscles (Kalin and Hirsch 1987). The first plantar interosseous muscle may extend into the dorsal part of the second interosseous space (Manter 1945). The second and third plantar interossei may originate from the sheath of the fibularis longus tendon (Ochiltree 1912). The second plantar interosseus may take partial origin from adductor hallucis (Kalin and Hirsch 1987). Accessory slips may be present connecting the plantar and dorsal interossei (Manter 1945). The plantar and dorsal interossei may also be fused (Manter 1945). The tendons of the interossei may be bifurcated upon insertion and attach to two separate digits (Hallisy 1930; Manter 1945). The insertions into the dorsal digital expansions may be missing in some cases (Manter 1945; Oukouchi et al. 1992).

Prevalence

Manter (1945) studied the variations of the interosseous muscles in 149 cadaveric feet. In 23 cases (15.4%), the origin of the first plantar interosseous muscle extended into the dorsal part of the second interosseous space. It occupied the full length of this space in 8 feet, three-fourth the length of the space in 8 feet, and half the length of the space in 7 feet. An accessory slip originating from the third dorsal interosseous muscle and joining the first plantar interosseous muscle was found in 17 cases (11.4%). The first plantar and second dorsal interosseous muscles were fused in two cases (1.4%). The second plantar and third dorsal interosseous muscles were fused in four cases (2.7%). Manter (1945) also found that the tendon of the first plantar interosseous split to insert onto digits two and three in one case (0.7%). The tendon of the second plantar interosseous split to insert

onto digits three and four in one case (0.7%). The tendon of the third plantar interosseous split to insert onto digits four and five in two cases (1.4%).

Edama et al. (2020) studied the insertion of fibularis longus in 104 feet from 52 Japanese cadavers. The anterior frenular ligament was present in 33 feet (31.7%), and it attached to the second plantar interosseous muscle in 13 feet (12.5%) and the third plantar interosseous muscle in 29 feet (27.9%).

Anomalies

N/A

Clinical Implications

N/A

INTEROSSEI DORSALES (DORSAL INTEROSSEI) (FIGURE 5.13)

Synonyms

N/A

Typical Presentation

Description

The dorsal interossei are comprised of four bipennate muscles that occupy the spaces in between the metatarsals (Standring 2016). Each muscle originates via two heads from adjacent metatarsals and inserts into the base of the proximal phalanx and dorsal digital expansion of its target digit (Standring 2016). The first dorsal interosseous muscle originates from the sides of the first and second metatarsals and inserts onto the medial aspect of digit two (Standring 2016). The second dorsal interosseous muscle originates from the sides of the second and third metatarsals and inserts into the lateral aspect of digit two (Standring 2016). The third dorsal interosseous muscle originates from the sides of the third and fourth metatarsals and inserts into the lateral aspect of digit three (Standring 2016). The fourth dorsal interosseous muscle originates from the sides of the fourth and fifth metatarsals and inserts into the lateral aspect of digit four (Standring 2016).

Innervation

The dorsal interossei are innervated by the lateral plantar nerve (Standring 2016).

Comparative Anatomy

While the functional axis of the foot is digit two in humans, in the apes, the digit around which the interosseous muscles are arranged is typically digit three (Champneys 1872; Dwight 1895; Boyer 1935; Sonntag 1924; Raven 1950; Miller 1952; Gibbs 1999; Diogo et al. 2010, 2012, 2013a,b, 2017; Hirasaki and Oishi 2018). In the apes, the dorsal interossei are bipennate, with the exception of the first dorsal interosseous muscle in some gibbons (Brooks 1887; Gibbs 1999; Diogo et al. 2012). Typically, the first dorsal interosseous muscle originates from the first and second

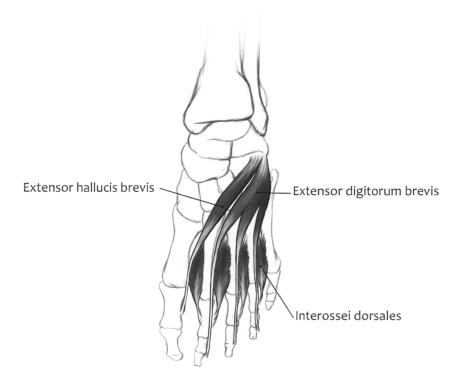

Extensor hallucis brevis

Extensor digitorum brevis

Interossei dorsales

FIGURE 5.13   Short extensors of the foot and the dorsal interossei in dorsal (superior) view of the foot.

metatarsal and inserts onto the medial side of digit two, the second originates from the second and third metatarsal and inserted onto the medial side of digit three, the third originates from the third and fourth metatarsals and inserts onto the lateral side of digit three, and the fourth originates from digits four and five and inserts onto the lateral side of digit four (Champneys 1872; Brooks 1887; Dwight 1895; Boyer 1935; Sonntag 1924; Raven 1950; Miller 1952; Gibbs 1999; Diogo et al. 2010, 2012, 2013a,b, 2017; Hirasaki and Oishi 2018). In gorillas and orangutans, the first dorsal interosseus muscle may originate from the medial cuneiform and second metatarsal (Brooks 1887; Boyer 1935; Raven 1950; Diogo et al. 2010, 2013b). Two accessory dorsal interossei on the lateral side of a common chimpanzee foot were observed by Dwight (1895). Hirasaki and Oishi (2018) found that the interossei exhibited the human presentation and were thus arranged around digit two in two out of ten chimpanzees (20%), one out of three gorillas (33.3%), and in one bonobo.

Variations

Description

Any one of the dorsal interossei may be unipennate as a variation (Macalister 1875; Manter 1945). The interossei may have accessory origins from the plantar ligaments and/or the fascia of adjacent muscles (Kalin and Hirsch 1987). Accessory slips may be present connecting the plantar and dorsal interossei (Manter 1945). The plantar and dorsal interossei may also be fused (Manter 1945). The

plantar portion of the second dorsal interosseous muscle may course plantarly and extend laterally over the first plantar interosseous muscle without directly attaching to it (Manter 1945). The second dorsal interosseous muscle may be doubled (Manter 1945). The tendons of the interossei may be bifurcated upon insertion and attach to two separate digits (Hallisy 1930; Manter 1945). The insertions into the dorsal digital expansions may be missing in some cases (Manter 1945; Oukouchi et al. 1992).

The fourth interosseous muscle may originate from the fusion of the fibularis tertius and fibularis brevis tendons (Olewnik 2019). Fibularis tertius may send an accessory tendon to the fascia that covers the fourth interosseus muscle (the fourth interosseous space) (Macalister 1875; Manter 1945; Joshi et al. 2006; Lambert 2016; Olewnik 2019). Fibularis longus may have insertions into the first, second, or fourth dorsal interossei (Kalin and Hirsch 1987; Edama et al. 2020). The first dorsal interosseous muscle may also originate from the fibularis longus tendon (Harbeson 1933, 1938; Manter 1945; Kalin and Hirsch 1987). The dorsal interosseous muscles may also receive slips or originate from fibularis brevis, extensor digitorum brevis, or flexor hallucis brevis (Wood 1867b; Macalister 1875; Manter 1945; Kalin and Hirsch 1987; Kafka et al. 2016).

An accessory slip deep to adductor hallucis between the first dorsal interosseous muscle and the first metatarsal may be present (Manter 1945). A well-developed fibrous band extending from the plantar aspect of the first dorsal interosseous to the proximal hallucal phalanx may also be present (Manter 1945). These variations may represent the "missing" plantar interosseous muscle in humans (Manter 1945).

Prevalence

Harbeson (1933) studied the origin of the first dorsal interosseous muscle in 27 feet from 15 subjects. In 20 cases, the medial head of the muscle originated via a tendinous slip from the fibularis longus tendon (74.1%). Harbeson (1938) provides the prevalence of this variation for two subsequent dissections in 1934 and 1937. In 1934, 24 feet from 13 subjects were dissected and the first dorsal interosseous muscle had an origin from the fibularis longus tendon in 11 feet (45.8%). In 1937, 24 feet from 12 subjects were dissected and the first dorsal interosseous muscle had an origin from the fibularis longus tendon in 15 feet (62.5%). The overall prevalence of this variation from Harbeson's research is therefore 46 out of 75 feet (61.3%).

Manter (1945) studied the variations of the interosseous muscles in 149 cadaveric feet. The first dorsal interosseous muscle originated as a single head from the second metatarsal in 17 cases (11.4%). The second dorsal interosseous muscle originated as single head from the second metatarsal in 11 cases (7.4%). The third dorsal interosseous muscle originated as a single head from the fourth metatarsal in five cases (3.4%). The fourth dorsal interosseous muscle originated as a single head from the fourth metatarsal in two cases (1.3%) and from the fifth metatarsal in 34 cases (22.8%).

Manter (1945) found an accessory slip originating from the third dorsal interosseous muscle that joined the first plantar interosseous muscle in 17 cases (11.4%). In four cases (2.7%), the plantar portion of the second dorsal interosseous muscle extended laterally over the first plantar interosseous muscle but did not directly attach to it. The first plantar and second dorsal interosseous muscles were fused in two cases (1.4%). The second plantar and third dorsal interosseous muscles were fused in four cases (2.7%). The second dorsal interosseous was doubled in two cases (1.4%). The first dorsal interosseous muscle received a tendinous slip of origin from the fibularis longus tendon in about 95 feet (63.5%). An accessory slip deep to adductor hallucis between the first dorsal interosseous muscle and the first metatarsal was present in three cases (2%). A well-developed fibrous band extending from the plantar aspect of the first dorsal interosseous to the proximal hallucal phalanx was present in 30 out of 54 feet (55.6%). Manter (1945) also found that the tendon of the second dorsal interosseous split to insert onto digits two and three in five cases (3.4%). The tendon of the third dorsal interosseous split to insert onto digits three and four in two cases (1.4%). The tendon of the fourth dorsal interosseous split to insert onto digits four and five in one case (0.7%).

Olewnik (2019) studied fibularis tertius in a sample of 106 cadaveric lower limbs. Out of the 91 limbs in which the muscle was present, the tendon had a single, broad insertion onto the base and shaft of the fifth metatarsal and the fascia

over the fourth interosseous space in 15 limbs (16.5%). In two limbs (2.2%), the tendon was fused with a slip from the fibularis brevis tendon, and the fourth interosseous muscle originated from this fusion. Edama et al. (2020) studied the insertion of fibularis longus in 104 feet from 52 Japanese cadavers. Insertions onto the first dorsal interosseous muscle were found in 38 feet (36.5%). The anterior frenular ligament was present in 33 feet (31.7%), and it attached to the fourth dorsal interosseous muscle in 20 feet (19.3%).

Anomalies

N/A

Clinical Implications

N/A

Extensor digitorum brevis (Figure 5.13)

Synonyms

This muscle may also be referred to as the extensor brevis digitorum pedis (Macalister 1875).

Typical Presentation

Description

Extensor digitorum brevis originates from the superolateral surface of the distal calcaneus, from the interosseous talo-calcaneal ligament, and from the inferior extensor retinaculum (Standring 2016). It ends in three tendons that insert onto the extensor digitorum longus tendons for digits two, three, and four (Standring 2016).

Innervation

Extensor digitorum brevis is innervated by the deep fibular nerve (Standring 2016).

Comparative Anatomy

Extensor digitorum brevis has a similar typical presentation in the apes, originating from the calcaneus and sending tendons to the dorsal aponeurosis of digits two, three, and four (Champneys 1872; Hepburn 1892; Beddard 1893; Sonntag 1924; Boyer 1935; Raven 1950; Miller 1952; Lewis 1966; Gibbs 1999; Vereecke et al. 2005; Diogo et al. 2010, 2012, 2013a,b, 2017). A tendon for digit five may be present in about half of gibbons (Lewis 1966) and in some common chimpanzees and bonobos (Miller 1952; Diogo et al. 2013a, 2017). An accessory slip attaching to digit two has been found in gibbons (Diogo et al. 2012). An origin from the base of the third metatarsal as well as a split insertion of the digit two tendon has been observed in orangutans (Gibbs 1999; Diogo et al. 2013b).

Variations

Description

One or more tendons, or even the entire muscle, may be absent (Flower and Murie 1867; Macalister 1875; Bergman et al. 1988; Sirasanagandla et al. 2013b; Standring 2016). The muscle belly or tendon going to digits two or three may be doubled (Wood 1867b, 1868; Macalister 1875; Sirasanagandla et al. 2013b; Won and Oh 2018). Sirasanagandla et al. (2013b) report a case where the tendon for digit two was tripled, having attachments to the proximal phalanx of digit two, the extensor digitorum longus tendon for digit two, and the fascia over the shaft of the third metatarsal.

Accessory bundles of extensor digitorum brevis may be present (Bergman et al. 1988; Kura et al. 1997; Sirasanagandla et al. 2013b; Won and Oh 2018). There may be an extra tendon of extensor digitorum brevis that joins the tendon of extensor digitorum longus going to digit five (Macalister 1875; Knott 1883b; Le Double 1897; Bergman et al. 1988; Chaney et al. 1996; Standring 2016). Extensor digitorum brevis may send slips to the dorsal interossei (Wood 1867b, 1868; Macalister 1875; Knott 1883b; Bergman et al. 1988; Sirasanagandla et al. 2013b; Standring 2016). The muscle bellies of extensor digitorum brevis may receive slips from tendons of extensor digitorum longus (Macalister 1875). It may also receive accessory slips from the talus, navicular, cuboid, lateral cuneiform, and/or third metatarsal (Macalister 1875; Bergman et al. 1988; Standring 2016).

Won and Oh (2018) report a case in which the extensor digitorum muscle belly to digit three was doubled and associated with an accessory muscle in the right foot of a cadaver. The extra muscular head originated from the cuboid and then joined with the extensor digitorum brevis tendon going to digit three. The accessory muscle was covered by extensor hallucis brevis, originated from the calcaneus, and inserted onto the lateral third of the transverse retinacular band.

Prevalence

Wood (1868) found that the extensor digitorum brevis tendon for digit two was doubled in 6 out of 40 males (15%) and 3 out of 30 females (10%). A slip to the first interosseous muscle was found in 3 out of 40 males (7.5%) and 1 out of 30 females (3.3%). Knott (1883b) found an extensor digitorum brevis tendon going to digit five in 2 out of 40 cases (5%).

Out of 291 cases, Chaney et al. (1996) found that both the extensor hallucis brevis tendon to digit one and the extensor digitorum tendons to digits two through four were present in 186 cases (63.9%). Tendons to the second, third, and fourth digits were present without the extensor hallucis brevis tendon in 50 cases (17.2%). In 11 subjects (3.8%), there were only two tendons present to various digits. There were more than four tendons present in 44 cases (15.1%). In a subsample of 284 limbs, Chaney et al. (1996) found an extensor digitorum brevis tendon to digit five in 51 limbs (18%). In a sample of 11 feet from 8 cadavers, Kura et al. (1997) found accessory muscles medial to extensor digitorum brevis going to digit two in 4 feet (36.4%).

Sirasanagandla et al. (2013b) studied extensor digitorum brevis in 44 limbs. In 36 limbs (81.8%) both the extensor hallucis brevis tendon to digit one and the extensor

digitorum tendons to digits two through four were present. In four limbs (9.1%), the tendon to the fourth digit was absent. In one limb (2.3%), there was an accessory bundle present that originated from extensor hallucis brevis and the extensor digitorum brevis belly going to digit two that merged with the first dorsal interosseous muscle. The extensor digitorum brevis tendon for digit two was doubled in two cases (4.5%) and tripled in one case (2.3%). In one case (2.3%), the extensor digitorum brevis tendon for digit three was doubled.

Anomalies

Description

Mieden (1982) describes an infant with median cleft lip, hypotelorism, and alobar holoprosencephaly. The tendon of extensor digitorum brevis to the second digit was absent on the left side (Mieden 1982). On the left side, the tendons of extensor digitorum brevis and longus were attached to the metatarsophalangeal joints (Mieden 1982). In a male infant with triploidy studied by Moen et al. (1984), extensor digitorum brevis was absent bilaterally. On the left foot of a male neonate with Meckel syndrome, Pettersen (1984) found that the extensor digitorum brevis tendons to digits five and six were absent and the tendon to digit two was diminutive.

On both sides of the fetus with craniorachischisis dissected by Alghamdi et al. (2017), extensor digitorum brevis did not send a tendon to the fourth digit. In the right foot of a fetus with trisomy 18 and cyclopia dissected by Smith et al. (2015), the extensor digitorum brevis tendon to the second digit bifurcated and attached onto digits two and three. In the female fetus with trisomy 18 dissected by Alghamdi et al. (2018), there was a supernumerary muscle situated lateral to the right extensor digitorum brevis. This muscle arose from the cuboid and sent a tendon to the dorsum of digit five. Furthermore, extensor hallucis brevis fused proximally with extensor digitorum brevis on both sides of the body.

Prevalence

N/A

Clinical Implications

Hypertrophy of the extensor digitorum brevis bundles may simulate ganglia (Montgomery and Miller 1988).

EXTENSOR HALLUCIS BREVIS (FIGURE 5.13)

Synonyms

N/A

Typical Presentation

Description

Extensor hallucis brevis is regarded as a distinct medial slip of extensor digitorum brevis (Standring 2016). This muscle thus originates from the superolateral surface of the distal calcaneus, from the interosseous talocalcaneal ligament, and from the deep aspect of the base of the inferior extensor retinaculum (Standring 2016). Its tendon inserts onto the dorsal surface of the base of the proximal hallucal phalanx (Standring 2016).

Innervation

Extensor hallucis brevis is innervated by the deep fibular nerve (Standring 2016).

Comparative Anatomy

Extensor hallucis brevis has a similar typical presentation in the apes, originating from the calcaneus and/or extensor digitorum brevis and inserting onto the base of the proximal hallucal phalanx (Champneys 1872; Hepburn 1892; Beddard 1893; Sonntag 1924; Boyer 1935; Raven 1950; Miller 1952; Lewis 1966; Gibbs 1999; Vereecke et al. 2005; Diogo et al. 2010, 2012, 2013a,b, 2017). In orangutans, there may be an origin from the navicular and the muscle may be fused with the extensor hallucis longus tendon (Boyer 1935; Gibbs 1999; Diogo et al. 2013a). An accessory slip attaching to digit two has been found in gorillas (Raven 1950).

Variations

Description

Extensor hallucis brevis may be absent (Macalister 1875; Knott 1883b; Bergman et al. 1988; Chaney et al. 1996). It may receive a slip from or be joined with extensor hallucis longus (Macalister 1875; Knott 1883b; Hallisy 1930; Bergman et al. 1988; Al-Saggaf 2003; Hill and Gerges 2008). Accessory bundles may be present (Bergman et al. 1988; Sirasanagandla et al. 2013b; Won and Oh 2018). Won and Oh (2018) report a case in which the extensor digitorum muscle belly to digit three was doubled and associated with an accessory muscle in the right foot of a cadaver. The accessory muscle was covered by extensor hallucis brevis, originated from the calcaneus, and inserted onto the lateral third of the transverse retinacular band.

Prevalence

Knott (1883b) found that the extensor hallucis brevis tendon was absent in 1 out of 40 cases (2.5%). Hallisy (1930) found that in 3 out of 290 feet (1%), the tendon of extensor hallucis longus sent a slip to the most medial tendon of extensor digitorum brevis (extensor hallucis brevis). Out of 291 cases, Chaney et al. (1996) found that both the extensor hallucis brevis tendon to digit one and the extensor digitorum tendons to digits two through four were present in 186 cases (63.9%). Tendons to the second, third, and fourth digits were present without the extensor hallucis brevis tendon in 50 cases (17.2%). In 11 subjects (3.8%), there were only two tendons present to various digits. There were more than four tendons present in 44 cases (15.1%).

Al-Saggaf (2003) studied the insertions of extensor hallucis longus in 60 cadaveric lower limbs. In three cases (5%), an accessory tendon of extensor hallucis longus inserted with extensor hallucis brevis onto the base of the proximal hallucal phalanx. In two cases (3.3%), the accessory tendon joined the tendon of extensor hallucis brevis, forming a common tendon that inserted onto the base of the proximal hallucal phalanx. Sirasanagandla et al. (2013b) studied extensor digitorum brevis and extensor hallucis brevis in 44 limbs. In 36 limbs (81.8%) both the extensor hallucis brevis tendon to digit one and the extensor digitorum tendons to digits two through four were present. In one limb (2.3%), there was an accessory bundle present that originated from extensor hallucis brevis and the extensor digitorum brevis belly going to digit two that merged with the first dorsal interosseous muscle.

Anomalies

Description

In a male fetus with triploidy studied by Moen et al. (1984), extensor hallucis brevis was absent on the right side. On the left foot of a male neonate with Meckel syndrome, Pettersen (1984) found that the extensor hallucis brevis tendon was rudimentary. In the female fetus with trisomy 18 dissected by Alghamdi et al. (2018), extensor hallucis brevis fused proximally with extensor digitorum brevis on both sides of the body.

Prevalence

N/A

Clinical Implications

Hypertrophy of extensor hallucis brevis may cause anterior tarsal tunnel syndrome (Tennant et al. 2014).

References

Aasar, Y.H. 1947. *Anatomical Anomalies*. Cairo: Fouad I University Press.

Abe, S., Lida, T., Ide, Y., Saitoh, C. 1997. An anatomical study of a muscle bundle separated from the medial pterygoid muscle. *CRANIO* 15(4):341–344.

Abe, M., Murakami, G., Noguchi, M., Kitamura, S., Shimada, K., Kohama, G.I. 2004. Variations in the tensor veli palatini muscle with special reference to its origin and insertion. *Cleft Palate Craniofac J* 41(5):474–484.

Abraham, P.S. 1883. Note on the occurrence of the musculus sternalis in human anencephalous fetuses. *Trans Acad Med Ireland* 1:301–304.

Adachi, B. 1909. Beitrage zur anatomie der Japaner. Die statistik der muskelvarietaten zweite mitteilung. *Zeitschr Morphol Anthropol* 12:261–312.

Adebonojo, F.O. 1973. Dysplasia of the anterior abdominal musculature with multiple congenital anomalies: Prune belly or triad syndrome. *J Nat Med Assoc* 65:327–333.

Agawany, A.E., Meguid, E.A. 2010. Mode of insertion of the abductor hallucis muscle in human feet and its arterial supply. *Folia Morphol (Warsz)* 69(1):54–61.

Aggarwal, A., Kaur, H., Sahni, D., Aggarwal, A. 2009. Four-headed biceps brachii muscle with variant course of musculocutaneous nerve: Anatomical and clinical insight. *Int J Anat Var* 2:127–130.

Agha, M., Abdelgawad, M.S., Aldeen, N.G. 2018 Lateral ankle anatomical variants predisposing to peroneal tendon impingement. *Alexandria J Med* 54(4):619–626.

Agrawal, K., Khair Mulla, R.U., Srivastava, R., Sharma, S. 2014. Congenital trilobe tongue associated with cleft palate: A rare anomaly. *Cleft Palate Craniofac J* 51(6):707–710.

Aguado-Henche, S., de Arriba, C.C., Cristóbal-Aguado, S. 2018. A right sternalis muscle: Clinical and surgical significance. *J Hum Anat* 2:000126.

Ahmad, I. 1975. Articular muscle of the knee – articularis genus. *Bull Hosp Joint Dis* 36:58–60.

Aiello, L., Dean, C. 1990. *An Introduction to Human Evolutionary Anatomy*. San Diego, CA: Academic Press.

Akcan, A.B., Akcan, M., Ozkiraz, S. 2016. Depressor anguli oris in IVF twins. *Iran J Pediatr* 26(4):e3810.

Akita, K., Sakamoto, H., Sato, T. 1992. Innervation of an aberrant digastric muscle in the posterior thigh: Stratified relationships between branches of the inferior gluteal nerve. *J Anat* 181:503–506.

Akita, K., Sakamoto, H., Sato, T. 1993. Innervation of the anteromedial muscle bundles of the gluteus medius. *J Anat* 182:433–438.

Akita, K., Sakamoto, H., Sato, T. 1994. Arrangement and innervation of the glutei medius and minimus and the piriformis: A morphological analysis. *Anat Rec* 238:125–130.

Akita, K., Ibukuro, K., Yamaguchi, K., Heima, S., Sato, T. 2000. The subclavius posticus muscle: A factor in arterial, venous or brachial plexus compression? *Surg Radiol Anat* 22:111–115.

Akita, K., Shimokawa, T., Sato, T. 2001. Aberrant muscle between the temporalis and the lateral pterygoid muscles: m. pterygoideus proprius (Henle). *Clin Anat* 14:288–291.

Akita, K., Nimura, A. 2016a. Arm muscles. In *Bergman's Comprehensive Encyclopedia of Human Anatomic Variation*, first edition, ed. Tubbs, R.S., Shoja, M.M., Loukas, M., 293–297. Hoboken, NJ: Wiley-Blackwell.

Akita, K., Nimura, A. 2016b. Forearm muscles. In *Bergman's Comprehensive Encyclopedia of Human Anatomic Variation*, first edition, ed. Tubbs, R.S., Shoja, M.M., Loukas, M., 298–314. Hoboken, NJ: Wiley-Blackwell.

Akita, K., Sakaguchi-Kuma, T., Fukino, K., Ono, T. 2019. Masticatory muscles and branches of mandibular nerve: Positional relationships between various muscle bundles and their innervating branches. *Anat Rec* 302:609–619.

Aktekin, M., Kurtoğlu, Z., Öztürk, A.H. 2003. A bilateral and symmetrical variation of the anterior belly of the digastric muscle. *Acta Med Okayama* 57:205–207.

Alamo, L., Meyrat, B.J., Meuwly, J.Y., Meuli, R.A., Gudinchet, F. 2013. Anorectal malformations: Finding the pathway out of the labyrinth. *Radiographics* 33:491–512.

Albay, S., Candan, B. 2017. Evaluation of fibular muscles and prevalence of accessory fibular muscles on fetal cadavers. *Surg Radiol Anat* 39:1337–1341.

Alberch, P. 1989. The logic of monsters: Evidence for internal constraint in development and evolution. *Geobios Mem Spec* 12:21–57.

Alberch, P., Gale, E.A. 1985. A developmental analysis of an evolutionary trend: Digital reduction in amphibians. *Evolution* 39:8–23.

Albinus, B.S. 1758. De extensore digitorum brevis manus. *Academicarum Annotationum* 4:28–29.

Albright, J.A., Linburg, R.M. 1978. Common variations of the radial wrist extensors. *J Hand Surg* 3:134–138.

Aleksandrova, J.N., Malinova, L., Jelev, L. 2013. Variations of the iliacus muscle. Report of two cases and review of the literature. *IJAV* 6:149–152.

Alexiou, D., Manolidis, C., Papaevangellou, G., Nicolopoulos, D., Papadatos, C. 1976. Frequency of other malformations in congenital hypoplasia of depressor anguli oris muscle syndrome. *Arch Dis Childhood* 51:891.

Alghamdi, M.A., Ziermann, J.M., Gregg, L., Diogo, R. 2017. A detailed musculoskeletal study of a fetus with anencephaly and spina bifida (craniorachischisis), and comparison with other cases of human congenital malformations. *J Anat* 230:842–858.

Alghamdi, M.A., Diogo, R., Izquierdo, R., Pastor, F.F., De La Paz F., Ziermann, J.M. 2018. Detailed musculoskeletal study of a fetus with Trisomy-18 (Edwards Syndrome) with Langer's axillary arch, and comparison with other cases of human congenital malformations. *J Anat Sci Res* 1:1–8.

Allen, L. 1950. Transpleural muscles. *J Thoracic Surg* 19:290–291.

Allouh, M., Mohamed, A., Mhanni, A. 2004. Complete unilateral absence of trapezius muscle. *McGill J Med* 8:31–33.

Al-Qattan, M.M., Duerksen, F. 1992. A variant of flexor carpi ulnaris causing ulnar nerve compression. *J Anat* 180:189–190.

Al-Saggaf, S. 2003. Variations in the insertion of the extensor hallucis longus muscle. *Folia Morphol (Warsz)* 62:147–155.

Alsharif, K.M.H., Alfaki, M.A., Elamin, A.Y., Manssor, E.H., Taha, K.M., Arafa, E.M., Aldosari, K.H.M. 2017. An accessory extensor pollicis longus tendon: A case report of rare anatomical variant. *Int J Morphol* 35:1276–1279.

Ammendolia, A. 2008. Extensor digitorum brevis manus associated with a dorsal wrist ganglion: Case report. *Clin Anat* 21:794–795.

Amonoo-Kuofi, H. S., Darwish, H. H. 1998. Accessory levator muscle of the upper eyelid: Case report and review of the literature. *Clin Anat Official J Am Assoc Clin Anat Br Assoc Clin Anat* 11(6):410–416.

Anderson, R.J. 1880. Vorkommen eines musculus tibio-tarsalis sive tensor fasciae plantaris. *Arch Pathol Anat Physiol Klin Med* 81:574–575.

Annerén, G., Sedin, G. 1981. Trisomy 9 Syndrome. *Acta Paediatr Scand* 70:125–128.

Anson, B.J., McVay, C.B. 1938. The anatomy of the inguinal region. *Surg Gyneocol Obstet* 66:186–191.

Anson, B.J., Beaton, L.E., McVay, C.B. 1938. The pyramidalis muscle. *Anat Rec* 72:405–411.

Antonopoulou, M., Latrou, I., Paraschos, A., Anagnostopoulou, S. 2013. Variations of the attachment of the superior head of human lateral pterygoid muscle. *J Craniomaxillofac Surg* 41(6):e91–e97.

Appleton, A.B., Ghey, P.H.R. 1929. An example of the cervicocosto-humeral muscle of Gruber. *J Anat* 63:434–436.

Arakawa, T., Tokita, K., Miki, A., Terashima, T. 2003. Anatomical study of human adductor hallucis muscle with respect to its origin and insertion. *Ann Anat* 185:585–592.

Arakawa, T., Murakami, G., Nakajima, F., Matsubara A., Ohtsuka, A., Goto, T., Teramoto, T. 2004. Morphologies of the interfaces between the levator ani muscle and pelvic viscera, with special reference to muscle insertion into the anorectum in elderly Japanese. *Anat Sci Int* 79:72–81.

Arakawa, T., Kondo, T., Tsutsumi, M., Watanabe, Y., Terashima, T., Miki, A. 2017. Multiple muscular variations including tenuissimus and tensor fasciae suralis muscles in the posterior thigh of a human case. *Anat Sci Int* 92:581–584.

Arican, R.Y., Coskun, N., Sarikcioglu, L., Sindel, M., Oguz, N. 2006. Co-existence of the pectoralis quartus and pectoralis intermedius muscles. *Morphologie* 90:157–159.

Arifoglu, Y., Sürüc, H.S., Sargon, M.F., Tanyeli, E., Yazar, F. 1997. Double superior gemellus together with double piriformis and high division of the sciatic nerve. *Surg Radiol Anat* 19:407–408.

Aristotle, S., Sundarapandian, S., Felicia, C. 2013. Accessory iliacus muscle with splitting of the femoral nerve: A case report. *OA Case Rep* 2:56.

Arnold, W.H., Nohadani, N., Koch, K.H.H. 2005. Morphology of the auditory tube and palatal muscles in a case of bilateral cleft palate. *Cleft Palate Craniofac J* 42(2):197–201.

Arora, J., Mehta, V., Kumar, H., Suri, R.K., Rath, G., Das, S. 2010. A rare bimuscular conglomeration gluteopiriformis case report. *Morphologie* 94(305):40–43.

Arora, A.K., Verma, P., Abrol, S. 2011. Study of extensor hallucis longus muscle in adult human cadavers of Punjab. *J Life Sci* 3(2):101–105.

Arthornthurasook, A., Gaew-Im, K. 1990. Anterior tibial tendon insertion: An anatomical study. *J Med Assoc Thai* 73:692–696.

Asakawa, H., Yanaka, K., Narushima, K., Meguro, K., Nose, T. 1999. Anomaly of the axis causing cervical myelopathy. Case report. *J Neurosurg* 91:121–123.

Ashaolu, J.O., Olorunyomi, O.I., Opabunmi, O.A., Ukwenya, V.O., Thomas, M.A. 2013. Surface anatomy and prevalence of fibularis tertius muscle in a south-western Nigerian population. *Forens Med Anat Res* 1(2):25–29.

Ashaolu, J.O., Oni-Orisan, O.P., Ukwenya, V.O., Alamu, O., Adeyemi, D.O. 2014. Variability of the morphology of gastrocnemius muscle in an African population. *Anat J Afr* 3(3):400–404.

Ashaolu, J.O., Abimbola, O.O., Ukwenya, V.O., Thomas, M.A. 2015. Aberrant rotator cuff muscles: Coexistence of triple-tailed teres minor and bi-formed infraspinatus (major and minor). *Forensic Med Anat Res* 3:20–24.

Ashley-Montagu, M.F. 1939. Anthropological significance of the musculus pyramidalis and its variability in man. *Am J Phys Anthropol* 25:435–490.

Asomugha, A.L., Chukwuanukwu, T.O., Nwajagu, G.I., Ukoha, U. 2005. An accessory flexor of the fifth toe. *Niger J Clin Pract* 8:130–132.

Astik, R.B., Dave, U.H. 2011. Anatomical variations in formation and branching pattern of the femoral nerve in iliac fossa: A study in 64 human lumbar plexuses. *People's J Sci Res* 4:14–19.

Astle, W.F., Hill, V.E., Ells, A.L., Chi, N.T., Martinovic, E. 2003. Congenital absence of the inferior rectus muscle--diagnosis and management. *J AAPOS* 7(5):339–344.

Athavale, S.A., Geetha, G.N., Swathi. 2012a. Morphology of flexor digitorum accessorius muscle. *Surg Radiol Anat* 34:367–372.

Athavale, S.A., Gupta, V., Kotgirwar, S., Singh, V. 2012b. The peroneus quartus muscle: Clinical correlation with evolutionary importance. *Anat Sci Int* 87(2):106–110.

Au, J., Webb, A.L., Buirsji, G., Smith, P.N., Pickering, M.R., Perriman, D.M. 2017. Anatomic variations of levator scapulae in a normal cohort: An MRI study. *Surg Radiol Anat* 39:337–343.

Aung, H.H., Sakamoto, H.H., Akita, K., Sato, T. 2001. Anatomical study of the obturator internus, gemelli and quadratus femoris muscles with special reference to their innervation. *Anat Rec* 263:41–52.

Aydoğ, S., Özçakar, L., Demiryürek, D., Bayramoğlu, A., Yörübulut, M. 2007. An intervening thoracic outlet syndrome in a gymnast with levator claviculae muscle. *Clin J Sport Med* 17:323–325.

Aziz, M.A. 1979. Muscular and other abnormalities in a case of Edwards' syndrome (18-Trisomy). *Teratology* 20:303–312.

Aziz, M.A. 1980. Anatomical defects in a case of Trisomy 13 with a D/D translocation. *Teratology* 22:217–227.

Aziz, M.A. 1981. Possible atavistic structures in human aneuploids. *Am J Phys Anthropol* 54:347–353.

Baba, M.A. 1954. The accessory tendon of the abductor pollicis longus muscle. *Anat Rec* 119:541–547.

Babinski, M.A., Machado, F.A., Costa, W.S. 2003. A rare variation in the high division of the sciatic nerve surrounding the superior gemellus muscle. *Eur J Morph* 41:41–42.

Babst, D., Steppacher, S.D., Ganz, R., Siebenrock, K.A., Tannast, M. 2011. The iliocapsularis muscle: An important stabilizer in the dysplastic hip. *Clin Ortho Rel Res* 469:1728–1734.

Backhouse, K.M., Churchill-Davidson, D. 1975. Anomalous palmaris longus muscle producing carpal tunnel-like compression. *The Hand* 7:22–24.

Bae, J. H., Choi, D. Y., Lee, J. G., Seo, K. K., Tansatit, T., Kim, H. J. 2014. The risorius muscle: Anatomic considerations with reference to botulinum neurotoxin injection for masseteric hypertrophy. *Dermatol Surg* 40(12):1334–1339.

Bahnsen, G. 1868. *Zeitschrift fur rationelle medicin, dritte reihe.* Leipzig and Heidelberg: Verlag.

Bakkum, B.W., Miller, N. 2016. Back muscles. In *Bergman's Comprehensive Encyclopedia of Human Anatomic Variation*, first edition, ed. Tubbs, R.S., Shoja, M.M., Loukas, M., 262–288. Hoboken, NJ: Wiley-Blackwell.

Bale, L.S.W., Herrin, S.O. 2016. Unilateral absence of the sternothyroid muscle: A case report. *Int J Anat Var* 9:55–56.

Bale, L.S.W., Herrin, S.O. 2017. Bilateral tensor fasciae suralis muscles in a cadaver with unilateral accessory flexor digitorum longus muscle. *Case Rep Med* 2017:864272.

Bale, L.S.W., Herrin, S.O. 2019. Tensor fasciae suralis - prevalence study and literature review. *MedRxiv* 19010389.

Barash, B.A., Freedman, L., Opitz, J.M. 1970. Anatomic studies in the 18-Trisomy Syndrome. *Birth Def* 4:3–15.

Barcia, J.M., Genovés, J.M. 2009. Chondrofascialis versus pectoralis quartus. *Clin Anat* 22:871–872.

Bardeen, C.R. 1906. Development and variation of the nerves and the musculature of the inferior extremity and of the neighboring regions of the trunk in man. *Am J Anat* 6:259–390.

Bardeen, C.R. 1921. Muscles of the urogenital diaphragm. In *Morris's Human Anatomy*, sixth edition, ed. Jackson, C.M., 482–483. Philadelphia, PA: P. Blakiston's Son & Co.

Bareither, D.J., Schuberth, J.M., Evoy, P.J., Thomas, G.J. 1984. Peroneus digiti minimi. *Anat Anz* 155(1–5):11–15.

Barfred, T., Adamsen, S. 1986. Duplication of the extensor carpi ulnaris tendon. *J Hand Surg A* 11:423–425.

Barker, B.C.W. 1981. The pterygoideus proprius muscle. *Aust Dent J* 26:309–310.

Barkow, H.C.L. 1828. *Monstra animalium duplicia per anatomen indagata*. Liepzig: Sumptibus L. Vossii.

Barnard, W.S. 1875. Observations on the membral musculation of *Simia satyrus* (Orang) and the comparative myology of man and the apes. *Proc Amer Assoc Adv Sci* 24:112–144.

Barnes, J., Boniuk, M. 1972. Anencephaly with absence of the superior oblique tendons. *Surv Ophthalmol* 16:371–374.

Barnwell, Y. 1977. The morphology of musculus styloglossus in fifteen-week human fetuses. *Int J Oral Myol* 3:8–46.

Barry, D., Bothroyd, J.S. 1924. Tensor fasciae suralis. *J Anat* 58(Pt 4):382–383.

Barsoumian, R., Kuehn, D.P., Moon, J.B., Canady, J.W. 1998. An anatomic study of the tensor veli palatini and dilatator tubae muscles in relation to eustachian tube and velar function. *Cleft Palate Craniofac J* 35(2):101–110.

Bascho, P. 1906. Beobachtung eines restes des hautrumpf-muskels beim menschen, pars thoracalis lateralis desselben. *Gegenbaur's Morphol Jahrb* 33:374–378.

Bayer, T., Kolodziejski, N., Flueckiger, G. 2014. The extensor hallucis capsularis tendon—a prospective study of its occurrence and function. *Foot Ankle Surg* 20:192–194.

Beaton, L.E., Anson, B.J. 1937. The relation of the sciatic nerve and of its subdivisions to the piriformis muscle. *Anat Rec* 70:1–5.

Beaton, L.E., Anson, B.J. 1938. The sciatic nerve and the piriformis muscle: Their inter-relation possible cause of coccygodynia. *J Bone Joint Surg [Am]* 20:686–688.

Beaton, L.E, Anson, B.J. 1939. Pyramidalis muscle: Its occurrence and size in American whites and negroes. *Am J Phys Anthropol* 25:261–269.

Beattie, J., Horsfall, F.L. 1930. An anomalous facial muscle. *J Anat* 65(Pt 1):145–148.

Beatty, J.D., Remedios, D., McCullough, C.J. 2000. An accessory extensor tendon of the thumb as a cause of dorsal wrist pain. *J Hand Surg [Br]* 25:110–111.

Belbl, M., Kunc, V., Kachlik, D. 2020. Absence of flexor digitorum profundus muscle and variation of flexor digitorum superficialis muscle in a little finger: Two case reports. *Surg Radiol Anat* 42:945–949.

Beck, M., Sledge, J.B., Gautier, E., Dora, C.F., Ganz, R. 2000. The anatomy and function of the gluteus minimus muscle. *J Bone Joint Surg [Br]* 82B:358–363.

Becker, I., Woodley, S.J., Baxter, G.D. 2009. Gross morphology of the vastus lateralis muscle: An anatomical review. *Clin Anat* 22:436–450.

Beddard, F.E. 1893. Contributions to the anatomy of the anthropoid apes. *Trans Zool Soc Lond* 13:177–218.

Beger, O., Koc, T., Dinc, U., Altuncu, K., Uzmansel, D., Kurtoglu, Z. 2018a. An unusual bilateral variation of the splenius capitis muscle: A case report. *Int J Anat Var* 11:46–47.

Beger, O., Elvan, Ö., Keskinbora, M., Ün, B., Uzmansel, D., Kurtoğlu, Z. 2018b. Anatomy of Master Knot of Henry: A morphometric study on cadavers. *Acta Orthop Traumatol Turc* 52:134–142.

Beger, O., Koc, T., Beger, B., Ozalp, H., Hamazaoglu, V., Vayisoglu, Y., Umit Talas, D., Kurtoglu Olgunas, Z. 2019. Multiple muscular abnormalities in a fetal cadaver with CHARGE syndrome. *Surg Radiol Anat* 41:601–605.

Bello-Hellegouarch, G., Aziz, M.A., Ferrero, E.M., Kern, M., Francis, N., Diogo, R. 2012. "Pollical palmar interosseous muscle" (musculus adductor pollicis accessorius): attachments, innervation, variations, phylogeny, and implications for human evolution and medicine. *J Morph* 274:275–293.

Bender-Heine, A., Zdilla, M.J. 2018. Variation of the mylohyoid: Implications for Ludwig angina, cervical contouring, and digastric muscle transfer. *Surg Radiol Anat* 40:221–225.

Bergman, R.A., Thompson, S.A., Afifi, A.K., Saadeh, F.A. 1988. *Compendium of Human Anatomic Variation: Text, Atlas, and World Literature*. Baltimore, MD: Urban and Schwarzenberg.

Bergman, R.A., Walker, C.W., El-Khour, G.Y. 1995. The third head of gastrocnemius in CT images. *Ann Anat - Anatomischer Anzeiger* 177(3):291–294.

Bergman, R.A., Afifi, A.K., Miyauchi, R. 2008. Illustrated Encyclopedia of Human Anatomic Variation. Available at: http://www.anatomyatlases.org/AnatomicVariants/AnatomyHP.shtml (accessed November 1, 2019).

Berkowitz, Y., Mushtaq, N., Amiras, D. 2016. MRI of the tibioastragalus anticus of Gruber muscle: A rare accessory muscle and normal anatomical variant. *Skeletal Radiol* 45:847–849.

Bernhard, A., Miller, J., Keeler, J., Siesel, K., Bridges, E. 2013. Absence of the fourth tendon of the flexor digitorum brevis muscle: A cadaveric study. *Foot Ankle Spec* 6(4):286–289.

Bersu, E.T. 1980. Anatomical analysis of the developmental effects of ancuploidy in man: The Down syndrome. *Am J Med Gen* 5:399–420.

Bersu, E.T., Pettersen, J.C., Charboneau, W.J., Opitz, J.M. 1976. Studies of malformation syndrome of Man XXXXIA: Anatomical studies in the Hanhart syndrome: A pathogenetic hypothesis. *Europ J Pediat* 122:1–17.

Bersu, E.T., Ramirez-Castro, J.L. 1977. Anatomical analysis of the developmental effects of aneuploidy in man—the 18-Trisomy Syndrome: I. anomalies of the head and neck. *Am J Med Gen* 1:173–193.

Bertilsson, O., Ström, D. 1995. A literature survey of a hundred years of anatomic and functional lateral pterygoid muscle research. *J Orofac Pain* 9(1):17–23.

Best, A., Giza, E., Linklater, J., Sullivan, M. 2005. Posterior impingement of the ankle caused by anomalous muscles. A report of four cases. *J Bone Joint Surg [Am]* 87:2075–2079.

Bhansali, R.M., Bhansali, R.R. 1997. Accessory abductor hallucis causing entrapment of the posterior tibial nerve. *J Bone Joint Surg* 69:479–480.

Bharambe, V.K., Shevde, S.P., Puranam, V., Kanaskar, N.S. 2013. Additional heads of dorsal interosseous muscle in Caucasian cadavers and their clinical significance. *Sahel Med J* 16:174–77.

Bharambe, V., Shevade, S., Patel, D., Manvikar, P.R., Bajpayee, P.G. 2017. A study of the extensor tendons of the hand from point of view of evolution. *J Anat Ind* 66:112–117.

Bhashyam, A.R., Harper, C.M., Iorio, M.L. 2017. Reversed palmaris longus muscle causing volar forearm pain and ulnar nerve paresthesia. *J Hand Surg* 42:298.e1–298.e5.

Bhate, M., Martin, F.J. 2012. Unilateral inferior rectus hypoplasia in a child with Axenfeld-Rieger syndrome. *J Am Assoc Pediatr Ophthalmol Strabismus* 16:304–306.

Bhatt, C.R., Prajapati, B., Patil, D.S., Patel, V.D., Singh, B.G.B., Mehta, C.D. 2013. Variation in the insertion of the latissimus dorsi and its clinical importance. *J Orthop* 10:25–28.

Bhojwani, V., Ghabriel, M.N., Mihailidis, S., Townsend, G.C. 2017. The human medial pterygoid muscle: Attachments and distribution of muscle spindles. *Clin Anat* 30:1064–1071.

Bibbo, C., Arangio, G., Patel, D.V. 2004. The accessory extensor tendon of the first metatarsophalangeal joint. *Foot Ankle Int* 25:387–390.

Billings, H.J., Sherrill, W.C. 2015. A novel variant of the cleidocervicalis muscle with clinical implications for nerve compression/entrapment. *Surg Radiol Anat* 37(6):697–699.

Bing, R. 1902. Uber angeboren muskeldefekte. *Virchow's Arch Pathol Anat* 170:175–228.

Birmingham, A. 1889. Homology and innervation of the achselbogen and pectoralis quartus and the nature of the lateral-cutaneous nerve of the thorax. *J Anat* 23:206–223.

Bischoff, T.L.W. 1870. Beitrage zur Anatomie des *Hylobates leuciscus* and zueiner vergleichenden Anatomie der Muskeln der Affen und des Menschen. *Abh Bayer Akad Wiss München Math Phys Kl* 10:197–297.

Bischoff, T.L.W. 1880. Beitrage zur anatomie des gorilla. *Abh Bayer Akad Wiss München Math Phys Kl* 13:1–48.

Blitz, N.M., Eliot, D.J. 2007. Anatomical aspects of the gastrocnemius aponeurosis and its insertion: A cadaveric study. *J Foot Ankle Surg* 46(2):101–108.

Blodget, P.H., Blatt, I.M. 1966. Anomalous symptomatic transversalis nuchae muscle. *Arch Otolaryng* 83:254–255.

Bloome, D.M., Marymont, J.V., Varner, K.E. 2003. Variations on the insertion of the posterior tibialis tendon: A cadaveric study. *Foot Ankle Int* 24(10):780–783.

Bluth, B.E., Wu, B., Stark, M.E., Wisco, J.J. 2011. Variant of the extensor pollicis tertius: A case report on a unique extensor muscle to the thumb. *Anat Sci Int* 86:160–163.

Bochdalek, V.A. 1867. Ein anomaler musculus supracostalis anterior. *Arch Pathol Anat Physiol* 41:257–258.

Bochdalek, V.A. 1868. *Beitrag zu den anomalen Muskel in der Augenhöle.* Braunschweig: von Friedrich Vieweg und Sohn.

Bojsen-Møller, F. 1978. Extensor carpi radialis longus muscle and the evolution of the first intermetacarpal ligament. *Am J Phys Anthropol* 48:177–184.

Bonala, N., Kishan, T.V., Sri Pavani, B., Murthy, P.V. 2015. Accessory belly of digastric muscle presenting as a submandibular space mass. *Med J Armed Forces India* 71(Suppl 2):S506–S508.

Bonastre, V., Rodríguez-Niedenführ, M., Choi, D., Sañudo, J.R. 2002. Coexistence of a pectoralis quartus muscle and an unusual axillary arch: Case report and review. *Clin Anat* 15:336–370.

Bonney, G. 1965. The Scalenus Medius Band; a Contribution to the Study of the Thoracic Outlet Syndrome. *J Bone Joint Surg Br* 47:268–72.

Boothe, R.G., Quick, M.W., Joosse, M.V., Abbas, M.A., Anderson, D.C. 1990. Accessory lateral rectus orbital geometry in normal and naturally strabismic monkeys. *Invest Ophthalmol Vis Sci* 31(6):1168–1174.

Botros, K.G., Bondok, A.A., Gabr, O.M., el-Eishi, H.I., State, F.A. 1990. Anatomical variations in the formation of the human esophageal hiatus. *Anat Anz* 71:193–199.

Boupha, T., Wree, A. 1995. Occurrence of a musculus abductor digiti minimi longus. *Ann Anat - Anat Anz* 177:147–149.

Bowers, C.A., Mendicino, R.W., Catanzariti, A.R., Kernick, E.T. 2009. The flexor digitorum accessorius longus-a cadaveric study. *J Foot Ankle Surg* 48(2):111–115.

Bowman, P., Johnson, L., Chiapetta, A., Mitchell, A., Belusko, E. 2003. The clinical impact of the presence or absence of the fifth finger flexor digitorum superficialis on grip strength. *J Hand Ther* 16:245–8.

Boyd, G.I. 1934. Abnormality of subclavian artery associated with presence of the scalenus minimus. *J Anat* 68:280–281.

Boyd, N., Brock, H., Meier, A., Miller, R., Mlady, G., Firoozbakhsh, K. 2006. Extensor hallucis capsularis: Frequency and identification on MRI. *Foot Ankle Int* 27(3):181–184.

Boyer, E.L. 1935. The musculature of the inferior extremity of the orang-utan, *Simia satyrus. Am J Anat* 56:193–256.

Boyer, E.L. 1939. The cranio-mandibular musculature of the orang-utan, *Simia satyrus. Am J Phys Anthropol* 24:417–426.

Boyle, E.K., Mahon, V., Diogo, R. 2020. Muscles lost in our adult primate ancestors still imprint in us: On muscle evolution, development, variations, and pathologies. *Curr Mol Bio Rep* 6:32–50.

Bozant, J.G., Serletic, D.R., Phillips, R.D. 1994. Tibialis posterior tendon associated with hallux abducto valgus. A preliminary study. *J Am Podiatr Med Assoc* 84(1):19–25.

Bradley, F.M., Hoover, H.C., Hulka, C.A., Whitman, G.J., McCarthy, K.A., Hall, D.A, Moore, R., Kopans, D.B. 1996. The sternalis muscle: An unusual normal finding seen on mammography. *Am J Roentgenol* 166:33–36.

Breisch, E.A. 1986. A rare human variation: The relationship of the axillary and inferior subscapular nerves to an accessory subscapularis muscle. *Anat Rec* 216:440–442.

Brenner, E. 1999. Insertion of the abductor hallucis muscle in feet with and without hallux valgus. *Anat Rec* 254:429–434.

Brenner, E. 2002. Insertion of the tendon of the tibialis anterior muscle in feet with and without hallux valgus. *Clin Anat* 15:217–233.

Brenner, E., Tripoli, M., Scavo, E., Cordova, A. 2019. Case report: Absence of the right piriformis muscle in a woman. *Surg Radiol Anat* 41:845–848.

Brooks, H.S.J. 1887. On the short muscles of the pollex and hallux of the anthropoid apes, with special reference to the opponens hallucis. *J Anat Physiol* 22:78–95.

Brown, C.E. 1941. Complete absence of the posterior arch of the atlas. *Anat Rec* 81:499–503.

Brown, B. 1983. An evaluation of primate caudal musculature in the identification of the ischiofemoralis muscle. *Am J Phys Anthropol* 60:177–178.

Brown, B., Ward, S.C. 1988. Basicranial and facial topography in *Pongo* and *Sivapithecus*. In *Orang-utan Biology*, ed. Schwartz, J.H., 247–260. Oxford: Oxford University Press.

Browne, R.S., Paton, D.F. 1979. Anomalous insertion of the tibialis posterior tendon in congenital metatarsus varus. *J Bone Joint Surg Br* 61(1):74–76.

Buck, W.R. 2007. Letter to the Editor. *Clin Anat* 20:1000.

Budge, J. 1859. Beschreibung eines neuen Muskels und mehrerer Muskel und Knochenvariet.ten. *Zeitschrift für Rat Med* 3:273–278.

Buffoli, B., Ferrari, M., Belotti, F., Lancini, D., Cocchi, M.A., Labanca, M., Tschabitscher, M., Rezzani, R., Rodella, L.F. 2017. The myloglossus in a human cadaver study: Common or uncommon anatomical structure? *Folia Morphol (Warsz)* 76(1):74–81.

Burkitt, A.N., Lightoller, G.S. 1926. The facial musculature of the Australian aboriginal Part I. *J Anat* 61:14–39.

Burman, M. 1968. The high-bellied popliteus muscle. An anomaly of the popliteus muscle. *J Bone Joint Surg [Am]* 50:761–762.

Burrows, A.M., Waller, B.M., Parr, L.A., Bonar, C.J. 2006. Muscles of facial expression in the chimpanzee (*Pan troglodytes*): Descriptive, comparative and phylogenetic contexts. *J Anat* 208:153–167.

Buschmann, W.R, Cheung, Y., Jahss, M.H. 1991. Magnetic resonance imaging of anomalous leg muscles: Accessory soleus, peroneus quartus, and the flexor digitorum longus accessorius. *Foot Ankle* 12(2):109–116.

Cachel, S. 1984. Growth and allometry in primate masticatory muscles. *Arch Oral Bio* 29(4):287–29.

Caetano, E.B., Sabongi Neto, J.J., Angelo Viera, L., Caetano, M.F., Moraes, D.V. 2015. Gantzer muscle. An anatomical study. *Acta Ortop Bras* 23:72–75.

Caetano, E.B., Nakamichi, Y., Alves de Andrade, R., Sawada, M.M., Nakasone, M.T., Vieira, L.A., Sabongi, R.G. 2017. Flexor pollicis brevis muscle. Anatomical study and clinical implications. *Open Orthop J* 11:1321–1329.

Caetano, A.P., Seeger, L.L. 2019. A rare anatomical variant of unilateral piriformis muscle agenesis: A case report. *Cureus* 11(6):e4887.

Calori, L. 1867. Di alcone variet. muscolari dell'avambraccio. Memorie dell'Acc. *delle Scienze dell'Inst di Bologna* 7:359–381.

Calori, L. 1870. Degli usi del muscolo pronatore quadrato e di un muscolo sopranumerario cubito-radio-carpeo nell'uomo. *Mem R Accad Sci Instituto di Bologna S2.* 10:647–657.

Campos, D., Nazer, M.B., Vieira, F.N., Bartholdy, L.M., Souza, P.L. 2011. Supranumerary muscle of the extensor indicis. *J Morphol Sci* 28:132–134.

Canter, D.E., Siesel, K.J. 1997. Flexor digitorum accessorius longus muscle: An etiology of tarsal tunnel syndrome? *J Foot Ankle Surg* 36(3):226–229.

Cardoso Souza, C.F., Soares, M., Lopes, J., Ráfare, A., Babinski, M. 2019. Pectoralis quartus: A case report. *Acta Sci Anat* 1:119–121.

Carlos, J.S., Goubran, E., Ayad, S. 2011. The presence of extensor digiti medii muscle—anatomical variant. *J Chiropr Med* 10:100–104.

Carmont, M., Bruce, C., Bass, A., Carty, H. 2002. An accessory abductor muscle of the fifth toe? An unusual cause of a lump in the foot. *Foot Ankle Surg* 8:125–128.

Carroll, M.A., Lebron, E.M., Jensen, T.E., Cooperman, T.J. 2019. Chondroepitrochlearis and a supernumerary head of the biceps brachii. *Ant Sci Int* 94:330–334.

Cash, C.J.C., MacDonald, K.J., Dixon, A.K., Bearcroft, P.W.P., Constant, C.R. 2009. Variation in MRI appearance of the insertion of the tendon of subscapularis. *Clin Anat* 22:489–494.

Caskey, C.I., Zerhouni, E.A., Fishman, E.K., Rahmouni, A.D. 1989. Aging of the diaphragm: A CT study. *Radiology* 171:385–389.

Catli, M.M., Ozsoy, U., Kaya, Y., Hizay, A., Yildirim, F.G., Sarikcioglu, L. 2012. Four-headed biceps brachii, three-headed coracobrachialis muscles associated with arterial and nervous anomalies in the upper limb. *Anat Cell Biol* 45:136–139.

Cauldwell, E.W., Anson, B.J., Wright, R.R. 1943. The extensor indicis proprius muscle. A study of 263 consecutive specimens. *Q Bull NWest Univ Med Sch* 17:267–279.

Cave, A.J. 1933. A Note on the Origin of the M. Scalenus Medius. *J Anat.* 67:480–483.

Cecava, N.D., Campbell, S.E. 2015. Peroneus brevis tendon variant insertion on the calcaneus. *J Radiol Case Rep* 9(5):22–29.

Çelik, H.H., Yilmaz, E., Atasever, A., Durgun, B., Taner, D. 1992. Bilateral anatomical anomaly of anterior bellies of digastric muscles. *Kaibogaku Zasshi* 67(5):650–651.

Çelik, H.H., Yilmaz, E., Atasever, A., Durgun, B., Taner, D. 1993. Observation of anomalus triplication of unilateral anterior digastric muscle. *Clin Anat* 6:353–355.

Çelik, H.H., Aktekin, M., Sargon, M., Cumhur, M. 1997. Bilateral anomaly of the semispinalis capitis muscle. *Morphologie* 81:15.

Çelik, H.H., Aldur, M.M., Özdemir, B., Akşit, M.D. 2002. Abnormal digastric muscle with unilateral quadrification of the anterior belly. *Clin Anat* 15(1):32–34.

Çetkin, M., Orhan, M., Bahşi, I., Kervancioglu, P. 2017. A unique muscle bridge between sternohyoid and sternothyroid muscles. *Anat Int J Exper Clin Anat* 11. 161–163.

Ceyhan, O., Mavt, A. 1997. Distribution of agenesis of palmaris longus muscle in 12–18 years old age groups. *Indian J Med Sci* 51:156–160.

Chakravarthi, K.K. 2013. Unusual unilateral multiple muscular variations of back of thigh. *Ann Med Health Sci Res* 3:S1–S2.

Champneys, F. 1872. The muscles and nerves of a Chimpanzee (*Troglodytes Niger*) and a *Cynocephalus Anubis*. *J Anat Physiol* 6:176–211.

Chan, T.K., Demer, J.L. 1999. Clinical features of congenital absence of the superior oblique muscle as demonstrated by orbital imaging. *J AAPOS* 3(3):143–150.

Chaney, D., Lee, M., Khan, M., Krueger, W., Mandracchia, V., Yoho, R. 1996. Study of ten anatomical variants of the foot and ankle. *J Am Podiatr Med Assoc* 86(11):532–537.

Chaney, M.E., Dao, T.V., Brechtel, B.S., Belovich, S.J., Siesel, K.J., Fredieu, J.R. 2018. The fibularis digiti quinti tendon: A cadaveric study with anthropological and clinical considerations. *Foot (Edinb)* 34:45–47.

Chang, L., Blair, W.F. 1985. The origin and innervation of the adductor pollicis muscle. *J Anat* 140:381–388.

Chang, S.F. 1978. Pear-shaped bladder caused by large iliopsoas muscles. *Radiology* 128:349–350.

Chapman, H.C. 1878. On the structure of the gorilla. *Proc Acad Nat Sci Philad* 30:385–394.

Chapman, H.C. 1879. On the structure of the chimpanzee. *Proc Acad Nat Sci Philad* 31:52–63.

Chapman, H.C. 1880. On the structure of the oran outang. *Proc Acad Nat Sci Philad* 32:160–175.

Chapman, H.C. 1900. Observations upon the anatomy of *Hylobates leuciscus* and *Chiromys madagascariensis*. *Proc Acad Nat Sci Philad* 52:414–423.

Chaudhary, P., Singh, Z., Khullar, M., Arora, K. 2013. Levator glandulae thyroideae, a fibromusculoglandular band with absence of pyramidal lobe and its innervation: A case report. *J Clin Diagn Res* 7(7):1421–1424.

Chaudhary, N., Niranjan, R., Singh, A.K., Sinha, D.N., Prat, M.K. 2016. Pyramidal lobe and levator glandulae thyroidae in human fetal thyroid gland. *J Anat Sci* 24:31–37.

Chavan, N.N., Wabale, R.N. 2014. Langer's axillary arch: A case report. *Asian Pac J Health Sci* 1:174–176.

Chepuri, N.B., Jacobson, J.A., Fessell, D.P., Hayes, C.W. 2001. Sonographic appearance of the peroneus quartus muscle: Correlation with MR imaging appearance in seven patients. *Radiology* 218(2):415–419.

Cheung, Y.Y., Rosenberg, Z.S., Ramsinghani, R., Beltran, J., Jahss, M.H. 1997. Peroneus quartus muscle: MR imaging features. *Radiology* 202(3):745–750.

Cheung, Y.Y., Rosenberg, Z.S., Colon, E., Jahss, M. 1999. MR imaging of flexor digitorum accessorius longus. *Skel Radiol* 28:130–137.

Chhaparwal, R., Joshi, S.S., Joshi, S.D., Mittal, P.S. 2015. Variations in the insertion of peroneus longus muscle. *J Anat Soc India* 64(2):133–136.

Chiba, S. 1992. Multiple positional relationships of nerves arising from the sacral plexus to the piriformis muscle in humans. *Kaibogaku Zasshi* 67:691–724.

Chiba, S., Suzuki, T., Kasai, T. 1983. A rare anomaly of the pectoralis major—the chondroepitrochlearis. *Okajimas Folia Anat Jpn* 60:175–185.

Chittoria, R.K., Pratap, H., Yekappa, S.H. 2015. Abductor hallucis: Anatomical variation and its clinical implications in the reconstruction of chronic nonhealing ulcers and defects of foot. *Adv Wound Care* 4(12):719–723.

Choi, Y., Lim, J., Han, K., Lee, W., Kim, M. 2011. Ankyloglossia correction: Z-plasty combined with genioglossus myotomy. *J Craniofac Surg* 22:2238–2240.

Choi, D., Hur, M., Youn, Kim, J., Kim, H., Kim, S. 2014. Clinical anatomic considerations of the zygomaticus minor muscle based on the morphology and insertion pattern. *Dermatol Surg* 40:858–863.

Choi, D., Bae, J., Hu, K., Kim, H. 2020. Anatomical variations of the stylopharyngeus and superior constrictors in relation to their function. *Anat Cell Biol* 53(4):417–421.

Chotigavanichaya, C., Scaduto, A.A., Jadhav, A., Otsuka, N.Y. 2000. Accessory soleus muscle as a cause of resistance to correction in congenital clubfoot: A case report. *Foot Ankle Int* 21:948–950.

Chouke, K.S. 1927. Some interesting anomalies of the human body. *Anat Rec* 36:389–394.

Chouke, K.S. 1935. The constitution of the sheath of the rectus abdominis muscle. *Anat Rec* 61:341–349.

Chudzinski, T.H. 1875. Contributions a panatomie du negre. *Rev de Soc d'Anthrop De Paris* 2:398–414.

Chudzinski, T. 1898. Observations sur les variations musculaires dans les races humaines. *Mem soc d'anthrop Paris.* Paris: Compte.

Cihak, R. 1972. Ontogenesis of the skeleton and intrinsic muscles of the human hand and foot. *Ergebn d Anat u Entw Gesch Bd* 46:1–194.

Cingel, V., Bohac, M., Mestanova, V., Zabojnikova, L., Varga, I. 2013. Poland syndrome: From embryological basis to plastic surgery. *Surg Radiol Anat* 35:639–646.

Ciołkowski, M.K., Krajewsjki, P., Ciszek, B. 2014. A case of atlas assimilation: Description of bony and soft structures. *Surg Radiol Anat* 26:833–836.

Claassen, H., Wree, A. 2002. Multiple variations in the region of mm. extensores carpi radialis longus and brevis. *Ann Anat* 184:489–491.

Claassen, H., Wree, A. 2003. Isolated flexor muscles of the little toe in the feet of an individual with atrophied or lacking 4th head of the m. extensor digitorum brevis and lacking the 4th tendon of the m. extensor digitorum longus. *Ann Anat* 185:81–84.

Claassen, H., Schmitt, O., Schulze, M., Wree, A. 2013. Variation in the hypothenar muscles and its impact on ulnar tunnel syndrome. *Surg Radiol Anat* 35:893–89.

Clarkson, R.D., Rainy, H. 1889. Unusual arrangement of the psoas muscle. *J Anat Physiol* 23:504–506.

Clarkson, M.J., Fox, J.N., Atsas, S., Daney, B.T., Dodson, S.C., Lambert, H.W. 2013. Clinical implications of novel variants of the fibularis (peroneus) quartus muscle inserting onto the cuboid bone: Peroneocuboideus and peroneocalcaneocuboideus. *J Foot Ankle Surg* 52(1):118–121.

Clarys, J.P., Barbaix, E., Van Rompacy, H., Caboor, D., Van Roy, P. 1996. The muscular arch of the axilla revisited: Its possible role in the thoracic outlet and shoulder instability syndromes. *Man Ther* 1:133–139.

Clason, E. 1869. Om muskelanomalier. *Upsala Lakareforening Forhandlingar* 4:244–248.

Clemens, H.J. 1957. Zur morphologic des ligamentum epitrochleo-anconcum. *Anat Anz* 104:343–344.

Coats, D., Ou, R. 2001. Anomalous medial rectus muscle insertion in a child with craniosynostosis. *Binocul Vis Strabismus* 16(2):119–120.

Coban, I., Topkul, O., Ozturk, L. 2019. A rare variation of the longest striated muscle in humans. *Acta Sci Anatom* 1(3):190–194.

Cogar, A.C., Johnsen, P.H., Potter, H.G., Wolfe, S.W. 2015. Subclavius posticus: An anomalous muscle in association with suprascapular nerve compression in an athlete. *HAND* 10:76–79.

Colacino, S., Pettersen, J. 1978. Analysis of the gross anatomical variations found in four cases of Trisomy 13. *Am J Med Gen* 2:31–50.

Collett, D.J., Karovalia, S., Bokor, D.J. 2018. An unusual variant of the origin of the short head of biceps brachii. *Int J Anat Var* 11:134–135.

Collins, R.M., Bhana, J., Patricios, J.S., Du Plessis, A., Veller, M., Schultz, D., Janse van Rensburg, D.C. 2014. Thoracic outlet syndrome in a patient with absent scalenus anterior muscle. *Clin J Sport Med* 24:268–270.

Cornwall, J., Stringer, M.D., Duxson, M. 2011. Functional morphology of the thoracolumbar transversospinalis muscles. *Spine* 36:1053–1061.

Coskun, N., Yildirim F.B., Ozkan, O. 2002. Multiple muscular variations in the neck region — case study. *Folia Morphol* 61:317–319.

Cralley, J.C., Schuberth, J.M. 1979. The transverse head of adductor hallucis. *Anat Anz.* 146(4):400–409.

Crerar, J.W. 1892. Note on the absence of the subclavius muscle. *J Anat Physiol* 26:554.

Cromeens, B., Reeves, R. 2011. Anomalous peroneus (fibularis) longus muscle: An atypical insertion and incomplete distal tendon. *Clin Anat* 24(8):997–999.

Crompton, T., Lloyd, C., Kokkinakis, M., Norman-Taylor, F. 2014. The prevalence of bifid iliopsoas tendon on MRI in children. *J Child Orthop* 8:333–336.

Cruveilhier, J. 1837. *Anatomie Descriptive*, vols. 1–3. Paris: Bechet.

Cunningham, D.J., St. John Brooks, H. 1889-1901. The peroneus quinti digiti. *Proc Roy Irish Acad* 1:78–81.

Curnow, J. 1873. Notes of some irregularities in muscles and nerves. *J Anat Physiol* 7:304–310.

Curry, B., Kuz, J. 2000. A new variation of abductor digiti minimi accessorius. *J Hand Surg [Am]* 25:585–587.

Cutler, H.S., Tao, M.A., O'Brien, S.J., Taylor, S.A. 2018. Trifurcate origin of long head of biceps brachii: A case report and literature review. *J Orthop Case Rep* 8:70–73.

Cuttone, J., Brazis, P., Miller, M., Folk, S. 1979. Absence of the superior rectus muscle in Apert's syndrome. *J Pediatr Ophthalmol Strab* 16:349–354.

da Silva, T.K., Marchiori, E., da Rosa Silva, G., Lago, L.N., Bello, R.M. 2012. Accessory diaphragm associated with single pulmonary vein in an asymptomatic patient: 64-multidetector CT findings. *Lung* 190:353–354.

Dalmia, D., Behera, S.K. 2017. Congenital absence of stapedius muscle and tendon: Rare finding in two cases. *Indian J Otol* 23:43–45.

Darwin, C. 1871. *The Descent of Man: And Selection in Relation to Sex.* London: J. Murray.

Das, N., Singh, B. 1950. Iliacus minor; a report. *Ind Med Gaz* 85(11):492.

Das, S., Paul, S. 2006. An anomalous palmaris brevis muscle and its clinical implications. *Internet J Surg* 9(2):1–3.

Das, S., Suhaimi, F.H., Latiff, A.A., Othman, F. 2008. Anomalous pronator quadratus muscle: A case report. *Eur J Anat* 12:123–125.

Das, S.S., Saluja, S., Vasudeva, N. 2017. Biometrics of pyramidalis muscle and its clinical importance. *J Clin Diagn Res* 11:AC05–AC07.

Daseler, E.H., Anson, B.J. 1943. The plantaris muscle: An anatomical study of 750 specimens. *J Bone Joint Surg [Am]* 25(4):822–827.

Date, H., Hayakawa, K., Nakagawa, K., Yamada, H. 2012. Snapping knee due to the biceps femoris tendon treated with repositioning of the anomalous tibial insertion. *Knee Surg Sports Traumatol Arthrosc* 20:1581–1583.

Dave, M.R., Yagain, V.K., Anadkat, S. 2012. Unilateral third/accessory head of the gastrocnemius muscle: A case report. *Int J Morphol* 30(3):1061–1064.

Dawson, S., Barton, N. 1986. Anatomical variations of the extensor pollicis brevis. *J Hand Surg* 11B:378–381.

DeAngelis, D., Kraft, S.P. 2001. The double-bellied inferior oblique muscle: Clinical correlates. *J AAPOS* 5(2):76–81.

DeAngelis, D,. Makar, I., Kraft, S.P. 1999. Anatomic variations of the inferior oblique muscle: A potential cause of failed inferior oblique weakening surgery. *Am J Ophthalmol* 128(4):485–488.

de Castro, C. 1980. The anatomy of the platysma muscle. *Plast Reconstr Surg* 66:680–683.

Dc Mey, A., Van Hoof, I., De Roy, G., Lejour, M. 1989. Anatomy of the orbicularis oris muscle in cleft lip. *Brit J Plast Surg* 42:710–714.

De-Ary-Pires, B., Ary-Pires, R., Pires-Neto, M.A. 2003. The human digastric muscle: Patterns and variations with clinical and surgical correlations. *Ann Anat* 185:471–479.

Dean, M.C. 1984. Comparative myology of the hominoid cranial base, I, the muscular relationships and bony attachments of the digastric muscle. *Folia Primatol* 43:234–48.

Dean, M.C. 1985. Comparative myology of the hominoid cranial base, II, the muscles of the prevertebral and upper pharyngeal region. *Folia Primatol* 44:40–51.

Debeer, P., Brys, P., De Smet, L., Fryns, J. 2002. Unilateral absence of the trapezius and pectoralis major muscle: A variant of Poland syndrome. *Genet Coun* 13(4):449–453.

Del Sol, M., Olave, E. 2005. Elevator muscle of the tendon of latissimus dorsi muscle. *Clin Anat* 18:112–114.

DeLancey, J.O., Morgan, D.M., Fenner, D.E., Kearney, R., Guire. K., Miller, J.M., Hussain, H., Umek, W., Hsu, Y., Ashton-Miller, J.A. 2007. Comparison of levator ani muscle defects and function in women with and without pelvic organ prolapse. *Obstet Gynecol* 109:295–302.

Demir, B.T., Gümüşalan, Y., Üzel, M., Çevik, H.B. 2015. The variations of peroneus digiti quinti muscle and its contribution to the extension of the fifth toe. A cadaveric study. *Saudi Med J* 36(11):1285–1289.

Deniker, J. 1885. Recherches anatomiques et embryologiques sur les singes anthropoïdes—foetus de gorille et de gibbon. *Arch Zool Exp Gén* 3(suppl 3):1–265.

Depuydt, K.H., Schuurman, A.H., Kon, M. 1998. Reversed palmaris longus muscle causing effort-related median nerve compression. *J Hand Surg Br* 23:117–119.

Dergin, G., Kiliç, C., Gozneli, R., Yildirim, D., Garip, H., Moroglu, S. 2012. Evaluating the correlation between the lateral pterygoid muscle attachment type and internal derangement of the temporomandibular joint with an emphasis on MR imaging findings. *J Craniomaxillofac Surg* 40(5):459–463.

De Smet, L. 2002. Median and ulnar nerve compression at the wrist caused by anomalous muscles. *Acta Orthop Belg* 68:431–438.

Diamond, G., Katowicz, J., Whitaker, L., Quinn, G., Shaffer, D. 1980. Variations in extraocular muscle number and structure in craniofacial dysostosis. *Am J Ophthalmol* 90:416–418.

Dickson, M.J. 1999. The pyramidalis muscle. *J Obst Gynecol* 19:300.

Didia, B., Loveday, O., Christian, I. 2009. Variation and incidence of agenesis of the pyramidalis muscles in Nigerian males. *J Exp Clin Anat* 8(1). doi:10.4314/jeca.v8i1.48031.

DiDio, L.J.A., Zappal, A., Carney, W.P. 1967. Anatomico-functional aspects of the musculus articularis genus in man. *Acta Anat (Basel)* 67:1–23.

DiDio, L.J.A., Zappal. A., Cardoso, A.D., Diaz, R.A. 1969. Muscularis articularis genus in human fetuses, newborn and young individuals. *Anat Anz* 124:121–32.

Diogo, R. 2004a. Muscles versus bones: Catfishes as a case study for a discussion on the relative contribution of myological and osteological features in phylogenetic reconstructions. *Animal Biology* 54:373–391.

Diogo, R. 2004b. *Morphological Evolution, Adaptations, Homoplasies, Constraints, and Evolutionary Trends: Catfishes as a Case Study on General Phylogeny & Macroevolution.* Boca Raton, FL: CRC Press.

Diogo, R. 2005. *Adaptations, Homoplasies, Constraints, and Evolutionary Trends: Catfish Morphology, Phylogeny and Evolution, A Case Study on Theoretical Phylogeny and Macroevolution.* Enfield: Science Publishers Inc.

Diogo, R. 2007. *On the Origin and Evolution of Higher-Clades: Osteology, Myology, Phylogeny and Macroevolution of Bony Fishes and the Rise of Tetrapods.* Enfield: Science Publishers Inc.

Diogo, R., Abdala, V. 2007. Comparative anatomy, homologies and evolution of the pectoral muscles of bony fish and tetrapods: A new insight. *J Morphol* 268:504–517.

Diogo, R., Abdala, V. 2010. *Muscles of Vertebrates: Comparative Anatomy, Evolution, Homologies and Development.* Oxford: Taylor & Francis.

Diogo, R., Abdala, V., Lonergan, N., Wood, B.A. 2008a. From fish to modern humans–comparative anatomy, homologies and evolution of the head and neck musculature. *J Anat* 213:391–424.

Diogo, R., Hinits, Y., Hughes, S.M. 2008b. Development of mandibular, hyoid and hypobranchial muscles in the zebrafish: Homologies and evolution of these muscles within bony fishes and tetrapods. *BMC Dev Biol* 8:1–22.

Diogo, R., Abdala, V., Aziz, M.A., Lonergan, N., Wood, B.A. 2009a. From fish to modern humans–comparative anatomy, homologies and evolution of the pectoral and forelimb musculature. *J Anat* 214:694–716.

Diogo, R., Wood, B.A., Aziz, M.A., Burrows, A. 2009b. On the origin, homologies and evolution of primate facial muscles, with a particular focus on hominoids and a suggested unifying nomenclature for the facial muscles of the Mammalia. *J Anat* 215:300–319.

Diogo, R., Potau, J.M., Pastor, J.F., De Paz, F., Barbosa, M.M., Ferrero, E.M., Bello, G., Wood, B.A. 2010. *Photographic and Descriptive Atlas of Gorilla - With Notes on the Attachments, Variations, Innervation, Synonymy and Weight of the Muscles.* Oxford: Taylor & Francis.

Diogo, R., Tanaka, E.M. 2014. Development of fore- and hindlimb muscles in GFP-transgenic axolotls: Morphogenesis, the tetrapod Bauplan, and new insights on the forelimb-hindlimb enigma. *J Exp Zool B Mol Dev Evol* 322:106–127.

Diogo, R., Ziermann, J.M. 2014. Development of fore- and hindlimb muscles in frogs: Morphogenesis, homeotic transformations, digit reduction, and the forelimb-hindlimb enigma. *J Exp Zool B Mol Dev Evol* 322:86–105.

Diogo, R., Wood, B.A. 2011. Soft tissue anatomy of the primates: Phylogenetic analyses based on the muscles of the head, neck, pectoral region and upper limb, with notes on the evolution of these muscles. *J Anat* 219:273–359.

Diogo, R., Wood, B.A. 2012a. *Comparative Anatomy and Phylogeny of Primate Muscles and Human Evolution.* New York: CRC Press.

Diogo, R., Wood, B. 2012b. Violation of Dollo's Law: Evidence of muscle reversions in primate phylogeny and their implications for the understanding of the ontogeny, evolution and anatomical variations of modern humans. *Evolution* 66:3267–3276.

Diogo, R., Wood, B. 2016. Origin, development, and evolution of primate muscles, with notes on human anatomical variations and anomalies. In *Developmental Approaches to Human Evolution*, eds. Boughner J.C., Rolian, C., 167–204. Hoboken, NJ: John Wiley & Sons, Inc.

Diogo, R., Potau, J.M., Pastor, J.F., De Paz, F., Barbosa, M.M., Ferrero, E.M., Bello, G., Aziz, M.A., Burrows, A., Wood, B.A. 2012. *Photographic and Descriptive Atlas of Gibbons and Siamangs (Hylobates) - With Notes on the Attachments, Variations, Innervation, Synonymy and Weight of the Muscles.* Oxford: Taylor & Francis.

Diogo, R., Potau, J.M., Pastor, J.F., De Paz, F., Barbosa, M.M., Ferrero, E.M., Bello, G., Aziz, M.A., Burrows, A., Wood, B.A. 2013a. *Photographic and Descriptive Atlas of Chimpanzees (Pan) - With Notes on the Attachments, Variations, Innervation, Synonymy and Weight of the Muscles.* Oxford: Taylor & Francis.

Diogo, R., Potau, J.M., Pastor, J.F., De Paz, F., Barbosa, M.M., Ferrero, E.M., Bello, G., Aziz, M.A., Burrows, A., Wood, B.A. 2013b. *Photographic and Descriptive Atlas of Orangutans (Pongo) - With Notes on the Attachments, Variations, Innervation, Synonymy and Weight of the Muscles.* Oxford: Taylor & Francis.

Diogo, R., Smith, C.M. and Ziermann, J.M. 2015. Evolutionary developmental pathology and anthropology: A new field linking development, comparative anatomy, human evolution, morphological variations and defects, and medicine. *Dev Dyn* 244:1357–1374.

Diogo, R., Noden, D., Smith, C.M., Molnar, J.A., Boughner, J., Barrocas, C., Bruno, J. 2016. *Learning and Understanding Human Anatomy and Pathology: An Evolutionary and Developmental Guide for Medical Students.* Oxford: Taylor & Francis.

Diogo, R., Shearer, B., Potau, J.M, Pastor, J.F, De Paz, F.J., Arias-Martorell, J., Turcotte, C., Hammond, A., Vereecke, E., Vanhoof, M., Nauwelaerts, S., Wood, B. 2017. *Photographic and Descriptive Musculoskeletal Atlas of Bonobos - With Notes on the Weight, Attachments, Variations, and Innervation of the Muscles and Comparisons with Common Chimpanzees and Humans.* New York: Springer.

Diogo, R., Ziermann, J.M., Molnar, J.A., Siomava, N., Abdala, V. 2018. *Muscles of Chordates: Development, Homologies and Evolution.* Oxford: Taylor & Francis.

Diogo, R., Siomava, N., Gitton, Y. 2019. Development of human limb muscles based on whole-mounted immunostaining and the links between ontogeny and evolution. *Development* 146:dev180349.

Dodds, S.D. 2006. A flexor carpi radialis brevis muscle with an anomalous origin on the distal radius. *J Hand Surg* 31(A):1507–1510.

Donley, B.G., Leyes, M. 2001. Peroneus quartus muscle. A rare cause of chronic lateral ankle pain. *Am J Sports Med* 29(3):373–375.

Doral, M.N., Atay, A.O., Bozkurt, M., Ayvaz, M., Tetik, O., Leblebicioglu, G. 2006. Three-bundle popliteus tendon: A nonsymptomatic anatomical variation. *The Knee* 13(4):342–343.

DosRemedios, E.T., Jolly, G.P. 2000. The accessory soleus and recurrent tarsal tunnel syndrome: Case report of a new surgical approach. *J Foot Ankle Surg* 39(3):194–197.

Doyle, J.R., Botte, M.J. 2003. *Surgical Anatomy of the Hand and Upper Extremity.* Philadelphia, PA: Lippincott Williams & Wilkins.

Dragieva, P., Zaharieva, M., Kozhuharov, Y., Markov, K., Stoyanov, G.S. 2018. Psoas minor muscle: A cadaveric morphometric study. *Cureus* 10(4):e2447.

Driver, J.R., Denison, A.B. 1914. The morphology of the long accessorius muscle. *Anat Rec* 8:341–347.

Drummond, G., Keech, R. 1989. Absent and anomalous superior oblique and superior rectus muscles. *Can J Ophthalmol* 24(6):275–279.

Dsouza, R., Shankar N., Gurubatham, R., Rajaleelan, W., Menon, N. 2017. Absent external oblique musculo-aponeurotic complex during inguinal hernioplasty: A case report and review of literature. *Surg Radiol Anat* 39:1045–1048.

DuBrul, E.L. 1958. *Evolution of the Speech Apparatus.* Springfield: Thomas.

Duc, S.R., Wentz, K.U., Käch, K.P., Zollikofer, C.L. 2004. First report of an accessory popliteal muscle: Detection with MRI. *Skeletal Radiol* 33:429–431.

Duda, G.N., Brand, D., Freitag, S., Lierse, W., Schneider, E. 1996. Variability of femoral muscle attachments. *J Biomech* 29:1185–1190.

Dudgeon, S.N., Marcotte, K.M., Fox, G.M., Alsup, B.K. 2017. A previously unclassified variant of sternalis muscle. *Surg Radiol Anat* 39:1417–1419.

Dunlap, S.S., Aziz, M.A., Rosenbaum, K.N. 1986. Comparative anatomical analysis of human trisomies 13, 18, and 21: I. The forelimb. *Teratology* 33:159–186.

Dunlap, S.S., Aziz, M.A., Ziermann, J.M. 2017. Anatomical variations of the deep head of Cruveilhier of the flexor pollicis brevis and its significance for the evolution of the precision grip. *PloS One* 12:e0187402.

Dunn, G.F., Hack, G.D., Robinson, W.L., Koritzer, R.T. 1996. Anatomical observation of a craniomandibular muscle originating from the skull base: The sphenomandibularis. *Cranio* 14(2):97–105.

Duparc, F., Thomine, J.M., Dujardin, F., Durand, C., Lukaziewicz, M., Muller, J.M., Freger, P. 1997. Anatomic basis of the transgluteal approach to the hip-joint by anterior hemimyotomy of the gluteus medius. *Surg Radiol Anat* 19:61–67.

Duranoğlu, Y., Gözkaya, O. 2005 Bifid right lateral rectus: A case report. *Strabismus* 13:89–92.

du Plessis, M., Loukas, M. 2016. Thigh muscles. In *Bergman's Comprehensive Encyclopedia of Human Anatomic Variation*, first edition, ed. Tubbs, R.S., Shoja, M.M., Loukas, M., 410–420. Hoboken, NJ: Wiley-Blackwell.

Duque-Parra, J.E., Barco-Ríos, J., Vélez-García, J.F. 2019. Incidence of sternalis muscle in the Caldas population (Colombia): Anatomical variations. *Int J Morphol* 37:1342–1346.

Duran-Stanton, A.M., Bui-Mansfield, L.T. 2010. Magnetic resonance diagnosis of tarsal tunnel syndrome due to flexor digitorum accessorius longus and peroneocalcaneus internus muscles. *J Comput Assist Tomogr* 34(2):270–272.

Dwight, T. 1887. Muscular abnormalities (notes on muscular abnormalities). *J Anat Physiol* 22:96–102.

Dwight, T. 1895. Notes on the dissection and brain of the chimpanzee 'Gumbo'. *Mem Boston Soc Nat Hist* 5:31–51.

Ebenezer, D.A., Rathinam, B.A.D. 2013. Rare multiple variations in brachial plexus and related structures in the left upper limb of a Dravidian male cadaver. *Anat Cell Biol* 46:163–166.

Eberle, C.F., Moran, B., Gleason, T. 2002. The accessory flexor digitorum longus as a cause of flexor hallucis syndrome. *Foot Ankle Intl* 23(1):51–55.

Ebrahimi, A., Nejadsarvari, N., Motamedi, M., Rezaee, M., Koushki, E. 2012. Anatomic variations found on dissection of depressor septi nasi muscles in cadavers. *Arch Facial Plast Surg* 14:31–33.

Edama, M., Takabayashi, T., Inai, T., Kikumoto, T., Hirabayashi, R., Ito, W., Nakamura, E., Ikezu, M., Kaneko, F., Kageyama, I. 2019. The relationships between the quadratus plantae and the flexor digitorum longus and the flexor hallucis longus. *Surg Radiol Anat* 41(6):689–692.

Edama, M., Takabayashi, T., Hirabayashi, R., Yokota, H., Inani, T., Sekine, C., Matsukawa, K., Otsuki, T., Maruyama, S., Kageyama, I. 2020. Anatomical variations in the insertion of the peroneus longus tendon. *Surg Radiol Anat* 42:1141–1144.

Edwards, W.G., Lincoln, C.R., Bassett 3rd, F.H., Goldner, J.L. 1969. The tarsal tunnel syndrome. Diagnosis and treatment. *JAMA* 207(4):716–720.

Eisler, P. 1912. *Die muskeln des stammes*. Jena: Gustav Fischer.

Eladoumikdachi, F., Valkov, P.L., Thomas, J., Netscher, D.T. 2002a. Anatomy of the intrinsic hand muscles revisited: Part I - interossei. *Plast Reconstr Surg* 110:1211–1224.

Eladoumikdachi, F., Valkov, P.L., Thomas, J., Netscher, D.T. 2002b. Anatomy of the intrinsic hand muscles revisited: Part II - lumbricals. *Plast Reconstr Surg* 110:1225–1231.

el-Badawi, M.G. 1987. An anomalous bifurcation of the sartorius muscle. *Anatomischer Anzeiger* 163(1):79–82.

el-Badawi, M.G., Butt, M.M., al-Zuhair, A.G., Fadel, R.A. 1995. Extensor tendons of the fingers: Arrangement and variations—II. *Clin Anat* 8:391–398.

El-Beshbishy, R.A., Abdel-Hamid, G.A. 2013. Variations of the abductor pollicis longus tendon: An anatomic study. *Folia Morphol* 72:161–166.

Elftman, H.O. 1932. The evolution of the pelvic floor of primates. *Am J Anat* 51:307–346.

El-Naggar, M.M., Zahir, F.I. 2001. Two bellies of the coracobrachialis muscle associated with a third head of biceps brachii muscle. *Clin Anat* 14:379–382.

El-Naggar, M.M., Al-Saggaf, S. 2004. Variant of the coracobrachialis muscle with a tunnel for the median nerve and brachial artery. *Clin Anat* 17:139–143.

Elsayed, S.M., Elsayed, G.M. 2009. Phenotype of apoptopic lymphocytes in children with Down Syndrome. *Immun Ageing* 6:2.

Elvan, Ö., Beger, O., Karagül, M.İ., Uzmansel, D., Yılmaz, N.Ş., Kurtoğlu Olgunus, Z. 2019. Anatomic and histological analyses of chiasma plantare and long flexor tendons of the foot on human fetuses. *Surg Radiol Anat* 41:775–784.

Elvan, Ö., Bobuş, Ö., Alev, M., Tezer, M. 2020. Anatomical evaluation of zygomaticus major muscle with relation to orbicularis oculi muscle and parotid duct. *J Craniofac Surg* 31(6):1844–1847.

Emsley, J., Davis, M. 2001. Partial unilateral absence of the trapezius muscle in a human cadaver. *Clin Anat* 14:383–386.

Erić, M., Krivokuća, D., Savović, S., Lekšan, I., Vučinić, N. 2010. Prevalence of the palmaris longus through clinical evaluation. *Surg Radiol Anat* 32:357–361.

Erić, M., Yammine, K., Gosh, V., Feigl, G., Marić, D. 2019. Prevalence of the Linburg–Comstock variation through clinical evaluation. *Surg Radiol Anat* 41:1307–1314.

Erickson, J., Kwart, A., Steven Yang, S. 2019. Extensor carpi ulnaris tendon anatomy may mimic tears. *J Hand Surg (Asian-Pacific Vol)* 24:175–179.

Fabrizio, P.A., Clemente, F.R. 1997. Variation in the triceps brachii muscle: A fourth muscular head. *Clin Anat* 10:259–263.

Farahvash, M., Abianeh, S., Farahvash, B., Farahvash, Y., Yagoobi, A., Nazparvar, B. 2010. Anatomic variations of midfacial muscles and nasolabial crease: A survey on 52 hemifacial dissections in fresh Persian cadavers. *Aesthet Surg J* 30(1):17–21.

Farfán, C.E., Inzunza, H.O., Echeverría, M.M., Inostroza, R.V. 2019. The dorsoepicondylar medial muscle, a clinically relevant anatomical variation. *Int J Morphol* 37:600–605.

Farias, M.C.G., Oliveira, B.D.R., Rocha, T.D.S., Caiaffo, V. 2012. Morphological and morphometric analysis of psoas minor muscle in cadavers. *J Morphol Sci* 29:202–205.

Favril, A., Vanhoenacker, F., Goubau, Y., Jager, T. 2019. Camptodactyly resulting from anatomical variation of lumbrical muscles: Imaging findings. *Skeletal Radiol* 48:2009–2014.

Fawcett, E. 1896. What is Sibson's Muscle (Scalenus pleuralis)? *J Anat Physiol* 30(Pt 3):433–436.

Feigl, G.C., Pixner, T. 2011. The cleidoatlanticus muscle: A potential pitfall for the practice of ultrasound guided interscalene brachial plexus block. *Surg Radiol Anat* 33:823–825.

Feipel, V., Simonnet, M.L., Rooze, M. 2003. The proximal attachments of the popliteus muscle: A quantitative study and clinical significance. *Surg Radiol Anat* 25:58–63.

Fernandes, S.J., Singh, A., Prakash, S., D'souza, P.A. 2016. Bilateral absence of extensor indicis proprius associated with presence of unilateral extensor indicis brevis: A cadaveric study. *Int J Sci Res* 5:480–482.

Fernández-de-Luna, M., Rodríguez-Martínez, A., Mohamed-Noriega, J. et al. 2020. Double-bellied medial rectus muscle in a patient with Down syndrome and congenital esotropia. *Surg Radiol Anat* 42:859–861.

Ferreira Arquez, H. 2017. An anatomical study of the musculus flexor digitorum brevis. *Intl Arch Med* 10:216.

Ferreli, F., Mercante, G., Spriano, G. 2019. Levator claviculae muscle: Anatomic variation found during neck dissection. *Laryngoscope* 129(3):634–636.

Ferrero, E.M. 2011. Anatomía comparada del sistema muscular de la extremidad posterior en primates superiores. PhD Thes., The Univ. of Valladolid, Spain.

Ferrero, E.M., Pastor, J.F., Fernandez, F.P., Barbosa, M., Diogo, R., Wood, B. 2012. Comparative anatomy of the lower limb muscles of hominoids: Attachments, relative weights, innervation and functional morphology. In *Primates: Classification, Evolution and Behavior*, ed. Hughes, E.F., Hill, M.E., Hauppauge: Nova Science Publishers.

Fetto, J.F., Marshall, J.L., Ghelman, B. 1977. An anomalous attachment of the popliteus tendon to the lateral meniscus. *J Bone Joint Surg [Am]* 59:548–549.

Fick, R. 1925. Beobachtungen an den muskeln einger schimpansen. *Z Anat Entwicklungsgesch* 76:117–141.

Flack, N.A.M.S., Nicholson, H.D., Woodley, S.J. 2012. A review of the anatomy of the hip abductor muscles, gluteus medius, gluteus minimus, and tensor fascia lata. *Clin Anat* 25(6):697–708.

Flack, N.A.M.S., Nicholson, H.D., Woodley, S.J. 2014. The anatomy of the hip abductor muscles. *Clin Anat* 27(2):241–253.

Flaherty, G., O'Neill, M.N., Folan-Curran, J. 1999. Case report: Bilateral occurrence of a chondroepitrochlearis muscle. *J Anat* 194:313–315.

Flower, W.H., Murie, J. 1867. Account of the dissection of a Bushwoman. *J Anat Physiol* 1:189–208.

Forcada, P., Rodriguez-Niedenfuhr, M., Liusa, M., Carrera, A. 2001. Subclavius posticus muscle: Supernumerary muscle as a potential cause for thoracic outlet syndrome. *Clin Anat* 14:55–57.

Fraser, P.R., Wood, A.R., Rosales, A.A. 2013. Anatomical variation of the semitendinosus muscle origin. *Int J Anat Var* 6:225–227.

Fraser, P.R., Thomas, J., Guttmann, G.D., Rosales, A.A. 2014. Rare accessory slip of the deltoid muscle conjoined with teres minor. *Eur J Anat* 18:195–197.

Freeman, A.J., Jacobson, N.A., Fogg, Q.A. 2008. Anatomical variations of the plantaris muscle and a potential role in patellofemoral pain syndrome. *Clin Anat* 21(2):178–181.

Frey, H. 1913. Der musculus triceps surae in der primatenreihe. *Morph Jahrb* 47:1–192.

Frey, H. 1919. Musculus gastrocnemius tertius. *Gegenbaurs Morphol Jahrbuch* 50:517–530.

Frohse, F., Frankel, M. 1908. Die Muskeln des menschlichen armes. In *Handbuchs der anatomie des menschen*, ed. Bardeleben, K.V., 160–161. Jena: Gustav Fischer.

Fujimura, A., Onodera, M., Feng, X., Osawa, T., Nara, E., Nagato, S., Matsumoto, Y., Sasaki, N., Nozaka, Y. 2003. Abnormal anterior belly of the digastric muscle: A proposal for the classification of abnormalities. *Anat Sci Intl* 78:185–188.

Fujita, S., Lizuka, T., Dauber, W. 2001. Variation of heads of lateral pterygoid muscle and morphology of articular disc of human temporomandibular joint–anatomical and histological analysis. *J Oral Rehabil* 28(6):560–571.

Furnas, D.W. 1965. Muscle tendon variations in the flexor compartment of the wrist. *Plast Reconstr Surg* 36:320–324.

Futamura, R. 1906. Uber die entwicklung der facialismuskulatur des menschen. *Anat Hefte* 30:433–516.

Gahhos, F.N., Ariyan, S. 1983. Extensor indicis brevis: A rare anatomical variation. *Ann Plast Surg* 10:326–328.

Gale, N.C., Kuxhaus, L., Ciani, M.J. 2016. Erector spinae muscle – iliocostalis anatomic variation. *J Musculoskel Res* 19:165007.

Galis, F., Metz, J.A.J. 2007. Evolutionary novelties: The making and breaking of pleiotropic constraints. *Integr Comp Biol* 47:409–419.

Galton, J.C. 1874 Note on the epitrochleo-anconeus or. anconeus sextus (Gruber). *J Anat Physiol* 9:168–75.

Gama, C. 1983. Extensor digitorum brevis manus: A report on 38 cases and a review of the literature. *J Hand Surg [Am]* 8:578–582.

Gandhi, S., Gupta, N., Thakur, A., Anshu, A., Mehta, V., Suri, R.K., Rath, G. 2013. Anatomical and clinical insight of variation morphologies of psoas minor muscle: A case report. *Int J Cur Res Rev* 5:106–110.

Garbelotti, S., Fernando de Sousa Rodrigues, C., Sgrott, E., et al. 2001, Unilateral absence of the thoracic part of the trapezius muscle. *Surg Radiol Anat* 23:131–133.

Garbelotti, S.A., Marques, S.R., Rocha, P.R., Pereira, V.R., Carvalo de Moraes, L.O. 2017. An unusual case of accessory head of coracobrachialis muscle involving lateral cord of brachial plexus and its clinical significance. *Folia Morphol* 76:762–765.

Gasser, R.F. 1967. The development of the facial muscles in man. *Am J Anat* 120:357–376.

Gaughran, G.R. 1957. Fasciae of the masticator space. *Anat Rec* 129(4):383–400.

Gaughran, G.R. 1963. Mylohyoid boutonniere and sublingual bouton. *J Anat* 97(Pt4):565–568.

Gebo, D.L. 1985. The nature of the primate grasping foot. *Am J Phys Anthropol* 67:269–277.

Geers, C., Nyssen-Behets, C., Cosnard, G., Lengelé, B. 2005. The deep belly of the temporalis muscle: An anatomical, histological and MRI study. *Surg Radiol Anat* 27(3):184–191.

George, B.M., Nayak, S.B., Marpalli, S. 2019. Clinical importance of tensor fasciae suralis arising from linea aspera along with short head of biceps femoris: A rare anomaly. *Anat Cell Biol* 52(1):90–92.

George, R. 1953. Co-incidence of palmaris longus and plantaris muscles. *Anat Rec* 116:521–523.

George, T.N., Kotlarek, K.J., Kuehn, D.P., Sutton, B.P., Perry, J.L. 2018. Differences in the tensor veli palatini between adults with and without cleft palate using high-resolution 3-dimensional magnetic resonance imaging. *Cleft Palate Craniofac J* 55(5):697–705.

Georgiev, G.P., Jelev, L. 2007. Variant triple origin of the flexor digiti minimi brevis (manus) muscle in relation to ulnar nerve and artery compression at the wrist. *Clin Anat* 20:976–977.

Georgiev, G.P., Jelev, L. 2009. Bilateral fibrous replacement of subclavius muscle in relation to nerve and artery compression of the upper limb. *Int J Anat Var* 2:57–59.

Georgiev, G.P., Jelev, L., Kinov, P., Vidiknov, N.K. 2009. A rare instance of an accessory long flexor to the second toe. *Intl J Anat Var* 2:108–110.

Georgiev, G.P., Jelev, L. 2011. An aberrant flexor digiti minimi brevis manus muscle. *J Hand Surg* 36:1965–1967.

Georgiev, G.P., Jelev, L., Surchev, L. 2007. Axillary arch in Bulgarian population: Clinical significance of the arches. *Clin Anat* 20:286–291.

Georgiev, G.P., Landzhov, B., Tubbs, R.S. 2017a. A novel type of coracobrachialis muscle variation and a proposed new classification. *Cureus* 9:e1466.

Georgiev, G.P., Iliev, A.A., Dimitrova, I.N., Kotov, G.N., Malinova, L.G., Landzhov, B.V. 2017b. Palmaris longus muscle variations: Clinical significance and proposal of new classifications. *Folia Medica* 59:289–297.

Georgiev, G.P., Tubbs, R.S., Landzhov, B. 2018a. Coracobrachialis longus muscle: Humeroepitrochlearis. *Cureus* 10:e2615.

Georgiev, G.P., Tubbs, R.S., Iliev, A., Kotov, G., Landzhov, B. 2018b. Extensor indicis proprius muscle and its variants together with the extensor digitorum brevis manus muscle: A common classification. Clinical significance in hand and reconstructive surgery. *Surg Radiol Anat* 40:271–280.

Ghormley, R.K., Spear, I.M. 1953. Anomalies of the posterior tibial tendon: A cause of persistent pain about the ankle. *AMA Arch Surg* 66(4):512–516.

Gibbs, S. 1999. Comparative soft tissue morphology of the extant hominoidea, including man. PhD Thesis, The University of Liverpool, Liverpool.

Gibbs, S., Collard, M., Wood, B.A. 2002. Soft-tissue anatomy of the extant hominoids: A review and phylogenetic analysis. *J Anat* 200:3–49.

Giles, K.W. 1960. Anatomical variations affecting the surgery of de Quervain's disease. *J Bone Joint Surg* 42(B):352–355.

Ginsberg, L.E., Eicher, S.A. 1999. Levator claviculae muscle presenting as a neck mass: CT imaging. *J Comput Assist Tomogr* 23:538–539.

Girolami, M., Tonetti, L., Pipola, V., Rimondi, E., Albisinni, U., Ricci, A., Gasbarrini, A. 2019. Quadratus femoris muscle causing deep gluteal syndrome: A rare cause of refractory sciatica of extraspinal origin in the presence of an anatomic variation. *J Back Musculoskel Rehab* 32:667–670.

Godwin, Y., Ellis, H. 1992. Distribution of the extensor tendons on the dorsum of the hand. *Clin Anat* 5:394–403.

Goktan, C., Orguc, S., Serter, S., Ovali, G.Y. 2006. Musculus sternalis: A normal but rare mammographic finding and magnetic resonance imaging demonstration. *Breast J* 12:488–489.

Göllner, K. 1982. Untersuchungen über die vom n. trigeminus innervierte kiefermusculatur des schimpansen (*Pan troglodytes*, Blumenbach 1799) und des gorilla (*Gorilla gorilla gorilla*, Savage and Wyman 1847). *Gegen Morphol Jahrb* 128:851–903.

Gonzales, J.R., Iwanaga, J., Oskouian, R.J., Tubbs, R.S. 2017. Variant prevertebral muscle: Unique cadaveric findings. *Cureus* 9:e1515.

Gonzalez, M.A., Netscher, D.T. 2016. Hand intrinsic muscles. In *Bergman's Comprehensive Encyclopedia of Human Anatomic Variation*, first edition, ed. Tubbs, R.S., Shoja, M.M., Loukas, M., 315–334. Hoboken, NJ: Wiley-Blackwell.

Gordon, S., Matheson, D. 1973. The accessory soleus. *Clin Orthop* 97:129–132.

Goubran, E., Carlos, J., Ayad, S. 2010. A bifurcated anterior scalene muscle: A case report. *Clin Chiropr* 13:153–155.

Gould, S.J. 1977. *Ontogeny and Phylogeny*. Cambridge: Harvard University Press.

Gould, S.J. 2002. *The Structure of Evolutionary Theory*. Belknap: Harvard.

Grand, T. I. 1968. The functional anatomy of the lower limb of the howler monkey (*Alouatta caraya*). *Am J Phys Anthropol* 28(2):163–181.

Gratiolet, L.P., Alix, P.H.E. 1866. Recherches sur l'anatomie du *Troglodytes aubryi*. *Nouv Arch Mus Hist Nat Paris* 2:1–264.

Gray, D.J. 1945. Some anomalous hamstring muscles. *Anat Rec* 91:33–38.

Graziano, P., Dell'Aversana Orabona, G., Astarita, F., Ponzo, L.M., Nunziata, R., Salzano, G., Maglitto, F., Solari, D., Santella, A., Cappabianca, M., Laconetta, G., Califano, L. 2016. Bilateral hypertrophy of masseteric and temporalis muscles, our fifteen patients and review of literature. *Eur Rev Med Pharmacol Sci* 20(1):7–11.

Green, H.L. 1931. The occurrence of a tenuissimus muscle in a human adult. *J Anat* 65 (Pt 2):266–271.

Gregory, W.K., Camp, L. 1918. Review and identification of muscles connected with the pelvis and sacrum in placentals, monotremes, sphenodon, and other reptiles, with inferred conditions in cynognathus. In *Bulletin of the American Museum of Natural History*, ed. Lutz, F.E., 450–514. New York: New York.

Gregory, J., Guse, D. 2007. Unique variant of levator glandulae thyroideae muscle. *Clin Anat* 20(8):966–967.

Greiner, T.M., Bedford, M.E., Walker, R.A. 2004. Variability in the human m. spinalis capitis and cervicis: Frequencies and definitions. *Ann Anat* 186:185–191.

Grider-Potter, N. 2017. Supernumerary rectus capitis posterior muscle in *Hylobates agilis*. *The FASEB J* 31:901.11.

Grob, K., Gilbey, H., Manestar, M., Ackland, T., Kuster, M.S. 2017. The anatomy of the articularis genus muscle and its relation to the extensor apparatus of the knee. *J Bone Joint Surg Open Access* 2(4):e0034.

Grönroos, H. 1903. Die musculi biceps brachii und latissimocondyloideus bei der affengattung *Hylobates* im vergleich mit den enprechenden gebilden der anthropoiden und des menschen. *Abh Kön Preuss Akad Wiss Berlin 1903*:1–102.

Gruber, W. 1844. Neue anomalien als beitroege der menschen. *Phys Chirurg u Path Anat* 6:31.

Gruber, W. 1859. Die musculi subscapulares (major et minor) und die neuen supernumerären schulter-muskeln des menschen. *Mem Acad Imp Sci St Petersberg* 8:219–58.

Gruber, W. 1860. Die supernumiraren brustmuskeln des menschen. *Mem Acad Imp Sci St Petersberg* 3:1–3.

Gruber, W. 1865. Neue supernumer.re schüsselbeinmuskeln. *Archiv Anat Phys Wissen Med* 2:703–718.

Gruber, W. 1867a. Ueber den anomalen verlauf des nervus ulnaris vor dem epitrochleus. *Reicherts Arch* 1867:560–564.

Gruber, W. 1867b. Uber die varietaten des musculus brachioradialis. *Bull Acad Imp Sci St Petersbourg* 12:527–528.

Gruber, W. 1867c. Ber den Musculus atlantico-mastoideus. *Arch Anat Physiol Wissen Med* 1867:733–738.

Gruber, W. 1868a. Über die muskeln des unteren schildknorpelrandes (musculi thyroeoidei marginales inferiors). *Arch Anat Physiol Wissen Med* 12:635–639.

Gruber, W. 1868b. Über den seltenen schildknorpelhorn-gie. beckenknorpelmuskel (musculus keratoarytaenoideus). *Arch Anat Physiol Wissen Med* 12:640–641.

Gruber, W. 1868c. Über eine neue variante des muculus thyreotrachealeis und über den musculus hyo-trachealis. *Arch Anat Physiol Wissen Med* 12:642–645.

Gruber, W. 1872. Mangel der mittlern portion des musculus deltoideus. *Archiv Anat Physiol Klin Med* 54:186–187.

Gruber, W. 1873a. Sur quelques muscles surnumeraires de l'abdomen chez l'homme. *Bull l'Acad Imp Sci St Petersbourg* 18:142–147.

Gruber, W. 1873b. Un cas de muscle oblique interne de l'abdomen, prive completement de sa portion inguinal. *Bull l'Acad Imp Sci St Petersbourg* 18:157–158.

Gruber, W. 1873c. Sur une variante du muscle tenseur de l'aponeurose surale, partant du muscle demi-tendinex. *Bull l'Acad Imp Sci St Petersbourg* 18:184–186.

Gruber, W. 1875a. Zwei neue falle eines rudimentaren musculus obliquus externus abdominis II. *Arch Path Anat Physiol Klin Med* 65:16–21.

Gruber, W. 1875b. Uber den musculus popliteus biceps. *Arch Anat Physiol Wissen Med* 1875:599–605.

Gruber, W. 1876. Ein musculus cleido-cervicalis s. trachelo-clavicularis imus. *Archiv Anat Phys Wissen Med* 1876:757–758.

Gruber, W. 1879. *Bcobachtungen aus der menschlichen und vcrgleichenden anatomie*, 2, 56–58. Berlin: Heft.

Gruber, W. 1886. About the abnormal abductor metatarsi quinti muscle, its substitution by a tendon cord (new) and its appearance as m. abductor metatarsi quinti circumflexus (new) in humans, as well as constant homologies for it in mammals. *Arch Patholo Anat* 106:489–501.

Gruber, W. 1887. Ueber einen musculus glutaeus quartus bei dem menschen (1. u. 2. fall) und einen homologen muskel bei *Säugethieren. Archiv für pathologische Anatomie und Physiologie und für Klinische Medicin* 107:480–484.

Gruen, P., Carranza, A., Karmody, C., Bachor, E. 2005. Anomalies of the ear in the Pierre Robin triad. *Ann Otol Rhinol Laryngol* 114(8):605–613.

Guelfguat, M., Nurbhai, N., Solounias, N. 2001. Median accessory digastric muscle: Radiological and surgical correlation. *Clin Anat* 14(1):42–46.

Guerra, D.R., Reis, F.P., Bastos, A.D.A., Brito, C.J., Silva, R.J.D.S., Aragão, J.A. 2012. Anatomical study on the psoas minor muscle in human fetuses. *Int J Morphol* 30:136–139.

Gugapriya, T.S. 2012. Morphology of flexor digitorum brevis muscle in northern Tamil Nadu region–an anatomical study with phylogenetic perspective. *Nat J Clin Anat* 1:129–132.

Gümüşalan, Y., Kalaycioğlu, A. 2000. Bilateral accessory flexor digitorum longus muscle in man. *Ann Anat - Anat Anz* 182:573–576.

Gunal, I., Sahinoglu, K., Bergman, R.A. 1994. Anomalous tibialis posterior muscle as an etiologic factor of hallux valgus. *Clin Anat* 7(1):21–25.

Guo-Hua, W., Xiao-Ling, J., Rong, W., Wei-Qiong, Z., Ting-Wei, B., Jian-Hua, L. 2009. Doubled omohyoid muscle in human: A case report and literature review. *Clin Anat* 22(8):868–70.

Gupta, R.K., Bhagwat, S.S. 2006. An anomalous muscle in the region of the popliteal fossa: A case report. *J Anat Soc India* 55(2):65–68.

Gupta, U.K., Nasir, N. 2013. A rare instance of a tendinous interconnection between flexor hallucis longus and flexor digitorum accessorius. *Int J Anat Var* 6:18–19.

Hack, G., Hallgren, R. 2004. Chronic headache relief after section of suboccipital muscle dural connections: A case report. *Headache* 44:84–89.

Hack, G., Koritzer, R., Robinson, W., Hallgren, R., Greenman, P. 1995. Anatomic relation between the rectus capitis posterior minor muscle and the dura mater. *Spine* 20:2484–2486.

Hahn, H.J., Shim, J.C., Kim, K.H., Lee, K.E., Hwang, D.H., Lee, G.J., Kim, H.K. 2019. MRI findings of accessory popliteus muscle: A case report. *J Korean Soc Radiol* 80:574–578.

Haładaj, R. 2019. Normal anatomy and anomalies of the rectus extraocular muscles in human: A review of the recent data and findings. *Biomed Rest Int* (6):1–9.

Haładaj, R., Wysiadecki, G., Polguj, M., et al. 2018. Bilateral muscular slips between superior and inferior rectus muscles: Case report with discussion on classification of accessory rectus muscles within the orbit. *Surg Radiol Anat* 40:855–862.

Haładaj, R., Wysiadecki, G., Clarke, E., Polguj, M., Topol, M. 2019. Anatomical variations of the pectoralis major muscle: Notes on their impact on pectoral nerve innervation patterns and discussion on their clinical relevance. *Biomed Res Intl* 2019:6212039.

Haładaj. R., Wysiadecki, G., Tubbs, R., Topol, M. 2020a. Anatomical variations of the levator palpebrae superioris, including observations on its innervation and intramuscular nerves' distribution pattern. *Ann Anat* 228:151439.

Haładaj, R., Polguj, M., Tubbs, R. 2020b. Comparison of the superior and inferior rectus muscles in humans: An anatomical study with notes on morphology, anatomical variations, and intramuscular innervation patterns. *BioMed Res Int* 2020:9037693.

Haładaj, R., Tubbs, R., Brzezinski, P., Olewnik, Ł., Polguj, M. 2020c. Anatomical variations and innervation patterns of the superior oblique muscle. *Ann Anat* 230:151522.

Hall, B.K. 1984. Developmental mechanisms underlying the formation of atavisms. *Biol Rev* 59:89–124.

Hallett, C.H. 1848. An account of the anomalies of the muscular system met within the dissecting-room of the University during the years 1846–1847; with general remarks. *Edinburgh Med Surg J* 69:1–32.

Halliburton, W.D. 1881. Remarkable abnormality of the musculus biceps flexor cruris. *J Anat Physiol* 15:296–299.

Hallisy, J.E. 1930. The muscular variations in the human foot: A quantitative study. *Am J Anat* 45(3):411–442.

Hammad, R.B., Mohamed, A. 2006. Unilateral four-headed pectoralis muscle major. *McGill J Med* 9:28–30.

Hamming, J.J. 1959. Intermittent claudication at an early age, due to an anomalous course of the popliteal artery. *Angiology* 10(5):369–371.

Haninec, P., Tomás, R., Kaiser, R., Cihák, R. 2009. Development and clinical significance of the musculus dorsoepitrochlearis in men. *Clin Anat* 22:481–488.

Hanson, P., Magnusson, S.P., Sorensen, H., Simonsen, E.B. 1999. Anatomical differences in the psoas muscles in young black and white men. *J Anat* 194:303–307.

Harbeson, A.E. 1933. The origin of the first dorsal interosseous muscle of the foot. *J Anat* 68(Pt 1):116–118.

Harbeson, A.E. 1938. Further studies on the origin of the first dorsal interosseous muscle of the foot from the tendon of the peroneus longus. *J Anat* 72(Pt 3):463–464.

Harrison, R. 1848. *A Text-Book of Practical Anatomy*, ed. Watts, R., 61. New York: S.S. and W. Wood.

Harry, W., Bennett, J., Guha, S. 1997. Scalene muscles and the brachial plexus: Anatomical variations and their clinical significance. *Clin Anat* 10:250–252.

Hartz, C.R., Linscheid, R.L., Gramse, R.R., Daube, J.R. 1981. The pronator teres syndrome: Compressive neuropathy of the median nerve. *J Bone Joint Surg* 63(A):885–890.

Harvey, J.A., Call, Z., Peterson, K., Wisco, J.J. 2015. Weave pattern of accessory heads to the anterior digastric muscle. *Surg Radiol Anat* 37:1001–1004.

Hatipoğlu, E., Kervancioğlu, P., Tuncer, M. 2006. An unusual variation of the omohyoid muscle and review of literature. *Ann Anat* 188(5):469–72.

Hatzantonis, C., Agur, A.M.R., Naraghi, A., Gautier, S., McKee, N. 2011. Dissecting the accessory soleus muscle: A literature review, cadaveric study, and imaging study. *Clin Anat* 24(7):903–910.

Hecker, P. 1923. Study on the peroneus of the tarsus. *Anat Rec* 26:79–82.

Hecker, P. 1924. Etude sur le pèronier du tarse: Variations des pèroniers latèraux. *Arch Anat Histol Embryol* 3:327–359.

Heidsieck, D.S.P., Smarius, B.J.A., Oomen, K.P.Q., et al. 2016. The role of the tensor veli palatini muscle in the development of cleft palate-associated middle ear problems. *Clin Oral Invest* 20:1389–1401.

Heimkes, B., Posel, P., Bolkart, M. 1992. The transgluteal approaches to the hip. *Arch Orthop Trauma Surg* 111:220–223.

Helveston, E., Giangiacomo, J., Ellis, F. 1981. Congenital absence of the superior oblique tendon. *Trans Am Ophthalmol Soc.* 79:123–135.

Henle, J. 1858. *Handbuch der systematichen anatomie des menschen.* Brunswick: Druck und Verlag von Friedrich Vieweg und Sohn.

Henle J. 1871. *Handbuch der eingeweidelehre des menschen*, vol. 1. Braunschweig: Friedrich Vieweg und Sohn.

Heo, Y., Kim, J., Lee, J. 2020. Variation of the sternocleidomastoid muscle: A case report of three heads and an accessory head. *Surg Radiol Anat* 42:711–713.

Hepburn, D. 1892. The comparative anatomy of the muscles and nerves of the superior and inferior extremities of the anthropoid apes: I—myology of the superior extremity. *J Anat Physiol* 26:149–186.

Hernandez, J.A., Rius, M., Noonan, K.J. 1996. Snapping knee from anomalous biceps femoris tendon insertion: A case report. *Iowa Orthop J* 16:161–163.

Herring, S., Rowlatt, U., Pruzansky, S. 1979. Anatomical abnormalities in mandibulofacial dysostosis. *Am J Med Gen* 3(3):225–259.

Herzog, R.J. 2011. Accessory plantaris muscle: Anatomy and prevalence. *HSSJ* 7(1):52–56.

Hetherington, J. 1934. The kerato-cricoid muscle in the American white and negro. *Am J Phys Anthropol* 19:203–212.

Hildebrand, R. 1978. Discovery of a variant in the region of the adductor magnus and the short head of the biceps femoris. *Anat Anz* 144:48–50.

Hill, R.V., Gerges, L. 2008. Unusual accessory tendon connecting the hallucal extensors. *Anato Sci Int* 83:298–300.

Hinchliffe, J.R., Johnson, D.R. 1980. *The Development of the Vertebrate Limb: An Approach through Experiment, Genetics, and Evolution.* Cambridge: Oxford University Press.

Hirai, Y., Yoshida, K., Yamanaka, K., Inoue, A., Yamaki, K., Yoshizuka, M. 2001. An anatomic study of the extensor tendons of the human hand. *J Hand Surg Am* 26:1009–1015.

Hirasaki, E., Kumakura, H. 2010. Estimating the functional axis of the primate foot using the distribution of plantar muscles. *Int J Primatol* 31:239–261.

Hirasaki, E., Oishi, M. 2018. Arrangement of foot interosseous muscles in African great apes. *Am J Phys Anthropol* 167:924–929.

Hirasawa, T., Kuratani, S. 2015. Evolution of the vertebrate skeleton - morphology, embryology and development. *Zool Lett* 1:2.

Hirsch, B.E., Vekkos, L.E. 1984. Anomalous contrahentes muscles in human feet. *Anat Anz* 155:123–9.

Hoban, K.J, Holcomb, K.J., Holst, G., Ibezim, K.O., Sakthi-Velavan, S. 2019. Bilateral variant hamstring musculature with unilateral variant sciatic nerve. *Eur J Anat* 3:227–232.

Hodin, J. 2000. Plasticity and constraints in development and evolution. *J Exp Zool B Mol Dev Evol* 288:1–20.

Holibková, A., Machálek, L. 1999. A report on anomalies of digastric muscle. *Acta Univ Palacki Olomuc Fac Med* 142:57–59.

Hollinshead, H. 1956. *Anatomy for Surgeons, vol 2: The Thorax, Abdomen and Pelvis.* New York: Hoeber-Harper.

Holt, G., Nunn, T., Allen, R.A., Forrester, A.W., Gregori, A. 2008. Variation of the vastus medialis obliquus insertion and its relevance to minimally invasive total knee arthroplasty. *J Arthroplasty* 23:600–604.

Hong, M. K.Y., Hong, M.K.H. 2005. An uncommon form of the rare extensor carpi radialis accessorius. *Ann Anat - Anat Anz* 187:89–92.

Hongsmatip, P., Smitaman, E., Delgado, G., Resnick, D.L. 2019. Flexor carpi radialis brevis: A rare accessory muscle presenting as an intersection syndrome of the wrist. *Skel Radiol* 48:457–460.

Hoogbergen, M.M., Schuurman, A.H., Rijnders, W., Kon, M. 1996. Auricular hypermobility due to agenesis of the extrinsic muscles. *Plast Reconstr Surg* 98:869–871.

Hootnick, D.R., Packard Jr., D.S., Levinsohn, E.M., Cady, R.B. 1987. Soft tissue anomalies in a patient with congenital tibial aplasia and talo-calcaneal synchrondrosis. *Teratology* 36:153–162.

Hosokawa, H., Kamiya, T. 1961–1962. Anatomical sketches of visceral organs of the mountain gorilla (*Gorilla gorilla beringei*). *Primates* 3:1–28.

Hough, J.V.D. 1958. Malformations and anatomical variations seen in the middle ear during the operation for mobilization of the stapes. *Laryngoscope* 68:1337–1379.

Houston, W. 1831. Two newly discovered muscles for compressing the dorsal vein of the penis of man and other animals. *Am J Med Sci* 8:477–478.

Howe, L. 1923. Variations in the primary insertions of the ocular muscles. *Trans Am Ophthalmol Soc* 21:124.

Howe, B.M., Murthy, N.S. 2012. An accessory peroneocalcaneus internus muscle with MRI and US correlation. *J Radiol Case Rep* 6(10):20–25.

Howell, A.B., Straus, W.L. 1932. The brachial flexor muscles in primates. *Proc US Natl Mus* 80:1–31.

Howell, A.B., Straus, W.L. 1933. The muscular system. In *The Anatomy of the Rhesus Monkey (Macaca mulatta)*, ed. Hartman, C.G., Straus, W.L., 89–175. Baltimore: Williams & Wilkins.

Hoshino, T., Paparella, M. 1971. Middle Ear Muscle Anomalies. *Arch Otolaryng* 94:235–239.

Hoyte, L., Jakab, M., Warfield, S.K., Shott, S., Flesh, G., Fielding, J.R. 2004. Levator ani thickness variations in symptomatic and asymptomatic women using magnetic resonance-based 3-dimensional color mapping. *Am J Obst Gynecol* 191:856–861.

Hsiao, T.H., Chang, H.P. 2019. Anatomical variations in the digastric muscle. *Kaohsiung J Med Sci* 35:83–86.

Hu, K., Jin, G., Youn, K., Kwak, H., Koh, K., Fontaine, C., Kim, H. 2008. An anatomic study of the bifid zygomaticus major muscle. *J Craniofac Surg* 19:534–536.

Huber, E., Hughson, W. 1926. Experimental studies on the voluntary motor innervation of the facial musculature. *J Comp Neurol* 42:113–163.

Huber, K.M., Boyd, T.G., Quillo, A.R., Wilhelmi, B.J. 2012. Implications of anomalous pectoralis muscle in reconstructive breast surgery: The oblique pectoralis anterior. *Eplasty* 12:e44.

Humphry, G.M. 1873. Lectures on varieties in the muscles of man. *Br Med J* 2:33–37.

Hung, L.Y., Lucaciu, O.C., Wong, J.J. 2012. Back to the debate: Sternalis muscle. *Int J Morphol* 30:330–336.

Hunt, J.D. 2017. Bilateral pectoralis major and pectoralis quartus variants: A conjoined tendon passing through the intertubercular groove. *Int J Anat Var* 10(S1):88–90.

Huntington, G.S. 1904. The derivation and significance of certain supernumerary muscles of the pectoral region. *J Anat Physiol* 39:1–68.

Hur, M., Hu, K., Cho, J., et al. 2008. Topography and location of the depressor anguli oris muscle with a reference to the mental foramen. *Surg Radiol Anat* 30:403–407.

Hur, M., Hu, K., Park, J., Youn, K., Kim, H. 2010. New anatomical insight of the levator labii superioris alaeque nasi and the transverse part of the nasalis. *Surg Radiol Anat* 32:753–756.

Hur, M., Hu, K., Kwak, H., Lee, K., Kim, H. 2011a. Inferior bundle (Fourth Band) of the Buccinator and the incisivus labii inferioris muscle. *J Craniofac Surg* 22:289–292.

Hur, M.S., Kim, J.H., Woo, J.S., Choi, B.Y., Kim, H.J., Lee, K.S. 2011b. An anatomic study of the quadratus plantae in relation to tendinous slips of the flexor hallucis longus for gait analysis. *Clin Anat* 24:768–773.

Hur, M., Kim, H., Choi, B., Hu, K., Kim, H., Lee, K. 2013. Morphology of the mentalis muscle and its relationship with the orbicularis oris and incisivus labii inferioris muscles. *J Craniofac Surg* 24:602–604.

Hur, M., Kim, H., Lee, K. 2014. An anatomic study of the medial fibers of depressor anguli oris muscle passing deep to the depressor Labii Inferioris Muscle. *J Craniofac Surg* 25:614–616.

Hur, M.S., Won, H.S., Chung, I.H. 2015a. A new morphological classification for the fibularis quartus muscle. *Surg Radiol Anat* 37(1):27–32.

Hur, M., Kim, J., Gil, Y., Kim, H., Lee, K. 2015b. New insights into the origin of the lumbrical muscles of the foot: Tendinous slip of the flexor hallucis longus muscle. *Surg Radiol Anat* 37:1161–1167.

Hur, M. 2018. Anatomical features of the incisivus labii superioris muscle and its relationships with the upper mucolabial fold, labial glands, and modiolar area. *Sci Rep* 8:12879.

Hussaini, S.A., Deshmukh, A.G. 2018. Clinical assessment of absence of palmaris longus muscle in Marathwada region. *Indian J Anat* 7:115–119.

Hwang, K., Lee, D., Chung, I., Chung, R., Lee, S. 2002. Identity of "orbitozygomatic muscle". *J Craniofac Surg* 13(2):202–204.

Iamsaard, S., Thunyaharn, N., Chaisiwamongkol, K., Boonruangsri, P., Uabundit, N., Hipkaeo, W. 2012. Variant insertion of the teres major muscle. *Anat Cell Biol* 45:211–213.

Ikidag, M.A. 2019. Ectopic appendix vermiformis located in the right deep gluteal region due to unilateral piriformis agenesis. *Surg Radiol Anat* 41:141–142.

Ikiz, Z.A.A., Üçerler, H.A. 2005. Previously unreported variation related to the insertion of the tibialis anterior muscle and the superficial fibular (peroneal) nerve. *Anato Sci Int* 80:172–175.

Ingalls, N.W. 1913. Musculi sternales and infraclavicularis. *Anat Rec* 7:203–206.

Ingham, P., McGovern, S., Crompton, J. 1986. Congenital absence of the inferior rectus muscle. *Aust N Z J Ophthalmol* 14(4):355–358.

Inoue, R. 1934. Relationship among muscles, blood vessels and nerves of forearm in Japanese. *Acta Anat Nippon* 7:1155–1207.

Ilaslan, H., Wenger, D.E., Shives, T.C., Unni, K.K. 2003. Unilateral hypertrophy of tensor fascia lata: A soft tissue tumor simulator. *Skeletal Radiol* 32:628–632.

Ilayperuma, I. 2012. On the variations of the muscle flexor digitorum brevis: Anatomical insight. *Int J Morphol* 30:337–340.

Ishimi, S. 1950. Studies on the musculature of the upper extremities of the Japanese fetus. Report on the muscles of the brachium. *Igaku Kenkyu* 20:766–778.

Isomura, G. 1977. Nerve supply for anomalous ocular muscle in man. *Anatomischer Anzeiger* 142(3):255–265.

Ito J, Moriyama, H., Shimada, K. 2006. Morphological evaluation of the human facial muscles. *Okajimas Folia Anat Jpn* 83(1):7–14.

Itoh, K., Yokoyama, N., Ishihara, A., Kawai, S., Takada, S., Nishino, M., Lee, Y., Negishi, H., Itoh, H. 1991. Two cases of fetal akinesia/hypokinesia sequence. *Pediatr Pathol* 11(3):467–477.

Iwai, T., Sato, S., Yamada, T., Muraoka, Y., Sakurazawa, K., Kinoshita, H., Inoue, Y., Endo, M., Yoshida, T., Suzuki, S. 1987. Popliteal vein entrapment caused by the third head of the gastrocnemius muscle. *Brit J Surg* 74(11):1006–1008.

Iwanaga, J., Watanabe, K., Schmidt, C.K., et al. 2017. Anatomical study and comprehensive review of the incisivus labii superioris muscle: Application to lip and cosmetic surgery. *Cureus* 9(9):e1689.

Iwanaga, J., Watanabe, K., Kikuta, S., et al. 2021. Anatomical study of the incisivus labii superioris and inferioris muscles in non-human primates. *Anat Rec* 304:366–371.

Jackson, C.M. (ed.) 1921. *Morris's Human Anatomy. 6th edition.* Philadelphia, PA: P. Blakiston's Son & Company.

Jadhav, S.D., Gosavi, S.N., Zambare, B.R. 2013. Study of Peroneus digiti minimi quinti in Indian population: A cadaveric study. *Rev Arg de Anat Clin* 5(2):67–72.

Jaijesh, P., Shenoy, M., Anuradha, L., Chithralekha, K.K. 2005. A bilateral case of a long flexor accessorius muscle of the foot. *Eur J Anat* 9:157–160.

Jaijesh, P., Shenoy, M., Anuradha, L., Chithralekha, K.K. 2006. Flexor accessorius longus: A rare variation of the deep extrinsic digital flexors of the leg and its phylogenetic significance. *Indian J Plast Surg* 39:169–171.

Jain, A., Sikka, A., Goyal, N. 2013. Tibiofascialis anticus – a rare variation. *Indian J Med Case Rep* 2(2):8–10.

Jain, M., Shukla, L., Kaur, D. 2012. Extended insertion of teres minor muscle: A rare case report. *Eur J Anat* 16:224–225.

Jain, R.K., Mantri, N., Mandlecha, P. 2018. Variation of abductor pollicis longus tendons in cadavers. *Int J Res Orthop* 4:417–420.

Jan, S.V.S., Rooze, M. 1994. Anatomical variations of the intrinsic muscles of the thumb. *Anat Rec* 238:131–146.

Jana, R., Roy, T.S. 2011. Variant insertion of the fibularis tertius muscle is an evidence of the progressive evolutionary adaptation for the bipedal gait. *Clin Pract* 1(4):e81.

Janis, J.E., Ghavami, A., Lemmon, J.A., Leedy, J.E., Guyuron, B. 2007. Anatomy of the Corrugator supercilii muscle: Part I. Corrugator topography. *Plast Reconstr Surg* 120(6):1647–1653.

Janis, J.E., Ghavami, A., Lemmon, J.A., Leedy, J.E., Guyuron, B. 2008. The anatomy of the corrugator supercilii muscle: Part II. Supraorbital nerve branching patterns. *Plast Reconstr Surg* 121(1):233–240.

Jayakumari, S., Suri, R.K., Rath, G., Arora, J. 2006. Accessory tendon and tripartite insertion pattern of fibularis longus muscle. A case report. *Int J Morphol* 24:633–636.

Jazuta, K.M. 1931. Glutaeus medius accessories. *Anat Anz* 72:10–11.

Jelev, L., Georgiev, G., Surchev, L. 2001. The sternalis muscle in the Bulgarian population: Classification of sternales. *J Anat* 199:359–63.

Jelev, L., Shivarov, V., Surchev, L. 2005. Bilateral variations of the psoas major and the iliacus muscles and presence of an undescribed variant muscle-accessory iliopsoas muscle. *Ann Anat* 187:281–286.

Jelev, L., Hristov, S., Ovtscharoff, W. 2011. Variety of transversus thoracis muscle in relation to the internal thoracic artery: An autopsy study of 120 subjects. *J Cardiovasc Surg* 27:6–11.

Jelev, L., Landzhov, B. 2012–2013. A rare muscular variation: The third of the rhomboids. *Anatomy* 6–7:63–64.

Johnson, R.K., Shrewsbury, M.M. 1976. The pronator quadratus in motions and in stabilization of the radius and ulna at the distal radioulnar joint. *J Hand Surg* 1:205–209.

Jordan, J. 1971a. Studies on the structure of the organ of voice and vocalization in the chimpanzee, Part 1. *Folia Morphol* 30:99–117.

Jordan, J. 1971b. Studies on the structure of the organ of voice and vocalization in the chimpanzee, Part 2. *Folia Morphol* 30:222–248.

Jordan, J. 1971c. Studies on the structure of the organ of voice and vocalization in the chimpanzee, Part 3. *Folia Morphol* 30:323–340.

Joshi, S.D., Joshi, S.S., Athavale, S.A. 2006. Morphology of peroneus tertius muscle. *Clin Anat* 19(7):611–614.

Joshi, S.D., Waghmode, P.S., Joshi, S.S. 2007. Bilateral presence of muscle 'Stylochondrohyoideus' - A rare anomaly. *J Anat Soc India* 56:39–40.

Joshi, S.D., Joshi, S.S., Dandekar, U.K., Daini, S.R. 2010. Morphology of psoas minor and psoas accessorius. *J Anat Soc India* 59:31–34.

Jouffroy, F.K. 1971. Musculature des membres. In *Traité de Zoologie, XVI: 3 (Mammifères)*, ed. Grassé, P.P., 1–475. Paris: Masson et Cie.

Jovanovski, T., Umek, N., Cvetko, E. 2020. Transversus nuchae muscle fused with risorius muscle: A case report. *Int J Morphol* 38(5):1208–1211.

Jung, J., Kyang Ahn, H., Huh, Y. 2012. Clinical and functional anatomy of the urethral sphincter. *Int Neurourol J* 16:102–106.

Kafka, R.M., Aveytua, I.L., Fiacco, R.C., Ream, G.M., DiLandro, A.C., D'Antoni, A. 2016. Intrinsic muscles of the foot. In *Bergman's Comprehensive Encyclopedia of Human Anatomic Variation*, first edition, ed. Tubbs, R.S., Shoja, M.M., Loukas, M., 438. Hoboken, NJ: Wiley-Blackwell.

Kakizaki, H., Zako, M., Nakano, T. et al. 2006. An anomalous muscle linking superior and inferior rectus muscles in the orbit. *Anat Sci Int* 81:197–199.

Kale, S.S., Herrmann, G., Kalimuthu, R. 2006. Sternomastalis: A variant of the sternalis. *Ann Plast Surg* 56(3):340–341.

Kallner, M. 1956. Die muskulatur und die funktion des schultergurtels und der vorderextremitat des orang-utans. *Morphol Jahrb* 97:554–665.

Kalniev, M.A., Krastev, N.S., Krastev, D.S., Mileva, M.M. 2014. An unusual variation of an additional plantaris originating from the soleus. *Int J Anat Var* 7:93–95.

Kalpana, R., Usha, K. 2010. Three unilateral recti sternalis muscles – an unusual variation and its clinical significance. *Eur J Anat* 14:99–103.

Kamburoğlu, H.O., Boran, O.F., Sargon, M.F., Kecik, A. 2008. An unusual variation of deltoid muscle. *Int J Shoulder Surg* 2:62–63.

Kameda, Y. 1976. An anomalous muscle (accessory subscapularisteres-latissimus muscle) in the axilla penetrating the brachial plexus in man. *Acta Anat (Basel)* 96:513–533.

Kamibayashi, L.K., Richmond, F.J.R. 1998. Morphometry of human neck muscles. *Spine* 23:1314–1323.

Kampan, N., Tsutsumi, M., Okuda, I., et al. 2018. The malaris muscle: Its morphological significance for sustaining the intraorbital structures. *Anat Sci Int* 93:364–371.

Kaneff, A. 1979. Évolution morphologique des musculi extensores digitorum et abductor pollicis longus chez l'homme. I. Introduction, méthodologie, m. extensor digitorum. *Gegenbaurs Morphol Jahrb* 125:818–873.

Kaneff, A. 1980a. Évolution morphologique des musculi extensores digitorum et abductor pollicis longus chez l'homme. II. Évolution morphologique des m. extensor digiti minimi, abductor pollicis longus, extensor pollicis brevis et extensor pollicis longus chez l'homme. *Gegenbaurs Morphol Jahrb* 126:594–630.

Kaneff, A. 1980b. Évolution morphologique des musculi extensores digitorum et abductor pollicis longus chez l'homme. III. Évolution morphologique du m. extensor indicis chez l'homme, conclusion générale sur l'évolution morphologique des musculi extensores digitorum et abductor pollicis longus chez l'homme. *Gegenbaurs Morphol Jahrb* 126:774–815.

Kang, D.W., Byeon, Y., Yoon, S.P. 2015. An accessory belly of the sternothyroid muscle on the anterior neck. *Surg Radiol Anat* 37:215–217.

Kanthack, A.A. 1892. The myology of the larynx. *J Anat Physiol* 26(3):279–294.

Kaplan, E.B. 1965. *Functional and Surgical Anatomy of the Hand.* Second edition. Philadelphia, PA: JB Lippincott.

Kaplan, E.B. 1969. Muscular and tendinous variations of the flexor superficialis of the fifth finger of the hand. *Bull Hosp Joint Dis* 30:59–67.

Kaplan, K.M., Patel, A., Stein, D.A. 2008. Peroneal nerve compression secondary to an anomalous biceps femoris muscle in an adolescent athlete. *Am J Orthop (Belle Mead NJ)* 37(5):268–271.

Kasai, T., Chiba, S. 1977. True nature of the muscular arch of the axilla and its nerve supply. *Kaibogaku Zasshi* 52:309–336.

Katsuki, S., Terayama, H., Tanaka, R., Qu, N., Tanaka, O., Umemoto, K., Suyama, K., Sakabe, K. 2018. Variation in the origin of the long head of the biceps brachii tendon in a cadaver: a case report. *Medicine (Baltimore)* 97:e10708.

Kaur, D., Jain, M., Shukla, L. 2013. Six heads of origin of sternocleidomastoid muscle: A rare case. *Internet J Med Update* 8:62–64.

Kayikçioglu, A., Celik, H.H., Yilmaz, E. 1993. An anatomic variation of the deltoid muscle (case report). *Bull Assoc Anat (Nancy)* 77:15–16.

Kedzia, A., Walek, E., Podlesry, K., Dudek, K. 2011. Muscular sartorius metrology in the fetal period. *Adv Clin Exp Med* 20:567–574.

Keeling, J.W., Hansen, B.F., Kjær, I. 1997. Pattern of malformations in the axial skeleton in human trisomy 21 fetuses. *Am J Med Genet* 68:466–471.

Keith, A. 1894. Note on the supracostalis anterior. *J Anat Physiol* 28:333–334.

Kelch, W.G. 1813. Abweichung des biceps femoris. *Beiträge z pathol anatomie* 8:42.

Kelemen, G. 1943. Malformation involving external, middle and internal ear, with otosclerotic focus. *Arch Otolaryngol* 37:183–198.

Keyes, E.L. 1940. Demonstration of the nerve to the levator glandulae thyreoideae muscle. *Anat Rec* 77:293–295.

Khaledpour, C., Schindelmeiser, J. 1994. Atypical course of the rare accessory extensor carpi radialis muscle. *J Anat* 184:161–163.

Khalid, S., Iwanaga, J., Loukas, M., Tubbs, R.S. 2017. Split femoral nerve due to psoas tertius muscle: A review with other cases of variant muscles traversing the femoral nerve. *Cureus* 9:e1555.

Khan, M.M., Darwish, H.H., Zaher, W.A. 2008. Axillary arch: A rare variation. *Eur J Anat* 12:169–173.

Khan, A.S., Pilavakis, Y., Batty, V., et al. 2017. Eustachian tube communicating with sphenoid sinus: Report of a novel anatomical variant. *Surg Radiol Anat* 39:461–465.

Khizer Hussain Afroze, M., Yuvaraj, M., Veenapai, Lakshmi Prabha, S., Shivaleela, C. 2015. Study on sterno-costo-coracoidian (pectoralis minimus). *Res J Pharm Biol Chem Sci* 6:1087–1091.

Khona, P., Kulkarni, D.U., Kulkarni, U.K. 2017. A study of variations of anterior belly of digastric muscle. *Nat J Clin Anat* 6:101–104.

Kida, M.Y., Izumi, A., Tanaka, S. 2000. Sternalis muscle: Topic for debate. *Clin Anat* 13:138–40.

Kikuta, S., Iwanaga, J., Kusukawa, J., et al. 2019. Untreated incomplete isolated cleft palate: Cadaveric findings. *Anat Sci Int* 94:154–157.

Kikuta, S., Iwanaga, J., Watanabe, K., Kusukawa, J., Tubbs, R.S. 2020. Correction of the topographic relationship between the depressor septi nasi and incisivus labii superioris: Application to cosmetic surgery on the lip and nose. *Plast Reconstr Surg* 145:524e–529e.

Kiliç, C., Dergin, G., Yazar, F., Kurt, B., Kutoğlu, T., Ozan, H., Balcioğlu, H.A. 2010. Insertions of the lateral pterygoid muscle to the discecapsule complex of the temporomandibular joint and condyle. *Turk J Med Sci* 40:435e441.

Kim, B.S., Kim, S.H., Cho, S.S., Yoon, S.P. 2014. A rare muscular variation in the superficial region of the popliteal fossa. *Surg Radiol Anat* 36:721–723.

Kim, D.I., Kim, H.J., Park, J.Y., Lee, K.S. 2009a. Appearance of the cleidohyoideus muscle combined with the multiple variations of the infrahyoid muscle. *Korean J Anat* 42:65–67.

Kim, D., Kim, H., Shin, C., Lee, K.S. 2009b. An abnormal muscle in the superficial region of the popliteal fossa. *Anat Sci Int* 84:61–63.

Kim, D.I., Kim, H.J., Park, J.Y., Lee, K.S. 2010. Variation of the infrahyoid muscle: Duplicated omohyoid and appearance of the levator glandulae thyroideae muscles. *Yonsei Med J* 51(6):984–986.

Kim, H.J., Hu, K.S., Kang, M.K., Chung, I.H., Hwang, K. 2001. Decussation patterns of the platysma in Koreans. *Brit J Plast Surg* 54:400–402.

Kim, H.S., Pae, C., Bae, J.H., Hu, K.S., Chang, B.M., Tansatit, T., Kim, H.J. 2015a. An anatomical study of the risorius in Asians and its insertion at the modiolus. *Surg Radiol Anat* 37(2):147–151.

Kim, J.S., Hong, K.H., Hong, Y.T., Han, B.H. 2015b. Sternohyoid muscle syndrome. *Am J Otolaryngol* 36(2):190–194.

Kim, J., Lee, J. 2019. A unique case of an accessory sartorius muscle. *Surg Radiol Anat* 41:323–325.

Kim, Y.C., Yoo, W.K., Chung, I.H., Seo, J.S., Tanaka, S. 1997. Tendinous insertion of semimembranosus muscle into the lateral meniscus. *Surg Radiol Anat* 19:365–369.

Kim, Y.J., Lee, J.H. Baek, J.H. 2016. Variant course of extensor pollicis longus tendon in the second wrist extensor compartment. *Surg Radiol Anat* 38:497–499.

Kimura, K., Takahashi, Y. 1987. M. articularis genus. Observations on arrangement and consideration of function. *Surg Radiol Anat* 9:231–239.

King, R.L., Tucker, A.S., Persky, L. 1961. Congenital hypoplasia of the abdominal muscles and associated genitourinary tract abnormalities. *Radiol* 77:228–236.

Kinoshita, M., Okuda, R., Morikawa, J., Abe, M. 2003. Tarsal tunnel syndrome associated with an accessory muscle. *Foot Ankle Intl* 24(2):132–136.

Kirici, Y., Ozan, H. 1999. Double gluteus maximus muscle with associated variations in the gluteal region. *Surg Radiol Anat* 21:397–400.

Kirici, Y., Yazar, F., Ozan, H. 2000. The neurovascular and muscular anomalies of the gluteal region: An atypical pudendal nerve. *Surg Radiol Anat* 21:393–396.

Klaatsch, H. 1900. Der kurze kopf des musculus biceps femoris. Seine morphologische und stammgeschichtliche bedeutung. *Sitz Ber Akad Wiss* 1900:852–858.

Klasen, M., Hansmann, I., Schmid, M., Schmidtke, J. 1981. A female with XO/XY mosaicism and partial trisomy 9p. *J Med Genet* 18:482.

Knott, J.F. 1880. Muscular anomalies. *J Anat Physiol* 15:139–140.

Knott, J.F. 1883a. Abnormalities in human myology. *Proc Roy Irish Acad* 3:407–427.

Knott, J.F. 1883b. Muscular anomalies, including those of the diaphragm, and subdiaphragmatic regions of the human body. *Proc Roy Irish Acad* 3:627–641.

Kocabiyik, N. 2016. Orbital muscles. In *Bergman's Comprehensive Encyclopedia of Human Anatomic Variation*, first edition, ed. Tubbs, R.S., Shoja, M.M., Loukas, M., 207–211. Hoboken, NJ: Wiley-Blackwell.

Kodama, K. 1986. Morphological significance of the supracostal muscles, and the superficial intercostal nerve: A new definition. *Acta Anat Nippon* 61:107–129.

Kohda, E., Fujioka, M., Ikawa, H., Yokoyama, J. 1985. Congenital anorectal anomaly: CT evaluation. *Radiology* 157:349–352.

Kohlbrügge, J.H.F. 1890–1892. Versuch einer anatomie des genus *Hylobates*. In *Zoologische ergebnisse einer reise in niederländisch Ost-Indien*, ed. Weber, M., 211–354 (vol. 1), 138–208 (vol. 2). Leiden: E.J. Brill.

Koizumi, K. 1934. Studies on the shoulder and brachial muscle. *JNMS* 5:1063–1083.

Kolpattil, S., Harland, R., Temperley, D. 2009. Case report: A case of subclavius posticus muscle mimicking a mass on mammogram. *Clin Radiol* 64:738–740.

Koplas, M.C., Grooff, R., Piraino, D., Recht, M. 2009. Third head of the gastrocnemius: An MR imaging study based on 1039 consecutive knee examinations. *Skeletal Radiol* 38(4):349–354.

Kopuz, C., Tetik, S., Özbenli, S. 1999. A rare anomaly of the abductor digiti minimi muscle of the foot. *Cells Tissues Organs* 164:174–176.

Kopuz, C., Turgut, S., Kale, A., Aydin, M.E. 2006. Absence of both stapedius tendon and muscle. *Neurosciences* 11:112–114.

Koritzer, R. T., Suarez, F. 1980. Accessory medial pterygoid muscle. *Cells Tissues Organs* 107(4):467–473.

Kosugi, K., Fujishima, A., Koda, M., Tokudome, M. 1984. Anatomical study on the variation of the extensor muscles of the forearm. 2. m. extensor digitorum manus brevis. *Tokyo Jikekai Med J* 99:877–883.

Kotby, M.N., Kirchner, J.A., Kahane, J.C., Basiouny, S.E., El-Samaa, M. 1991. Histo-anatomical structure of the human laryngeal ventricle. *Acta Oto-laryngologica* 111(2):396–402.

Kotian, S.R., Sachin, K.S., Bhat, K.M.R. 2013. Bifurcated plantaris with rare relations to the neurovascular bundle in the popliteal fossa. *Anat Sci Int* 88:239–241.

Kotlarek, K.J., Perry, J.L., Fang, X. 2017. Morphology of the levator veli palatini muscle in adults with repaired cleft palate. *J Craniofac Surg* 28(3):833–837.

Krammer, E.B., Lischka, M.F., Gruber, H. 1979. Gross anatomy and evolutionary significance of the human peroneus III. *Anat Embryol* 155:291–302.

Krasny, A., Lutz, S., Gramsch, C., Diepenbruck, S., Schlamann, M. 2011. Accessory eye muscle in a young boy with external ophthalmoplegia. *Clint Anat* 24(8):948–949.

Krishnan, J.V., Brittain, J., Gabriel, J., Murphy, T., Reid, M.D., Shaw, V., Smith, C.F. 2017. The sternalis – more common than we believe? A cadaveric study. *J Anat* 231:463.

Kristensen, G., Nielsen, K., Blyme, P.J.H. 1989. Snapping knee from biceps femoris tendon. A case report. *Acta Orthop Scand* 60:621.

Kshirsagar, R., Gilde, J., Cruz, R. 2019. Duplicate omohyoid muscle causing progressive dysphagia and dyspnea: A case report. *Perm J* 23:18.316.

Kubota, H., Noguchi, Y., Urabe, K., Itokawa, T., Nakashima, Y., Iwamoto, Y. 2001. Flexor digitorum longus accessorius in the club foot of an infant with Nager syndrome. *Arch Orthop Trauma Surg* 121:95–96.

Kudo, K., Otobe, I. 1952. Statistics on the anatomy of Northern Chinese. The lateral abdominal muscles and others. *Hirosaki Igaku* 3:103–108.

Kuehn, D.P., Azzam, N.A. 1978. Anatomical characteristics of palatoglossus and the anterior faucial pillar. *Cleft Palate J* 15(4):349–359.

Kuiper, J.W.P., Nellensteijn, J.M., Burger, B.J. 2014. A painful swelling above the clavicle caused by a musculus levator claviculae. *Nederlands Mijdschrift voor Orthopaedie* 21(2):49–51.

Kulkarni, V., Ramesh, B.R., Prakash, B.S. 2014. Gantzer's muscle: A case report. *Dr. B.R. Ambedkar Intl J Med Sci* 1:10–13.

Kumar, H., Rath, G., Sharma, M., Kohli, M., Rani, B. 2003. Bilateral sternalis with unusual left-sided presentation: A clinical perspective. *Yonsei Med J* 44:719–722.

Kumar, S., Tiwary, S.K., Khanna, A.K. 2009. An accessory tongue. *Singapore Med J* 50(5):e172.

Kunc, V., Stulpa, M., Feigl, G., Kachlik, D. 2019. Accessory flexor carpi ulnaris muscle with associated anterior interosseous artery variation: Case report with the definition of a new type and review of concomitant variants. *Surg Radiol Anat* 41:1315–1318.

Kura, H., Luo, Z.P., Kitaoka, H.B., An, K.N. 1997. Quantitative analysis of the intrinsic muscles of the foot. *Anat Rec* 249(1):143–151.

Kutluk, A.C., Metin, M. 2017. Congenital chest wall deformities. *J Turk Spin Surg* 28:195–204.

Kwak, H., Kim, H., Youn, K., Park, H., Chung, I. 2003. An anatomic variation of the trapezius muscle in a Korean: The cleidooccipitalis cervicalis. *Yonsei Med J* 44(6):1098–1100.

Kwinter, D.M., Lagrew, J.P., Kretzer, J., Lawrence, C., Malik, D., Mater, M., Brueckner, J.K. 2010. Unilateral double plantaris muscle: A rare anatomical variation. *Int J Morphol* 28(4):1097–1099.

Kyung, D., Lee, J., Lee, Y., Kim, D., Choi, I. 2011. Bilateral variations of the head of the digastric muscle in Korean: A case report. *Anat Cell Biol* 44(3):241–243.

Labranche, L., Quinette, J., Hendryx, J.T., et al. 2017. Dissection of spinalis capitis and implications for osteopathic treatment. *Int J Anat Var* 10(4):73–74.

Laidlaw, P.P. 1902. A supraclavicularis proprius (Gruber). *J Anat Physiol* 36:417–418.

Lamb, C. 2016. Scapulohumeral muscles. In *Bergman's Comprehensive Encyclopedia of Human Anatomic Variation*, first edition, ed. Tubbs, R.S., Shoja, M.M., Loukas, M., 289–292. Hoboken, NJ: Wiley-Blackwell.

Lambert, H.W., Atsas, S. 2010. An anterior fibulocalcaneus muscle: An anomalous muscle discovered in the anterior compartment of the leg. *Clin Anat* 23(8):911–914.

Lambert, H.W., Atsas, S., Dayton, T.A. 2010. Discovery of a novel variant of the stylochondrohyoideus muscle. *Int J Anat Var* 3:197–199.

Lambert, H.W., Atsas, S., Fox, J.N. 2011a. The fibulocalcaneus (peroneocalcaneus) internus muscle of MacAlister: Clinical and surgical implications. *Clin Anat* 24:1000–1004.

Lambert, H.W., Atsas, S., Dodson, S.C., Daney, B.T., Billings, H.J., Campbell, F.R. 2011b. The anterior fibulocalcaneus muscle: Confirmation of its presence in the anterior leg compartment. *Clin Anat* 24(8):1029.

Lambert, H.W. 2016. Leg muscles. In *Bergman's Comprehensive Encyclopedia of Human Anatomic Variation*, first edition, ed. Tubbs, R.S., Shoja, M.M., Loukas, M., 421–437. Hoboken, NJ: Wiley-Blackwell.

Lamont, J.C. 1908. Note on a tendon found in association with the insertion of the peroneus longus, and origin of the first dorsal interosseous muscles. *J Anat Physiol* 42(Pt 2):236.

Langer, C. 1846. Zur anatomie des musculus latissimus dorsi. *Oester Med Wochenschrift* 15:454–458.

Larsson, S.G., Lufkin, R.B. 1987. Anomalies of digastric muscles: CT and MR demonstration. *J Comput Assist Tomogr* 11:422–425.

LaRue, B.G., Anctil, É.P. 2006. Distal anatomical relationship of the flexor hallucis longus and flexor digitorum longus tendons. *Foot Ankle Int* 27(7):528–532.

Last, R.J. 1950. The popliteus muscle and the lateral meniscus. *J Bone Joint Surg Br* 32(B):93–99.

Lauth, E.A. 1830. Varietes dans la distribution des muscles de l'homme. *Mem de la Soc d'Histoire Naturelle de Strasbourg* 1:65–69.

Lawrence, D.L., Bersu, E.T. 1984. An anatomical study of human otocephaly. *Teratology* 30:155–165.

Leal-Blanquet, J., Ginés-Cespedosa, A., Monllau, J.C. 2009. Bifurcated popliteus tendon: A descriptive arthroscopic study. *Int Orthop* 33(6):1633–1635.

Le Double, F. 1897. *Traité des variations du systéme musculaire de l'homme et de leur signification au point de vue de l'anthropologie zoologique, I et II*. Paris: Librairie C. Reinwald.

Lee, Y.H., Chun, S. 1991. Congenital absence of pectoralis major: A case report and isokinetic analysis of shoulder motion. *Yonsei Med J* 32:87–90.

Lee, J., Jung, W. 2015. A pair of atypical rhomboid muscles. *Korean J Phys Anthropol* 28:247–251.

Lee, S.C., Kim, U. 2009. Accessory medial rectus muscle in strabismus fixus convergens. *Eye (Lond)* 23:2119.

Lee, H.Y., Yang, H.J. 2016. Anterior neck muscles. In *Bergman's Comprehensive Encyclopedia of Human Anatomic Variation*, first edition, ed. Tubbs, R.S., Shoja, M.M., Loukas, M., 228–235. Hoboken, NJ: Wiley-Blackwell.

Lee, J.Y., Hur, M.S. 2017. The tendinous slip of the flexor digitorum longus for the great toe: An anatomic variation. *Korean J Phys Anthropol* 30(2):61–65.

Lee, D., Lee, S., Ahn, M. 2013. Congenital bilateral medial rectus muscle aplasia. *J Pediatr Ophthalmol Strabismus* 50:134–135.

Lee, S., Koh, K., Song, W. 2018. Oblique thyroarytenoid muscle in humans: An independent muscle or an accessory belly? *Laryngoscope* 128:1634–1638.

Lee, G.B., Kholinne, E., Kwak, J., Sun, Y., Alhazmi, A.M., Jeon, I. 2019a. Infraglenoid muscle as an anatomic variation of the anterior rotator cuff. *Case Rep Surg* 2019:6938252.

Lee, D.H., Lee, J.H., Woo, R.S., Song, D.Y., Baik, T.K., Yoo, H.I. 2019b. A rare bilateral variation on the dorsum of the hand: Extensor digitorum brevis manus and extensor medii proprius. *Anat Cell Biol* 52:97–99.

Legg, J.W. 1880. Enlargement of the temporal and masseter muscles on both sides. *Trans Pathol Soc Lond* 31:361–365.

Lehr, R.P. 1979. Musculus levator glandulae thyroideae: An observation. *Anat Anz* 146(5):494–496.

Lei, T., Cui, L., Zhang, Y., Shi, G., Peng, P., Wang, X., Xu, D., Gao, J. 2010. Anatomy of the transversus nuchae muscle and its relationship with the superficial musculoaponeurotic system. *Plast Reconstr Surg* 126:1058–1062.

Leon, X., Maranillo, E., Quer, M., Sañudo, J.R. 1995. Case report: Cleidocervical or levator claviculae muscle. A new embryological explanation as to its origin. *J Anat* 187:503–504.

Leppi, T.J. 1962. An anomalous infrahyoid muscle. *Yale J Biol Med* 34(5):522–523.

Levi, D. 1948. Anomalous insertion of the scalenus medius muscle with forearm pain. *Postgrad Med J* 24:259–260.

Levin, S.E., Trummer, M.J. 1973. Agenesis of the serratus anterior muscle: A cause of winged scapula. *JAMA* 225:748.

Levinton, J.S. 2001. *Genetics, Paleontology and Macroevolution.* New York: Cambridge University Press.

Lew, V.K., Gray, A.T. 2012. An unusual transversus abdominis plane block: Anatomic variation in the internal oblique muscle. *Anesthesiology* 119:1209.

Lewin, M.L., Croft, C.B., Shprintzen, R.J. 1980. Velopharyngeal insufficiency due to hypoplasia of the musculus uvulae and occult submucous cleft palate. *Plast Reconstr Surg* 65:585–591.

Lewis, O.J. 1962. The comparative morphology of m. flexor accessorius and the associated long flexor tendons. *J Anat* 96:321–333.

Lewis, O.J. 1964. The tibialis posterior tendon in the primate foot. *J Anat* 98(Pt2):209–218.

Lewis, O.J. 1966. The phylogeny of the cruropedal extensor musculature with special reference to the primates. *J Anat* 100:865–880.

Lewis, O.J. 1989. *Functional Morphology of the Evolving Hand and Foot.* Oxford: Clarendon Press.

Lewis, W.H. 1910. The development of the muscular system. In *Manual of Human Embryology*, vol. 1, ed. Keibel, F., Mall, F.P., 454–522. Philadelphia, PA: Lippin-cott.

Li, Y., Qiu, Q., Watson, S.S., Schweitzer, R., Johnson, R.L. 2010. Uncoupling skeletal and connective tissue patterning: Conditional deletion in cartilage progenitors reveals cell-autonomous requirements for Lmx1b in dorsal-ventral limb patterning. *Development* 137:1181–1188.

Liao, Y.J., Hwang, J.J. 2014. Accessory lateral rectus in a patient with normal ocular motor control. *Neuro-Ophthalmol* 34:153–154.

Lightoller, G.H. 1925. Facial muscles: The modiolus and muscles surrounding the rima oris with some remarks about the panniculus adiposus. *J Anat* 60(Pt 1):1–85.

Lightoller, G.S. 1928. The facial muscles of three orang utans and two cercopithecidae. *J Anat* 63:19–81.

Lim, T.A., Spanier, S.S., Kohut, R.I. 1979. Laryngeal clefts: A histopathologic study and review. *Ann Otol Rhinol Laryngol* 88(6):837–845.

Lima, G.V., Cabra, R.H., Andrade, D.L., Lacerda, N.S.O., Araujo, V.F., Masuko, T.S. 2012. An unusual anatomical variation of the levator scapulae muscle. *Int J Morphol* 30:866–869.

Lin, C. 1988. Contracture of the chondroepitrochlearis and the axillary arch muscles. *J Bone Joint Surg [Am]* 70:1404–1406.

Linburg, R.M., Comstock, B.E. 1979. Anomalous tendon slips from the flexor pollicis longus to the digitorum profundus. *J Hand Surg* 4:79–83.

Lindman, R., Paulin, G., Stål, P.S. 2001. Morphological characterization of the levator veli palatini muscle in children born with cleft palates. *Cleft Palate Craniofac J* 38(5):438–448.

Lindman, R., Stål, P.S. 2002. Abnormal palatopharyngeal muscle morphology in sleep-disordered breathing. *J Neurol Sci* 195(1):11–23.

Liquidato, B.M., Barros, M.D., Alves, A.L., Pereira, C.S.B. 2007. Anatomical study of the digastric muscle: Variations in the anterior belly. *Int J Morphol* 25(4):797–800.

Liu, H., Fletcher, J., Garrison, M.K., Holmes, C. 2011. Bilateral absence of quadratus femoris and semimembranosus. *Intl J Anat Var* 4:40–42.

Liu, H., Salem, Y. 2016. Pelvic diaphragm and external anal sphincter. In *Bergman's Comprehensive Encyclopedia of Human Anatomic Variation*, first edition, ed. Tubbs, R.S., Shoja, M.M., Loukas, M., 381–383. Hoboken, NJ: Wiley-Blackwell.

Liu, P.T., Moyer, A.C., Huettl, E.A., Fowl, R.J., Stone, W.M. 2005. Popliteal vascular entrapment syndrome caused by a rare anomalous slip of the lateral head of the gastrocnemius muscle. *Skeletal Radiol* 34:359–363.

Lobo, S.W., Menezes, R.G., Mamata, S., Baral, P., Hunnargi, S.A., Kanchan, T., Bodhe, A.V., Bhat, N.B. 2008. Phylogenetic variation in flexor digitorum brevis: A Nepalese cadaveric study. *Nepal Med Coll J* 10:230–232.

Lohrmann, S., Flöel, H., Christ, B. 1997. Insertion of musculus tibialis posterior into musculus peroneus (fibularis) longus. *Ann Anat* 179(2):161–163.

Lorentzon, R., Wirell, S. 1987. Anatomic variations of the accessory soleus muscle, *Acta Radiologica* 28(5):627–629.

Loth, E. 1912. *Beiträge zur anthropologie der negerweichteile (muskelsystem).* Stuttgart: Strecker Schroder.

Loth, E. 1931. *Anthropologie des parties molles (muscles, intestins, vaisseaux, nerfs peripheriques).* Paris: Mianowski-Masson et Crobie.

Lotito, G., Pruvost, J., Collado, H., et al. 2011. Peroneus quartus and functional ankle instability. *Ann Phys Rehabil Med* 54(5):282–292.

Loukas, M., Tubbs, R.S. 2007. An accessory muscle within the suboccipital triangle. *Clin Anat* 20:962–963.

Loukas, M., Bowers, M., Hullett, J. 2004. Sternalis muscle: A mystery still. *Folia Morphol (Warsz)* 63:147–149.

Loukas, M., Louis Jr., R.G., Merbs, W. 2006a. A case of atypical insertion of the levator scapulae. *Folia Morphol* 65:232–235.

Loukas, M., South, G., Louis Jr., R.G., Fogg, Q.A., Davis, T. 2006b. A case of an anomalous pectoralis major muscle. *Folia Morphol* 65:100–103.

Loukas, M., Louis Jr., R.G., South, G., Alsheik, E., Christopherson, C. 2006c. A case of an accessory brachialis muscle. *Clin Anat* 19:550–553.

Loukas, M., Merbs, W., Tubbs, R.S., Curry, B., Jordan, R. 2008a. Levator glandulae thyroideae muscle with three slips. *Anat Sci Int* 83(4):273–276.

Loukas, M., Sullivan, A., Tubbs, R.S., Shoja, M.M. 2008b. Levator claviculae: A case report and review of the literature. *Folia Morphol* 67:307–310.

Loukas, M., Louis Jr., R.G., Wartmann, C.T., Tubbs, R.S., Gupta, A.A., Apaydin, N., Jordan, R. 2008c. An anatomic investigation of the serratus posterior superior and serratus posterior inferior muscles. *Surg Radiol Anat* 30:119–123.

Low, S.C.S., Tan, S.C. 2010. Ectopic insertion of the pectoralis minor muscle with tendinosis as a cause of shoulder pain and clicking. *Clin Radiol* 65:254–256.

Lucas, D.E., Hyer, C.F., Berlet, G.C., Shockley, J.A. 2013. Anomalous peroneal tendon insertion masquerading as a retracted tendon tear: Case report. *Foot Ankle Int* 34(4):603–606.

Luck, M.D., Gordon, A.G., Blebea, J.S., Dalinka, M.K. 2008. High association between accessory soleus muscle and achilles tendonopathy. *Skeletal Radiol* 37:1129–1133.

Lundeen, R.O., Latva, D., Yant, J. 1983. The secondary tendinous slip of the extensor hallucis longus (extensor ossis metatarsi halluces). *J Foot Surg* 22:142–144.

Luschka, H.V. 1869. Die cartilage interarytenodea des menschlichen stimmorganes. *Arch Anat Physiol* 12:432–439.

Ma, L., Wang, G., Chen, R. 1999. Palatoglossus anomaly and speech disorder. *Int J Oral Maxillofac Surg* 28(suppl 1):90.

Macalister, A. 1866. Notes on muscular anomalies in human anatomy. *Proc Roy Irish Acad* 9:444–469.

Macalister, A. 1867a. Notes on an instance of irregularity in the muscles around the shoulder joint. *J Anat Physiol* 1:316–319.

Macalister, A. 1867b. Further notes on muscular anomalies in human anatomy, and their bearing upon homotypical myology. *P Roy Irish Acad* 10:121–164.

Macalister, A. 1871. On some points in the myology of the chimpanzee and others of the primates. *Ann Mag Nat Hist* 7:341–351.

Macalister, A. 1873. The muscular anatomy of the gorilla. *Proc Royal Irish Acad, Ser 2* 1:501–506.

Macalister, A. 1875. Additional observations on the muscular anomalies in the human anatomy. Third Series with a catalogue of principal muscular variations hitherto published. *Trans Royal Irish Acad Sci* 25:1–134.

MacDonald, K., Bridger, J., Cash, C., Parkin, I. 2007. Transverse humeral ligament: Does it exist? *Clin Anat* 20:663–667.

Macdonald Brown, J. 1880. Variations in myology. *J Anat Physiol* 14:512–513.

MacDowell, E.C. 1910. Notes on the myology of *Anthropopithecus niger* and *Papio-thoth ibeanus*. *Am J Anat* 10:431–460.

Machida, N. 1961. Studoj pri la double nervoprovizitaj muskoloj ĉe homa supra membro: La braka muskolo. *J NUMA* 20:7–16.

Neves, L.M.A., Curi, I. 2019. Increased restriction from an accessory lateral rectus in exotropic Duane syndrome. *J AAPOS* 23(3):174–176.

Mack, P.J. 1984. Sphenotemporalis: A new muscle in man. *J Anat* 139:587–591.

Mackinnon, S.E., Dellon, A.L (eds.). 1998. *Ulnar Nerve Entrapment at the Wrist. Surgery of the Peripheral Nerve.* New York: Thieme Medical Publishers.

Madhavi, C., Holla, S.J. 2003. Anomalous flexor digiti minimi brevis in Guyon's canal. *Clin J Anat* 16:340–343.

Malpas, P. 1926. Anomalies of the mylohyoid muscle. *J Anat* 61(Pt 1):64–67.

Manohar, K. 1939. Congenital absence of the right femur. *Brit J Surg* 27:158–161.

Manter, J.T. 1945. Variations of the interosseous muscles of the human foot. *Anat Rec* 93:117–124.

Maranillo, E., Sanudo, J. 2016. Laryngeal muscles. In *Bergman's Comprehensive Encyclopedia of Human Anatomic Variation*, first edition, ed. Tubbs, R.S., Shoja, M.M., Loukas, M., 254–261. Hoboken, NJ: Wiley-Blackwell.

Maranillo, E., Vázquez, T., Mirapeix, R., León, X., McHanwell, S., Quer, M., Sañudo, J.R. 2009. Ceratocricoid muscle: An embryological and anatomical study. *Clin Anat* 22(4):463–470.

Maranillo, E., Rodriguez-Niedenführ, M., Hernandez-Morato, I., Pascual-Font, A., Donat, E., McHanwell, S., Vázquez, T. 2011. The clinical interest of the ary-thyro-cricoid fascicle. *Clin Anat* 24(6):706–710.

Marques, E.F., Souza, J.A., Graziano, L., Bitencourt, A.G.V., Senaga, C., Fontes, C.E.M. 2009. Sternalis muscle simulating a breast nodule. *Rev Bras Ginecol Obstet* 31:492–495.

Martin, B.F. 1964. Observations on the muscles and tendons of the medial aspect of the sole of the foot. *J Anat* 98:437–453.

Martin, A. 1994. Spinalis capitis, or an accessory paraspinous muscle? *J Anat* 185:195–198.

Martinelli, B., Bernobi, S. 2002. Peroneus quartus muscle and ankle pain. *Foot Ankle Surg* 8:223–225.

Martinoli, C., Miguel Perez, M., Padua, L., Valle, M., Capaccio, E., Altafini, L., Michaud, J., Tagliafico, A. 2010. Muscle variants of the upper and lower limb (with anatomical correlation). *Semin Musculoskelet Radiol* 14:106–121.

Masada, K., Yasuda, M., Takeuchi, E., Mizusawa, K. 2003. Duplicate extensor tendons of the thumb mimicking rupture of the extensor pollicis longus tendon. *Scand J Plast Reconstr Surg Hand Surg* 37:18–19.

Masear, V.R., Hill Jr., J.J., Cohen, S.M. 1988. Ulnar compression neuropathy secondary to the anconeus epitrochlearis muscle. *J Hand Surg Am* 13:720–724.

Matsumae, G., Motomiya, M., Iwasaki, N. 2018. Failed reconstruction of the extensor pollicis longus in a patient with a major variation of the extensor indicis proprius tendon: A case report. *J Hand Surg (Asian-Pacific Vol)* 23:132–136.

Matsuo, T., Ohtsuki, H., Sogabe, Y., Konishi, H., Takenawa, K., Watanabe, Y. 1988. Vertical abnormal retinal correspondence in three patients with congenital absence of the superior oblique muscle. *Am J Ophthalmol* 106:341–345.

Matsuo, T., Watanabe, T., Furuse, T., Hasebe, S., Ohtsuki, H. 2009. Case report and literature review of inferior rectus muscle aplasia in 16 Japanese patients. *Strabismus* 17(2):66–74.

Matsune, S., Sando, I., Takahashi, H. 1991. Insertion of the tensor veli palatini muscle into the eustachian tube cartilage in cleft palate cases. *Ann Otol Rhinol Laryngol* 100(6):439–446.

May, C.A. 2020. Long abductor digiti minimi muscle: Variation of the hypothenar muscles and clinical consequences. *Clin Anat* 33:643–645.

Mazza, D., Marini, M., Impara, L., Cassetta, M., Scarpato, P., Barchetti, F., Di Paolo, C. 2009. Anatomic examination of the upper head of the lateral pterygoid muscle using magnetic resonance imaging and clinical data. *J Craniofac Surg* 20:1508–1511.

McCarthy, F.P. 1941. A clinical and pathologic study of oral disease: Based on 2,300 consecutive cases. *J Am Med Assoc* 116(1):16–21.

McFarlane, R.M., Classen, D.A., Porte, A.M., Botz, J.S. 1992. The anatomy and treatment of camptodactyly of the small finger. *J Hand Surg [Am]* 17:35–44.

McKenzie, J. 1955. The morphology of the sternomastoid and trapezius muscles. *J Anat* 89:526–531.

McKinley, L.M., Hamilton, L.R. 1976. Torticollis caused by absence of the right sternocleidomastoid muscle. *South Med J* 69:1099–1101.

McMurtry, J.G., Yahr, M.D. 1966. Extracranial carotid artery occlusion by an anomalous digastric muscle. *J Neurosurg* 24(1):108–110.

McVay, C.B., Anson, B.J. 1940. Composition of the rectus sheath. *Anat Rec* 77:213–225.

Mehta, V., Arora, J., Yadav, Y., Suri, R.K., Rath, G. 2010. Rectus thoracis bifurcalis: A new variant in the anterior chest wall musculature. *Rom J Morphol Embryol* 51:799–801.

Mehta, V., Suri, R.K., Arora, J., Dave, V., Rath, G. 2011a. Supernumerary peronei in the leg musculature-utility for reconstruction. *Chang Gung Med J* 34:62–65.

Mehta, V., Gupta, V., Arora, J., Kumar, A., Yadav, Y., Kumar Suri, R., Rath, G. 2011b. Clinico-anatomical revelation of a rare bilaminar constitution of the Geniohyoid muscle: Unique disposition of suprahyoid musculature. *Asian J Oral Maxillofacial Surg* 23:150–152.

Mellado, J.M., Rosenberg, Z.S., Beltran, J., Colon, E. 1997. The peroneocalcaneus internus muscle: MR imaging features. *Am J Roentgenol* 169:585–588.

Melling, M., Zweymüller, K. 1996. Musculus sartorius bicaudatus. *Acta Anat* 155:215–218.

Mérida Velasco, J.R., Rodríguez Vázquez, J.F., Arraez Aybar, L., Jiménez Collado, J. 1994. Study of pterygospinosus muscle in human fetuses. *Acta Anat* 151:14–19.

Mérida Velasco, J.R., Rodríguez-Vazquez, J.F., De La Cuadra Blanco, C., Sánchez-Montesinos, I., Mérida-Velasco, J.A. 2006. Origin of the styloglossus muscle in the human fetus. *J Anat* 208:649–653.

Mestdagh, H., Bailleul, P., Vilette, B., Bocquet, F., Depreux, R. 1985. Organization of the extensor complex of the digits. *Anat Clin* 7:49–53.

Michaelis, P. 1903. Beiträge zur vergleichenden myologie des *Cynocephalus babuin, Simia satyrus*, und *Troglodytes niger. Arch Anat Physiol Anat Abt* 1903:205–256.

Michilsens, F., Vereecke, E.E., D'Août, K., Aerts, P. 2009. Functional anatomy of the gibbon forelimb: Adaptations to a brachiating lifestyle. *J Anat* 215:335–354.

Michna, H. 1989. Anatomical anomaly of human digastric muscles. *Cells Tissues Organs* 134:263–264.

Mieden, G.D. 1982. An anatomical study of three cases of alobar holoprosencephaly. *Teratology* 26(2):123–133.

Miguel, M., Llusa, M., Ortiz, J.C., Porta, N., Lorente, M., Gotzens, V. 2001. The axillopectoral muscle (of Langer): Report of three cases. *Surg Radiol Anat* 23:341–343.

Miller, R.A. 1952. The musculature of *Pan paniscus. Am J Anat* 91:182–232.

Mitsuyasu, H., Yoshida, R., Shah, M., Patterson, R. M., Viegas, S.F. 2004. Unusual variant of the extensor carpi radialis brevis muscle: A case report. *Clin Anat* 17:61–63.

Miyauchi, R. 1976. Statistical observations on the musculi interspinales of the Japanese. *Okajimas Folia Anat Jpn* 53:231–244.

Miyauchi, R. 1982a. A case of the latissimus dorsi muscle with an accessory insertion into the first rib. *Acta Med Nagasaki* 27:21–29.

Miyauchi, R. 1982b. On the musculus supracostalis anterior. *Okajimas Folia Anat Jpn* 59:45–64.

Miyauchi, R., Kurihara, K., Tachibana, G. 1985. A case of tensor fasciae suralis muscle. *Acta Med Nagasaki* 30:285–288.

Miyauchi, R., Kurihara, K., Tachibana, G. 1986. On the human obliquus abdominis externus profundus. *Acta Med Nagasaki* 31:59–75.

Moen, D.W., Werner, J.K., Bersu, E.T. 1984. Analysis of gross anatomical variations in human triploidy. *Am J Med Gen* 18:345-356.

Moineau, G., Cikes, A., Trojani, C., Boileau, P. 2008. Ectopic insertion of the pectoralis minor: implication in the arthroscopic treatment of shoulder stiffness. *Knee Surg Sports Traumatol Arthrosc* 16:869–871.

Molina, C.R., Pinochet, J.A., Heras, A.A., Taunton, M.J., Letelier, R.G., Letelier, R.F. 2017. Prevalence of the sternalis muscle in Chilean population: A computed tomography study. *Ital J Anat Embryol* 122:173–178.

Molloy, A.P., Lyons, R., Bergin, D., Kearns, S.R. 2015. Flexor digitorum accessorius causing tarsal tunnel syndrome in a paediatric patient: A case report and review of the literature. *Foot Ankle Surg* 21(2):e48–e50.

Moncayo, V.M., Carpenter, W.A., Pierre-Jerome, C., Smitson, R.D., Terk, M.R. 2010. Congenital absence of the semimembranosus muscle: Case report. *Surg Radiol Anat* 32:519–523.

Monkhouse, W.S., Khalique, A. 1986. Variations in the composition of the human rectus sheath: A study of the anterior abdominal wall. *J Anat* 145:61–66.

Montet, X., Sandoz, A., Mauget, D., Martinoli, C., Bianchi, S. 2002. Sonographic and MRI appearance of tensor fasciae suralis muscle, an uncommon cause of popliteal swelling. *Skeletal Radiol* 31:536–538.

Montgomery, F., Miller, R. 1998. Hypertrophic extensor digitorum brevis muscles simulating pseudotumors: A case report. *Foot Ankle Int* 19(8):566–567.

Moore, A.T. 1922. An anomalous connection of the piriformis and biceps femoris muscles. *Anat Rec* 23:306–309.

Moore, C.W., Rice, C.L. 2018. Rare muscular variations identified in a single cadaveric upper limb: A four-headed biceps brachii and muscular elevator of the latissimus dorsi tendon. *Anat Sci Int* 93:311–316.

Mori, M. 1964. Statistics on the musculature of the Japanese. *Okajimas Folia Anat Jap* 40:195–300.

Morimoto, N. 2018. What could hominoid fetuses tell us about human evolution? *Anat Rec* 301:970–972.

Mortensen, O.A., Pettersen, J.C. 1966. The musculature. In *Morris' Human Anatomy*, 12th edition, ed. Anson, B.J., 421–611. New York: McGraw-Hill Book Co.

Moss, A.L.H. 1988. Is there an association between an absence of palmaris longus tendon and an absence of plantaris tendon? *Eur J Plast Surg* 11(1):32–34.

Mossallam, I., Nasser Kotby, M., Abd-el-Rahman, S., el-Samma, M. 1987. Attachment of some internal laryngeal muscles at the base of the arytenoid cartilage. *Acta Otolaryngol* 103:649–656.

Motabagani, M.A., Sonalla, A., Abdel-Meguid, E., Bakheit, M.A. 2004. Morphological study of the uncommon rectus sterni muscle in German cadavers. *East Afr Med J* 81:130–133.

Moyano, P.J., Capurro, M., Apa, S.N., Albanese, E.F. 2018. Subclavius posticus muscle with anomalous posterior insertion: Case report. *Int J Morphol* 36:22–25.

Mu, L., Sanders, I. 2008. The human cricothyroid muscle: Three muscle bellies and their innervation pattern. *J Voice* 23(1):21–28.

Muñoz, M. 1996. Congenital absence of the inferior rectus muscle. *Am J Ophthalmol* 121(3):327–329.

Murakami, S., Horiuchi, K., Yamamoto, C., Ohtsuka, A., Murakami, T. 2003. Absence of scalenus anterior muscle. *Acta Med Okayama* 57:159–161.

Murata, K., Tamai, M., Gupta, A. 2004. Anatomic study of variations of hypothenar muscles and arborization patterns of the ulnar nerve in the hand. *J Hand Surg* 29:500–509.

Murugan, M.S., Sudha, R., Bhargavan, R. 2016. Clinical significance of an unusual variation: Anomalous additional belly of the sternothyroid muscle. *Sultan Qaboos Univ Med J* 16(4):e491–e494.

Mustafa, A.Y.A.E., Mohammed, W.A., Alkushi, A.A.G., Sakran, A.M.E.A. 2017. Peroneus quartus muscle: Its incidence and clinical importance. *Int J Anat Res* 5(4.3):4691–4694.

Naidoo, L.C. 1996. Lateral pterygoid muscle and its relationship to the meniscus of the temporomandibular joint. *Oral Surg Oral Med Oral Pathol Oral Radiol Endod* 82(1):4–9.

Nair, V., Nair, R.V., Mookambika, R.V., Mohandas, Rao, K.G., Krishnaraja Somayaji, S. 2011. Persistent sacrococcygeus ventralis muscle in an adult human pelvic wall: A variation for surgeons to note. *J Chinese Med Ass* 74:567–569.

Nakahashi, T., Izumi, R. 1987. Anomalous interconnection between flexor and extensor carpi radialis brevis tendons. *Anat Rec* 218:94–97.

Nakajima, K., Nakamura, M. 2008. Rare case of myloglossus in Japanese cadaver: Anatomical and developmental considerations. *Anato Sci Int* 83:1.

Nakamura, E., Masumi, S., Muara, M., Kato, S., Miyauchi, R. 1992. A supernumerary muscle between the adductors brevis and minimus in humans. *Okajimas Folia Anat Jpn* 69:89–98.

Nakano, T. 1923. Beitrage zur anatomie der Chinesen. Die statistik der muskelvarietaten. *Folia Anat Jpn* 1:273–282.

Nakatani, T., Tanaka, S., Mizukami, S. 1998. Bilateral four-headed biceps brachii: The median nerve and brachial artery passing through a tunnel formed by a muscle slip from the accessory head. *Clin Anat* 11:209–212.

Nakayama, T., Okuda S. 1952. On the m. obliquus abdominis externus profundus. *Kaibogaku Zasshi* 27:89–94.

Naldaiz-Gastesi, N., Bahri, O.A., López de Munain, A., McCullagh, K.J., Izeta, A. 2018. The panniculus carnosus muscle: An evolutionary enigma at the intersection of distinct research fields. *J Anat* 233:275–288.

Namking, M., Mo-thong, W., Chaijaroonkhanarak, W., Khamanarong, K., Woraputtaporn, W. 2013. A rare variation of the posterior cord brachial plexus branching coexisting with the intercalated ectopic muscle. *Anat Sci Int* 88:115–117.

Nascimento, S.R.R., Costa, R.W., Ruiz, C.R., Wafae, N. 2012. Analysis on the incidence of the fibularis quartus muscle using magnetic resonance imaging. *Anat Res Int* 2012:485149.

Nascimento, S.R.R., Ruiz, C.R., 2018. A study on the prevalence of the anconeus epitrochlearis muscle by magnetic resonance imaging. *Rev Bras Ortop* 53:373–377.

Nathan, H., Gloobe, H. 1974. Flexor digitorum brevis: Anatomical variations. *Ann Anat* 135:295–301.

Nathan, H., Gloobe, H., Yosipovitch, Z. 1975 Flexor digitorum accessorius longus. *Clin Orthop Relat Res* 113:158–161.

Nathan, H., Luchansky, E. 1985. Sublingual gland herniation through the mylohyoid muscle. *Oral Surg Oral Med Oral Pathol.* 59(1):21–23.

Nathan, H. 1989. The pterygo-spinous muscle–an aberrant (atavic) remnant. *Anatomischer Anzeiger* 169(2):97–99.

Nation, H.L., Jeong, S.Y., Jeong, S.W., Occhialini, A.P. 2019. Anomalous muscles and nerves in the hand of a 94-year-old cadaver—A case report. *Int J Surg Case Rep* 65:119–123.

Natsis, K., Asouchidou, I., Vasileiou, M., Papathanasiou, E., Noussios, G., Paraskevas, G. 2009. A rare case of bilateral supernumerary heads of sternocleidomastoid muscle and its clinical impact. *Folia Morphol* 68(1):52–54.

Natsis, K., Vlasis, K., Totlis, T., Paraskevas, G., Noussios, G., Skandalakis, P., Koebke, J. 2010. Abnormal muscles that may affect axillary lymphadenectomy: Surgical anatomy. *Breast Cancer Res Treat* 120:77–82.

Natsis, K., Totlis, T., Sofidis, G. 2012. Chondroepitrochlearis: An abnormal muscle that may affect axillary lymphadenectomy. *Anz J Surg* 82:286–287.

Natsis, K., Totlis, T., Didagelos, M., Tsakotos, G., Vlassis, K., Skandalakis, P. 2013. Scalenus minimus muscle: Overestimated or not? An anatomical study. *Am Surg* 79:372–374.

Natsis, K., Totlis, T., Konstantindis, G.A., Paraskevas, G., Piagkou, M., Koebke, J. 2014. Anatomical variations between the sciatic nerve and the piriformis muscle: A contribution to surgical anatomy in piriformis syndrome. *Surg Radiol Anat* 36(3):273–280.

Natsis, K., Piagkou, M., Repousi, E., Apostolidis, S., Kotsiomitis, E., Apostolou, K., Skandalakis, P. 2016. Morphometric variability of pyramidalis muscle and its clinical significance. *Surg Radiol Anat* 38:285–292.

Natsis, K., Konstantinidis, G.A., Symeonidis, P.D., Totlis, T., Anastasopoulos, N., Stavrou, P. 2017. The accessory tendon of extensor hallucis longus muscle and its correlation to hallux valgus deformity: A cadaveric study. *Surg Radiol Anat* 39:1343–1347.

Nayak, G. 2017. A morphometric analysis of fibularis tertius muscle in Eastern Indian Population. *Intl J Anat Radiol Surg* 6(4): AO23–AO25.

Nayak, S.R., Krishnamurthy, A. 2007. An unusually large palmaris brevis muscle and its clinical significance. *Clin Anat* 20:978–979.

Nayak, S.R., Krishnamurthy, A., Madhan Kumar, S.J., Pai, M.M., Prabhu, L.V., Jetti, R. 2006. A rare case of bilateral sternocleidomastoid muscle variation. *Morphologie* 90:203–204.

Nayak, S.R., Madhan Kumar, S.J., Krishnamurthy, A., Prabhu, L.V., Vinod Ranade, A., Rai, R., Ramanathan, L. 2007. An additional radial wrist extensor and its clinical significance. *Ann Anat - Anat Anz* 189:283–286.

Nayak, S.R., Rai, R., Krishnamurthy, A., Prabhu, L.V., Potu, B.K. 2009a. An anomalous belly of sternothyroid muscle and its significance. *Rom J Morphol Embryol* 50(2):307–308.

Nayak, S.R., Hussein, M., Krishnamurthy, A., Mansur, D.I., Prabhu, L.V., D'Souza, P., Potu, B.K., Chettiar, G.K. 2009b. Variation and clinical significance of extensor pollicis brevis: A study in South Indian cadavers. *Chang Gung Med J* 32:600–604.

Nayak, S.R., Krishnamurthy, A., Ramanathan, L., Ranade, A.V., Prabhu, L.V., Jiji, P.J., Rai, R., Chettiar, G.K., Potu, B.K. 2010. Anatomy of plantaris muscle: A study in adult Indians. *La Clin Terapeutica* 161(3):249–252.

Nayak, S.R., Swamy, R., Krishnamurthy, A., Dasgupta, H. 2011. Bilateral anomaly of rectus capitis posterior muscles in the suboccipital triangle and its clinical implication. *La Clin Terapeutica* 162:355–356.

Nayak, V.S., Priya, A., Bhat, N., Nayak, S.S., D'Souza, A.S., Bangera, H., Sumalatha, S. 2016. Cadaveric study on morphology of dorsal interossei of hand and its anatomical variation. *J Clin Diagn Res* 10:AC04–AC06.

Nayak, S.B., Shetty, S.D., Kumar, N., et al. 2019. Double-bellied superior rectus muscle. *Surg Radiol Anat* 41:713–715.

Nayyar, A., Mehta, V., Gupta, V., Suri, R.K., Rath, G. 2010. Clinico-anatomical considerations of unilateral bipartite abductor digiti minimi muscle of the foot: A case report. *Anat* 4:72–75.

Nazarian, S., Tisserand, P., Brunet, C., Müller, M.E. 1987. Anatomic basis of the transgluteal approach to the hip. *Surg Radiol Anat* 9:27–35.

Nebot-Cegarra, J., Perez-Berruezo, J., Reina de la Torre, F. 1991–1992. Variations of the pronator teres muscle: Predispositional role to median nerve entrapment. *Arch Anat Histol Embryol* 74:35–45.

Nelimarkka, O., Lehto, M., Järvinen, M. 1988. Soleus muscle anomaly in a patient with exertion pain in the ankle. *Arch Orthop Trauma Surg* 107:120–121.

Nelson, M.L., Burkle, C., Ricardo, R., Shibao, S. 1992. Observation of the anterior supracostal muscles. *Anat Rec* 232:318–321.

Newell, R.L.M. 1991. An anomalous muscle crossing the supraclavicular triangle: The cleidotrachelian muscle. *Surg Radiol Anat* 13(3):231–233.

Newman, R.M., Cogen, M.S. 1997. Congenital absence of the superior oblique tendon in a patient with neurofibromatosis. *J Pediatr Ophthalmol Strabismus* 34(3):192–194.

Nguyen, M.S., Kheyfits, V., Giordano, B.D., Dieudonne, G., Monu, J.U.V. 2013. Hip anatomic variants that may mimic pathologic entities on MRI: Nonlabral variants. *Am J Roentgenol* 201:W401–W408.

Nicholson, H., Woodley, S., Flack, N. 2016. Gluteal muscles and lateral rotators of the hip. In *Bergman's Comprehensive Encyclopedia of Human Anatomic Variation*, first edition, ed. Tubbs, R.S., Shoja, M.M., Loukas, M., 386–409. Hoboken, NJ: Wiley-Blackwell.

Nievelstein, R.A.J., Vos, A., Valk, J. 1998. MR imaging of anorectal malformations and associated anomalies. *Eur Radiol* 8:573–581.

Niikura, H., Zin, Z.W., Cho, B.H., Murakami, G., Yaegashi, N., Lee, J.K., Li, C.A. 2010. Human fetal anatomy of the coccygeal attachments of the levator ani muscle. *Clin Anat* 23:566–574.

Nishi, S. 1966. Kelkaj muskolvarioj cirka u la kubutartiko. *Acta Anat Nippon* 41:246.

Novakov, S., Yotova, N., Fusova, A., Petleshkova, T., Timonov, P. 2012. Variable position of some structures in the neck. A case report. *Acta Morphol Et Anthropol* 19:153–159.

Nussbaum, M. 1893. Vergleichend-anatomische Beiträge zur Kenntnis der Augenmuskeln. *Anat Anz* 8:208–210.

Ochiltree, A.B. 1912. Some muscular anomalies in the lower limb. *J Anat Physiol* 47:31–34.

Odate, T., Kawai, M., Lio, K., Funayama, S., Futamata, H., Takeda, A. 2012. Anatomy of the levator claviculae, with an overview and a literature survey. *Anat Sci Int* 87:203–211.

Oelrich, T.M. 1983. The striated urogenital sphincter muscle in the female. *Anat Rec* 2015:223–232.

Ogata, S., Mine, K., Tamatsu, Y., Shimada, K. 2002. Morphological study of the human chondroglossus muscle in Japanese. *Ann Anat - Anat Anz* 184:493–499.

Ogura, T., Inoue, H., Tanabe, G. 1987. Anatomic and clinical studies of the extensor digitorum brevis manus. *J Hand Surg [Am]* 12:100–107.

Oh, C.S., Chung, I.H., Koh, K.S. 2000. Anatomical study of the accessory head of the flexor pollicis longus and the anterior interosseous nerve in Asians. *Clin Anat* 13:434–438.

O'Hara, J.J., Stone, J.H. 1988. Ulnar neuropathy at the wrist associated with aberrant flexor carpi ulnaris insertion. *J Hand Surg* 13:370–372.

Ohtsuka, H. 2005. Hypertrophy of the depressor septi nasi muscle. *Plast Reconstr Surg* 116:1817.

Oishi, M., Ogihara, N., Endo, H., Ichihara, N., Asari, M. 2009. Dimensions of forelimb muscles in orangutans and chimpanzees. *J Anat* 215:373–382.

Okamoto, K., Wakebe, T., Saiki, K., Nagashima, S. 2004. An anomalous muscle in the superficial region of the popliteal fossa, with special reference to its innervation and derivation. *Ann Anat* 186:555–559.

Okuda, S., Abe, S., Kim, H.J., Agematsu, H., Mitarashi, S., Tamatsu, Y., Ide, Y. 2008. Morphologic characteristics of palatopharyngeal muscle. *Dysphagia* 23(3):258–266.

Olewnik, Ł., Podgórski, M., Polguj, M., Wysiadecki, G., Topol, M. 2018a. Anatomical variations of the pronator teres muscle in a Central European population and its clinical significance. *Anat Sci Int* 93:299–306.

Olewnik, Ł., Wysiadecki, G., Podgórski, M., Polguj, M., Topol, M. 2018b. The plantaris muscle tendon and its relationship with the achilles tendinopathy. *BioMed Res Int* 2018:9623579.

Olewnik, Ł. 2019. Fibularis tertius: Anatomical study and review of the literature. *Clin Anat* 32:1082–1093.

Olewnik, Ł., Podgórski, M., Polguj, M., Topol, M. 2019a. A cadaveric and sonographic study of the morphology of the tibialis anterior tendon - A proposal for a new classification. *J Foot Ankle Res.* 12:9.

Olewnik, Ł., Podgórski, M., Ruzik, K., Polguj, M., Topol, M. 2019b. New classification of the distal attachment of the fibularis brevis — anatomical variations and potential clinical implications. *Foot Ankle Surg* 26:208–313.

O'Neill, M.N., Folan-Curran, J. 1998. Case report: Bilateral sternalis muscles with a bilateral pectoralis major anomaly. *J Anat* 193:289–292.

Opdam, K.T., van Dijk, P.A., Stufkens, S.A., van Dijk, C.N. 2017. The peroneus quartus muscle in a locking phenomenon of the ankle: A case report. *J Foot Ankle Surg* 56(1):108–111.

Orthaber, S., Pritsch, A., Zach, A.J.L., Feigl, G.C. 2020. Gluteus medius accessorius and gluteus quartus scansorius in one specimen: Case report of two rare variations. *Eur J Anat* 24:161–163.

Ortega, M., Doll, J.E., Pascoe, P.A. 2013. Duplication of the gemellus superior and misplacement of gemelli-obturator internus complex. *Int J Anat Var* 6:182–183.

Ortug, G., Sipahi, B., Ortug, A., Ipsalali, H.O. 2020. Variations of the digastric muscle and accessory bellies - a study of gross anatomic dissections. *Morphologie* 104(345):125–132.

O'Sullivan, E., Carare-Nnadi, R., Greenslade, J., Bowyer, G. 2005. Clinical significance of variations in the interconnections between flexor digitorum longus and flexor hallucis longus in the region of the knot of Henry. *Clin Anat* 18(2):121–125.

Otto, A.W. 1830. *Lehrbuch der pathologisches anatomie des menschen und der thiere*, first edition. Berlin: A Rücher.

Ottone, N.E., Medan, C. 2009. A rare muscle anomaly: The supraclavicularis proprius muscle. *Folia Morphol* 68:55–57.

Oukouchi, H., Murakami, T., Kikuta, A. 1992. Insertions of the lumbrical and interosseous muscles in the human foot. *Okajimas Folia Anat Jpn* 69(2–3):77–83.

Owen, R. 1868. *The Anatomy of Vertebrates, vol. 3: Mammals*. London: Longmans, Green and Co.

Ozgur, Z., Govsa, F., Ozgur, T. 2007. Bilateral quadrification of the anterior digastric muscles With variations of the median accessory digastric muscles. *J Craniofac Surg* 18(4):773–775.

Ozgur, Z., Govsa, F., Celik, S., Ozgur, T. 2010. An unreported anatomical finding: Unusual insertions of the stylohyoid and digastric muscles. *Surg Radiol Anat* 32:513–517.

Ozgursoy, O.B., Kucuk, B. 2006. Unique variation of digastric muscle: A confusing landmark for head and neck surgeons. *Acta Otolaryngol* 126(8):881–883.

Pác, L., Malinovský Jr., L., 1985. M. flexor digitorum longus accessorius in the lower limb of man. *Anat Anz* 159(1–5):253–257.

Pacífico, F.A., Filho, G.C.S., Marinho, A.J.P., et al. 2019. A variant topography of levator glandulae thyroideae: A case report. *Int J Anat Var* 12:10–11.

Pai, M.M., Nayak, S.R., Vadgaonkar, R., Ranade, A.V., Prabhu, L.V., Thomas, M., Sugavasi, R. 2008a. Accessory brachialis muscle: A case report. *Morphologie* 92:47–49.

Pai, M.M., Nayak, S.R., Krishnamurthy, A., Vadgaonkar, R., Prabhu, L.V., Ranade, A.V., Janardhan, J.P., Rai, R. 2008b. The accessory heads of flexor pollicis longus and flexor digitorum profundus: Incidence and morphology. *Clin Anat* 21:252–258.

Paik, D.J., Shin, S.Y. 2009. An anatomical study of the inferior oblique muscle: The embalmed cadaver vs the fresh cadaver. *Am J Ophthalmol* 147(3):544–549.e1.

Palagama, S.P., Tedman, R.A., Barton, M.J., Forwood, M.R. 2016. Bilateral chondroepitrochlearis muscle: Case report, phylogenetic analysis, and clinical significance. *Anat Res Int* 2016:5402081.

Palatty, B.U., Veeramani, R., Manjunath, K.Y. 2018. Variations in extensor tendons of the thumb—a cadaveric study. *Ind J Clin Anat Phys* 5:383–388.

Palomo-López, P., Losa-Iglesias, M.E., Calvo-Lobo, C., Rodríguez-Sanz, D., Navarro-Flores, E., et al. 2019. Fibularis tertius muscle in women & men: A surface anatomy cross-sectional study across countries. *PLOS One* 14(4):e0215118.

Pandey, V., Madi, S., Maddukuri, S., Deepika, N., Hafiz, N., Acharya, K. 2016. A case of bilateral aberrant pectoralis minor insertion with absent coracohumeral ligament: Clinical relevance and controversies. *J Clin Orthop Trauma* 7(Suppl 1):76–79.

Paraskevas, G., Papaziogas, B., Spanidou, S., Papadopoulos, A. 2002. Unusual variation of the extensor digitorum brevis manus: A case report. *Eur J Orthop Surg Traumatol* 12:158–160.

Paraskevas, G., Ioannidis, O., Papaziogas, B., Natsis, K., Spanidou, S., Kitsoulis, P. 2007. An accessory middle scalene muscle causing thoracic outlet syndrome. *Folia Morphol (Warsz)* 66:194–197.

Paraskevas, G.K., Raikos, A., Ioannidis, O. 2010. Supernumerary semitendinosus muscle: A rare case presentation and its clinical significance. *Clin Anat* 23(8):909–910.

Paraskevas, G.K., Natsis, K., Ioannidis, O. 2013. Accessory cleido-occipitalis muscle: Case report and review of the literature. *Rom J Morphol Embryol* 54(3 Suppl):893–895.

Paraskevas, G., Koutsouflianiotis, K., Iliou, K., Bitsis, T., Kitsoulis, P. 2016. Accessory coracobrachialis muscle with two bellies and abnormal insertion – case report. *Acta Med Acad* 45:163–168.

Paria, P., Roy, S., Gayen, S., Mondal, P.C., Biswas, P., Ghosh, S. 2015. Congenital absence of ribs: A rare association in infant of diabetic mother. *Int J Res Med Sci* 3:3416–3419.

Park, C.Y., Oh, S.Y. 2003. Accessory lateral rectus muscle in a patient with congenital third-nerve palsy. *Am J Ophthalmol* 136(2):355–356.

Park, S.W., Heo, H., Park, Y.G. 2009a. Brown syndrome with bifid scleral insertion of the superior oblique. *J Pediatr Ophthalmol Strabismus* 46(3):171–172.

Park, S.W., Kim, H.G., Heo, H., Park, Y.G. 2009b. Anomalous scleral insertion of superior oblique in Axenfeld-Rieger syndrome. *Korean J Ophthalmol* 23(1):62–64.

Park, J., Youn, K., Hur, M., Hu, K., Kim, H., Kim, H. 2011. Malaris muscle, the lateral muscular band of orbicularis oculi muscle. *J Craniofac Surg* 22:659–662.

Park, J., Youn, K., Lee, J., Kwak, H., Hu, K., Kim, H. 2012. Medial muscular band of the orbicularis oculi muscle. *J Craniofac Surg* 23(1):195–197.

Parsons, F.G. 1898a. The muscles of mammals, with special relation to human myology. *J Anat* 32:428–450.

Parsons, F.G. 1898b. The muscles of mammals, with special relation to human myology: A course of lectures delivered at the Royal College of Surgeons of England - lecture II, the muscles of the shoulder and forelimb. *J Anat Physiol* 32:721–752.

Parsons, F.G. 1919–1920. Note an abnormal muscle in popliteal space. *J Anat Physiol* 54:170.

Pasick, C., McDonald-McGinn, D.M., Simbolon, C., Low, D., Zackai, E., Jackson, O. 2013. Asymmetric crying facies in the 22q11.2 deletion syndrome: Implications for future screening. *Clin Pediatr* 52(12):1144–1148.

Patel, M.R., Desai, S.S., Bassini-Lipson, L., Namba, T., Sahoo, J. 1989. Painful extensor digitorum brevis manus muscle. *J Hand Surg* 14:674–678.

Patel, S., Loukas, M. 2016. Soft palate and tongue muscles. In *Bergman's Comprehensive Encyclopedia of Human Anatomic Variation*, first edition, ed. Tubbs, R.S., Shoja, M.M., Loukas, M., 240–244. Hoboken, NJ: Wiley-Blackwell.

Patil, V., Frisch, N.C., Ebraheim, N.A. 2007. Anatomical variations in the insertion of the peroneus (fibularis) longus tendon. *Foot Ankle Int* 28:1179–1182.

Patten, C.J. 1935. Proceedings of the anatomical society of Great Britain and Ireland. *J Anat* 69:147.

Paul, S., Das, S. 2007. Variant abductor pollicis longus muscle: A case report. *Acta Medica (Hradec Kralove)* 50:213–215.

Peddity, S., Velichety, S.D. 2013. Bilateral variations in tendons of dorsum or foot. *Int J Anat Res* 3:132–35.

Peikert, K., Platzek, I., Bessède, T., Albrecht May, C. 2015. The male bulbospongiosus muscle and its relation to the external anal sphincter. *J Urol* 193:1433–1440.

Peker, T., Turgut, H.B., Anil, A. 2000. Bilateral anomaly of anterior bellies of digastric muscles. *Surg Radiol Anat* 22:119–21.

Pellatt, A. 1979. The facial muscles of three African primates contrasted with those of *Papio ursinus*. *S Afr J Sci* 75:436–440.

Penhall, B., Townsend, G., Tomo, S., Nakajima, K. 1998. The pterygoideus proprius muscle revisited. *Clin Anat* 11:332–337.

Percy, E.C., Telep, G.N. 1984. Anomalous muscle in the leg: Soleus accessorium. *Am J Spor Med* 12(6):447–450.

Pérez, J., Pérez-Gumá, J.E., Correa, R., Rivera, M., Castro, A., Cedeño, J., López, M., Nazario, L., Otero, K, Quiles, J., et al. 2008. Breast mass or sternalis muscle? *PR Health Sci J* 27:185.

Perez Carro, L., Sumillera Garcia, M., Gracia, C.S. 1999. Bifurcate popliteus tendon. *Arthroscopy* 15(6):638–639.

Perkins, J.D. 1914. An anomalous muscle of the leg: Peronaeocalcaneus internus. *Anat Rec* 8:21–25.

Perkins, R.E., Hast, M.H. 1993. Common variations in muscles and tendons of the human hand. *Clin Anat* 6:226–331.

Perry, J.L., Chen, J.Y., Kotlarek, K.J., Haenssler, A., Sutton, B.P., Kuehn, D.P., Sitzman, T.J., Fang, X. 2019. Morphology of the musculus uvulae in vivo using MRI and 3D modeling among adults with normal anatomy and preliminary comparisons to cleft palate anatomy. *Cleft Palate Craniofac J* 56(8):993–1000.

Perry, J.L., Kotlarek, K.J., Spoloric, K., Baylis, A., Kollara, L., Grischkan, J.M., Kirschner, R., Bates, D.G., Smith, M., Findlen, U. 2020. Differences in the tensor veli palatini muscle and hearing status in children with and without 22q11.2 deletion syndrome. *Cleft Palate Craniofac J* 57(3):302–309.

Perumal, A., Shanthi, K.C., Srinivasan, K.R. 2018. Scalenus anterior muscle with two heads associated with variation in the branches of subclavian artery: A rare presentation. *Int J Anat Res* 6:4939–4942.

Pessa, J.E., Zadoo, V.P., Adrian, E.K., Yuan, C.H., Aydelotte, J., Garza, J.R. 1998. Variability of the midfacial muscles: Analysis of 50 hemifacial cadaver dissections. *Plast Reconstr Surg* 102:1888–1893.

Peterson, D.A., Stinson, W., Lairmore, J.R. 1995. The long accessory flexor muscle: An anatomical study. *Foot Ankle Int* 16(10):637–640.

Petleshkova, P., Krasteva, M., Gencheva, D., Anesteva Ivanova, N., Grozdanova, L., Parahuleva, N., Mihaylova, A. 2019.

Poland syndrome: Two cases of new-borns with left-sided chest defect and dextrocardia. *Biomed Res* 30:362–365.

Pettersen, J.C. 1979. Anatomical studies of a boy trisomic for the distal portion of 13q. *Am J Med Gen* 4:383–400.

Pettersen, J.C., Koltis, G.G., White, M.G. 1979. An examination of the spectrum of anatomic defects and variations found in eight cases of Trisomy 13. *Am J Med Gen* 3:183–210.

Pettersen, J.C. 1984. Gross anatomical studies of a newborn infant with the Meckel syndrome. *Am J Med Gen* 18:649–659.

Phan, K., Onggo, J. 2019. Prevalence of bifid zygomaticus major muscle. *J Craniofac Surg* 30:758–760.

Philippon, M.J., Devitt, B.M., Campbell, K.J., Michalski, M.P., Espinoza, C., Wijdicks, C.A., Laprade, R.F. 2014. Anatomic variance of the iliopsoas tendon. *Am J Sports Med* 42:807–811.

Piagkou, M., Totlis, T., Anastasopoulos, N., Lazaridis, N., Natsis, K. 2019. An atypical biceps brachii and coracobrachialis muscles associated with multiple neurovascular aberrations: A case report with clinical significance. *Folia Morphol* 78:444–449.

Pınar, Y., Gövsa, F., Bilge, O., Celik, S. 2012. Accessory tendon slip arising from the extensor carpi ulnaris and its importance for wrist pain. *Acta Orthop Traumatol Turc* 46:132–135.

Pinchoff, B.S., Sandall, G. 1985. Congenital absence of the superior oblique tendon in craniofacial dysostosis. *Ophthalmic Surg* 16(6):375–377.

Pine, J., Binns, M., Wright, P., Soames, R. 2011. Piriformis and obturator internus morphology: A cadaveric study. *Clin Anat* 24:70–76.

Pineles, S.L., Velez, F.G. 2015. Accessory fibrotic lateral rectus muscles in exotropic Duane syndrome with severe retraction and upshoot. *J AAPOS* 19:549–550.e1

Pira, A. 1913. Beiträge zür anatomie des gorilla, I, das extremitätenmuskelsystem. *Morphol Jahrb* 47:309–354.

Pirani, S., Beauchamp, R.D., Li, D., Sawatzky, B. 1991. Soft tissue anatomy of proximal femoral focal deficiency. *J Pediatr Ortho* 11:563–570.

Pires, L.A.S., Souza, C.F.C., Teixeira, A.R., Leite, T.F.O., Babinski, M.A., Chagas, C.A.A. 2017. Accessory subscapularis muscle - a forgotten variation? *Morphologie* 101:101–104.

Plaass, C., Abuharbid, G., Waizy, H., Ochs, M., Stukenborg-Colsman, C., Schmiedl, A. 2013. Anatomical variations of the flexor hallucis longus and flexor digitorum longus in the chiasma plantare. *Foot Ankle Int* 34(11):1580–1587.

Playfair McMurrich, J. 1906. The phylogeny of the plantar musculature. *Am J Anat* 6:407–437.

Plochocki, J.H., Bodeen M. 2010. Unusual supernumerary muscle in the anterior compartment of the leg. *Clin Anat* 23(1):104–105.

Plock, J., Contaldo, C., von Ludin-Ghausen, M. 2005. Levator palpebrae superioris muscle in human fetuses: Anatomical findings and their clinical relevance. *Clin Anat* 18:473–480.

Plock, J., Contaldo, C., Von Lüdinghausen, M. 2007. Extraocular eye muscles in human fetuses with craniofacial malformations: Anatomical findings and clinical relevance. *Clin Anat* 20(3):239–245.

Poland, J. 1890. Variations of the external pterygoid muscle. *J Anat Physiol* 24:567–572.

Pollard, Z.F. 1988. Bilateral superior oblique muscle palsy associated with Apert's syndrome. *Am J Ophthalmol* 106:337–340.

Polster, J.M., Elgabaly, M., Lee, H., Klika, A., Drake, R., Barsoum, W. 2008. MRI and gross anatomy of the iliopsoas tendon complex. *Skel Radiol* 37:55–58.

Pompei Filho, H., Guimaraes, A.S., Suazo, G.I.C. 2009. Prevalence of the third head of the lateral pterygoid muscle a magnetic resonance image study. *Int J Morphol* 27(4):1043–1046.

Pontell, M.E., Scali, F., Marshall, E., Enix, D. 2013. The obliquus capitis inferior myodural bridge. *Clin Anat* 26:450–454.

Porter, R.W. 1996. An anomalous muscle in children with congenital talipes. *Clin Anat* 9(1):25–27.

Posey, W.C. 1923. Concerning some gross structural anomalies of eye and its adnexa. *Trans Amer Acad Ophthal* 28:243–257.

Potau, J.M., Arias-Martorell, J., Bello-Hellegouarch, G., Casado, A., Pastor, J.F., de Paz, F., Diogo, R. 2018. Inter- and intraspecific variations in the pectoral muscles of common chimpanzees (*Pan troglodytes*), bonobos (*Pan paniscus*), and humans (*Homo sapiens*). *BioMed Res Int* 2018:9404508.

Potu, B.K., Kumar, V., Annam, S., Salem, A.H., Abu-Hijleh, M. 2016. Prevalence of fibularis tertius muscle in Southeastern Indian population: A surface anatomical study. *Eur J Gen Med* 13:27–30.

Poveda, C.A., Muñoz, E.J., Camargo, D.C. 2013. Músculo esternalis: Variante anatómica que simula neoplasia en mamografía. *Rev Colomb Cancerol* 17:46–49.

Prabhu, L.V., Asif, M., Murlimanju, B.V., Anup Rao, K., Shivaprakash, S. 2012. Anomalous fascicle of triceps brachii muscle and its clinical importance in relation to radial nerve entrapment. *Clin Ter* 163:123–124.

Prakash, P., Nayak, B.K., Menon, V. 1983. Abnormal insertion of inferior oblique. *Indian J Ophthalmol* 31(1):21–22.

Prakash, Narayanswamy, C., Singh, D.K., Rajini, T., Venkatiah, J., Singh, G. 2011. Anatomical variations of peroneal muscles: A cadaver study in an Indian population and a review of the literature. *J Am Podiatr Med Assoc* 101(6):505–508.

Prasad, A.M., Nayak, B.S., Deepthinath, R., Vallala, V.R., Bhat, S. 2005. Clinically important variations in the lower limb: A case report. *Eur J Anat* 9:167–169.

Pretterklieber, B. 2017. The high variability of the chiasma plantare and the long flexor tendons: Anatomical aspects of tendon transfer in foot surgery. *Ann Anat - Anat Anz* 211:21–32.

Pretterklieber, B. 2018. Morphological characteristics and variations of the human quadratus plantae muscle. *Ann Anat* 216:9–22.

Preuschoft, H. 1965. Muskeln und gelenk der vorderextremitat des gorillas. *Morphol Jahrb* 107:99–183.

Pribyl, C.R., Moneim, M.S. 1994. Anomalous hand muscle found in the Guyon's canal at exploration for ulnar artery thrombosis. A case report. *Clin Orthop Relat Res* 306:120–123.

Primrose, A. 1899. The anatomy of the orang-outang (*Simia satyrus*), an account of some of its external characteristics, and the myology of the extremities. *Trans Royal Can Inst* 6:507–594.

Primrose, A. 1900. *The Anatomy of the Orang Outan*. Toronto: University of Toronto Studies, Anatomical Series 1.

Priyadharshini, N.A., Kumar, V.D., Rajprasath, R. 2019. Unilateral and isolated absence of opponens pollicis and adductor pollicis: Could it be Cavanagh's syndrome? *J Curr Res Sci Med* 5:62–64.

Protas, M., Voin, V., Wang, J. M., Iwanaga, J., Loukas, M., Tubbs, R.S. 2017. A rare case of double-headed psoas minor muscle with review of its known variants. *Cureus* 9(6):e1312.

Puig, S., Dupuy, D.E., Sarmiento, A., et al. 1996. Articular muscle of the knee: A muscle seldom recognized on MR imaging. *Am J Roentgenol* 166:1057–1060.

Raheja, S., Choudhry, R., Singh, P. Tuli, A., Kumar, H. 2005. Morphological description of combined variation of distal attachments of fibulares in a foot. *Surg Radiol Anat* 27:158–160.

Rahman, H.A., Yamadori T. 1994. An anomalous cleido-occipitalis muscle. *Acta Anat* 150:156–158.

Rai, R., Nayak, S.R., Ranade, A.V., Prabhu, L.V., Vadgaonkar, R. 2007. Duplicated omohyoid muscle and its clinical significance. *Rom J Morphol Embryol* 48(3):295–297.

Rai, R., Ranade, A.V., Prabhu, L.V., Prakash, Rajanigandha, V., Nayak, S.R. 2008. Unilateral pectoralis minimus muscle. A case report. *Int J Morphol* 26:27–29.

Rai, R., Iwanaga, J., Loukas, M., Oskouian, R.J., Tubbs, R.S. 2018. The role of the axillary arch variant in neurovascular syndrome of brachial plexus compression. *Cureus* 10:c2875.

Raikos, A., Paraskevas, K., Tzika, M., Faustmann, P., Triaridis, S., Kordali, P., Kitsoulis, P., Brand-Saberi, B. 2011. Sternalis muscle: An underestimated anterior chest wall anatomical variant. *J Cardiothorac Surg* 6:73.

Raikos, A., Paraskevas, G.K., Triaridis, S., Kordali, P., Psillas, G., Brand-Saberi, B. 2012. Bilateral supernumerary sternocleidomastoid heads with critical narrowing of the minor and major supraclavicular fossae: Clinical and surgical implications. *Int J Morphol* 30(3):927–933.

Raikos, A., English, T., Agnihotri, A., Yousif, O.K., Sandhu, M., Bennetto, J., Stirling, A. 2014. Supraclavicularis proprius muscle associated with supraclavicular nerve entrapment. *Folia Morphol* 73:527–530.

Rajanigandha, V., Ranade, A.V., Pai, M.M., Rai, R., Prabhu, L.V., Nayak, S.R. 2008. The scalenus accessorius muscle. *Int J Morphol* 26:385–388.

Raju, S., Kanchana, L., Venu, M.N., Raghu, J., Srinivasa, R.S. 2014. A rare bilateral asymmetric variation of the anterior belly of digastric muscle. *Surg Acad* 4:29–31.

Ramirez, D., Gajardo, C., Caballero, P., Zavando, D., Cantin, M., Galdames, I.S. 2010. Clinical evaluation of fibularis tertius muscle prevalence. *Int J Morphol* 28(3):759–764.

Ramirez-Castro, J.L., Bersu, E.T. 1978. Anatomical analysis of the developmental effects of aneuploidy in man—the 18 trisomy syndrome: II. Anomalies of the upper and lower limbs. *Am J Med Gen* 2:285–306.

Ramsay, A. 1812. An account of unusual conformation of some muscles and vessels. *Edinburgh Med Surg J* 8:281–283.

Rana, K.K., Das, S. 2006. Anomalous attachment of the flexor digiti minimi muscle of the foot: An anatomical study with clinical implications. *Eur J Anat* 10:153–155.

Rana, K.K., Das, S., Verma, R. 2006. Double plantaris muscle: A cadaveric study with clinical importance. *Int J Morphol* 24(3):495–498.

Ranade, A.V., Rai, R., Prabhu, L.V., Rajanigandha, V., Janardhanan, J.P., Ramanathan, L., Prameela, M.D. 2008. Incidence of extensor digitorum brevis manus muscle. *HAND* 3:320–323.

Ranade, A.V., Rai, R., Murlimanju, B.V., Eladl, M.A. 2017. Atypical insertion of the abductor pollicis longus muscle, an anatomical case report. *Ital J Anat Embryol* 122:147–150.

Ramesh Rao, T., Vishnumaya, G., Prakashchandra, S.K., Suresh, R. 2007. Variation in the origin of sternocleidomastoid muscle. A case report. *Int J Morphol* 25(3):621–623.

Ramesh Rao, T., Rao, S.R. 2017. Variation in the origin of flexor digitorum brevis – a case report. *J Appl Life Sci Int* 11(4):1–4.

Rask, M.R. 1980. Superior gluteal nerve entrapment syndrome. *Muscle Nerve* 3(4):304–307.

Raveendran, S.S., Anthony, D.J. 2021. Classification and morphological variation of the frontalis muscle and implications on the clinical practice. *Aesth Plast Surg* 45:164–170.

Raven, H.C. 1950. Regional anatomy of the gorilla. In *The Anatomy of the Gorilla*, ed. Gregory, W.K., 15–188. New York: Columbia University Press.

Ravi, P.K., Gaikwad, M.R., Tirpude, A.P., Panda, M., Mishra, P.R. 2020. Morphological variations of biceps brachii muscle in Eastern Indian population: A cadaveric study. *Nat J Clin Anat* 9(1):31–35.

Ravindra, S.S., Somayaji, S.N., Nayak, S.B., Rao, M.K.G. 2012. External jugular vein passing through triangle formed by tendon of cleido-occipitalis cervicalis muscle, trapezius muscle and clavicle – a case report. *Int J Anat Var* 5:51–53.

Ravindranath, Y., Manjunath, K.Y., Ravindranath, R. 2008. Accessory origin of the piriformis muscle. *Singapore Med J* 49:217–218.

Redler, L.H., Kim, H.M., Tang, P., Ahmad, C.S. 2012. An anomalous accessory pectoralis major muscle: A case report. *Am J Sports Med* 40:2149–2153.

Reimann, A.F., Daseler, E.H., Anson, B.J., Beaton, L.E. 1944. The palmaris longus muscle and tendon. A study of 1600 extremities. *Anat Rec* 89:495–505.

Reina-de la Torre, F., Nebot-Cegarra, J., Pérez-Berruezo, J. 1994. Biceps brachii muscle attached to the extensor carpi radialis brevis muscle: An unreported anatomical variation in humans. *Ann Anat – Anat Anz* 176:319–321.

Rex, H. 1887. Über einen abnormen Augenmuskel (Musc. obliquus accessorius inferior). *Anat Anz* 2:624–630.

Richardson, D.R., Gadzala, L.A., Bonsall, D.J., Hogg, J.P., Williams, H.J., Nguyen, J. 2017. Congenital paradoxical lower eyelid retraction with upgaze due to an anomalous extraocular muscle. *Ophthalmic Plast Reconstr Surg* 33(4):e101–e102.

Rickenbacher J., Landolt, A.M., Theiler, K., Scheier, H., Siegfried, J., Wagenhäuser, F.J., Wilson, R.R., Winstanley, D.P. 1985. The musculature of the back. In *Applied Anatomy of the Back*, ed. Rickenbacher, J., Landolt, A.M., Theiler, K., 54–100. Berlin, Heidelberg: Springer.

Roberts, J.A., Seibold, H.R. 1971. The histology of the primate urethra. *Folia Primatol* 14:59–69.

Roberts, W., Zurada, A., Zurada-Zielinska, A., Gielecki, J., Loukas, M. 2016. Anatomy of Trisomy 18. *Clin Anat* 29:628–632.

Rochier, A.L., Sumpio, B.E. 2009. Variant of popliteal entrapment syndrome involving the lateral head of the gastrocnemius muscle: A case report. *Ann Vasc Surg* 23:535.e5–535.e9.

Rodrigues, V., Rao, M.K., Nayak, S. 2016. Multiple heads of gastrocnemius with bipennate fiber arrangement - a clinically significant variation. *J Clin Diagn Res* 10(8):AD01–AD02.

Rodríguez-Niedenführ, M., Vázquez, T., Parkin, I., Nearn, L., Sañudo, J.R. 2001. Incidence and morphology of the brachioradialis accessorius muscle. *J Anat* 199:353–355.

Rodríguez-Niedenführ, M., Vázquez, T., Golanó, P., Parkin, I., Sañudo, J.R. 2002. Extensor digitorum brevis manus: Anatomical radiological and clinical relevance. A review. *Clin Anat* 15:286–292.

Rodríguez-Vázquez, J.F. 2016. Middle ear muscles. In *Bergman's Comprehensive Encyclopedia of Human Anatomic Variation*, first edition, ed. Tubbs, R.S., Shoja, M.M., Loukas, M., 212–216. Hoboken, NJ: Wiley-Blackwell.

Rodríguez-Vázquez, J.F., Mérida-Velasco, J.R., Verdugo-López, S. 2010. Development of the stapedius muscle and unilateral agenesia of the tendon of the stapedius muscle in a human fetus. *Anat Rec* 293:25–31.

Rodríguez-Vázquez, J.F., Mérida-Velasco, J.R., Verdugo-López, S., de la Cuadra-Blanco, C., Sanz-Casado, J.V. 2009. Anatomical relationships of the cleidoatlanticus muscle. Interpretation about its origin. *Anat Sci Int* 84:47–52.

Rogawski, K.M. 1990. The rhomboideus capitis in man – correctly named rare muscular variation. *Okajimas Folia Anat Jpn* 67:161–164.

Rohrich, R.J., Huynh, B., Muzaffar, A.R., Adams, W.P., Robinson, J.B. 2000. Importance of the depressor septi nasi muscle in rhinoplasty: Anatomic study and clinical application. *Plast Reconstr Surg* 105(1):376–383.

Rončević, R. 1986. Masseter muscle hypertrophy: Aetiology and therapy. *J Maxillofac Surg* 14:344–348.

Roos, D.B. 1976. Congenital anomalies associated with thoracic outlet syndrome: Anatomy, symptoms, diagnosis, and treatment. *Am J Surg* 132:771–778.

Rosenberg, Z.S., Beltran, J., Cheung, Y.Y., Colon, E., Herraiz, F. 1997. MR features of longitudinal tears of the peroneus brevis tendon. *Am J Roentgenol* 168(1):141–147.

Ross, J.A., Troy, C.A. 1969. The clinical significance of the extensor digitorum brevis manus. *J Bone Joint Surg* 51B:473–478.

Rosser, B.W.C., Salem, A.H., Gbamgbola, S.A., Mohamed, A. 2019. Bilateral tripartite insertion of the fibularis (peroneus) brevis muscle: A case report. *Int J Morphol* 37(2):481–485.

Rourke, K., Dafydd, H., Parkin, I.G. 2007. Fibularis tertius: Revisiting the anatomy. *Clin Anat* 20(8):946–949.

Rubin, G., Wolovelsky, A., Rinott, M., Rozen, N. 2011. Anomalous course of the extensor pollicis longus: Clinical relevance. *Ann Plast Surg* 67:489–492.

Rubinstein, D., Escott, E.J., Hendrick, L.L. 1999. The prevalence and CT appearance of the levator claviculae muscle: A normal variant not to be mistaken for an abnormality. *J Neuroradiol* 20:583–586.

Rüdisüli, T. 1995. Demonstration of the musculus levator claviculae. *Surg Radiol Anat* 17:85–87.

Ruge G. 1887b. Die vom facialis innervirten muskeln des halses, nackens und des schädels einen jungen Gorilla. *Morphol Jahrb* 12:459–529.

Ruiz Santiago, F., Ruiz Tristan, A., Butani, P. 2019. Anomalous insertion of the pectoralis minor tendon at the greater tuberosity. *J Ultrasound* 23:407–410.

Rusnak-Smith, S., Moffat, M., Rosen, E. 2001. Anatomical variations of the scalene triangle: Dissection of 10 cadavers. *J Orthop Sports Phys Ther* 31:70–80.

Saadeh, F.A., El-Sabban, M., Hawi, J.S. 2001. Rare variations of the mylohyoid muscle: Case study. *Clin Anat* 14:285–287.

Saban, R. 1968. Musculature de la tête. In *Traité de zoologie, XVI, 3 (mammifères)*, ed. Grassé, P.P., 229–472. Paris: Masson et Cie.

Sacks, J.G. 1985. The levator-trochlear muscle: A supernumerary orbital structure. *Arch Ophthalmol* 103(4):540–541.

Saeed, M., Murshid, K.R., Rufai, A.A., Elsayed, S.E., Sadiq, M.S. 2002. Sternalis. An anatomic variant of chest wall musculature. *Saudi Med J* 23:1214–1221.

Saga, T., Takahashi, N. 2016. Abdominal wall muscles. In *Bergman's Comprehensive Encyclopedia of Human Anatomic Variation*, first edition, ed. Tubbs, R.S., Shoja, M.M., Loukas, M., 369–380. Hoboken, NJ: Wiley-Blackwell.

Sainsbury, J.R., Wagget, J. 1984. An absent gracilis: A case report. *Br J Clin Pract* 38:72.

Sakamoto, Y. 2009. Classification of pharyngeal muscles based on innervations from glossopharyngeal and vagus nerves in human. *Surg Radiol Anat* 31(10):755–761.

Sakamoto, Y. 2012. Spatial relationships between the morphologies and innervations of the scalene and anterior vertebral muscles. *Ann Anat* 194:381–388.

Sakamoto, Y. 2013. Interrelationships between the innervations from the laryngeal nerves and the pharyngeal plexus to the inferior pharyngeal constrictor. *Surg Radiol Anat* 35:721–728.

Sakamoto, Y. 2014. Gross anatomical observations of attachments of the middle pharyngeal constrictor. *Clin Anat* 27:603–609.

Sakamoto, Y. 2015. Spatial relationship between the palatopharyngeus and the superior constrictor of the pharynx. *Surg Radiol Anat* 37:649–655.

Sakamoto, Y. 2016a. Pharyngeal muscles. In *Bergman's Comprehensive Encyclopedia of Human Anatomic Variation*, first edition, ed. Tubbs, R.S., Shoja, M.M., Loukas, M., 236–239. Hoboken, NJ: Wiley-Blackwell.

Sakamoto, Y. 2016b. Prevertebral and craniocervical junction muscles. In *Bergman's Comprehensive Encyclopedia of Human Anatomic Variation*, first edition, ed. Tubbs, R.S., Shoja, M.M., Loukas, M., 245–253. Hoboken, NJ: Wiley-Blackwell.

Sakamoto, Y., Akita, K. 2004. Spatial relationships between masticatory muscles and their innervating nerves in man with special reference to the medial pterygoid muscle and its accessory muscle bundle. *Surg Radiol Anat* 26:122–127.

Sakamoto, K., Nasu, H., Nimura, A., Hamada, J., Akita, K. 2015. An anatomic study of the structure and innervation of the pronator quadratus muscle. *Anat Sci Int* 90:82–88.

Sakthivel, S., Verma, S. 2017. Accessory flexor carpi ulnaris and bilaterally variant vascular anatomy of upper limb: An unusual presentation. *Int J Appl Basic Med Res* 7:143–145.

Sakuma, E., Kato, H., Honda, N., Mabuchi, Y., Soji, T. 2004. A rare anomaly of the extensor digitorum longus. *Anat Sci Int* 79:235–238.

Sakuma, E., Omi, K., Takeda, N., Hasegawa, H., Mori, K., Mabuchi, Y., Soji, T. 2007. Bilaterally existing sternoclavicularis anticus muscles. *Ant Sci Int* 82:237–241.

Sakuma, E., Sasaki, Y., Yamada, N., et al. 2014. Morphological characteristics of the deep layer of articularis genus muscle. *Folia Morphol* 73:309–313.

Salem, A.H., Abdel, Kader, G., Almallah, A.A., Hussein, H.H., Abdel Badie, A., Behbehani, N., Nedham, F.N., Nedham, A.N., Almarshad, R., Alshammari, M., Amer, H., Hasan, W.A., Alyaseen, F.A., Mohammed, E.A. 2018. Variations of peroneus tertius muscle in five Arab populations: A clinical study. *Transl Res Anat* 13:1–6.

Sammarco, G.J., Stephens, M.M. 1990. Tarsal tunnel syndrome caused by the flexor digitorum accessorius longus. *J Bone Joint Surg [Am]* 72:453–454.

Sammarco, G.J., Brainard, B.J.A. 1991. Symptomatic anomalous peroneus brevis in a high-jumper. A case report. *J Bone Joint Surg* 73(1):131–133.

Sammarco, G.J., Conti, S.F. 1994. Tarsal tunnel syndrome caused by an anomalous muscle. *J Bone Joint Surg [Am]* 76(9):1308–1314.

Sandall, G.S., Morrison, J.W. 1979. Congenital absence of lateral rectus muscle. *J Pediatr Ophthalmol Strabismus* 16(1):35–39.

Sanders, I., Wu, B.L., Mu, L., Biller, H.F. 1994. The innervation of the human posterior cricoarytenoid muscle: Evidence for at least two neuromuscular compartments. *Laryngoscope* 104(7):880–884.

Santiago, F.R., Milena, G.L., Santos, C.C., Fernandez, J.M.T. 2001. Levator claviculae muscle presenting as a hard clavicular mass: Imaging study. *Eur Radiol* 11:2561–2563.

Sañudo, J.R., Mirapeix, R.M., Ferreira, B. 1993. A rare anomaly of abductor digiti minimi. *J Anat* 182:439–442.

Sargon, M.F., Çelik, H.H. 1994. An abnormal digastric muscle with three bellies. *Surg Radiol Anat* 16(2):215–216.

Sargon, M.F., Onderoğlu, S., Sürücü, H.S., Bayramoğlu, A., Demiryürek, D.D., Oztürk, H. 1999. Anatomic study of complex anomalies of the digastric muscle and review of the literature. *Okajimas Folia Anat Jpn* 75(6):305–313.

Sataloff, R.T., Selber, J.C. 2003. Phylogeny and embryology of the facial nerve and related structures. Part II: Embryology. *Ear Nose Throat J* 82:764–779.

Sato, K. 1980. A morphological analysis of the nerve supply of the sphincter ani externs, levator ani and coccygeus. *Kaibogaku Zasshi* 55:187–223.

Sato, S. 1968a. Statistical studies on the exceptional muscles of the Kyushu-Japanese. 1. The muscles of the head (the facial muscles). *Kurume Med J* 15:69–82.

Sato, S. 1968b. Statistical studies on the exceptional muscles of the Kyushu-Japanese. 2. The muscles of the neck. *Kurume Med J* 15:83–95.

Sato, S. 1968c. Statistical studies on the anomalous muscles of the Kyushu Japanese. 3. The muscles of the back, breast and abdomen. *Kurume Med J* 15:209–220.

Sato, S. 1969. Statistical studies on the anomalous muscles of the Kyushu-Japanese. 4. The muscles of the upper limb. *Kurume Med J* 16:69–81.

Sato, S. 1970. Statistical studies on the anomalous muscles of the Kyushu-Japanese. 5. The muscles of the lower limb. *Kurume Med J* 17:39–48.

Sato, I., Ueno, R., Sato, T. 1987. A consideration of the normal and abnormal human suprahyoid and infrahyoid musculature. *Okajimas Folia Anat Jpn* 64:17–38.

Satoh, J. 1969. The m. serratus posterior superior in certain catarrhine monkeys and man, in particular the structure of the muscular digitations and their nerve supply. *Okajimas Folia Anat Jpn* 46:65–122.

Satoh, J. 1970. The m. serratus posterior inferior in monkey and man, in particular the structure of the digitations and their nerve supply. *Okajimas Folia Anat Jpn* 47:19–61.

Satoh, J. 1971. The m. transversus thoracis in man and monkey. *Okajimas Folia Anat Jpn* 48:103–137.

Satoh, J. 1974. The mm. subcostales in man and monkeys. *Okajimas Folia Anat Jpn* 50:345–358.

Satoh, J., Shu, T. 1968. On the mm. levatores costarum in man and monkey. *Okajimas Folia Anat Jpn* 45:35–50.

Saupe, N., Mengiardi, B., Pfirrmann, C.W., Vienne, P., Seifert, B., Zanetti, M. 2007. Anatomic variants associated with peroneal tendon disorders: MR imaging findings in volunteers with asymptomatic ankles. *Radiology* 242(2):509–517.

Sauser, G. 1935. Beobachtung zweier muskelvarietaten an lebenden. *Wien Klin Wochenschrift* 48:430–432.

Sawada, M., Ishibashi, Y., Suzuki, T., Chiba, S. 1991. Case reports on the pectoralis quartus and the pectoralis intermedius muscles. *Kaibogaku Zasshi* 66:99–105.

Sawaizumi, T., Nanno, M., Ito, H. 2003. Supernumerary extensor pollicis longus tendon: A case report. *J Hand Surg [Am]* 28:1014–1017.

Saxena, A., Bareither, D. 2000. Magnetic resonance and cadaveric findings of the incidence of the plantaris tendon. *Foot Ankle Int* 21(7):570–572.

Sayson, S.C., Ducey, J.P., Maybrey, J.B., Wesley, R.L., Vermillion, D. 1994. Sciatic entrapment neuropathy associated with an anomalous piriformis muscle. *Pain* 59:149–152.

Scali, F., Marsili, E.S., Pontell, M.E. 2011. Anatomical connection between the rectus capitis posterior major and the dura mater. *Spine* 36:E1612–1614.

Scali, F., Pontell, M.E., Enix, D.E., Marshall, E. 2013. Histological analysis of the rectus capitis posterior major's myodural bridge. *Spine J* 13:558–563.

Schaeffer, J. P. 1913. On two muscle anomalies of the lower extremity. *Anat Rec* 7(1):1–7.

Schaumann, B.F., Peagler, F.D., Gorlin, R.J. 1970. Minor craniofacial anomalies among a Negro population. *Oral Surg Oral Med Oral Pathol* 29(5):729–734.

Schmidt, H.M. 1982. Transversus nuchae muscle: Two observations of hitherto unknown deviations of its nerve supply. *Anat Anz* 151:144–150.

Schnyder, H. 1984. The innervation of the monkey accessory lateral rectus muscle. *Brain Res* 296:139–144.

Schön Ybarra, M.A., Bauer, B. 2001. Medial portion of m. temporalis and its potential involvement in facial pain. *Clin Anat* 14:25–30.

Schück, A.C. 1913. Beiträge zur myologie der primaten, I – der m. lat. dorsi und der m. latissimo-tricipitalis. *Morphol Jahrb* 45:267–294.

Schweizer, V., Dörfl, J. 1997. The anatomy of the inferior laryngeal nerve. *Clin Otolaryngol* 22:362–369.

Sehirli, Ü., Çavdar, S. 1996. An accessory mylohyoid muscle. *Surg Radiol Anat* 18:57–59.

Seib, G.A. 1934. Incidence of the m. psoas minor in man. *Am J Phys Anthropol* 19:229–246.

Seif, S., Dellon, A.L. 1978. Anatomic relationships between the human levator and tensor veli palatini and the eustachian tube. *Cleft Palate J* 15:329–336.

Seiler, R. 1976. Die Gesichtsmuskeln. In *Primatologia, Handbuch der Primatenkunde, Bd. 4, Lieferung 6*, eds. Hofer, H., Schultz, A.H., Starck, D., 1–252. Basel: Karger.

Seipel, R., Linklater, J., Pitsis, G., Sullivan, M. 2005. The peroneocalcaneus internus muscle: An unusual cause of posterior ankle impingement. *Foot Ankle Int* 26:890–893.

Sekine, J., Hamada, N., Toh, H., Ohmori, T. 1988. An anomalous case of the risorius arising from the masseter tendon. *Okajimas Folia Anat Jpn* 65:29–33.

Sekiya, S., Kumaki, K., Yamada, T. K., Horiguchi, M. 1994. Nerve supply to the accessory soleus muscle. *Cells Tissues Organs* 149(2):21–127.

Senoo, H., Kogo, M., Mukai, N., Otani, T., Nomura, K., Matsuya, T. 2001. A case of congenital dysplasia of the soft palate. *J Jpn Soc Oral Surg* 47:316–319.

Serpell, J.W., Baum, M. 1991. Significance of Langer's axillary arch in axillary dissection. *Aust New Zeal J Surg* 61:310–312.

Sevinç, Ö., Çetin, Z., Barut, Ç., Büken, B., Arïfoğlu, Y. 2009. A complex variation of the digastric muscle: A case report. *Anatomy* 3:72–74.

Sevivas, N., Kalouche, I., Roulot, E. 2009. Double extensor pollicis longus tendon in independent extensor compartments: A case report of an anatomical variation requiring alteration of surgical strategy. *Chirurgie de La Main* 28:180–182.

Shapiro, B.L., Hermann, J., Opitz, J.M. 1983. Down syndrome—a disruption of homeostasis. *Am J Med Genet* 14:241–269.

Sharma, R., Narang, P., Reddy, Y.G., Sharma, A.K. 2013. A triad of developmental anomalies-an unusual case. *J Clin Diagn Res* 7:1264–1265.

Sharp, J.F. 1990. The ceratocricoid muscle. *Clin Otolaryngol* 5:257–261.

Shepherd, F.J. 1889. Some vascular anomalies observed during the session 1888–89. *J Anat Physiol* 24:69–71.

Shetty, P., Pai, M.M., Prabhu, L.V., Vadgaonkar, R., Nayak, S.R., Shivanandan, R. 2006. The subclavius posticus muscle:

Its phylogenetic retention and clinical significance. *Int J Morphol* 24:599–600.

Shinohara, H. 1995. Gemelli and obturator internus muscles: Different heads of one muscle? *Anat Rec* 243:145–150.

Shimada, K., Gasser, R.F. 1989. Morphology of the pterygomandibular raphe in human fetuses and adults. *Anat Rec* 224:117–122.

Shimada, K., Yokoi, A., Ozawa, H., Kitagawa, T., Tezuka, M. 1991. Observation of the petropharyngeal muscle in Japanese. *Anat Anz* 173(4):193–198.

Shore, L.R. 1926. An example of the muscle scalenus minimus. *J Anat* 60:418–419.

Shpizner, B.A., Holliday, R.A. 1993. Levator scapulae muscle asymmetry presenting as a palpable neck mass: CT evaluation. *Am J Neuroradiol* 14:461–464.

Shprintzen, R.J., Schwartz, R.H., Daniller, A., Hoch, L. 1985. Morphologic significance of bifid uvula. *Pediatr* 75(3):553–561.

Shrewsbury, M.M., Kuczynski, K. 1974. Flexor digitorum superficialis tendon in the fingers of the human hand. *Hand* 6:121–130.

Shrewsbury, M.M., Marzke, M.M., Linscheid, R.L., Reece, S.P. 2003. Comparative morphology of the pollical distal phalanx. *Am J Phys Anthropol* 121:30–47.

Shu, B., Safran, M.R. 2011. Case report: Bifid iliopsoas tendon causing refractory internal snapping hip. *Clin Ortho Rel Res* 469:289–293.

Shved, I.A., Lazjuk, G.I., Cherstvoy, E.D., Opitz, J.M., Reynolds, J.F. 1985. Elaboration of the phenotypic changes of the upper limbs in the Neu-Laxova syndrome. *Am J Med Gen* 20:1–11.

Shyamsundar, S., Wazir, A., Allen, P.E. 2012. Variations in the insertion of peroneus longus tendon - a cadaver study. *Foot Ankle Surg* 18(4):293–295.

Siddiqui, A.U., Satapathy, B.C., Siddiqui, A.T., Gill, S.S. 2017. Anatomical insight into the muscle petropharyngeus-a supernumerary muscle of the posterior pharyngeal wall. *Anat Physiol* 7:S6–004.

Sigmon, B.A. 1974. A functional analysis of pongid hip and thigh musculature. J Hum Evol 3:161–185.

Silawal, S., Rayan Galal, K., Schulze-Tanzil, G. 2018. A rare variation of intrinsic and extrinsic hand muscles represented by a bi-ventered first lumbrical extending into the carpal tunnel combined with bilateral fifth superficial flexor digitorum tendon regression. *Morphologie* 102:294–301.

Singh, N., Kathole, M., Kaur, J., Mehta, V., Suri, R.K., Rath, G., Kohli, M. 2018. Bilateral clavicular attachment of omohyoid muscle. *Morphologie* 102:87–90.

Sinha, D.N., Kumar, V. 1985. Study of human pyramidalis muscle in Indian subjects. *Anthro Anz* 43:173–177.

Sirasanagandla, S.R., Potu, B.K., Nayak, B.S., Bhat, K.M.R. 2013a. Popliteal vessels entrapment by a variant accessory belly of medial head of gastrocnemius. *Anat Physiol* 3(1):116–117.

Sirasanagandla, S.R., Swamy, R.S., Nayak, S.B., Somayaji, N.S., Rao, M.K., Bhat, K.M. 2013b. Analysis of the morphometry and variations in the extensor digitorum brevis muscle: An anatomic guide for muscle flap and tendon transfer surgical dissection. *Anat Cell Biol* 46(3):198–202.

Sirasanagandla, S.R., Bhat, K.M., Nayak, S.B., Shetty, P., Thangarajan, R. 2014. A rare case of variant morphology of peroneus tertius muscle. *J Clin Diagn Res* 8(10):AD01–AD02.

Smith, C.M., Ziermann, J.M., Molnar, J., Gondre-Lewis, M.C., Sandone, C., Bersu, E.T., Aziz, M.A., Diogo, R. 2015. Muscular and skeletal anomalies in human trisomy in an evo-devo context: Description of a T18 cyclopic fetus and comparison between Edwards (T18), Patau (T13) and Down (T21) Syndromes using 3-D imaging and anatomical illustrations. Boca Raton, FL: CRC Press.

Smith, E.B. 1896. Some points in the anatomy of the dorsum of the hand, with special reference to the morphology of the extensor brevis digitorum manus. *J Anat Physiol* 31:45–58.

Smith Jr., R., Nyquist-Battie, C., Clark, M., Rains, J. 2003. Anatomical characteristics of the upper serratus anterior: Cadaver dissection. *J Orthop Sports Phys Ther* 33:449–454.

Smith-Petersen, M.N. 1949. Approach to and exposure of the hip joint for mold arthroplasty. *J Bone Joint Surg* 31A:40–46.

Snider, C.C., Amalfi, A.N., Hutchinson, L.E., Sommer, N.Z. 2017. New insights into the anatomy of the midface musculature and its implications on the nasolabial fold. Aesth Plast Surg 41:1083–1090.

Snosek, M., Loukas, M. 2016. Thoracic wall muscles. In *Bergman's Comprehensive Encyclopedia of Human Anatomic Variation*, first edition, ed. Tubbs, R.S., Shoja, M.M., Loukas, M., 335–368. Hoboken, NJ: Wiley-Blackwell.

Sobel, M., Levy, M.E., Bohne, W.H. 1990. Congenital variations of the peroneus quartus muscle: An anatomic study. *Foot Ankle* 11(2):89–90. [published correction appears in Foot Ankle 11(5):342].

Sodre, H., Bruschini, S., Magalhaes, A.A.C., Lourenco, A. 1994. Anomalous muscles in clubfeet. In *The Clubfoot*, ed. Simons, G.W., 42–48. New York: Springer.

Soldado-Carrera, F., Vilar-Coromina, N., Rodríguez-Baeza, A. 2000. An accessory belly of the abductor digiti minimi muscle: A case report and embryologic aspects. *Surg Radiol Anat* 22:51–54.

Sommer, A. 1907. Das muskelsystem des gorilla. *Jena Z Naturwiss* 42:181–308.

Soni, S., Rath, G., Suri, R., Kumar, H. 2008. Anomalous pectoral musculature. *Anat Sci Int* 83:310–313.

Sonne, J.W.H. 2020. Prevalence of the sternalis muscle in a sample of routinely dissected human cadavers. *Surg Radiol Anat* 42:87–90.

Sonntag, C.F. 1923. On the anatomy, physiology, and pathology of the chimpanzee. *Proc Zool Soc Lond* 23:323–429.

Sonntag, C.F. 1924. On the anatomy, physiology, and pathology of the orang-utan. *Proc Zool Soc Lond* 24:349–450.

Sontakke, Y., Joshi, S.S., Joshi, S.D. 2013. Sternoclavicularis - a variant of pectoralis major muscle. *People's J Sci Res* 6:33–35.

Somayaji, S.N., Vincent, R., Bairy, K.L. 1998. An anomalous muscle in the region of the popliteal fossa: Case report. *J Anat* 192:307–308.

Sookur, P.A., Naraghi, A.M., Bleakney, R.R., Jalan, R., Chan, O., White, L.M. 2008. Accessory muscles: Anatomy, symptoms, and radiographic evaluation. *Radiographics* 28:481–499.

Spears, J., Kim, D.C., Saba, S.C., Mitra, A., Schneck, C., Mitra, A. 2011. Anatomical relationship of Roos' type 3 band and the T1 nerve root. *Plast Reconstr Surg* 128:1257–1262.

Spinner, M. 1968. The arcade of Frohse and its relationship to posterior interosseous nerve paralysis. *J Bone Joint Surg Br* 50:809–812.

Spinner, R.J., Carmichael, S.W., Spinner, M. 1991. Infraclavicular ulnar nerve entrapment due to a chondroepitrochlearis muscle. *J Hand Surg* 16:315–317.

Spinner, R.J., Spinner, M. 1996. Superficial radial nerve compression at the elbow due to an accessory brachioradialis muscle: A case report. *J Hand Surg [Am]* 21:369–372.

Spinner, R.J., Lins, R.E., Spinner, M. 1996. Compression of the medial half of the deep branch of the ulnar nerve by an anomalous origin of the flexor digiti minimi. *J Bone Joint Surg [Am]* 78:427–430.

Spratt, J.D., Logan, B.M., Abrahams, P.H. 1996. Variant slips of psoas and iliacus muscles, with splitting of the femoral nerve. *Clin Anat* 9:401–404.

Sripanidkulchai, K., Chaisiwamongkol, K., Iamsaard, S. 2013. Transversus menti muscle in a Thai cadaver. *Int J Morphol* 31(4):1399–1400.

Stanchev, S., Iliev, A., Malinova, L., Landzhov, B. 2017. A rare case of bilateral occipitoscapular muscle. *Acta morpholo et anthropol* 24:74–77.

Standring, S (ed.). 2005. *Gray's Anatomy. The Anatomical Basis of Clinical Practice.* 39th ed. New York: Elsevier Churchill Livingstone.

Standring, S (ed.). 2016. *Gray's Anatomy. The Anatomical Basis of Clinical Practice.* 41st ed. New York: Elsevier Limited.

Staniek, M., Brenner, E. 2012. Variations in the anatomy of the anterior-inferior rotator cuff: The "infraglenoid muscle". *Ann Anat* 194:373–380.

Starck, D., Schneider, R. 1960. Respirationsorgane. In *Primatologia III/2*, ed. Hofer, H., Schultz, A.H., Starck, D., 423–587. Basel: Karger.

Starck, D. 1973. The skull of the fetal chimpanzee. In *The Chimpanzee*, vol. 6, ed. Bourne, G.H., 1–33. Basel: Karger.

Stark, H.H., Otter, T.A., Boyes, J.H., Rickard, T.A. 1979. Atavistic contrahentes digitorum and associated muscle abnormalities of the hand: A cause of symptoms. *J Bone Joint Surg* 61A:286–289.

Stark, M.E., Wu, B., Bluth, B.E., Wisco, J.J. 2009. Bilateral accessory cleidohyoid in a human cadaver. *Int J Anat Var* 2:122–123.

Stein, A.H. 1951. Variations of the tendons of insertion of the abductor pollicis longus and the extensor pollicis brevis. *Anat Rec* 110:49–55.

Steinbach, K. 1923. Uber Varietation der Unterzungenbeinund Brustmuskulatur. *Anat Anz* 15:488–506.

Stern, J.T. 1972. Anatomical and functional specializations of the human gluteus maximus. *Am J Phys Anthropol* 36:315–340.

Stevens, K., Platt, A., Ellis, H. 1993. A cadaveric study of the peroneus tertius muscle. *Clin Anat* 6(2):106–110.

Stevenson, P.H. 1921. On an unusual anomaly of the peroneus tertius in a Chinese. *Anat Rec* 22(1):81–83.

Stevenson, A., McCarthy, S., Kalmey, J., Kuleza, R. 2014. Anatomical dissection of a cadaver with congenital scoliosis. *Folia Morphol* 73:389–394.

Stevenson, R. 2006. *Human Malformations and Related Anomalies.* Oxford: Oxford University Press, Inc.

Stewart, T.D. 1936. The musculature of the anthropoids, I, neck and trunk. *Am J Phys Anthropol* 21:141–204.

Still, J.M., Kleinert, H.E. 1973. Anomalous muscles and nerve entrapment in the wrist and hand. *Plast Reconstr Surg* 52:394–400.

Stöckle, M., Fanghänel, J., Knüttel, H., Alamanos, C., Behr, M. 2019. The morphological variations of the lateral pterygoid muscle: A systematic review. *Ann Anat* 222:79–87.

Stott, C.F. 1928. A note on the scalenus minimus muscle. *J Anat* 62:359–361.

Straus, W.L. 1941. The phylogeny of the human forearm extensors. *Hum Biol* 13:23–50.

Stringer, M.D., Kano, M., Fausett, C., Samallia, L. 2012. Unilateral short rectus femoris muscle belly. *Int J Anat Var* 5:56–58.

Stuart, T.P. 1879. Note on a variation in the course of the popliteal artery. *J Anat Physiol* 13:162.

Suda, M., Takahashi, 1957. A rare case of an anomalous digastric muscle in the thigh. *Sapporo Med J* 14:134–137.

Sugavasi, R., Latha, K., Indira Devi, Jetti, R., Sirasanagandla, S.R., Gorantla, V.R. 2013. A case report of variant insertion of plantaris muscle and its morphological and clinical implications. *J Morphol Sci* 30:304–305.

Sujata, M., Raju, S., Sirisha, B., Indira, B., Kanchana, G., Raghu, J. 2013. A thyreotrachealis muscle: A case report. *Eur J Anat* 17(2):127–128.

Sukekawa, R., Itoh, I. 2006. Anatomical study of the human omohyoid muscle: Regarding intermediate morphologies between normal and anomalous morphologies of the superior belly. *Anat Sci Int* 81(2):107–114.

Sullivan, W.E., Osgood, C.W. 1925. The facialis musculature of the orang, *Simia satyrus. Anat Rec* 29:195–343.

Sullivan, W.E., Osgood, C.W. 1927. The musculature of the superior extremity of the orang-utan, *Simia satyrus. Anat Rec* 35:193–239.

Sultan, A.H., Kamm, M.A., Hudson, C.N., Nichols, J.R., Bartram, C.I. 1994. Endosonography of the anal sphincters: Normal anatomy and comparsion with manometry. *Clin Radiol* 49:368–374.

Sultana, S.Z., Khalil, M., Khan, M.K., Shamim, R., Parveen, S., Ara, Z.G. 2009. Morphological study of levator glandulae thyroidea in Bangladeshi cadaver. *Mymensingh Med J* 18(2):179–183.

Sumida, K., Yamashita, K., Kitamura, S. 2012. Gross anatomical study of the human palatopharyngeus muscle throughout its entire course from origin to insertion. *Clin Anat.* 25(3):314–323.

Sumida, K., Ando, Y., Seki, S., Yamashita, K., Fujimura, A., Baba, O., Seiichiro, K. 2017. Anatomical status of the human palatopharyngeal sphincter and its functional implications. *Surg Radiol Anat* 39:1191–1201.

Sundaram, V., Chen, S.D., Colley, S., Hundal, K., Elston, J. 2005. Bifid medial rectus muscle insertion associated with intermittent distance exotropia. *Arch Ophthalmol* 123:1453.

Surendran, S., Nayak, S.B., Reghunathan, D., Nelluri, V.M. 2016. Sternocleiodomastoid muscle with five fleshy bellies and thirteen heads of origin. *Online J Health Allied Sci* 15(3):11.

Susman, R.L., Jungers, W.L., Stern, J.T. 1982. The functional morphology of the accessory interosseous muscle in the gibbon hand: Determination of locomotor and manipulatory compromises. *J Anat* 134:111–20.

Sussmann, A.R. 2019. Congenital bilateral absence of the semimembranosus muscles. *Skeletal Radiol* 48:1651–1655.

Sutton, J.B. 1883. On some points in the anatomy of the chimpanzee (*Anthropopithecus troglodytes*). *J Anat Physiol* 18:66–85.

Sutton, J.B. 1888. Nature of ligaments: Part V. *J Anat Physiol* 22(Pt 4):542–553.

Suwannakhan, A., Tawonsawatruk, T., Meemon, K. 2016. Extensor tendons and variations of the medial four digits of hand: A cadaveric study. *Surg Radiol Anat* 38:1083–1093.

Suwannakhan, A., Nontunha, N., Meemon, K. 2020. Complete extensor digitorum profundus complex: A deep hand extensor muscle to the medial four digits. *Surg Radiol Anat* 42:935–938.

Suzuki, C., Sando, I., Kitagawa, M., Balaban, C.D., Takasaki, K. 2003. Difference in Attachment of the tensor veli palatini muscle to the eustachian tube cartilage with age. *Ann Otol Rhinol Laryngol* 112(5):439–443.

Swindler, D.R., Wood, C.D. 1973. *An Atlas of Primate Gross Anatomy: Baboon, Chimpanzee and Men.* Seattle: University of Washington Press.

Tachibana, G., Miyauchi, R. 1989. Nerve supply to and the true nature of anterior supracostal muscle: Three cases of the anterior supracostal muscle innervated by the external muscular branch of the first intercostal nerve having lateral cutaneous branch. *Anat Anz* 169:235–245.

Tadaki, T., Kamiyama, R., Okamura, H., Ohtani, I. 2003. Anomalies of the auditory organ in trisomy 18 syndrome: Human temporal bone histopathological study. *J Laryngol Otol* 117(7):580–583.

Tagil, S.M., Özçakar, L. and Bozkurt, M.C. 2005. Insight into understanding the anatomical and clinical aspects of supernumerary rectus capitis posterior muscles. *Clin Anat* 18:373–375.

Tagliapietra, J.C., Robles, J.M., Iturralde, N.G., Alonson, F.J. 1989. Gluteus maximus agenesia. *Eur J Plast Surg* 12:41–42.

Takase, K., Imakita, S., Kuribayashi, S., Onishi, Y., Takamiya, M. 1997. Popliteal artery entrapment syndrome: Aberrant origin of gastrocnemius muscle shown by 3D CT. *J Comp Ass Tomol* 2:523–528.

Takashima, M., Kitai, N., Murakami, S., Furukawa, S., Kreiborg, S., Takada, K. 2003. Volume and shape of masticatory muscles in patients with hemifacial microsomia. *Cleft Palate Craniofac J* 40(1):6–12.

Takeshige, A., Okinaga, H., Shirai, N., Tanaka, M. 1960. Variation of the origin of the m. quadriceps femoris. *Kurume Igakkai Zasshi* 23:861–864.

Tanaka, T., Moran, S.L., Zhao, C., Zobitz, M.E., An, K.N., Amadio, P.C. 2007. Anatomic variation of the 5th extensor tendon compartment and extensor digiti minimi tendon. *Clin Anat* 20:677–682.

Tansatit, T., Apinuntrum, P., Phetudom, T., Phanchart, P. 2013. New insights into the pelvic organ support framework. *Eur J Obst Gynecol Reprod Biol* 166:221–225.

Tanyeli, E., Pestemalci, T., Uzel, M., Yildirim, M. 2006. The double deep gluteal muscles. *Saudi Med J* 27:385–386.

Taskaya-Yilmaz, N., Ceylan, G., Incecu, L., Muglali, M. 2005. A possible etiology of the internal derangement of the temporomandibular joint based on the MRI observations of the lateral pterygoid muscle. *Surg Radiol Anat* 27:19–24.

Tate, R., Pachnik, R.L. 1976. The accessory tendon of extensor hallucis longus: Its occurrence and function. *J Am Podiatr Assoc* 66:899–907.

Tatu, L., Parratte, B., Vuillier, F., Diop, M., Monnier, G. 2002. Descriptive anatomy of the femoral portion of the iliopsoas muscle. Anatomical basis of anterior snapping of the hip. *Surg Radiol Anat* 23:371–374.

Taylor, V., Guttmann, G.D., Reeves, R.E. 2015. A variant accessory muscle of the gluteus maximus. *Int J Anat Var* 8:10–11.

Taylor, R.H., Kraft, S.P. 1997. Aplasia of the inferior rectus muscle. A case report and review of the literature. *Ophthalmology* 104(3):415–418.

Teixeira, Á., Ráfare, A., Chagas, C., Pires, L. 2019. A supernumerary variation of the pharyngeal muscles - a case report. *Acta Scientiae Anatom* 1(3):161–163.

Tekelioglu, U.Y., Demirhan, A., Ozlu, Y., Kocoglu, H. 2015. Anatomic variation of the internal oblique muscle detected during transversus abdominis plane block. *Gen Meg (Los Angel)* 3:187.

Tennant, J.N., Rungprai, C., Phisitkul, P. 2014. Bilateral anterior tarsal tunnel syndrome variant secondary to extensor hallucis brevis muscle hypertrophy in a ballet dancer: A case report. *Foot Ankle Surg* 20(4):e56–e58.

Terry, R.J. 1942. Absence of superior gemellus muscle in American Whites and Negroes. *Am J Phys Anthropol* 29:47–56.

Testut, L. 1884. Les anomalies musculaires chez l'homme expliquèes par l'anatomie comparée et leur importance en anthropologie. Paris: Masson.

Testut, L. 1892. Les anomalies musculaires considres du point de due de la ligature des artres. Paris: Doin.

Tewari, J., Mishra, P.R., Tripathy, S.K. 2015. Anatomical variation of abductor pollicis longus in Indian population: A cadaveric study. *Indian J Orthop* 49:549–553.

Tezer, M., Cicekcibasi, A.E. 2012. A variation of the extensor hallucis longus muscle (accessory extensor digiti secundus muscle). *Anat Sci Int* 87:111–114.

Thomas, G.I., Jones, T.W., Stavney, L.S., Manhas, D.R. 1983. The middle scalene muscle and its contribution to the thoracic outlet syndrome. *Am J Surg* 145(5):589–592.

Thompson, N.W., Mockford, B.J., Cran, G.W. 2001. Absence of the palmaris longus muscle: A population study. *Ulster Med J* 70:22–24.

Thomson, A. 1885. Notes on some unusual variations in human anatomy. *J Anat Physiol* 19(Pt 3):328–332.

Tichý, M., Grim, M. 1985. Morphogenesis of the human gluteus maximus muscle arising from two muscle primordia. *Anat Embryol* 173:275–277.

Tiengo, C., Macchi, V., Stecco, C., Bassetto, F. and De Caro, R. 2006. Epifascial accessory palmaris longus muscle. *Clin Anat* 19:554–557.

Todd, N.W., Krueger, B.L. 1992. Minuscule submucous cleft palate: Cadaver study. *Ann Otolo Rhinolo Laryngolo* 101(5):417–422.

Todd, R.B. 1839. *The Cyclopaedia of Anatomy and Physiology*, vol. 2. London: Longman, Brown, Green, Longmans, & Roberts.

Tokat, A.O., Atınkaya, C., Esmer, A.F., Apaydın, N., Tekdemir, I., Güngör, A. 2011. Cadaver analysis of thoracic outlet anomalies. *Turkish J Thorac Cardiovasc Surg* 19:72–76.

Tomo, S., Toh, H., Hirakawa, T., Tomo, I., Kobayashi, S. 1994. Case report: The cleidocervical muscle with speculation as to its origin. *J Anat* 184:165–169.

Tonkin, M.A., Lister, G.D. 1985. The palmaris brevis profundus. An anomalous muscle associated with ulnar nerve compression at the wrist. *J Hand Surg* 10:862–864.

Torres, R., Levitt, M.A., Tovilla, J.M., Rodriguez, G., Peña, A. 1998. Anorectal malformations and Down's syndrome. *J Pediatr Surg* 33:194–197.

Toscano, A.E., Moraes, A.S.R., Almeida, S.K.S. 2004. The articular muscle of the knee: Morphology and disposition. *Int J Morphol* 22:303–306.

Tountas, C.P., Bergman, R.A. 1993. *Anatomic Variations of the Upper Extremity.* New York: Churchill Livingstone.

Touré, G., Anzouan-Kacou, E. 2016. The styloauricular muscle: Clinical relevance and literature review of this rare muscle. *Surg Radiol Anat* 38:983–986.

Trackler, R.T., Koehler, P.R. 1968. The radiographic findings in posterior perineal hernia. *Radiology* 91:950–951.

Traini, M. 1983. Bilateral accessory digastric muscles. *Anat Clin* 5(3):199–200.

Trono, M., Tueche, S., Quintart, C., Libotte, M., Baillon, J.M. 1999. Peroneus quartus muscle: A case report and review of the literature. *Foot Ankle Int* 20:659–662.

Trudel, M., Laframboise, R., Leclerc, J.E. 2018. Musculo-mucous web velum and velopharyngeal dysfunction associated with 8q22.1–22.2 microduplication. *Int J Pediatr Otorhinolaryngol* 104:134–137.

Tsuneki, M., Maruyama, S., Yamazaki, M., Niimi, K., Kobayashi, T., Nishiyama, H., Hayshi, T., Tanuma, J. 2019. Masseter muscle hypertrophy: A case report. *J Oral Maxillofac Surg Med Pathol* 31:428–431.

Tubbs, R.S., Salter, E.G., Oakes, W.J. 2004a. Unusual origin of the omohyoid muscle. *Clin Anat* 17:578–582.

Tubbs, R.S., Salter, G., Oaks, W.J. 2004b. Femoral head of the rectus femoris muscle. *Clin Anat* 17:276–278.

Tubbs, R.S., Oakes, W.J., Salter, E.G. 2005a. Unusual attachment of the pectoralis minor muscle. *Clin Anat* 18:302–304.

Tubbs, R.S., Salter, E.G., Oakes, W.J. 2005b. Contrahentes digitorum muscle. *Clin Anat* 18:606–608.

Tubbs, R.S., Zehren, S. 2006. Popliteal vein aneurysm due to an anomalous slip of the adductor magnus. *Clin Anat* 19:722–723.

Tubbs, R.S., Salter, E.G. 2006a. The iliacus minimus muscle. *Clin Anat* 19:720–721.

Tubbs, R.S., Salter, E.G. 2006b. A variant gluteal muscle. *Clin Anat* 19:729.

Tubbs, R.S., Oakes, W.J., Salter, E.G. 2006a. The subanconeus muscle. *Folia Morphol (Warsz)* 65:22–25.

Tubbs, R.S., Salter, E.G., Oakes, W.J. 2006b. Triceps brachii muscle demonstrating a fourth head. *Clin Anat* 19:657–660.

Tubbs, R.S., Oakes, W.J., Salter, E.G. 2006c. The psoas quartus muscle. *Clin Anat* 19:678–680.

Tubbs, R.S., Stetler, W., Jr., Savage, A.J., et al. 2006d. Does a third head of the rectus femoris muscle exist? *Folia Morphol (Warsz)* 65:377–380.

Tubbs, R.S., Salter, E.G., Oakes, W.J. 2006e. Dissection of a rare accessory muscle of the leg: The tensor fasciae suralis muscle. *Clin Anat* 19:571–572.

Tubbs, R.S., Stetler, W., Shoja, M.M., Loukas, M., Salter, E.G., Oakes, W.J. 2007. An unusual muscular variation of the infratemporal fossa. *Folia Morphol* 66:200–202.

Tubbs, R.S., Shoja, M.M., Shokouhi, G., Loukas, M., Oakes, W.J. 2008a. Insertion of the pectoralis major into the shoulder joint capsule. *Anat Sci Int* 83:291–293.

Tubbs, R.S., May, W.R., Shoja, M.M., Loukas, M., Salter, E.G., Oakes, W.J. 2008b. Peroneotalocalcaneus muscle. *Anat Sci Int* 83(4):280–282.

Tubbs, R.S., Jones, V.L., Loukas, M., Shoja, M.M., Cohen-Gadol, A.A. 2010. Quantification and anatomy of the sinus of morgagni at the skull base. *Biomed Int* 1:16–18.

Tubbs, R.S., Griessenauer, C.J., Marshall, T., Dennison, C.P., Shoja, M.M., Loukas, M., Apaydin, N., Cohen-Gadol, A.A. 2011. The adductor minimus muscle revisited. *Surg Radiol Anat* 33:429–432.

Tubbs, R.S., Watanabe, K. 2016. Perineal muscles. In *Bergman's Comprehensive Encyclopedia of Human Anatomic Variation*, first edition, ed. Tubbs, R.S., Shoja, M.M., Loukas, M., 384–385. Hoboken, NJ: Wiley-Blackwell.

Tuite, D., Finegan, P., Saliaris, A., Renström, P.A.F.M., Donne, B., O'Brien, M. 1998. Anatomy of the proximal musculotendinous junction of the adductor longus muscle. *Knee Surg* 6:134–137.

Tuncel, U., Gumus, M., Kurt, A., Güzel, N. 2017. An extremely rare condition: Unilateral and isolated temporalis muscle hypertrophy. *Plast Reconstr Surg Glob Open* 5(6):e1383.

Tunn, R., Delancey, J.O., Howard, D., Ashton-Miller, J.A., Quint, L.E. 2003. Anatomic variations in the levator ani muscle, endopelvic fascia, and urethra in nulliparous evaluated by magnetic resonance imaging. *Am J Obst Gynecol* 188:116–121.

Turan-Özdemir, S., Cankur, N.S. 2004. Unusual variation of the inferior attachment of the pectoralis minor muscle. *Clin Anat* 17:416–417.

Turan-Özdemir, S., Oygucu, I.H., Kafa, I. 2004. Bilateral abnormal anterior bellies of digastric muscles. *Anat Sci Int* 79:95–97.

Turgut, H.B., Anil, A., Peker, T., Barut, C. 2000. Insertion abnormality of bilateral pectoralis minimus. *Surg Radiol Anat* 22:55–57.

Turgut, H.B., Peker, T., Gulekon, N., Anil, A., Karakose, M. 2005. Axillopectoral muscle (Langer's muscle). *Clin Anat* 183:220–223.

Türker, T., Robertson, G.A., Thirkannad, S.M. 2010. A classification system for anomalies of the extensor pollicis longus. *Hand (NY)* 5:403–407.

Turki, M.A., Adds, P.J. 2017. Langer's axillary arch: A rare variant, and prevalence among Caucasians. *Folia Morphol* 76:536–539.

Turkof, E., Puig, S., Choi, M.S.S., Schilhan, R., Millesi, H., Firbas, W. 1994. The superficial branch of the radial nerve emerging between two slips of a split brachioradialis muscle tendon: A variation of possible clinical relevance. *Acta Anat* 3:217–219.

Turkof, E., Puig, S., Choi, S.S., Zöch, G. 1995. The radial sensory nerve entrapped between the two slips of a split brachioradialis tendon: A rare aspect of Wartenberg's syndrome. *J Hand Surg* 20A:676–678.

Turner, W. 1860. Remarks on the musculus kerato-cricoideus, a muscle of the larynx (Merkel's Muscle). *Edinb Med J* 5(8):744–746.

Turner, W. 1884–1885. Absence of extensor carpi ulnaris and presence of an accessory sural muscle. *J Anat Physiol* 19:333–334.

Türp, J.C., Cowley, T., Stohler, C.S. 1997. Media hype: Musculus sphenomandibularis. *Cells Tissues Organs* 158:150–154.

Tyrie, C.C.B. 1894. Musculus saphenous. *J Anat Physiol* 28:288–290.

Tyson, E. 1699. *Orang-Outang sive Homo Sylvestris, or the Anatomy of a Pygmie Compared to that of a Monkey, an Ape and a Man*. London: T. Bennet.

Ucerler, H., Ikiz, Z.A., Pinar, Y. 2005. Clinical importance of the muscular arch of the axilla (axillopectoral muscle, Langer's axillary arch). *Acta Chir Belg* 105:326–328.

Ullah, M., Khan, T. 2006. Anomalous muscle adjacent to temporalis. *Clin Anat* 19:648–650.

Upadhyay, B., Amiras, D. 2015. MRI appearances of the anterior fibulocalcaneus muscle: A rare anterior compartment muscle. *Skeletal Radiol* 44(5):723–726.

Upasna, Kumar, A. 2011. Bicipital origin of plantaris muscle: A case report. *Int J Anat Var* 4:177–179.

Upasna, Kumar, A., Sharma, T. 2011. Rare variation of flexor digitorum longus muscle of leg – a case report. *Int J Anat Var* 4:69–71.

Upasna, Kumar, A., Kalyan, G.S. 2013. Variant adductor muscle complex of thigh - a case report. *Int J Anat Var* 6:36–40.

Upasna, Kumar, A., Singh, B., Kaushal, S. 2015. Muscular variations during axillary dissection: A clinical study in fifty patients. *Niger J Surg* 21:60–62.

Urban, B., Bersu, E.T. 1987. Chromosome 18 aneuploidy: Anatomical variations observed in cases of full and mosaic trisomy 18 and a case of deletion of the short arm of chromosome 18. *Am J Med Gen* 27(2):425–434.

Uzel, A.P., Bertino, R., Caix, P., Boileau, P. 2008. Bilateral variation of the pectoralis minor muscle discovered during practical dissection. *Surg Radiol Anat* 30:679–682.

Vadgaonkar, R., Rai, R., Ranade, A.V., Nayak, S.R., Pai. M.M., Lakshmi, R. 2008. A case report on accessory brachialis muscle. *Romanian J Morph Embryol* 49:581–583.

Vaida, M.A., Gug, C., Jianu, A.M., et al. 2021. Bilateral anatomical variations in the extensor compartment of forearm and hand. *Surg Radiol Anat* 43:697–702.

Vajramani, A., Witham, F., Richards, R.H. 2010. Congenital unilateral absence of sternocleidomastoid and trapezius muscles: A case report and literature review. *J Pediatr Orthop B* 19(5):462–464.

Valenti, G. 1926. Sur un muscle mandibulo-glosse (m. myloglossus Wood). *Arch Ital Biol* 75:77.

Valenzuela, J.J., Orellana, M., Gold, M., Garcia, G., Santana, A. 2020. Anatomy of the lateral pterygoid muscle and its relationship with temporomandibular disorders. A literature review. *Eur J Anat* 24:249–256.

Valmaggia, C., Zaunbauer, W., Gottlob, I. 1996. Elevation deficit caused by accessory extraocular muscle. *Am J Ophthalmol* 121(4):444–445.

Valtanen, R.S., Katrikh, A.Z., Chen, A.Y., Stark, M.E. 2017. Unilateral absence of ascending and transverse trapezius fibers accompanied by mild thoracic scoliosis: A case report. *Eur J Anat* 21:71–75.

Van den Broek, A.J.P. 1909. Ein doppelseitiger M.sternalis und ein M.pectoralis quartus bei *Hylobates syndactylus*. *Anat Anz* 35:591–596.

Van Dongen, G.K. 1968. Het temporo-mandibulaire gebied bij de mens in de stadia van 50 en 80 mm kop-stuitlengte. Drukkerij: Albani den Haag.

Vázquez, M.T., Murillo, J., Maranillo, E., Parkin, I. G., Sanudo, J. 2007. Femoral nerve entrapment: A new insight. *Clin Anat* 20:175–179.

Velasco-Nieves, N., Fakoya, A.O.J., Matthew, S., Zafar, W., Zafar, M., Milla, K.A., Yerra, S., Afolabi, A., McCracken, T. 2020. Anatomical variation of the thyroid gland - levator glandulae thyroideae: A case report. *J Health Sci* 10(2):173–175.

Venieratos, D., Samolis. A, Piagkou, M., Douvetzemis, S., Kourotzoglou, A., Natsis, K. 2017. The chondrocoracoideus muscle: A rare anatomical variant of the pectoral area. *Acta Med Acad* 46:155–161.

Venugopal, S.P., Mallula, S.B. 2010. Unique musculoaponeurotic attachment between two anterior bellies of digastric. *Int J Anat Var* 3:156–157.

Vereecke, E.E., D'Aout, K., Payne, R., Aerts, P. 2005. Functional analysis of the foot and ankle myology of gibbons and bonobos. *J Anat* 206:453–476.

Verma, P., Arora, A.K., Sharma, R.K., Bhatia, B.S., Agnihotri, G. 2011. A variation at the insertion of peroneus longus: A case report. *Case Study Case Rep* 1:99–103.

Verma, P., Arora, A.K. 2012. An anatomic variant insertion of peroneus longus in a cadaver: A case report. *Int J Anat Var* 5:18–19.

Verma, R., Hertle, R.W. 2014. An interesting case of bilateral bifid insertion of superior rectus muscle as an intra-operative finding in a patient with oculocutaneous albinism. *Surg Radiol Anat* 36(6):605–606.

Verma, V., Arora, J., Kohli, M. 2018. Flexor digitorum accessorius brevis muscle: A unique anomalous variation of quadratus plantae. *Int Med J* 25:273–274.

Vishal, K., Kavitha, K., Vinay, K.V., Raghavendra, A.Y. 2013. Unilateral rectus sternalis muscle: A case report. *Nitte Univ J Health Sci* 3:66–68.

von der Hellen, E. 1903. Beitrag zur anatomie des zwerchfelles: Das centrum tendineum. *Zeitschr Morphol Anthropol* 6:151–181.

Von Lüdinghausen, M. 1998. Bilateral supernumerary rectus muscles of the orbit. *Clin Anat* 11:271–277.

Von Lüdinghausen, M., Miura, M., Würzler, N. 1999. Variations and anomalies of the human orbital muscles. *Surg Radiol Anat* 21(1):69–76.

von Lüdinghausen, M., Kageyama, I., Miura, M., Alkhatib, M. 2006. Morphological peculiarities of the deep infratemporal fossa in advanced age. *Surg Radiol Anat* 28(3):284–292.

von Luschka, H. 1870. Der Musc. pubo-transversalis des menschen. *Arch Anat Physiol Wissen Med* 1870:227–231.

von Schroeder, H.P., Botte, M.J. 1995. Anatomy of the extensor tendons of the fingers: Variations and multiplicity. *J Hand Surg (Am)* 20:27–34.

Vymazalová, K., Vargová, L., Joukal, M. 2015. Variability of the pronator teres muscle and its clinical significance. *Rom J Morphol Embryol* 56:1127–1135.

Wagenseil, F. 1927. Muskelbefunde bei Chinesen. Anthropol Anz 4 Sonderheft Verhandlungen der Gesellschaft für Physische Anthropologie 2:42–51.

Wagenseil, F. 1937. Untersuchungen über die muskulatur der chinesen. *Zeitschr Morphol Anthropol* 36:39–150.

Wagstaffe, W.W. 1871. Two Cases showing a peculiar arrangement in the fibres of the external pterygoid muscle in man. *J Anat Physiol* 5:281–284.

Wall, C.E., Larson, S.G., Stern, J.T. 1994. EMG of the digastric muscle in gibbon and orangutan: Functional consequences of the loss of the anterior digastric in orangutans. *Am J Phys Anthropol* 94:549–567.

Wallace, D.K., von Noorden, G.K. 1994. Clinical characteristics and surgical management of congenital absence of the superior oblique tendon. *Am J Ophthalmol* 118(1):63–69.

Wang, B.H., , S.J., Wang, H., Olivero, W.C. 2013. Isolated unilateral temporalis muscle hypertrophy: Case report. *J Neurosurg Pediatr* 11:451–453.

Ward, W.T., Fleisch, I.D., Ganz, R. 2000. Anatomy of the iliocapsularis muscle: Relevance to surgery of the hip. *Clin Orthop Rel Res* 374:278–285.

Watanabe, K. 2016. Facial muscles and muscles of mastication. In *Bergman's Comprehensive Encyclopedia of Human Anatomic Variation*, first edition, ed. Tubbs, R.S., Shoja, M.M., Loukas, M., 217–227. Hoboken, NJ: Wiley-Blackwell.

Watanabe, K., Saga, T., Iwanaga, J., Tabira, Y., Yamaki, K. 2017. An anatomical study of the transversus nuchae muscle: Application to better understanding occipital neuralgia. *Clin Anat* 30:32–38.

Waterman, H.C. 1929. Studies on the evolution of the pelvis of man and other primates. *Bull Am Mus Nat Hist* 58:585–642.

Watson, M. 1880. The curvatores coccygis muscles of man. *J Anat Physiol* 14(Pt4):407–412.

Wayman, J., Miller, S., Shanahan, D. 1993. Anatomical variation of the insertion of scalenus anterior in adult human subjects: Implications for clinical practice. *J Anat* 183:165–167.

Weaver, C. 1978. Frequency of occurrence of the transversus menti muscle. *Plast Reconstr Surg* 61(2):231–233.

Wehrli, F., Bergmann, M., Nyffeler, R.W. 2017. Bilateral musculus infraclavicularis. *Glob J Arch Anthropol* 1:555572.

Wiedersheim, R. 1895. *The Structure of Man - and Index to His Past History*. London: MacMillan and Co.

Weinstock, F.J., Hardesty, H.H. 1965. Absence of superior recti in craniofacial dysostosis. *Arch Ophthalmol* 74:152–153.

Wells, L.H., Thomas, E.A. 1927. A Note on Two Abnormal Laryngeal Muscles in a Zulu. *J Anat* 61(Pt 3):340–343.

Wenning, M., Heitner, A.H., Ulrich, M., Paul, J., Rist, H.J. 2019. M. peroneus quartus causing chronic peroneal compartment syndrome in a runner treated by endoscopic fasciotomy: A case report. *J Foot Ankle Surg* 58(4):653–656.

West, C.T., Ricketts, D., Brassett, C. 2017. An anatomical study of additional radial wrist extensors including a unique extensor carpi radialis accessorius. *Folia Morphol* 76:742–747.

West-Eberhard, M.J. 2003. *Developmental Plasticity and Evolution*. Oxford: Oxford University Press.

Wheeler, T. 1918. *Study of a Human Spina Bifida Monster with Encephaloceles and Other Abnormalities*. Washington, D.C.: Carnegie Institution of Washington.

Whillis, J. 1930. A note on the muscles of the palate and the superior constrictor. *J Anat* 65(Pt 1):92–95.

White III, A.A., Johnson, D., Griswold, D.M. 1974. Chronic ankle pain associated with the peroneus accessorius. *Clin Orthop Relat Res* 103:53–55.

Whitnall, S.E. 1911. An instance of the retractor bulbi muscle in man. *J Anat Physiol* 46(Pt 1):36–40.

Whitnall, S.E. 1921. Some abnormal muscles of the orbit. *Anat Rec* 21:143–152.

Wijayaweera, C.J., Amaratunga, N.A., Angunawela, P. 2000. Arrangement of the orbicularis oris muscle in different types of cleft lips. *J Craniofac Surg* 11(3):232–235.

Wilde, S., Feneck, E.M., Mohun, T.J., Logan, M.P.O. 2021. 4D formation of human embryonic forelimb musculature. *Development* 148(4). doi:10.1242/dev.194746.

Wilder, B. 1862. Contributions to the comparative myology of the chimpanzee. *Boston J Nat Hist* 6:352–384.

Willan, P.L.T., Mahon, M., Golland, J.A. 1990. Morphological variations of the human vastus lateralis muscle. *J Anat* 168:235–239.

Willard, F. 1997. Movement, stability, & low back pain: The essential role of the pelvis, ed. Vleeming, A., Mooney, V., Snijders, C., Dorman, T., Stoeckart, R., 19–20. London: Churchill Livingstone.

Wille, L., Holthusen, W., Willich, E. 1975. Accessory diaphragm. Report of 6 cases and review of the literature. *Pediatr Radiol* 4:14–20.

Willis, R.A. 1958. The borderland of embryology and pathology. London: Butterworth & Co.

Wilson, R.S., Landers, J.H. 1982. Anomalous duplication of inferior oblique muscle. *Am J Ophthalmol* 93:521–522.

Wilson, P.S., Brown, A.M.S. 1990. Unilateral temporalis muscle hypertrophy: Case report. *Int J Oral Maxillofac Surg* 19:287–288.

Wilson, T.J., Tubbs, R.S., Yang, L.J.S. 2016. The anconeus epitrochlearis muscle may protect against the development of cubital tunnel syndrome: A preliminary study. *J Neurosurg* 125:1522–1538.

Windle, B.C. 1893. The Myology of the anencephalous foetus. *J Anat Physiol* 27:348–353.

Wingerter, S., Gupta, S., Le, S., Shamasunder, S., Bernstein, S., Rabitaille, W., Kukuyeva, Y., Downie, S. 2003. Unusual origin of the flexor digiti minimi brevis muscle. *Clin Anat* 16:531–533.

Winslow, J.B. 1732. Exposition anatomique de la structure du corps humain T. 1 and 2. Paris: Chez Guillaume Desprez et Jean Desessartz.

Witkop Jr., C.J., Barros, L. 1963. Oral and genetic studies of Chileans 1960. I. Oral anomalies. *Am J Phys Anthropol* 21:15–24.

Witvrouw, E., Borre, K.V., Willems, T.M., Huysmans, J., Broos, E., De Clercq, D. 2006. The significance of peroneus tertius muscle in ankle injuries: A prospective study. *Am J Sports Med* 34(7):1159–1163.

Wolpert, L. 1969. Positional information and the spatial pattern of cellular differentiation. *J Theor Biol* 25:1–47.

Wolpert, L. 2011. Positional information and patterning revisited. *J Theor Biol* 269:359–365.

Won, H.J., Oh, C.S. 2018. Muscular variations of extensor digitorum brevis muscle related with anterior tarsal tunnel syndrome. *Korean J Phys Anthropol* 31(1):35–39.

Wong, T.L., Kikuta, S., Iwanaga, J., Tubbs, R.S. 2019. A multiply split femoral nerve and psoas quartus muscle. *Anat Cell Biol* 52:208–210.

Wood, J. 1864. On some varieties in human myology. *Proc Roy Soc Lond B* 13:299–303.

Wood, J. 1865. Additional varieties in human myology. *Proc Royal Soc Lond* 14:379–393.

Wood, J. 1866. Variations in human myology observed during the winter session of 1865–6 at King's College, London. *Proc Royal Soc Lond* 15:229–244.

Wood, J. 1867a. On human muscular variations and their relation to comparative anatomy. J Anat Physiol 1867:44–59.

Wood, J. 1867b. Variations in human myology observed during the winter session of 1866–7 at King's College London. *Proc Royal Soc Lond* 15:518–545.

Wood, J. 1868. Variations in human myology observed during the winter session of 1867–68 at King's College, London. *Proc Royal Soc Lond* 16:483–525.

Wood, J. 1870. On a group of varieties of the muscles of the human neck, shoulder, and chest, with their transitional forms and homologies in the Mammalia. *Philos Trans R Soc Lond* 160:83–116.

Woodley, S.J. 2016. Articularis genus. In: *Gray's Anatomy. The Anatomical Basis of Clinical Practice*, 41st edition, e84–c86. New York: Elsevier.

Woodley, S.J., Latimer, C.P., Meikle, G.R., et al. 2012. Articularis genus: An anatomic and MRI study in cadavers. *J Bone Joint Surg Am* 94:59–67.

Woyski, D., Olinger, A., Wright, B. 2012. Incidence of gluteus quartus in human cadavers. *Fed Am Soc Exper Biol* 26(Suppl 1):57.

Wright, J.L.W., Etholm, B. 1973. Anomalies of the middle-ear muscles. *J Laryngol* 87:281–288.

Wright, C.G., Meyerhoff, W.L., Brown, O.E., Rutledge, J.C. 1986. Auditory and temporal bone abnormalities in CHARGE association. *Ann Otol Rhinol Laryng* 95(5):480–486.

Wylen, E.L., Brown, M.S., Rich, L.S., Hesse, R.J. 2001. Supernumerary orbital muscle in congenital eyelid retraction. *Ophthal Plast Reconstr Surg* 17(2):120–122.

Yadav, A., Yadav, M., Dixit, A. 2014. A morphological study of levator glanduleae thyroideae and pyramidal lobe in normal adult human thyroid gland. *Int J Res Health Sci* 2:1030–1033.

Yalçin, B., Ozan, H. 2005a. Insertional pattern of the inferior oblique muscle. *Am J Ophthalmol* 139:504–508.

Yalçin, B., Ozan, H. 2005b. Some variations of the musculus flexor digitorum brevis. *Anat Sci Int* 80:189–192.

Yalçin, B., Kocabiyik, N., Ozan, H., Kutoglu, T. 2004. Muscular bridge between the inferior oblique and inferior rectus muscles. *Am J Ophthalmol* 137:121–124.

Yalçin, B., Hurmeric, V., Loukas, M., Tubbs, R. S., Ozan, H. 2009. Accessory levator muscle slips of the levator palpebrae superioris muscle. *Clin Exper Ophthalmol* 37(4):407–411.

Yamamoto, C., Murakami, T., Ohtsuka, A. 1988. Homology of the adductor pollicis and contrahentes muscles: A study of monkey hands. *Acta Med Okayama* 42:215–226.

Yamazaki, Y., Shibata, M., Ushiki, T., Isokawa, K., Sato, N. 2011. Bilateral, asymmetric anomalies of the anterior bellies of digastric muscles. *J Oral Sci* 53:523–527.

Yammine, K. 2015a. The prevalence of the extensor indicis tendon and its variants: A systematic review and meta-analysis. *Surg Radiol Anat* 37:247–254.

Yammine, K. 2015b. The prevalence of extensor digitorum brevis manus and its variants in humans: A systematic review and meta-analysis. *Surg Radiol Anat* 37:3–9.

Yammine, K. 2015c. The accessory peroneal (fibular) muscles: Peroneus quartus and peroneus digiti quinti. A systematic review and meta-analysis. *Surg Radiol Anat* 37:617–627.

Yammine, K. 2015d. The fourth slip of the flexor digitorum brevis muscle of the human foot. A systematic review and meta-analysis. *Ital J Anat Embryolo* 120(1):59–70.

Yammine, K., Erić, M. 2017. The fibularis (peroneus tertius muscle in humans: A meta-analysis of anatomical studies with clinical and evolutionary implications. *Biomed Res Int* 2017:6021707.

Yammine, K., Erić, M. 2018. Agenesis, functional deficiency and the common type of the flexor digitorum superficialis of the little finger: A meta-analysis. *Hand Surg Rehabil* 37:77–85.

Yang, K., Choi, I., Lee, J. 2018. Accessory head of the extensor carpi radialis longus muscle merging with extensor carpi radialis brevis muscle. *Surg Radiol Anat* 40:1001–1003.

Yatsunami, M., Tai, T., Irie, Y., Ogawa, K., Miyauchi, R. 2004. A morphological study on the human obturator externus muscle with reference to anomalous muscle and anomalous fasciculus originating from the obturator externus muscle. *Okajimas Folia Anat Jpn* 80:103–114.

Yeh, H.C., Halton, K.P., Gray, C.E. 1990. Anatomic variations and abnormalities in the diaphragm seen with US. *Radio Graph* 10:1019–1030.

Yildirim, F.B., Sarikcioglu, L., Nakajima, K. 2011. The co-existence of the gastrocnemius tertius and accessory soleus muscle. *J Korean Med Sci* 26(10):1378–1381.

Yildiz, S., Yalcin, B. 2012. An unique variation of the peroneus tertius muscles. *Surg Radiol Anat* 34:661–663.

Yiyit, N., Işıtmangil, T., Oztürker, C. 2014. The abnormalities of trapezius muscle might be a component of Poland's syndrome. *Med Hypotheses* 83(5):533–536.

Yoshida, Y., Yasutaka, S., Seki, T. 1984. Studies on the extensor digitorum brevis manus muscle in man. *Acta Anat Nippon* 59:313–321.

Young Lee, B., Young Byun, J., Hee Kim, H., Sook Kim, H., Mee Cho, S., Hoon Lee, K., Sup Song, K., Soo Kim, B., Mun Lee, J. 2006. The sternalis muscles: Incidence and imaging findings on MDCT. *J Thorac Imaging* 21:179–183.

Yu, J., Resnick, D. 1994. MR imaging of the accessory soleus muscle appearance in six patients and a review of the literature. *Skel Radiol* 23(7):525–528.

Yuan, X.Y., Yu, S.B., Li, Y.F., et al. 2016. Patterns of attachment of the myodural bridge by the rectus capitis posterior minor muscle. *Anat Sci Int* 91:175–179.

Yun, S., Park, S., Kim, C.S. 2018. Absence of the subclavius muscle with contralateral subclavius posticus muscle: First imaging report. *Clin Imag* 49:54–57.

Yurasakpong, L., Meemon, K., Suwannakhan, A. 2018. Linburg–Comstock variation: Histoanatomy and classification of the connection between flexor pollicis longus and flexor digitorum profundus to the index finger. *Surg Radiol Anat* 40:297–301.

Zağyapan, R., Pelin, C., Mas, N. 2008. A rare muscular variation: The occipito-scapularis muscle: Case report. *Turkiye Klinikleri J Med Sci* 28:87–90.

Zammit, J., Singh, D. 2003. The peroneus quartus muscle: Anatomy and clinical relevance. *J Bone Joint Surg* 85:1134–1137.

Zawawi, F., Varshney, R., Schloss, M.D. 2014. Shortened stapedius tendon: A rare cause of conductive hearing loss. *J Laryngol Otol* 128:98–100.

Zdilla, M.J., Soloninka, H.J., Lambert, H.W. 2014a. Unilateral duplication of the anterior digastric muscle belly: A case report with implications for surgeries of the submental region. *J Surg Case Rep* 2014:rju131.

Zdilla, M.J., Soloninka, H.J., Lambert, H.W. 2014b. A fractal anterior digastric: A case report with surgical implications. *Int J Anat Var* 7:106–108.

Zdilla, M.J., Lambert, H.W. 2015. Mylohyoid insertion at the mid-belly of a combined geniohyoid via a fibrous pseudo-hyoid: An observation with implications for submental flap surgery. *J Plast Reconstr Aesthet Surg Open* 5:1–3.

Zdilla, M.J., Mangus, K.R., Swearingen, J.V., Miller, K.D., Lambert, H.W. 2018. The submental arrowhead variation of the mylohyoid and anterior belly of the digastric muscles. *Surg Radiol Anat* 40:1429–1436.

Zdilla, M.J., Pacurari, P., Celuck, T.J., Andrews, R.C., Lambert, H.W. 2019. A Gantzer muscle arising from the brachialis and flexor digitorum superficialis: Embryological considerations and implications for median nerve entrapment. *Ant Sci Int* 94:150–153.

Zemlin, W., Elving, S., Hull, L. 1984. The superior thyroarytenoid muscle in the human larynx. *Am Speech Hear Ass* 26:71.

Zenker, W. 1955. Ueber einige neue befunde am m. temporalis des menschen. *Z Anat Entwicklungsgeschichte* 118:355–368.

Zeren, B., Oztekin, H.H, Boya, H., Ozcan, O. 2009. Symptomatic entrapment of an anomalous semimembranosus muscle by the semitendinosus tendon in a professional soccer player: A case report. *Am J Sports Med* 37:2049–2052.

Zhao, W., Liu, J., Xu, J., et al. 2015. Duplicated posterior belly of digastric muscle and absence of omohyoid muscle: A case report and review of literature. *Surg Radiol Anat* 37:547–550.

Ziegler, A.C. 1964. Brachiating adaptations of chimpanzee upper limb musculature. *Am J Phys Anthropol* 22:15–32.

Zilber, S., Oberlin, C. 2004. Anatomical variations of the extensor tendons to the fingers over the dorsum of the hand: A study of 50 Hands and a review of the literature. *Plast and Reconstr Surg* 113:214–221.

Zöller, C.C., Gräf, M., Kaufmann, H. 2001. Einseitige aplasie eines musculus rectus lateralis. *Klin Monbl Augenheilkd* 218(1):55–60.

Zufferey, J.A. 2013. Is the malaris muscle the anti-aging missing link of the midface? *Eur J Plast Surg* 36(6):345–352.

Zumpano, M.P., Hartwell, S., Jagos, C.S. 2006. Soft tissue connection between rectus capitis posterior minor and the posterior atlanto-occipital membrane: A cadaveric study. *Clin Anat* 19:522–527.

Index

Note: *Italic* page numbers refer to figures.